Methods in Pharmacology and Toxicology

Series editor:
Y. James Kang
University of Louisville
School of Medicine
Prospect, Kentucky, USA

For further volumes:
http://www.springer.com/series/7653

Histamine Receptors as Drug Targets

Edited by

Ekaterini Tiligada

Department of Pharmacology, Medical School, National and Kapodistrian University of Athens, Athens, Greece

Madeleine Ennis

Centre for Experimental Medicine, School of Medicine, Dentistry and Biomedical Sciences, Queen's University Belfast, Belfast, Northern Ireland, UK

Humana Press

Editors
Ekaterini Tiligada
Department of Pharmacology
Medical School
National and Kapodistrian University of Athens
Athens, Greece

Madeleine Ennis
Centre for Experimental Medicine
School of Medicine
Dentistry and Biomedical Sciences
Queen's University Belfast
Belfast, Northern Ireland, UK

ISSN 1557-2153 ISSN 1940-6053 (electronic)
Methods in Pharmacology and Toxicology
ISBN 978-1-4939-6841-1 ISBN 978-1-4939-6843-5 (eBook)
DOI 10.1007/978-1-4939-6843-5

Library of Congress Control Number: 2017931656

Printed on acid-free paper

This Humana Press imprint is published by Springer Nature
The registered company is Springer Science+Business Media LLC
The registered company address is: 233 Spring Street, New York, NY 10013, U.S.A.

Preface

Histamine [2-(4-imidazolyl) ethylamine] is a biogenic amine that is synthesized from the amino acid L-histidine through the catalytic activity of histidine decarboxylase (HDC, EC 4.1.1.22) and catabolized by two enzymes, namely diamine oxidase (DAO, EC 1.4.3.6) and histamine N-methyltransferase (HNMT, EC 2.1.1.8) [1, 2].

The history of histamine and antihistamines reflects numerous pioneering moments in the development of pharmacology over the last 100 years, achieved by research groups led by outstanding scientists, including six Nobel Prize winners: Paul Ehrlich, Charles Richet, Adolf Windaus, Sir Henry Dale, Daniel Bovet, and Sir James Black (Fig. 1).

Histamine was chemically synthesized by Adolf Windaus and Karl Vogt in 1907 [3], and the investigation of its pharmacological actions started in the early twentieth century by Sir Henry H. Dale in the Wellcome Research Laboratories in south-east London [4]. One of the first described actions of histamine was its ability to mimic the anaphylactic reaction [4]. A few years earlier, Paul Portier and Charles R. Richet had coined the term "anaphylaxis" [5] and Clemens von Pirquet and Bela Schick the term "allergy" to describe the hypersensitivity reactions [6]. However, it was not until the early 1950s that James Riley and Geoffrey West associated histamine with the mast cell [7] which had been discovered more than 70 years earlier by Paul Ehrlich [8] and was linked to anaphylactic reactions in 1941 [9].

In addition to its pivotal role in hypersensitivity reactions [10], smooth muscle contraction [11], and vascular permeability [10, 12], we now know that histamine is produced and released from a variety of cells and modulates gastric acid secretion [13], neurotransmission [14], and immune cell chemotaxis [15]. Its regulatory properties are mediated through four types of G protein-coupled receptors (GPCR), designated as H_1, H_2, H_3, and H_4 [16, 17] which are differentially expressed in various tissues and cell types and show intra- and interspecies variations [18]. In general, the tissue distribution and localization in target cells associate the H_1, H_2, H_3, and H_4 receptors with allergy, gastric acid secretion, neurotransmission, and immunomodulation, respectively [15–18].

For more than 70 years, histamine has been one of the most exploited substances in medicine (Fig. 1). It has provided blockbuster drugs acting on H_1 and H_2 receptors for the treatment of allergies and gastrointestinal disorders, respectively. Interestingly, the high affinity H_4 receptor was identified in 2000, and since then it has been shown to be constitutively active and expressed mostly, but not exclusively, on cells of the immune system. This discovery revealed novel attractive perspectives for the translational potential of this new drug target in acute and chronic inflammation, autoimmune disorders, host defense, and neuropathic pain. Histamine also has profound effects in cancer. Claude Burtin found that cimetidine increased the survival of patients with advanced cancer [19]. However, the pharmacological diversity and complexity of histamine receptors (HRs) and their ligands, as well as their association with the recently described phenomenon of "biased agonism," justifies ongoing efforts to translate preclinical drug actions into promising therapies for pathologies with high economic and societal impact, such as asthma, dementias, dermatitis, and arthritis.

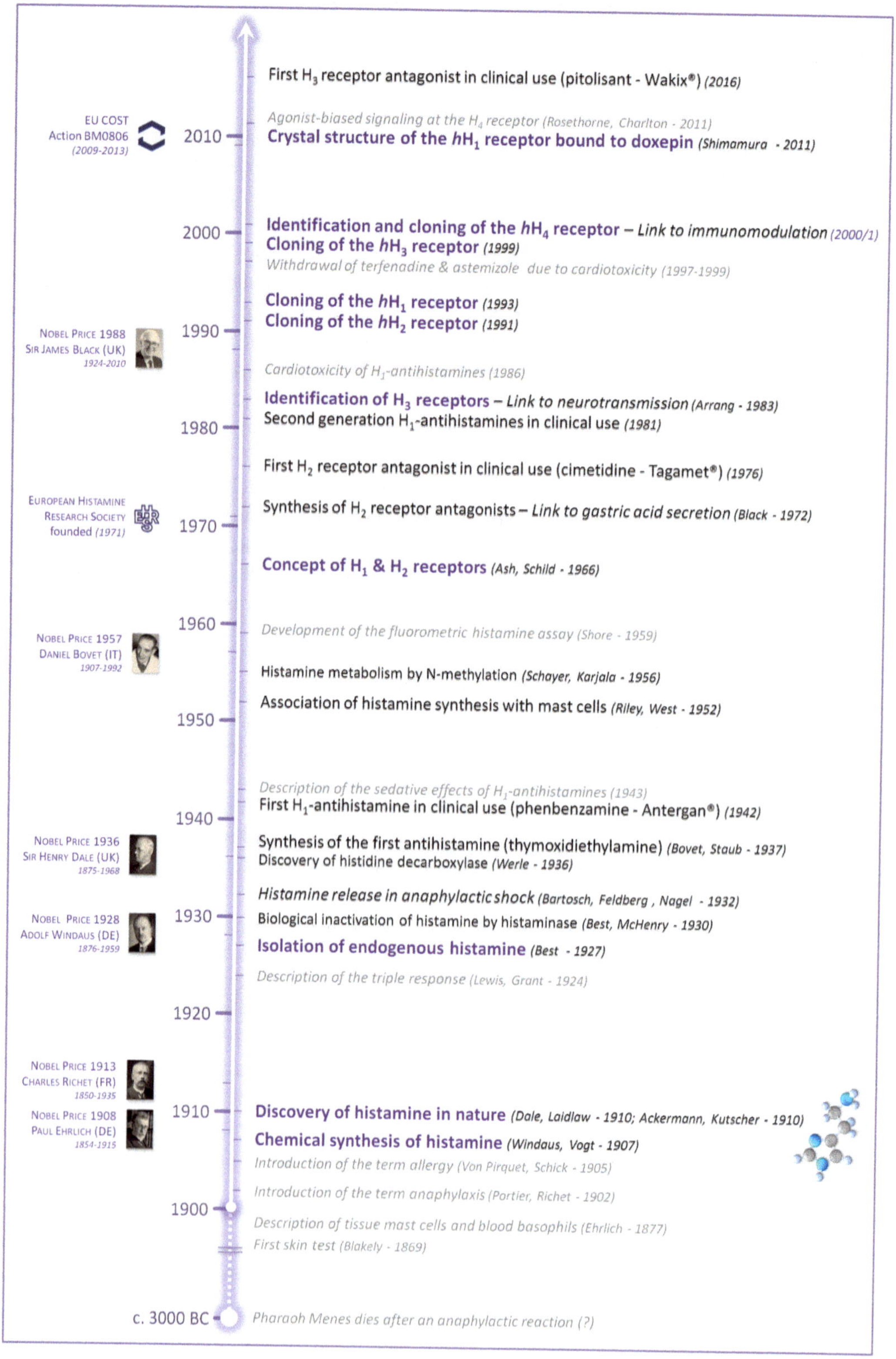

Fig. 1 Milestones in the pharmacology and the therapeutic exploitation of histamine and histamine receptors (H_1–H_4)

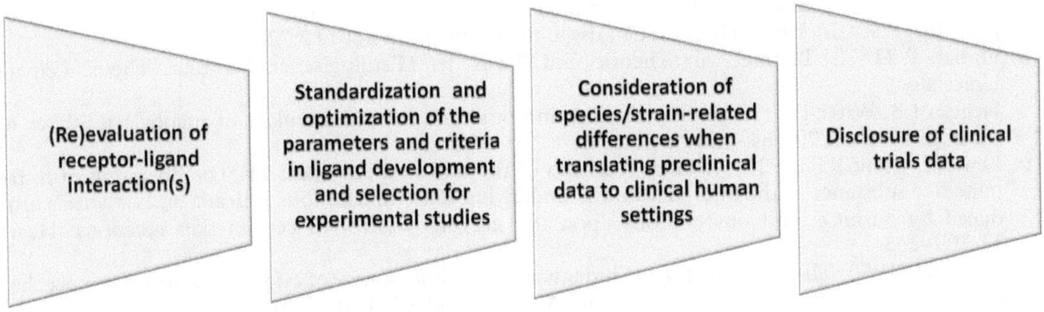

Fig. 2 Key perspectives directing future histamine and histamine receptor research towards the development of new drugs

This book illustrates the current state of the art in histamine research. It is designed to comprehensively present the most effective methods and protocols available in order to aid researchers around the world in pursuing the study of this vital scientific area (Fig. 2). It largely focuses on the appropriate methodologies to investigate the pharmacological properties and the therapeutic exploitation of HRs and their ligands. In addition, the range of techniques described in this volume also provides an introduction to complementary cross-methodological disciplines beyond these fields. This multidisciplinary approach is required to define the "decision gates" that determine the development of more effective and safer therapeutic options for many forms of highly prevalent and debilitating diseases.

Chapters that deal with critical discussions on both laboratory and clinical topics have mainly been contributed by members of the long-standing European Histamine Research Society (EHRS). In general, chapters contain an informative theoretical part and a detailed methods section, all supported by extensive bibliography. The aim is to help academic and industry drug discovery researchers and pharmacologists to deliver beneficial end points through basic and translational research (Fig. 2). The target audience includes pharmacologists, biochemists, drug discovery researchers, molecular biologists, chemists, toxicologists, lab scientists, medical doctors, principal investigators, research scientists, lab directors and technicians, as well as graduate students.

Athens, Greece — *Ekaterini Tiligada*
Belfast, UK — *Madeleine Ennis*

References

1. Bovet D (1950) Introduction to antihistamine agents and antergan derivative. Ann N Y Acad Sci 50:1089–1126
2. Moya-Garcia AA, Medina MA, Sanchez-Jimenez F (2005) Mammalian histidine decarboxylase: from structure to function. BioEssays 27:57–63
3. Windaus A, Vogt W (1907) Synthese des Imidazolyläthylamins. Ber Dtsch Chem Ges 40:3691–3695
4. Dale HH, Laidlaw PP (1910) The physiological action of β-imidazolylethylamine. J Physiol 41:318–341
5. Portier P, Richet CR (1902) De l'action anaphylactique de certains venins. C R Soc Biol 54:170–172

6. Von Pirquet CP, Schick B (1905) Die Serumkrankeit. F Deuticke, Wien
7. Riley JF, West GB (1952) Histamine in tissue mast cells. J Physiol 117:72–73
8. Ehrlich P (1878) Beiträge zur Theorie und Praxis der Histologischen Färbung. Thesis, Leipzig University
9. Jacques LB, Water ET (1941) The identity and origin of the anticoagulant of anaphylactic shock in the dog. J Physiol 99:454–466
10. Lewis T, Grant RT (1924) Vascular reactions of the skin to injury. Part 11. The liberation of histamine-like substance in the injured skin, the underlying cause of factitious urticaria and of wheals produced by burning: and observations upon the nervous control of certain skin reactions. Heart 11:209–265
11. Dale HH (1950) The pharmacology of histamine: with a brief survey of evidence for its occurrence, liberation, and participation in natural reactions. Ann NY Acad Sci 50:1017–1028
12. Best CH, Dale HH, Dudley HW et al (1927) The nature of the vasodilator constituents of certain tissues. J Physiol 62:397
13. Black JW, Duncan WAM, Durant CJ et al (1972) Definition and antagonism of histamine H_2-receptors. Nature 236:385–390
14. Arrang JM, Garbarg M, Schwartz JC (1983) Auto-inhibition of brain histamine release mediated by a novel class (H_3) of histamine receptor. Nature 302:832–837
15. Zampeli E, Tiligada E (2009) The role of histamine H_4 receptor in immune and inflammatory disorders. Br J Pharmacol 157:24–33
16. Parsons ME, Ganellin CR (2006) Histamine and its receptors. Br J Pharmacol 147:S127–S135
17. Panula P, Chazot PL, Cowart M et al (2015) International Union of Basic and Clinical Pharmacology. XCVIII. Histamine receptors. Pharmacol Rev 67:601–655
18. Leurs R, Chazot PL, Shenton FC et al (2009) Molecular and biochemical pharmacology of the histamine H_4 receptor. Br J Pharmacol 157:14–23
19. Burtin C, Noirot C, Scheinmann P et al (1988) Clinical improvement in advanced cancer disease after treatment combining histamine and H2-antihistaminics (ranitidine or cimetidine). Eur J Cancer Clin Oncol 24:161–167

Acknowledgements

We gratefully acknowledge the support from members of the European Histamine Research Society, EU COST Action BM0806, as well as members of *ImmuPhar*, the Immunopharmacology Section of the International Union of Basic and Clinical Pharmacology (IUPHAR).

Contents

Contributors

CARLOS ACOSTA-ANDRADE • *Departamento de Biología Molecular y Bioquímica, Andalucía Tech, Facultad de Ciencias, Universidad de Málaga, Campus Universitario de Teatinos, Málaga, Spain*
XENOPHON AGGELIDES • *Allergy Unit 'D. Kalogeromitros', 2nd Department of Dermatology and Venereology, Medical School, National and Kapodistrian University of Athens, University Hospital 'Attikon', Athens, Greece*
MARIA C. ANAGNOSTOULI • *Demyelinating Diseases Clinic, Immunogenetics Laboratory, A' Department of Neurology, Medical School, Aeginition Hospital, National and Kapodistrian University of Athens, Athens, Greece*
WOLFGANG BÄUMER • *Department of Molecular Biomedical Sciences, College of Veterinary Medicine, NC State University, Raleigh, NC, USA*
DIMITRIOS P. BESINIS • *Department of Ophthalmology, Evaggelismos General Hospital, Athens, Greece; Department of Ophthalmology, The Hillingdon Hospitals NHS Foundation Trust, Uxbridge, London, UK*
REGGIE BOSMA • *Faculty of Sciences, Division of Medicinal Chemistry, Amsterdam Institute for Molecules, Medicines and Systems, Vrije Universiteit Amsterdam, Amsterdam, The Netherlands*
PAUL L. CHAZOT • *Department of Biosciences, Durham University, Durham, UK*
CATERINA CHLIVA • *Allergy Unit 'D. Kalogeromitros', 2nd Department of Dermatology and Venereology, Medical School, National and Kapodistrian University of Athens, University Hospital 'Attikon', Athens, Greece*
URSZULA CICHOŃ • *Department of Technology and Biotechnology of Drugs, Faculty of Pharmacy, Jagiellonian University Medical College, Kraków, Poland*
MILAN ČÍŽ • *Institute of Biophysics, Czech Academy of Sciences, Brno, Czech Republic*
GRACIELA A. CREMASCHI • *Laboratory of Radioisotopes, School of Pharmacy and Biochemistry, University of Buenos Aires, Buenos Aires, Argentina; Neuroimmunomodulation and Molecular Oncology Division, Institute for Biomedical Research (BIOMED), School of Medical Sciences, Pontifical Catholic University of Argentina (UCA), and the National Scientific and Technical Research Council (CONICET), Buenos Aires, Argentina*
GRACIELA P. CRICCO • *Laboratory of Radioisotopes, School of Pharmacy and Biochemistry, University of Buenos Aires, Buenos Aires, Argentina*
CARLOS DAVIO • *Instituto de Investigaciones Farmacológicas, Facultad de Farmacia y Bioquímica, ININFA-UBA-CONICET, Ciudad Autónoma de Buenos Aires, Argentina*
MADELEINE ENNIS • *Centre for Experimental Medicine, School of Medicine, Dentistry and Biomedical Sciences, Queen's University Belfast, Belfast, Northern Ireland, UK*
IGNACIO FAJARDO • *Departamento de Biología Molecular y Bioquímica, Andalucía Tech, Facultad de Ciencias, Universidad de Málaga, Malaga, Spain; Instituto de Biomedicina de Málaga, Malaga, Spain; CIBER de Enfermedades Raras, Instituto de Salud Carlos III, Malaga, Spain*
NATALIA C. FERNÁNDEZ • *Instituto de Investigaciones Farmacológicas, Facultad de Farmacia y Bioquímica, ININFA-UBA-CONICET, Ciudad Autónoma de Buenos Aires, Argentina*

TOMOKI FUKUYAMA • *Department of Molecular Biomedical Sciences, College of Veterinary Medicine, NC State University, Raleigh, NC, USA*
CRISTINA GRANGE • *Department of Medical Sciences, University of Turin, Turin, Italy*
MAREK GROSICKI • *Department of Technology and Biotechnology of Drugs, Faculty of Pharmacy, Jagiellonian University Medical College, Kraków, Poland*
VIERA JANČINOVÁ • *Institute of Experimental Pharmacology and Toxicology, Slovak Academy of Sciences, Bratislava, Slovakia*
MARIA KAKOLYRI • *Department of Pharmacology, Medical School, National and Kapodistrian University of Athens, Athens, Greece*
TADEUSZ KARCZ • *Department of Technology and Biotechnology of Drugs, Faculty of Pharmacy, Jagiellonian University Medical College, Kraków, Poland*
KATARZYNA KIEĆ-KONONOWICZ • *Department of Technology and Biotechnology of Drugs, Faculty of Pharmacy, Jagiellonian University Medical College, Kraków, Poland*
MANFRED KIETZMANN • *Institute for Pharmacology, Toxicology and Pharmacy, University of Veterinary Medicine, Hannover, Germany*
HANNA KÖCHLING • *Institute for Pharmacology, Toxicology and Pharmacy, University of Veterinary Medicine, Hannover, Germany*
CHRYSOVALANTIS KORFITIS • *Department of Dermatology, 401 General Military Hospital of Athens, Athens, Greece*
CHRISTOPHER KOULIAS • *Allergy Unit 'D. Kalogeromitros', 2nd Department of Dermatology and Venereology, Medical School, National and Kapodistrian University of Athens, University Hospital 'Attikon', Athens, Greece*
NATASHA LETHBRIDGE • *Department of Biosciences, Durham University, Durham, UK*
ROB LEURS • *Faculty of Sciences, Division of Medicinal Chemistry, Amsterdam Institute for Molecules, Medicines and Systems, Vrije Universiteit Amsterdam, Amsterdam, The Netherlands*
MICHAEL MAKRIS • *Allergy Unit 'D. Kalogeromitros', 2nd Department of Dermatology and Venereology, Medical School, National and Kapodistrian University of Athens, University Hospital 'Attikon', Athens, Greece*
GABRIELA A. MARTIN • *Laboratory of Radioisotopes, School of Pharmacy and Biochemistry, University of Buenos Aires, Buenos Aires, Argentina; National Scientific and Technical Research Council (CONICET), Buenos Aires, Argentina*
DIEGO J. MARTINEL LAMAS • *Laboratory of Radioisotopes, School of Pharmacy and Biochemistry, University of Buenos Aires, Buenos Aires, Argentina; Laboratory of Tumor Biology and Inflammation, Institute for Biomedical Research (BIOMED), School of Medical Sciences, Pontifical Catholic University of Argentina (UCA), and the National Scientific and Technical Research Council (CONICET), Buenos Aires, Argentina*
VANINA A. MEDINA • *Laboratory of Radioisotopes, School of Pharmacy and Biochemistry, University of Buenos Aires, Buenos Aires, Argentina; Laboratory of Tumor Biology and Inflammation, Institute for Biomedical Research (BIOMED), School of Medical Sciences, Pontifical Catholic University of Argentina (UCA), and the National Scientific and Technical Research Council (CONICET), Buenos Aires, Argentina*
STEPHANY MICALLEF • *School of Pharmacy and Pharmaceutical Sciences, Panoz Institute, Trinity Biomedical Sciences Institute, Trinity College, Dublin, Ireland*
TAMARA A.M. MOCKING • *Faculty of Sciences, Division of Medicinal Chemistry, Amsterdam Institute for Molecules, Medicines and Systems, Vrije Universiteit Amsterdam, Amsterdam, The Netherlands*

Federico Monczor • *Instituto de Investigaciones Farmacológicas, Facultad de Farmacia y Bioquímica, ININFA-UBA-CONICET, Ciudad Autónoma de Buenos Aires, Argentina*

Melisa B. Nicoud • *Laboratory of Tumor Biology and Inflammation, Institute for Biomedical Research (BIOMED), School of Medical Sciences, Pontifical Catholic University of Argentina (UCA), and the National Scientific and Technical Research Council (CONICET), Buenos Aires, Argentina*

Radomír Nosáľ • *Institute of Experimental Pharmacology and Toxicology, Slovak Academy of Sciences, Bratislava, Slovakia*

Silvia Pažoureková • *Institute of Experimental Pharmacology and Toxicology, Slovak Academy of Sciences, Bratislava, Slovakia*

Tomáš Perečko • *Institute of Biophysics, Czech Academy of Sciences, Brno, Czech Republic; International Clinical Research Center, St. Anne's University Hospital, Brno, Czech Republic*

Alessandro Pini • *Department of Experimental and Clinical Medicine, University of Florence, Florence, Italy*

Efstathios Rallis • *Department of Dermatology, Veterans Administration Hospital of Athens, Athens, Greece*

Dimitrios Rigopoulos • *2nd Department of Dermatology and Venereology, Medical School, National and Kapodistrian University of Athens, University Hospital 'Attikon', Athens, Greece*

Elena S. Rivera • *Laboratory of Radioisotopes, School of Pharmacy and Biochemistry, University of Buenos Aires, Buenos Aires, Argentina*

Arianna Carolina Rosa • *Dipartimento di Scienza e Tecnologia del Farmaco, University of Turin, Turin, Italy*

Kristine Roßbach • *Institute for Pharmacology, Toxicology and Pharmacy, University of Veterinary Medicine, Hannover, Germany*

Francisca Sánchez-Jiménez • *Departamento de Biología Molecular y Bioquímica, Andalucía Tech, Facultad de Ciencias, Universidad de Málaga, Malaga, Spain; Instituto de Biomedicina de Málaga, Malaga, Spain; CIBER de Enfermedades Raras, Instituto de Salud Carlos III, Malaga, Spain*

Astrid Sasse • *School of Pharmacy and Pharmaceutical Sciences, Panoz Institute, Trinity Biomedical Sciences Institute, Trinity College, Dublin, Ireland*

Hubert G. Schwelberger • *Molecular Biology Laboratory, Department of Visceral, Transplant and Thoracic Surgery, Medical University Innsbruck, Innsbruck, Austria*

Carina Shayo • *Instituto de Biología y Medicina Experimental, IByME-CONICET, Ciudad Autónoma de Buenos Aires, Argentina*

Fiona C. Shenton • *Department of Biosciences, Durham University, Durham, UK*

Helena Sterle • *Neuroimmunomodulation and Molecular Oncology Division, Institute for Biomedical Research (BIOMED), School of Medical Sciences, Pontifical Catholic University of Argentina (UCA), and the National Scientific and Technical Research Council (CONICET), Buenos Aires, Argentina*

Ekaterini Tiligada • *Department of Pharmacology, Medical School, National and Kapodistrian University of Athens, Athens, Greece*

José L. Urdiales • *Departamento de Biología Molecular y Bioquímica, Andalucía Tech, Facultad de Ciencias, Universidad de Málaga, Málaga, Spain; Instituto de Biomedicina de Málaga, Málaga, Spain; CIBER de Enfermedades Raras, Instituto de Salud Carlos III, Málaga, Spain*

ONDŘEJ VAŠÍČEK • *Institute of Biophysics, Czech Academy of Sciences, Brno, Czech Republic; International Clinical Research Center, St. Anne's University Hospital, Brno, Czech Republic*

ELEONORA VEGLIA • *Dipartimento di Scienza e Tecnologia del Farmaco, University of Turin, Turin, Italy*

ELÉONORE W.E. VERWEIJ • *Faculty of Sciences, Division of Medicinal Chemistry, Amsterdam Institute for Molecules, Medicines and Systems, Vrije Universiteit Amsterdam, Amsterdam, The Netherlands*

HENRY F. VISCHER • *Faculty of Sciences, Division of Medicinal Chemistry, Amsterdam Institute for Molecules, Medicines and Systems, Vrije Universiteit Amsterdam, Amsterdam, The Netherlands*

JENNY WILZOPOLSKI • *Institute for Pharmacology, Toxicology and Pharmacy, University of Veterinary Medicine, Hannover, Germany*

Chapter 1

Methodologies to Identify and Analyze Genetic Polymorphisms for Human Histamine Receptors

Stephany Micallef and Astrid Sasse

Abstract

Histamine is a biogenic amine that has an inherent biological importance in many physiological functions. With the new genomic era we are facing, personalized care and treatment is becoming one of the major focal points in research. This chapter will focus on the tools available to assess polymorphisms and genetic variations in the human histamine receptor family. The genetic composition of this receptor family is discussed and explained. Methodologies in genetic analysis are described, the use of bioinformatics information available is explored, and the use of Hapmap data and how it can be used in genome-wide association studies and linkage analysis is explained. Bioinformatics and molecular biology prove to be essential tools in investigating genetic associations between genotype and disease. This area of research is of utmost importance for identification of biological markers and is essential in the search to develop personalized medication.

Key words Histamine, Histamine receptors, Polymorphisms, Genome-Wide Association Studies (GWAS), Linkage Disequilibrium (LD), Genetic variations

1 Introduction

Histamine is a biogenic amine that plays an essential role in controlling many physiological functions, both in the central nervous system (CNS) and in the peripheral nervous system (PNS). Most of these physiological effects are mediated through interactions with four histamine receptor subtypes, all of which are members of the larger family of rhodopsin-like class A G-protein coupled receptors (GPCRs) [1, 2]. This chapter looks into the human histamine receptor (HRH) genes and describes how bioinformatics data can be used in linkage and association studies.

1.1 Human Histamine Receptor Family

The first two GPCRs from this subtype, namely histamine H_1 and histamine H_2 receptors, were first cloned in 1991 [3]. The human histamine H_1 receptor (HRH1) is the largest protein of the histamine receptor family [3] and is expressed primarily in smooth muscle, endothelial cells, the adrenal medulla, the heart and also

Ekaterini Tiligada and Madeleine Ennis (eds.), *Histamine Receptors as Drug Targets*, Methods in Pharmacology and Toxicology, DOI 10.1007/978-1-4939-6843-5_1, © Springer Science+Business Media LLC 2017

the CNS. The HRH1 is predominantly involved in smooth muscle contraction and increased vascular permeability [4]. The main therapeutic targets for HRH1 antagonists are allergic conditions and sleep disorders [5]. The human histamine H_2 receptor (HRH2) is mostly expressed in gastric parietal cells, vascular smooth muscle, suppressor T cells, neutrophils, the CNS and the heart. Its main involvement is in stimulation of gastric acid secretion and hence an important therapeutic target for gastric ulcers [4]. The histamine 3 receptor (HRH3), first cloned in 1999 by Johnson & Johnson [6], is a presynaptic autoreceptor on histamine neurons and heteroreceptor on various neurotransmitter neurons, and is expressed in the CNS and peripheral nerves [4]. Homology and phylogenetic analysis of HRH3 suggested it to be markedly different from the previously cloned HRH1 and HRH2 receptors, which suggests that these histamine receptors evolved from different ancestor genes [3]. This discovery led to the identification of a fourth receptor, the human histamine H_4 receptor (HRH4), in the year 2000/2001 by several research groups [7–9, 4, 5]. The genomic organization of the HRH family is shown in Fig. 1, where the National Centre for Biotechnology Information (NCBI) Gene ID and the nucleotide number (NC) is represented for each gene respectively.

Comparing these four receptors, HRH1 is characterized by a large intron located between the 5′-untranslated region (UTR) with only one exon. On the other hand, HRH2 has two introns and two exons, where one large intron (intron 1) is located within

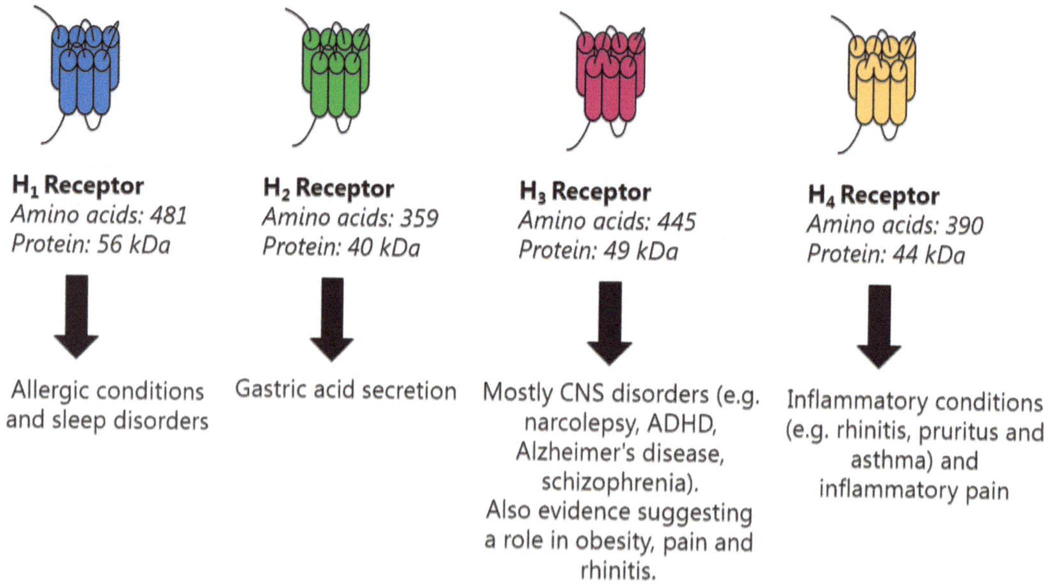

Fig. 1 Genomic organization of HRH family as per GRCH38.p2 Primary Assembly; where the darker boxes represent the exons, while the lighter boxes represent the UTRs at the 5′ and 3′ termini of the genes. (Image adapted from [10])

the 5′-UTR. Looking at the other two HRH members, it becomes evident that HRH3 and HRH4 share a similar genomic organization, consisting of three exons and two introns. Using a bioinformatics tool, the GenomeNet multiple sequence alignment CLUSTALW, homology for genes can be estimated (further information on bioinformatics tools is discussed further on in this chapter). Comparing the DNA sequence between all HRH genes the homology appears to be in the same range (18–20%) for all four HRHs [10].

The translated sequence of the HRH genes, however, results in four receptors with different functions and properties. The largest protein is histamine H_1 receptor with 481 amino acids, while the smallest protein is histamine H_2 receptor with 359 amino acids (Fig. 2) [11]. Considering the biological significance of histamine, polymorphisms of histamine-related genes are potential genetic factors likely to influence disease and therapy. Single nucleotide polymorphisms can show an effect at a phenotypic level. In humans, these SNPs occur in at least 1% of the population at a frequency of 1 every 100–300 bases along the 3 billion-base human genome [12].

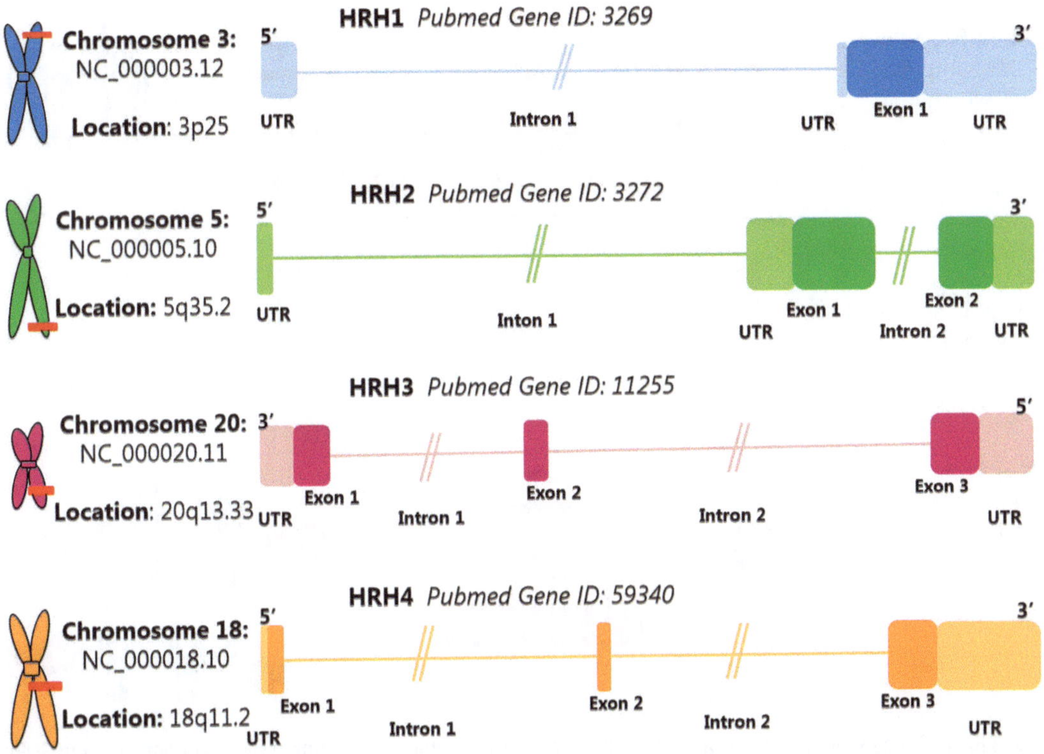

Fig. 2 Key characteristics of the histamine receptor family; the number of amino acids and protein weight is shown for each receptor and the respective main function is shown above (Image adapted from [10])

2 Basis of Association Studies and Linkage Analysis

2.1 The HapMap Project

The completion of the Human Genome Project in April 2003 opened a lot of doors for the "Genomic Era" which helped in understanding the genetic basis of many common phenotypes of biochemical importance. Several diseases have been studied and are now known to be caused by a combination of multiple genetic and environmental factors. Understanding and identifying these genetic factors can provide new insights into the pathogenesis, diagnosis, and treatment of human diseases [12]. In establishing an association between genotype and phenotype of a population, it is essential to understand the haplotypes in the human genome [13]. Haplotype is a series of polymorphisms that are close together in the genome (Fig. 3). The distribution of alleles at each polymorphic site is nonrandom, i.e., the base at one position predicts with some accuracy the base at the adjacent position [14], as adjacent SNPs tend to be inherited together. Hence, as shown in Fig. 3, a "Tag SNP" is a good marker to predict the haplotype of the individual.

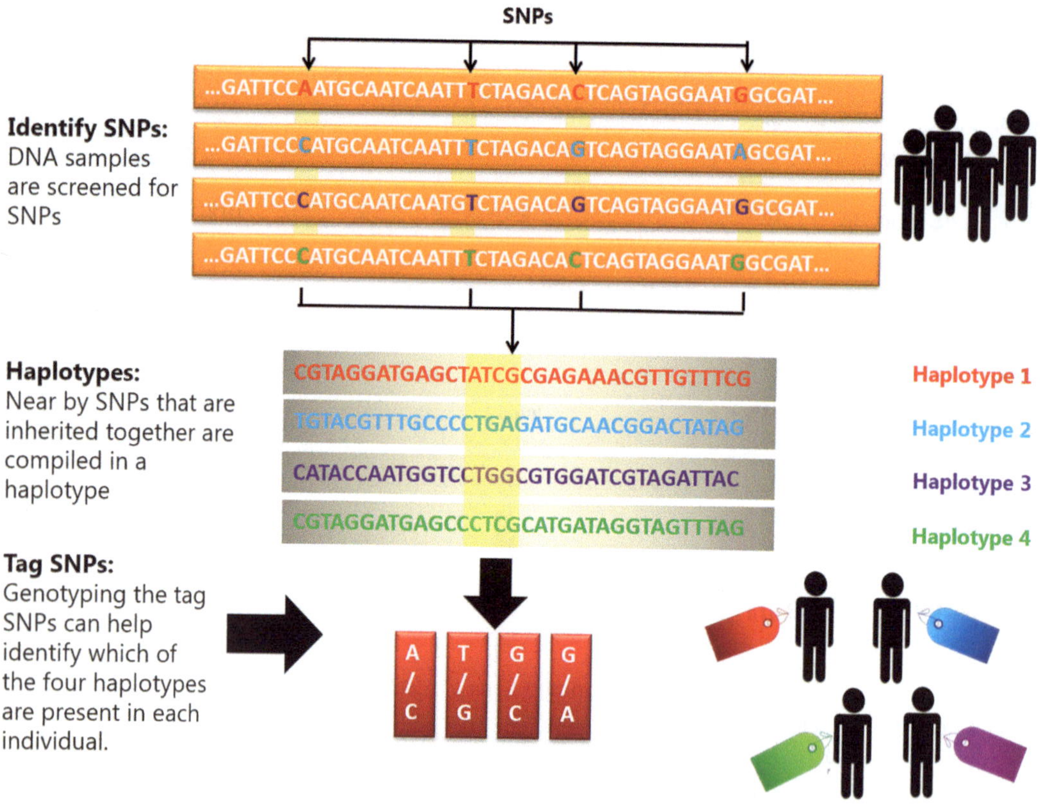

Fig. 3 Basic Concept of Haplotypes and Tag SNP; each chromosome of the sample DNA is genotyped and SNPs are identified. Adjacent SNPs are aligned next to each other to create a Haplotype profile for each DNA sample. The DNA variations within this haplotype profile are then used as Tag SNP for that haplotype. By genotyping a few Tag SNPs researchers are able to identify the haplotype profile for a patient [12]

The aim of the International HapMap Project is to determine the common patterns of DNA sequence variation in the human genome, by characterizing sequence variations, their frequencies, and correlations in DNA samples from populations with ancestry from parts of Africa, Asia, and Europe. This project therefore provides a tool that allows development of an indirect association to any functional gene in the genome. Using this indirect approach it is possible to use a set of sequence variants in the genome as genetic markers to detect association between a particular genomic region and the disease, irrespective of the markers themselves having functional effects. Hence, the HapMap is a valuable tool to reduce the number of SNPs required to be examined in the genome for association with a certain phenotype from the 10 million SNPs that exist to roughly 500,000 tag SNPs [12]. This approach in using tag SNPs throughout the genome makes the search for gene loci that affect diseases much more efficient and comprehensive, since effort is not wasted in genotyping more SNPs than necessary and all regions of the genome can be included. The HapMap therefore provides an important shortcut to carry out candidate-gene, linkage-based, and genome-wide association studies.

2.2 Genome-Wide Association Studies and Linkage Disequilibrium

A very popular approach in the age of high-throughput screening is running a genome-wide association study (GWAS). A GWAS is a test of association between genetic markers, such as SNPs, across the genome and disease. A large number of clear associations between specific chromosomal loci and a complex human disease, such as type 2 diabetes and rheumatoid arthritis, have been discovered by GWAS [14]. From the information collected on the International HapMap project, genetic variance at one locus can predict with high probability genetic variance at an adjacent locus in the human genome. By surveying the genome for common variability it can be associated with the risk of disease simply by genotyping approximately 500,000 carefully chosen markers in the genome of several thousand case and control subjects [14].

This approach is hypothesis free, i.e., there is no existing hypothesis about a particular gene or locus but the null hypothesis that no detectable association exists [14]. Conducting a GWAS analysis requires each individual in the sample population to be genotyped for a comprehensive set of markers. The two major technologies used to genotype samples contain 906,000 and 1,199,187 SNPs (Affymetrix 6.0 and Illumina 1 M, respectively) spaced across the 22 autosomes (chr1-22), the sex chromosomes (chrX and chrY), and the mitochondrial genome (chrM). The major concept for this association to a disease is logistic regression with the dependent variable case-control status and a SNP genotype as an independent variable (represented as the number of copies of minor allele frequency in a population). The output of a logistic regression is identity of the reference allele and an odds ratio with its standard error (or confidence intervals) along with a statistic and a *P* value that tests whether the odds ratio differs from unity. From various GWAS findings, it has emerged that to have a standard of evidence there has to be:

1. a strong association in an initial sample,
2. a precise replication in one or more independent samples,
3. a cumulative *P* value $<5 \times 10^{-8}$.

The *P* values that are smaller than expected by chance and that replicate well in other samples highlight a genomic region associated with a disorder [15].

The primary difference between linkage and association is that linkage analysis directly measures co-segregation within a pedigree, whereas association analysis indirectly measures co-segregation within populations. Within a family, linkage will identify a genomic region inherited with a trait in families. In association studies, the frequency of a specific genetic variant is analyzed in a population for a particular allele or genotype to determine if it is associated with the disease more often than expected by chance. Allelic association can be direct, due to a true biological mechanism of the susceptibility allele (e.g., in the case of APOE-4 allele in Alzheimer's disease, where the presence of this gene is directly linked to the condition), or indirect, due to linkage disequilibrium (e.g., Disruptive in Schizophrenia-1 (DISC-1) intron variations in Schizophrenia) [16–18].

Linkage disequilibrium (LD) is the nonrandom association between two alleles at different loci, i.e., the coinheritance of SNP alleles on haplotypes leads to associations between these alleles in the population [12]. In this manner, a nonfunctional allele can be indirectly associated with a disease phenotype if it is in LD with the biologically influential allele. This study of allelic association is a useful tool in identifying susceptibility alleles, particularly in complex diseases [16]. A perfect LD between alleles is therefore represented by $r^2 = 1.0$. A strong disequilibrium is generally more pronounced when the marker is closest to a mutation. With new generations and recombination the disequilibrium between the markers and the mutation decreases and eventually the mutation reaches equilibrium with the surrounding markers. When equilibrium is reached, the probability of identifying a combination of alleles occurring together becomes the individual allele frequency. Moreover, factors such as genetic drift, recombination patterns, chromosomal composition, and pattern of mating within a population can alter the pattern of LD significantly between populations [17].

2.3 Useful Bioinformatics Databases and Software

As a result of the human genome sequencing, a lot of attention was directed toward molecular targets and bioinformatics networks. Over the past decades the human genome, transcriptomes, proteomes, and resources from other biological sources are publicly available by data being deposited in databases [19].

NCBI. One of the main sources for bioinformatics data is NCBI. This resource includes multiple databases with more in-depth information for each molecular target. The Gene database provides information from gene positioning, intron and exon locations, SNPs with rs numbers, allele frequency, and isoforms of the gene.

OMIM. Another database in NCBI is the Online Mendelian Inheritance in Man (OMIM) that is a library of human genes and genetic disorders and traits, with particular focus on the molecular relationship between genetic variation and phenotypic expression.

1000genomes. As whole genome sequencing is still an expensive process, the goal of 1000genomes project is to find most genetic variants that have frequencies of at least 1% in the populations studied. By downloading this information, the data can be used without the need for researchers to genotype their own samples.

EMBL-EBI. Another useful site for gene analysis is provided by European Bioinformatics Institute (EBI) that is a part of European Molecular Biology lab (EMBL). This source provides multiple links to regularly updated databases that can help to search for genetic variants with functional impact or help to perform analyses such as multiple sequence alignments to study similarities between genes or within family groups.

Promoter 2.0. A useful tool in analyzing promoter regions of a gene is by using a specialized bioinformatics software (Promoter 2.0). Identifying the recognition start site of a promoter region requires analysis of various promoter lengths. This bioinformatics software takes advantage of genetic algorithms to discriminate between promoters and non-promoters on a given DNA stretch [20]. A proximal promoter controls gene expression, where the pre-initiation complex (PIC) determines the location of transcription initiation for protein-coded genes [21]. The PIC is a large complex of proteins which initiates RNA synthesis from a DNA template, and it includes RNA polymerase II and other general initiation factors such as TFIIA, TFIIB, TFIID, TFIIE, TFIIF, and TFIIH [21]. The arrangement of transcription factor-binding sites is specific for each gene; hence, a promoter region is characterized differently for each gene [20]. Using bioinformatics tools such as Promoter 2.0 gives an indication of where the promoter region is located.

Multiple databases and software provide a wide range of specific and mostly comprehensive resources for molecular research. They offer profound knowledge bases, and also provide significant support to genomic research in histamine-related disease development and drug targeting. Table 1 provides a list of different sources that can be used as tools in this area.

Table 1
Databases and software useful in bioinformatics analyses; this table shows resources that are found publicly available for genetic analysis and association studies

Database	Web link and description of tool
NCBI	http://www.ncbi.nlm.nih.gov/ The National Centre for Biotechnology Information provides access to biomedical and genomic information. Multiple resource pages are located in this database including gene, protein, blast, nucleotide, SNP, OMIM, and genome.
1000genomes	http://www.1000genomes.org/ A useful tool used in GWAS analysis where combining the data from 1000 Genomes with the genotype data in the targeted disease GWAS to impute the genotypes in the samples for millions of additional variants beyond those they genotyped directly. The additional genotype data will allow the researchers to localize the disease-associated regions more precisely.
International HapMap Project	http://hapmap.ncbi.nlm.nih.gov/index.html.en The information provided in the HapMap project will be able to provide researchers the tool to identify genes that affect health, disease, and individual responses to medications and environmental factors. The Project is collaboration among scientists and funding agencies from Japan, the United Kingdom, Canada, China, Nigeria, and the United States [12]. Haplotype can be downloaded from this website.
EMBL-EBI	http://www.ebi.ac.uk/ European Molecular Biology lab—European Bioinformatics Institute is a website that provides regularly updated molecular databases such as Ensembl (where genomic sequences can be screened for variants and prediction of functional consequence) and Uniport (where DNA can be subjected to blast and identify the origin and perform multiple sequence alignments).
Haploview	https://www.broadinstitute.org/scientific-community/science/programs/medical-and-population-genetics/haploview/haploview A software supported by the Board Institute that helps to process haplotype analysis such as LD & haplotype block analysis, haplotype population frequency estimation, single SNP, and haplotype association tests [42].
Sequence manipulation suite: Primer stats	http://www.bioinformatics.org/sms2/pcr_primer_stats.html A resource used to analyze newly designed PCR Primers and provides a report describing the properties of each primer, including melting temperature, percent GC content, hair-loop potential, and PCR suitability. This site is used to evaluate potential PCR primers.
Promoter 2.0	http://www.cbs.dtu.dk/services/Promoter/ This source helps researchers to predict transcription start sites of vertebrate PolII promoters in the DNA sequence. It simulates transcription factors that interact with sequences in promoter region and is built on principles of neural network and genetic algorithms [20].
A Plasmid Editor (ApE)	http://biologylabs.utah.edu/jorgensen/wayned/ape/ A useful program that can be downloaded freely that helps to text map showing DNA sequence, translation, and features as text-based graphics. This software can also help to create circular and linear DNA which can be annotated and also perform virtual restriction enzyme digest.

3 Analyzing Complex Polymorphisms on the Human Histamine Receptors

Microsatellite polymorphisms are normally two to four base-pair-long tandem repeats, and are spread throughout the whole genome and are used as genetic markers also in mapping of disease gene loci [22]. Microsatellites are very common in eukaryotes and are typical landmarks in genome mapping [23, 24]. Microsatellite instabilities have been associated with neurological disorders, where both "loss of function" and "gain of function" mechanisms can result from expanded trinucleotide repeats [25]. In the case of "loss of function," the gene product is either not produced or produced at a lower level. "Gain of function" can occur at RNA or protein level, and repeat expansions located in a translated part of the protein can affect protein structure or function. The translated variation can lead to a change in amino acids which makes either the protein work in a different way or potentially affecting binding of therapeutic drugs. If the repeat expansion is in a nontranslated region, it can affect the protein in an indirect method, where when the repeat is transcribed it can influence the function of the mRNA or other transcription factors [25]. These repeat instabilities are a product of DNA replication, where unpaired bases form loops resulting in expansions or contractions depending on whether the loops are in the synthesized or in the template strand [25] (Fig. 4). When the loop is present on the template strand, contraction occurs, while if the loop forms on the newly synthesized strand, expansion occurs.

3.1 Genotyping Complex Polymorphisms

Genetic polymorphisms are detected through popular molecular biology techniques such as polymerase chain reaction (PCR), DNA sequencing, SNaP-shot assay, gel and capillary electrophoresis. When facing microsatellite repeats however, running association studies can prove to be challenging as each SNP cannot be directly analyzed for association with a disease.

A repeat expansion located on the histamine H_4 receptor was studied by the authors [26–28]. One way of analyzing this type of variation is by genotyping the region by PCR and run on a capillary electrophoresis on an ABI 3700XL Genetic Analyzer using 6-Fam dye on the forward primer. The position of the peak when performing capillary electrophoresis (CE) represents the number of repeat expansions for the region. The position of the peak representing the number of repeats is validated by sequence analysis of selected samples and using these samples as control. When a sample is homozygous one peak is represented in the CE plot, similarly, when the sample is heterozygous two peaks are seen in the CE plot and the difference in migration time (between peaks) depends on the difference in allele repeats (Fig. 5). The migration time of the PCR product was assigned to each sample and an allele

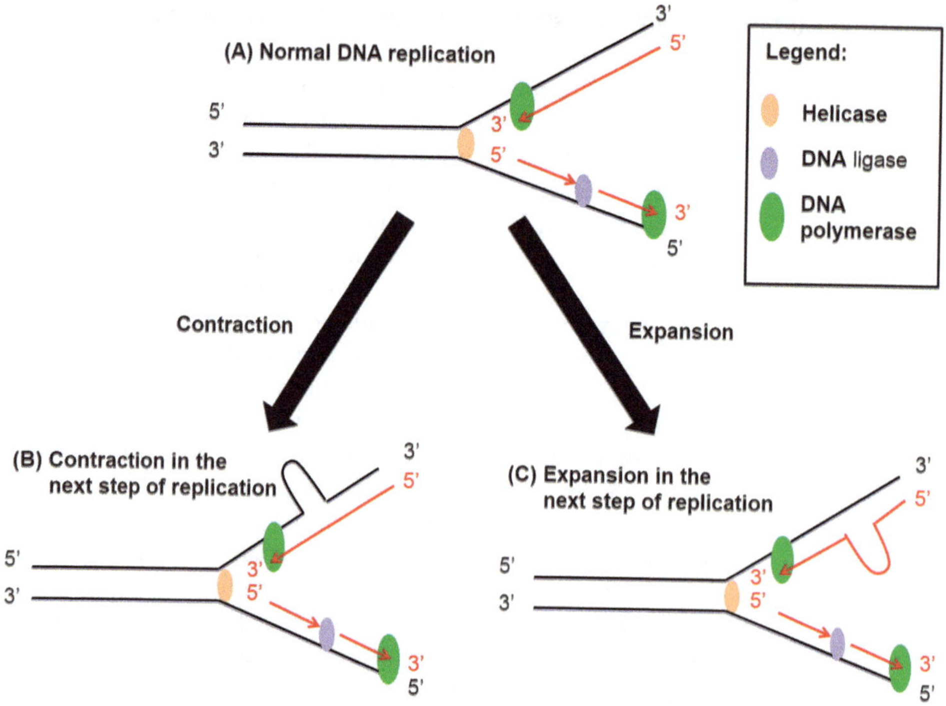

Fig. 4 Formation of microsatellites; (**a**) during DNA replication helicase opens up the double strand and DNA polymerase synthesizes the 5′–3′ strand. (**b**) When loops are formed in the template, contraction occurs in the next step of replication. (**c**) When loops are formed in the synthesized strand, expansion occurs in the next step of replication [25]

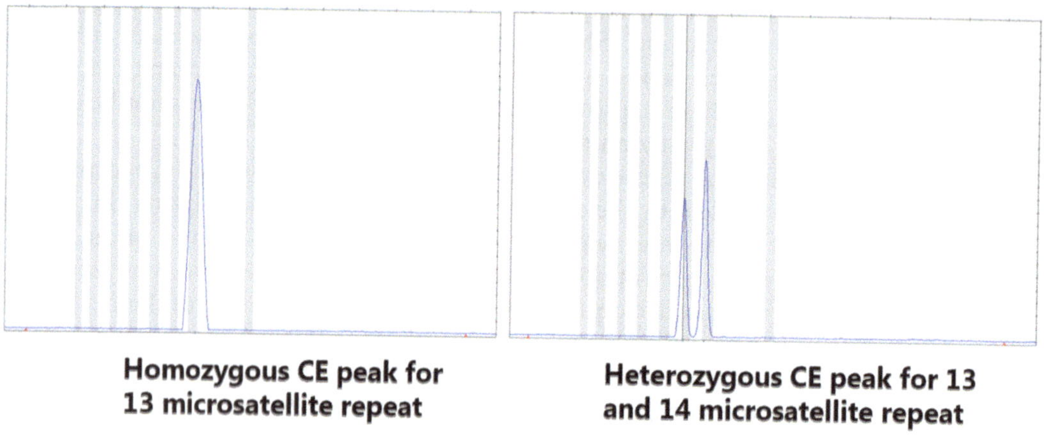

Fig. 5 Capillary Electrophoresis (CE) for a microsatellite repeat expansion located on the HRH4 gene; where the position of the peak represents the number of repeat expansions in the sample [26]

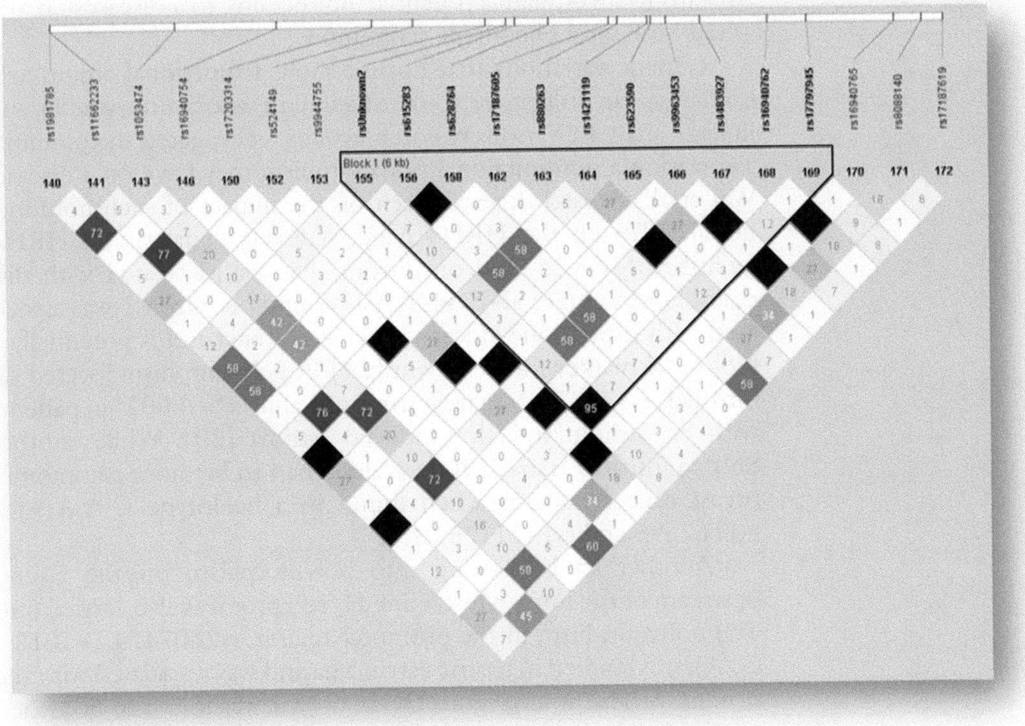

Fig. 6 LD plot a microsatellite repeat on HRH4 named rsunknown. Diagonal boxes represent an SNP, with each box representing a pairwise association of each SNP. Black squares indicate statistically significant allelic association between the pair of SNPs as measured by r^2 statistics; darker colors of black indicate higher values of r^2, max = 1. White squares indicate pairwise r^2 values of <1 with no statistically significant evidence of LD [26, 27]

image profile was developed for all genotypes in the sample group. Pedigree analysis was carried out and only individuals that followed a Mendelian trait of inheritance were used for further investigations [26].

3.2 Establishing Linkage Analysis

Once an allele image profile was created, each data set was considered one variation of the polymorphism. The data set was regarded as an SNP and given an rs identity code to be comparable to other SNPs. The rs number is a reference snp number that is used in databases as an accession and reference number. It stands for reference snp cluster ID assigned by NCBI. These genotype data sets are then integrated using the bioinformatics software Haploview. The online database of the International HapMap Project and 1000genomes was used to download genotypes, and by using Haploview an LD plot was constructed for all the data sets (Fig. 6). This plot was used to analyze the LD between one polymorphism and another. Figure 6 shows the LD between a microsatellite repeat named as "rsunknown" to another SNP where r^2 = 0.956, i.e., high LD between variations [26, 27]. This tool can be used as a means to investigate a potential indirect link to a disease and also as tag SNP for a phenotype/condition.

Genetic variations that do not show a functional amino acid exchange can still prove to be of value in association studies and linkage analysis. Various research groups investigated the potential association a nonfunctional polymorphism may have on a disease. Wei et al. focused their research on the impact of such nonfunctional SNPs on the HRH4 gene. A linkage analysis on HRH4 identified SNPs located on introns that are associated with diseases. For example, SNP rs4483927 found on intron 1 was associated with risperidone efficacy in schizophrenia and is potentially a biological marker for treatment [29]. A polymorphism located on intron 2, rs17187619, gave a strong *P* value ($P = 0.002$) in patients with or without infection-induced asthma [30]. While another SNP in intron 1, rs623590, was described to be more common in breast cancer patients when found in a haplotype C-A-A with rs1162595 and rs1421125 [31].

Another study looking into polymorphism on the 5′-end upstream of the human histamine H_2 receptor was also carried out. The polymorphism in the promoter region, rs2607474 (−1018--G/A), was studied in gastric carcinoma and was associated with the condition. The homozygous GG genotype was found to be associated with gastric mucosal atrophy ($P = 0.0052$) with a subsequent development of gastric cancer (mostly intestinal, $P = 0.0047$), especially at an advanced age [32]. Due to the location of this SNP in an important region for gene regulation, it seems like it has an important implication in gene transcription, but further analysis is needed to prove this biological significance.

Looking at a study on another family member, a promoter polymorphism present on the human histamine H_1 receptor was analyzed. Different variations located in this promoter region of H_1 receptor were investigated for association with psychiatric disorders. A significant Linkage Disequilibrium (LD) ($P < 10^{-6}$) was found in the excess of C allele, but no strong association with schizophrenia was identified in multiple testing. However, the polymorphism for G/C allele may represent a marker for more functional polymorphisms located further upstream [33]. Hence, polymorphisms that do not lie on a translation site (such as an exon) may still play a biological role and contribute to a disease or may influence treatment leading to personalized medicine.

4 Other Tools for Assessing Polymorphisms on Human Histamine Receptors

4.1 SNaP-Shot Assay

Genome sequencing is still considered a resource-intensive means to obtain data. Sequencing polymorphisms of interest can prove to be inexpensive by adopting other methods such as the SNaP-shot assay. This type of analysis enables simultaneous genotyping up to 10 SNPs with commercially available multiplex kits. This type of analysis makes use of polymerase chain reaction (PCR) and adopts a similar technique to Sanger's sequencing. The reaction is based on the dideoxy single-base extension using an unlabeled oligonucleotide primer (or primers). Each oligonucleotide binds to its complementary template in the presence of fluorescently labeled ddNTPs and DNA polymerase. The enzyme extends the primer by one nucleotide, adding only one ddNTP to its 3′ end. The fluorescent color readout reports which base was added. This type of analysis proved to be cost-effective and efficient in several studies such as identification of *KRAS* and *BRAF* mutations in advanced stage colorectal cancer [34] and identification and monitoring of increased theophylline clearance between a SNP (−3860G > A) and CYP1A2 in Korean nonsmoking asthmatics [35].

4.2 Taqman Assay

Other studies such as Taqman assays are also useful tools to analyze genetic variations. This technique uses a probe and unlabeled PCR primers with a fluorescent dye on the 5′-end and a non-fluorescent quencher on the 3′-end. The sample of interest, generally from the mRNA, is reverse transcribed into the cDNA and this cDNA serves as the template for the real-time PCR. A study on histamine N-methyltransferase (HNMT) used this technique to try and verify a functional polymorphism linked to alcoholism in German Caucasians. In this study, the genomic DNA was used with a probe for Thr105 and Ile105 variations using 6-Fam dye on the 5′-end and VIC quencher on the 3′-end. Once an allele profile was generated for the Thr105Ile variation, a statistical approach was adopted to analyze associations. In this study, the association between the polymorphism Thr105Ile with alcoholism could not be replicated but an association was found between Ile105 allele and family history of alcoholism supporting the protective role of the Ile105 allele against alcoholism [36].

4.3 Molecular Beacon

The use of oligonucleotide hybridization probes is highly specific and can be monitored by real-time PCR. Molecular beacons are single-stranded oligonucleotide hybridization probes in a hairpin formation that form a stem-and-loop structure. The probe contains the sequence that is complementary to a target sequence. The stem anneals on complementary arm sequences located on either side of the probe sequence. A fluorophore is linked at the end of one arm and a quencher is covalently linked to the end of the other arm. When the probe finds the target sequence a probe-target hybrid is formed, which is longer and more stable than the stem hybrid. As a result, the molecular beacon undergoes a conformational change that forces the stem hybrid to dissociate and the fluorophore and the quencher to separate from each other. This results in fluorescence of the probe which is recorded and analyzed for the target sequence [37]. This type of assay is not yet adopted in histamine research but may prove to be important in identifying molecular targets in future studies.

4.4 Promoter Identification

Identification of the promoter region of a gene is of biological significance since transcriptional control can have direct implications on human health. Recent publications on the histamine receptors identified the decreased expression of HRH1 and HRH4 in colorectal tumors, where the mRNA for these two receptors was significantly reduced when compared to healthy controls [38]. One of the latest studies on HRH4 shows that it is highly expressed in keratinocytes in patients suffering from atopic dermatitis and its stimulation might contribute to epidermal hyperplasia noticed in atopic dermatitis patients [39]. Promoter prediction is based on transcription-binding sites where algorithms are used to predict promoter length. However, no matter how extensive these predictions are, they can still vary from biological data, especially since not all identified binding sites are confirmed experimentally [40]. As mentioned in earlier in this chapter, the length of the promoter can be postulated by using a bioinformatics database Promoter 2.0, where the highly predictable area is taken from the maximum value achieved in relation to the length of the promoter.

4.5 Luciferase Assay

The basic components for the potentially functional active promoter can be cloned into a reporter vector and activity of the promoter can be determined. This type of assay can also be used to assess polymorphisms located in the promoter region and determine the impact on gene expression. A dual-luciferase assay on a mammalian cell line can be used to measure the activity of a promoter. For example, the putative promoter region can be introduced upstream of the ATG start codon on firefly luciferase and transiently transfected into a mammalian cell line; hence, transcription of the protein is recorded as a light signal and represents activity of the promoter. The renilla luciferase vector, pRL-SV40, can be used as an internal control that contains the SV40 enhancer elements and promoter and it can be used as a normalizing vector for transfection and luciferase activity. Optimization of co-transfection protocol for promoter-of-interest/firefly vector and control/renilla vector ratio is required to ensure independent genetic expression between experimental and control reporter genes [26, 27].

Firefly and renilla proteins are widely used as co-reporters, and the renilla luciferase can be used as a normalizing control vector. Normalizing the expression of an experimental reporter to the expression of a control vector can help differentiate between specific and nonspecific cellular responses. Gene expression of firefly luciferase is quantified as transcription activity for the promoter region. The firefly luciferase is commonly used as reporter gene for this type of analysis and tracks the physiological response, where the bioluminescence represents the immediate function upon translation. Thus, if the amount of luminescence from an experimental sample (promoter constructs) is greater than the luminescence from the control (such as pGL3-basic, promoter-less control vector) an increase in transcription or translation has occurred. The mechanism of the luciferase assay is shown in Fig. 7. The transcription or translation of the reporter molecules, such as firefly and renilla luciferase, is immediately recorded because they do not need posttranslational modification and thus are fully functional after translation. In order to activate firefly luciferase, beetle luciferin, ATP, magnesium, and oxygen are required, while renilla luciferase requires only coelenterazine and oxygen (Fig. 7). Running the assay requires the addition of luciferase substrate that lyses the cell and drives the reaction shown in Fig. 7. Bioluminescence produced by firefly luciferase is recorded. Following the firefly luciferase measurement, a second reagent is added which simultaneously quenches the firefly luminescence and generates renilla luminescence.

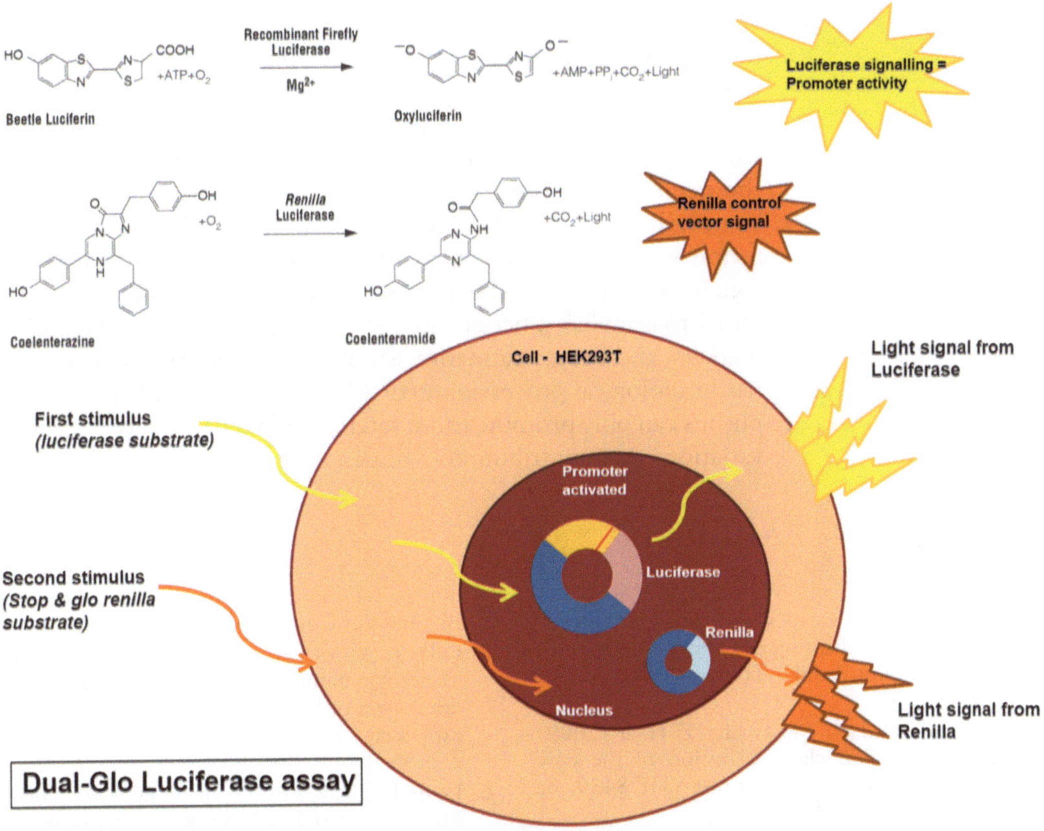

Fig. 7 Luciferase assay for promoter identification; the promoter-of-interest containing luciferase construct is transfected into a cell line, e.g., HEK293T and activated for transcription with the luciferase substrate containing beetle luciferin, ATP, and magnesium. The light emitted is recorded and normalized to the light emitted by the renilla luciferase, stimulated by coelenterazine

Various luciferase constructs (such as pGL3 or pGL4 vectors from promega, pMetLuc-2 vector from Clontech, pSelect zero plasmids from InvivoGen) are available commercially with their respective experimental assays. The putative promoter region can be cloned into the vector construct by using popular molecular biology techniques such as PCR and restriction enzyme digest. Care is also needed in choosing a suitable assay and the construct used to clone the promoter into as some vectors can produce some background luminescence without a promoter being present. Some commercially available kits also claim to contain promoter regions with the gene constructed in a vector; however, these are not necessarily biologically validated. Hence in-depth literature review and background reading is required to select the appropriate vector/plasmid for the assay.

5 Future Perspective

Molecular biology techniques are becoming progressively important in association studies and linkage analysis. With the development of the human genome project, the medical attention has been shifted toward the analysis of complex traits. The increase in studies toward the molecular biological aspect of diseases enhances the need to develop new approaches that take into account the complexity of the genetic basis of conditions and the possible interaction with other, nongenetic factors [41]. Development in this area benefits also genomic research on biogenic amines, here histamine, to establish a better association between diseases, biological markers, and drug treatments. Knowing the importance histamine has in biological processes, further knowledge on HRH polymorphisms can only promote more interest in identifying novel genetic variations that contribute to a disease.

References

1. Leurs R, Vischer HF, Wijtmans M et al (2011) En route to new blockbuster anti-histamines: surveying the offspring of the expanding histamine receptor family. Trends Pharmacol Sci 32:250–257
2. Lim HD, Adami M, Guaita E et al (2009) Pharmacological characterization of the new histamine H4 receptor agonist VUF 8430. Br J Pharmacol 157:34–43
3. Zhu Y, Michalovich D, Wu H et al (2001) Cloning, expression, and pharmacological characterization of a novel human histamine receptor. Mol Pharmacol 59:434–441
4. Nakamura T, Itadani H, Hidaka Y et al (2000) Molecular cloning and characterization of a new human histamine receptor, HH4R. Biochem Biophys Res Commun 279:615–620
5. Oda T, Morikawa N, Saito Y et al (2000) Molecular cloning and characterization of a novel type of histamine receptor preferentially expressed in leukocytes. J Biol Chem 275:36781–36786
6. Leurs R, Chazot PL, Shenton FC et al (2009) Molecular and biochemical pharmacology of the histamine H4 receptor. Br J Pharmacol 157:14–23
7. Coge F, Guenin SP, Rique H et al (2001) Structure and expression of the human histamine H4-receptor gene. Biochem Biophys Res Commun 284:301–309

8. Liu C, Ma X, Jiang X et al (2001) Cloning and pharmacological characterization of a fourth histamine receptor (H(4)) expressed in bone marrow. Mol Pharmacol 59:420–426
9. Morse KL, Behan J, Laz TM et al (2001) Cloning and characterization of a novel human histamine receptor. J Pharmacol Exp Ther 296:1058–1066
10. Micallef S, Stark H, Sasse A (2013) Polymorphisms and genetic linkage of histamine receptors. Life Sci 93:487–494
11. Panula P, Chazot PL, Cowart M et al (2015) International union of basic and clinical pharmacology. XCVIII. Histamine receptors. Pharmacol Rev 67:601–655
12. Consortium IH (2003) The international HapMap project. Nature 426:789–796
13. Gabriel SB, Schaffner SF et al (2002) The structure of haplotype blocks in the human genome. Science 296:2225–2229
14. Hardy J, Singleton A (2009) Genomewide association studies and human disease. N Engl J Med 360:1759–1768
15. Corvin A, Craddock N, Sullivan PF (2010) Genome-wide association studies: a primer. Psychol Med 40:1063–1077
16. Bush WS, Haines J (2010) Overview of linkage analysis in complex traits. Curr Protoc Hum Genet Chapter 1:Unit 1.9.1–18
17. Rosmond R (2003) Association studies of genetic polymorphisms in central obesity: a critical review. Int J Obes Relat Metab Disord 27:1141–1151
18. Schumacher J, Laje G, Abou Jamra R et al (2009) The DISC locus and schizophrenia: evidence from an association study in a central European sample and from a meta-analysis across different European populations. Hum Mol Genet 18:2719–2727
19. Teufel A (2015) Bioinformatics and database resources in hepatology. J Hepatol 62:712–719
20. Knudsen S (1999) Promoter2.0: for the recognition of PolII promoter sequences. Bioinformatics 15:356–361
21. Fickett JW, Hatzigeorgiou AG (1997) Eukaryotic promoter recognition. Genome Res 7:861–878
22. Toth-Petroczy A, Szilagyi A, Ronai Z et al (2006) Validation of a tentative microsatellite marker for the dopamine D4 receptor gene by capillary gel electrophoresis. J Chromatogr A 1130:201–205
23. Queller DC, Strassmann JE, Hughes CR (1993) Microsatellites and kinship. Trends Ecol Evol 8:285–288
24. Varela MA, Amos W (2010) Heterogeneous distribution of SNPs in the human genome: microsatellites as predictors of nucleotide diversity and divergence. Genomics 95:151–159
25. Brouwer JR, Willemsen R, Oostra BA (2009) Microsatellite repeat instability and neurological disease. Bioessays 31:71–83
26. Micallef S, Quinn E, Morris D, Sasse A (2012) Microsatellite repeat expansions in human histamine(4) receptor gene. Inflamm Res 61:S52–S52
27. Micallef S, Sasse A (2014) Characterisation of the promoter region of the human histamine H 4 receptor (hH4R). Inflamm Res 63:S21–S21
28. Micallef S (2013) PhD thesis, Characterization of polymorphisms on the promoter region of the human histamine H4 receptor (Trinity College, University of Dublin, Ireland).
29. Wei Z, Wang L, Yu T et al (2013) Histamine H4 receptor polymorphism: a potential predictor of risperidone efficacy. J Clin Psychopharmacol 33:221–225
30. Simon T, Semsei AF, Ungvári I et al (2012) Asthma endophenotypes and polymorphisms in the histamine receptor HRH4 gene. Int Arch Allergy Immunol 159:109–120
31. He GH, Lu J, Shi PP et al (2013) Polymorphisms of human histamine receptor H4 gene are associated with breast cancer in Chinese Han population. Gene 519:260–265
32. Arisawa T, Tahara T, Ozaki K et al (2012) Association between common genetic variant of HRH2 and gastric cancer risk. Int J Oncol 41:497–503
33. Mancama D, Arranz MJ, Munro J et al (2002) Investigation of promoter variants of the histamine 1 and 2 receptors in schizophrenia and clozapine response. Neurosci Lett 333:207–211
34. Magnin S, Viel E, Baraquin A et al (2011) A multiplex SNaPshot assay as a rapid method for detecting KRAS and BRAF mutations in advanced colorectal cancers. J Mol Diagn 13:485–492
35. Yim E-Y, Kang H-R, Jung J-W et al (2013) CYP1A2 polymorphism and theophylline clearance in Korean non-smoking asthmatics. Asia Pac Allergy 3:231–240
36. Reuter M, Jeste N, Klein T et al (2007) Association of THR105Ile, a functional polymorphism of histamine N-methyltransferase (HNMT), with alcoholism in German Caucasians. Drug Alcohol Depend 87:69–75
37. Nguyen LV, Giannetti S, Warren-Smith S et al (2014) Genotyping Single Nucleotide

Polymorphisms Using Different Molecular Beacon Multiplexed within a Suspended Core Optical Fiber. Sensors (Basel, Switzerland) 14:14488–14499

38. Boer K, Helinger E, Helinger A et al (2008) Decreased expression of histamine H1 and H4 receptors suggests disturbance of local regulation in human colorectal tumours by histamine. Eur J Cell Biol 87:227–236

39. Glatzer F, Gschwandtner M, Ehling S et al (2013) Histamine induces proliferation in keratinocytes from patients with atopic dermatitis through the histamine 4 receptor. J Allergy Clin Immunol 132:1358–1367

40. Pedersen AG, Baldi P, Chauvin Y et al (1999) The biology of eukaryotic promoter prediction—a review. Comput Chem 23:191–207

41. Forabosco P, Falchi M, Devoto M (2005) Statistical tools for linkage analysis and genetic association studies. Expert Rev Mol Diagn 5:781–796

42. Barrett JC, Fry B, Maller J et al (2005) Haploview: analysis and visualization of LD and haplotype maps. Bioinformatics 21:263–265

Chapter 2

Development, Characterization, and Validation of Anti-Human H_3 Receptor Isoform-Specific Antibodies

Fiona C. Shenton*, Natasha Lethbridge*, and Paul L. Chazot

Abstract

Generation of selective anti-G-protein coupled receptor (GPCR) antibodies is a challenging pursuit and the anti-histamine receptor antibodies are no exception. Furthermore, producing isoform-selective antibodies is even more of a challenge. The first anti-histamine H_3 receptor (H_3) antibodies were developed in 2001 and validated in 2007. The first two antibodies were raised against human H_3 receptor sequences common to most human and rodent isoforms. This chapter describes how a panel of anti-hH_3 receptor isoform-specific antibodies have been generated, characterized, and validated for selectivity [individual rH_3R and hH_3R isoform transient expression in human embryonic kidney (HEK) 293 cells, isoform peptide blockade, and the use of H_3R knock-out (KO) mice], and utility for a range of immunobiochemical techniques (immunoblotting, immunohistochemical, and immunofluorescence techniques).

Key words Antibodies, H_3R, Human, Immunobiochemistry, KO mice, Peptide-directed, Polyclonal, Splice-variants

1 Introduction

1.1 Cloning of the H_3 Receptor

Due to lower than expected homology with histamine receptors H_1 and H_2, the H_3 receptor was not cloned until 1999 [1] more than a decade after it was first described by seminal studies in France [2]. It was discovered as part of an effort to identify orphan G-protein coupled receptors (GPCRs).

Lovenberg and colleagues identified a partial clone (GPCR97) that had significant homology to a range of biogenic amine receptors. The GPCR97 clone was used to probe a human thalamus library, which resulted in the isolation of a full-length clone encoding a putative GPCR. Homology analysis showed the highest similarity to M_2 muscarinic acetylcholine receptors and overall low homology to all other biogenic amine receptors. Subsequent

*These authors contributed equally in this chapter.

Ekaterini Tiligada and Madeleine Ennis (eds.), *Histamine Receptors as Drug Targets*, Methods in Pharmacology and Toxicology, DOI 10.1007/978-1-4939-6843-5_2, © Springer Science+Business Media LLC 2017

analysis revealed a pharmacological profile practically indistinguishable from that for the histamine H_3 receptor. In two analyses of the human gene [3, 4] a 1063 base pair (bp) intron beginning 250 nucleotides downstream of the start codon (corresponding to aa 84) and another 1564 bp intron at position 417 (corresponding to aa 139) suggests a gene with three exons and two introns. By contrast, Cogé and colleagues [5] put forward a gene having a minimum of four exons and three introns. In their analysis, the coding region is interrupted by introns of 1062, 1565, and 240 bp. A further exon may result in an additional eight amino acids at the C-terminus, leading to a protein of 453 aa. The result of these diverse exon/intron junctions is the possibility of alternative splicing to generate multiple splice variants that may potentially lead to several receptor isoforms.

1.2 H_3 Receptor Isoforms

The cloning of the H_3 receptor initiated a new era in histamine research. The existence of multiple H_3 receptor isoforms could contribute to the pharmacological heterogeneity in H_3 receptors, within and across species, which has long been recognized but not understood. In all species tested so far the full-length H_3 receptor encodes a polypeptide of 445 amino acids (predicted polypeptide $M_{r.}$ 47,000). Shorter isoforms with deletions predominantly in the third intracellular loop domain have also been identified (predicted polypeptide $M_{r.}$ 20,000–45,000 range).

1.2.1 H_3 receptor Isoform Anatomical Topology

While the full-length clone is found in most abundance in the CNS in all species studied so far, there is regional variation in the distribution of the mRNAs encoding the different isoforms [5]; this has given rise to speculation that H_3 heterogeneity could underlie different activities and functions of H_3 receptors in specific tissues [6].

The evidence for heterogeneity in anatomical distribution was based initially on the distribution pattern of mRNA coding for the various isoforms. Note that these splicing events yield potentially different protein sequences in rodents and human H_3R orthologs. In order to define the importance of human and rodent H_3 receptor heterogeneity, specific immunological probes are required.

1.3 Anti-Histamine H_3 Receptor Antibodies

Generation of selective anti-GPCR antibodies is a challenging pursuit and the histamine receptors are no exception. Furthermore, producing isoform-selective antibodies is even more testing. The first anti-histamine H_3 receptor (H_3) antibodies were developed in 2001 and validated using knock-out (KO) mice in 2007 [7, 8]. The first two antibodies were raised against human H_3 receptor sequences common to most human and rodent isoforms: anti-hH_3 (349–358) and anti-hH_3 (175–187), respectively. They both detected two specific immunoreactive protein species (M_r 68,000 and 93,000) that were suppressed by prior incubation with their

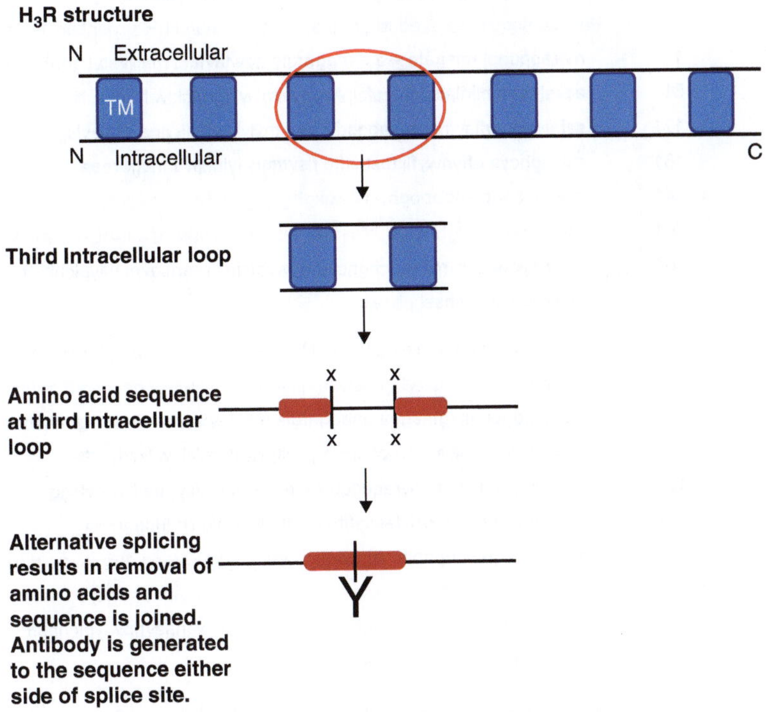

Fig. 1 Schematic showing how peptide sequences were selected in an attempt to produce isoform-specific antibodies against the distinctly spliced third intracellular loop of the human H$_3$R. Amino acid sequences were chosen that spanned either side of the splicing event so once the sequence was removed and the sequence at either side joined, the antibody generated would be predicted to detect the sequence. The sequence selected (10–15-mer) was long enough so that the antibody was specific but not too long that the antibody would detect other closely related isoforms

respective peptide antigens, in many adult rat and mouse brain regions. These protein species are most likely derived from the dimeric and/or glycosylation variants of the receptor.

In an attempt to generate an antibody specific to the rat $H_{3C\,(397)}$ isoform a peptide sequence was chosen which spanned the deletion within the third intracellular loop rat isoform sequences and should therefore be unique to this isoform (Fig. 1). However, when tested against three of the major human and rat isoforms heterologously expressed in HEK 293 cells namely $hH_{3\,(445)}$, $hH_{3\,(365)}$, and $hH_{3\,(329)}$; $rH3_{A\,(445)}$, $rH3_{B\,(413)}$, and $rH3_{C\,(397)}$, the antibody was found to be selective for both the full-length human and rat isoforms ($hH_{3\,(445)}$ and $rH_{3A\,(445)}$) as well as the expected $rH_{3C\,(397)}$ isoform. Using this same strategy, antibodies specific for three of the other major human H$_3$R isoforms, $hH_{3\,(415)}$, $hH_{3\,(365)}$, and $hH_{3\,(329)}$ ΔI3 (*see* Fig. 2, human isoform sequences), were also sought.

Peptide sequences chosen for each isoform:

(A) Human sequence showing the H_3R_{365} deletion / isoform 2 **(spliced deletion in red and bold)**

Peptide sequence used to generate: anti-human H_3R_{365} peptide 1 antibody, blue

1 merappdgpl nasgalagea aaaggargfs aawtavlaal mallivatvl gnalvmlafv
61 adsslrtqnn ffllnlaisd flvgafcipl yvpyvltgrw tfgrglcklw lvvdyllcts
121 safnivlisy drflsvtrav syraqqgdtr ravrkmllvw vlafllygpa ilsweylsgg
181 ssipeghcya effynwyfli tastlefftp flsvtffnls iylniqrrtr lrldgareaa
241 gpepppeaqp sppppgcwg cwqkghgeam plhrygvgea avgaeageat lgggggggsv
301 asptsssgss srgterprsl krgskpsass aslekrmkmv sqsftqrfrl srdrkvaksl
361 avivsifglcwapytllmii raachghcvp dywyetsfwl lwansavnpv lyplchhsfr
421 raftkllcpq klkiqphssl ehcwk

(B) Human sequence showing the H_3R_{365} deletion / isoform 2 **(spliced deletion in red and bold)**

Peptide sequence used generate: anti-human H_3R_{365} peptide 2 antibody, blue

1 merappdgpl nasgalagea aaaggargfs aawtavlaal mallivatvl gnalvmlafv
61 adsslrtqnn ffllnlaisd flvgafcipl yvpyvltgrw tfgrglcklw lvvdyllcts
121 safnivlisy drflsvtrav syraqqgdtr ravrkmllvw vlafllygpa ilsweylsgg
181 ssipeghcya effynwyfli tastlefftp flsvtffnls iylniqrrtr lrldgareaa
241 gpepppeaqp sppppgcwg cwqkghgeam plhrygvgea avgaeageat lgggggggsv
301 asptsssgss srgterprsl krgskpsass aslekrmkmv sqsftqrfrl srdrkvaksl
361 avivsifglcwapytllmii raachghcvp dywyetsfwl lwansavnpv lyplchhsfr
421 raftkllcpq klkiqphssl ehcwk

(C) Human sequence showing the H_3R_{329} deletion / isoform 2 **(spliced deletion in red and bold)**

Peptide sequence used to generate:anti-human H_3R_{329} antibody, blue

1 merappdgpl nasgalagea aaaggargfs aawtavlaal mallivatvl gnalvmlafv
61 adsslrtqnn ffllnlaisd flvgafcipl yvpyvltgrw tfgrglcklw lvvdyllcts
121 safnivlisy drflsvtrav syraqqgdtr ravrkmllvw vlafllygpa ilsweylsgg
181 ssipeghcya effynwyfli tastlefftp flsvtffnls iylniqrrtr lrldgareaa
241 gpepppeaqp sppppgcwg cwqkghgeam plhrygvgea avgaeageatlgggggggsv
301 asptsssgss srgterprsl krgskpsass aslekrmkmv sqsftqrfrl srdrkvaksl
361 avivsifglc wapytllmii raachghcvp dywyetsfwl lwansavnpv lyplchhsfr
421 raftkllcpq klkiqphssl ehcwk

(D) Human sequence showing the H_3R_{200} deletion / isoform 5 **(spliced deletion in red and bold).**

Peptide sequence used to generate: anti-human H_3R_{200} antibody, blue

1 merappdgpl nasgalagea aaaggargfs aawtavlaal mallivatvl gnalvmlafv
61 adsslrtqnn ffllnlaisd flvgafcipl yvpyvltgrw tfgrglcklw lvvdyllcts
121 safnivlisy drflsvtrav syraqqgdtr ravrkmllvw vlafllygpailsweylsgg
181 ssipeghcya effynwyfli tastlefftp flsvtffnls iylniqrrtr lrldgareaa
241 gpepppeaqp sppppgcwg cwqkghgeam plhrygvgea avgaeageatlgggggggsv
301 asptsssgss srgterprsl krgskpsass aslekrmkmv sqsftqrfrl srdrkvaksl
361 avivsifglc wapytllmii raachghcvp dywyetsfwl lwansavnpv lyplchhsfr
421 raftkllcpq klkiqphssl ehcwk paaprgalrg rahsrgapsr rrprprwrsa

Fig. 2 The amino acid sequences of the full-length human H_3R and its isoforms and the peptide sequences used to generate specific antibodies to isoforms. (**a**) H_3R_{365} amino acid sequence with the area spliced out highlighted in *red* and selected immunogen sequence in *blue*. (**b**) $H_3R_{(365)}$ amino acid sequence with the area spliced out highlighted in *red* and selected immunogen sequence in *blue*. (**c**) $H_3R_{(329)}$ amino acid sequence with the area spliced out highlighted in *red* and selected immunogen sequence in *blue*. (**d**) $H_3R_{(200)}$ amino acid sequence with the area spliced out highlighted in *red* and sequence highlighted to raise an antibody against selected immunogen sequence in *blue*

Finally, a peptide sequence unique to the heavily truncated $hH_{3(200)}$ was selected ([9], Isoform 5). $hH_{3(200)}$ has a 170–306 deletion plus a frame shift and a novel stop codon, so that the C terminus is unique to this isoform. Therefore, the last 10 amino acids of $hH_{3(200)}$ were selected as the immunogen. Herein, the rationale for peptide selection is described and methods for the preparation of the peptides for immunization, the immunization procedure, antibody purification, and the experiments performed to validate the individual antibody specificities. Results of immunohistochemical analysis using the human/rodent antibody in mouse brain slices from both wild-type (WT) and H_3R KO mice (kind gift of Dr. Tim Lovenberg, Janssens/Johnson & Johnson, USA) are also presented as exemplars.

2 Materials

2.1 Antibody Production

1. Synthetic peptides are purchased commercially (*see* **Note 1**).
2. Keyhole limpet hemocyanin (KLH) or thyroglobulin (Sigma-Aldrich, UK).
3. Imject® Maleimide activated mcKLH kit (Thermo Fisher Scientific, UK).
4. Female Dutch and New Zealand (NZ) white rabbits (suppliers include Harlan or Charles Rivers, UK).
5. Chromatography column with scintered disc (SLS, UK).
6. Phosphate buffered saline (PBS) (Sigma-Aldrich, UK).
7. Spectrophotometer (there are many suppliers, e.g., Jenway Genova).
8. Freund's complete and incomplete adjuvant (Sigma-Aldrich, UK).
9. 1 mL syringes (SLS, UK).
10. 25-gauge needle (SLS, UK).
11. Sterile scalpel blade (SLS, UK).
12. 15 mL and 50 mL falcon tubes (SLS, UK).
13. Microcentrifuge (12,000 × *g*) (e.g., Biofuge Fresco Heraeus, Kendro Laboratory Products).
14. Activated thiol-sepharose beads (Peirce, UK).
15. Rotary Shaker, Stuart™ Just Go SSL5 Shaker (Fisher Scientific laboratories, UK).
16. 0.1 M Tris-HCl pH 8.0, containing 0.3 M NaCl and 1 mM ethylenediamine tetra-acetic acid (EDTA) (Sigma-Aldrich, UK).

17. Tris pH 8.0 (Sigma-Aldrich, UK).
18. 0.1 M citric acid pH 4.5 (Sigma-Aldrich, UK).
19. 0.02% (w/v) sodium azide (Sigma-Aldrich, UK).

2.2 Transfection of Individual Human H_3R Isoforms in HEK 293 Cells

1. 75 cm^3 tissue culture flasks (SLS, UK).
2. Dulbecco's Modified Eagle Medium/F12 (DMEM/F12, 1:1 ratio) (Sigma-Aldrich, UK).
3. Mix powdered DMEM/F12 (15 g/L) and 15 mM N-2-hydroxyethylpoiperazine-N′-2-ethane sulfonic acid (HEPES) with 800 mL of sterile water (Sigma-Aldrich, UK). Supplement the media with 40 mL of 10% (v/v) fetal calf serum (FCS) (Cambrex BoioSciences, Belgium), 7.5% (w/v) $NaHCO_3$ (Sigma-Aldrich, UK) giving a final concentration 3 g/L, and 20 mL of penicillin (500 μg/mL)/streptomycin (500 μg/mL) solution (Sigma-Aldrich, UK).
4. 10 M NaOH (Sigma-Aldrich, UK).
5. 0.2 μm Sartorius Satolab-V150 filter unit (SLS, UK).
6. CO_2 incubator (e.g., Shel Lab, Sheldon Manufacturing Inc., USA).
7. Trypsin-EDTA (Sigma-Aldrich, UK).
8. Polyethyleneimine (PEI) (Sigma-Aldrich, UK).
9. pC DNA 3.1 (-) (Promega Corporation, UK) FLAG-tagged H_3R isoforms.
10. 3 mL Petri dish to 75 cm^3 TC flask depending on scale (SLS, UK).
11. Greiner cell scraper (SLS, UK).
12. Dounce glass/glass homogenizer (Sigma-Aldrich, UK).
13. Ice.

2.3 Immunoblotting of Cell Homogenates of HEK 293 Expressing H_3R Isoforms

1. Resolving gel buffer [50 mM Tris, 384 mM glycine, 1.8 mM EDTA and 0.1% (w/v) sodium dodecyl sulfate (SDS) pH 8.8] (Sigma-Aldrich, UK).
2. Tetramethylethylenediamine (TEMED) (Sigma-Aldrich, UK).
3. 30% (v/v) acrylamide (Sigma-Aldrich, UK).
4. 10% (w/v) ammonium persulfate (APS) (Sigma-Aldrich, UK).
5. Hoefer SE 245 dual gel caster (GE Healthcare Biosciences, UK).
6. Saturated water/butanol solution (Sigma-Aldrich, UK).
7. Electrode buffer [50 mM Tris, 384 mM glycine, 1.8 mM EDTA, and 0.1% (w/v) SDS pH 8.8] (Sigma-Aldrich, UK).

8. Chloroform (Sigma-Aldrich, UK).
9. Methanol (Sigma-Aldrich, UK).
10. Sample buffer [30 mM sodium hydrogen phosphate, pH 7.0, 30% (v/v) glycerol, 0.05% (v/v) bromophenol blue, and 7.5% (w/v) SDS] (Sigma-Aldrich, UK).
11. Stacking gel buffer [0.5 M Tris-glycine, pH 6.8, containing 8 mM EDTA and 0.4% (w/v) SDS] (Sigma-Aldrich, UK).
12. Prestained standards (protein molecular weight range of 200–6.5 kDa, e.g., Takara Bio Group, USA).
13. Hamilton syringe (SLS, UK).
14. Transfer buffer: 25 mM Tris pH 8.4, 192 mM glycine, 20% (v/v) methanol (Sigma-Aldrich, UK).
15. Hoefer TE 22 tank transfer unit (GE Healthcare, UK).
16. Nitrocellulose membrane (GE Healthcare, UK) cut to size, for 10 cm v 8 cm of gels.
17. PBS or Tris-buffered saline (TBS, 50 mM)/0.9% (w/v) NaCl pH 7.4, containing 5% (w/v) dried milk and 0.02% (v/v) Tween-20 (Sigma-Aldrich (UK).
18. PBS or TBS containing 2.5% (w/v) dried milk (Sainsburys supermarket, UK).
19. Wash buffer: PBS or TBS (50 mM)/0.9% (w/v) NaCl containing 2.5% (w/v) dried milk (Sainsburys supermarket, UK) and 0.02% (v/v) Tween-20 (Sigma-Aldrich, UK).
20. Horseradish peroxidise (HRP) labeled secondary antibody, either anti-rabbit or anti-mouse (GE Healthcare, UK) depending on the host species for primary antibody, at a dilution of 1/2000 in 10 mL of incubation buffer.
21. Chemiluminescence developing solution containing 100 μL of 68 mM p-coumaric acid, 10 mL of 1.25 mM luminal, and 6 μL of 30% (v/v) H_2O_2 (Sigma-Aldrich, UK).
22. Hyperfilm™ (GE Healthcare, UK).
23. Kodak D-19 Developer (Sigma-Aldrich, UK).
24. Kodak Unifix (Sigma-Aldrich, UK).

2.4 Immunohistochemistry (IHC) and Immunofluorescence of H_3R in Wild-Type and H_3R KO Mice

1. 4% (w/v) paraformaldehyde, 0.05% (v/v) glutaraldehyde in 0.1 M phosphate buffer (Sigma-Aldrich, UK).
2. Wild-type and H_3R KO Mice produced by Janssens/J&J, USA on a C5731/6 J mouse background (Lovenberg, Johnson and Johnson, US Patent no. 7151200).
3. 10%, 20%, and 30% (w/v) sucrose in 0.01 M phosphate buffer, pH 7.4 (Sigma-Aldrich, UK).

4. Isopentane (Sigma-Aldrich, UK).
5. Cryostat (e.g., Leica model CM3050S, set to −20C).
6. 10% (v/v) methanol and 3% (v/v) hydrogen peroxide in 50 mM TBS, pH 7.4 (Sigma-Aldrich, UK).
7. PBS, 0.2% (w/v) glycine, and 0.2% (v/v) Tween-20 (Sigma-Aldrich, UK).
8. 2% (v/v) FCS in PBS, 0.02% (v/v) Tween-20 (Sigma-Aldrich, UK).
9. Primary anti-H_3R antibody at a range of concentrations (0–5 μg/mL) (In house).
10. PBS/0.1% (v/v) Triton X 100 (Sigma-Aldrich, UK).
11. Vectastain ABC Elite kit (Promega Ltd., Southampton, UK) including biotin linked, anti-rabbit secondary antibody, and streptavidin-HRP complex (GE Healthcare, UK).
12. 3,3′-diaminobenzidine tetrahydrochloride as the HRP substrate (Sigma-Aldrich, UK).
13. PBS pH 7.4 containing 0.4% Triton X-100, 4% FCS or normal serum from the same species as the secondary antibodies are raised in and 1% bovine serum albumin (BSA) (Sigma-Aldrich, UK).
14. Primary anti-H_3R antibody at a range of concentrations (0–5 μg/mL) (In house).
15. Secondary antibodies: fluorophore linked anti-rabbit antibodies, e.g., Cy3 or Alexa 488, for 1 Citifluor AF4 mountant or equivalent (BDH Laboratories, UK).
16. Peptide is used in molar excess (500 μg/mL) (Cambridge Research Biochemicals, UK) for immunoblotting and IHC/immunofluorescence experiments.

3 Methods

3.1 Choice of Peptide Sequences

Specific peptide sequences are chosen to immunize rabbits to produce anti-peptide antibodies (Fig. 2). The peptides are chosen based on the peptide specificity being unique to the particular isoform and its likely immunogenicity using the rationale described herein and previously [10]. A cysteine residue is added to one end of each sequence so that the peptide could be *directionally* coupled to a carrier protein, KLH, or thyroglobulin to ensure the appropriate configuration of peptide is maintained.

3.2 Antibody Production

The 10-15-mer peptide alone is too small to stimulate an adequate immune response and is therefore conjugated to a large immunogenic carrier protein before being injected into the rabbit (female

Dutch and NZ white rabbits are commonly used breeds). The peptide is conjugated using Imject® Maleimide activated mcKLH kit to elicit an enhanced humoral immune response. The rabbit serum is collected and purified using peptide affinity chromatography.

3.2.1 The Imject Maleimide Activated mcKLH Method of Coupling Peptides to Carrier Proteins

The method is used to conjugate the peptide to the carrier protein KLH through its carboxyl-terminal cysteine residue. There are other coupling strategies available, including amino- and carboxy-terminal coupling described in other publications [10].

1. Dissolve one vial of maleimide-activated mcKLH by adding 200 μL of distilled water (dd.H_2O), making a 10 mg/mL solution. 200 μL of conjugation buffer is added to 5 mg synthetic peptide (*see* **Note 1**).
2. Immediately add the peptide solution to the reconstituted mcKLH. Incubate the carrier protein and peptide mixture for a further 2 h at room temperature (RT) with gentle agitation.
3. Separate the conjugated peptide from EDTA by desalting. Dissolve one bottle of purification buffer salts in 60 mL of d. H_2O (bottle supplied in Imject® Maleimide activated mcKLH kit). Remove the top and bottom caps from a desalting column and wash three times with 15 mL of purification buffer salts. Add the hapten-carrier mixture to the center of the column disc. Apply to the column and collect each of the fractions sequentially.
4. Read the absorbance of each fraction at 280 nm to detect the fractions containing the conjugate. Pool the peak fractions, and re-read the absorbance. Dilute the peptide protein conjugate with PBS to a final concentration of 1 mg/mL and store in 100 μL aliquots at −20C.

3.2.2 Inoculation Procedure

1. All procedures are performed in accordance with the UK Animals Scientific Procedures Act 1986, or equivalent.
2. Carefully mix 200 μL of sterile PBS with 100 μg of freshly thawed peptide-carrier protein conjugate, and emulsify with an equal volume of Freund's adjuvant (Sigma-Aldrich (UK) using a 1 mL syringe (*see* **Note 2**).
3. Inject the conjugate-adjuvant preparation equally using a 25-gauge needle intramuscularly into both hind legs of a Dutch or NZ White rabbit (*see* **Note 3**). Perform the primary immunization using complete Freund's adjuvant, while for subsequent immunizations (at 1 month intervals) use Freund's incomplete adjuvant.
4. Bleed rabbits (*see* **Note 3**) from the marginal ear vein 7–10 days following the booster injections, and collect 10–15 mL of blood. Allow blood to stand at RT for 2 h, and then for

16 h at 4 °C to complete clot formation and contraction, respectively.

5. Remove cellular material by centrifugation at 12,000 × *g* for 10 min at 4 °C, and store the serum in 1 mL aliquots at −20 °C.

In order to improve the quality and specificity of the antibodies, purification is recommended, particularly for use in immunohistochemical and quantitative immunoblotting experiments.

3.3 Affinity Purification

3.3.1 Coupling of Peptides to Sepharose Beads

The method is carried out largely as described previously [10] and is used to couple the peptide to activated thiol-sepharose beads via its C-terminal cysteine residue.

1. Allow 0.35 g of activated thiol-sepharose to swell in 100 mL dd. H_2O for 15 min at RT. Place the swollen sepharose beads in a 25 mL column containing a scinter filter and wash with 100 mL of 0.1 M Tris-HCl pH8.0, containing 0.3 M NaCl and 1 mM EDTA.
2. Drain the column until 0.7 mL of buffer remains. Dissolve 1 mL of 5 mg/mL peptide in the 0.1 M Tris-HCl pH 8.0, containing 0.3 M NaCl and 1 mM EDTA and add to the swollen sepharose beads and incubate for 2 h at RT with gentle agitation.
3. Terminate the reaction by draining the column and washing the sepharose beads with 25 mL of Tris pH 8.0 followed by 10 mL of 0.1 M citric acid pH 4.5. All remaining un-reacted thiol groups on the sepharose beads are blocked by incubation with 3 mL of 1 mM β-mercaptoethanol in 0.1 M citric acid pH 4.5 for 1 h at RT with gentle agitation.
4. Terminate the blocking reaction by washing the sepharose beads with 25 mL of 0.1 M citric acid pH 4.5. Finally, equilibrate the sepharose column with 25 mL PBS and store in 10 mL PBS containing 0.02% (w/v) sodium azide, at 4 °C until required.

3.3.2 Peptide Affinity Purification of Antibodies

Purification of the anti-peptide polyclonal antibody requires the use of a 1 mL sepharose column linked to the appropriate peptide (5 mg) as described above.

1. Equilibrate the column with 100 mL of PBS, and drain. Then apply 4 mL of the immune serum to the column followed by either a 2 h incubation period at RT or overnight at 4 °C with gentle agitation on a rotary shaker.
2. Drain unbound immune serum from the column (*see* **Note 4**), and then wash the column slowly with 100 mL of PBS. Elute the bound antibody from the column with 8 mL of 50 mM glycine/HCl pH 2.3. Collect the eluate in eight sequential 1 mL fractions, containing 15 μL of 1 M Tris to neutralize the

contents to a final approximate pH 7.4. For each fraction determine the optical density (OD) at $\lambda = 280$ nm using a standard bench spectrophotometer and pool the peak fractions (at least 0.1 OD unit). The protein concentration can be calculated using the Beer Lambert law:

C = A/ЄL, where

C is the protein concentration of the antibody.

A is the absorbance at $\lambda = 280$ nm.

L is the sample path length = 1 cm.

Є is the molar absorptivity or extinction coefficient of the chromophore at wavelength λ (the OD of a 1 cm thick sample of a 1 M solution). Є is a property of the material and the solvent = 1.35.

3. Pool the fractions containing the highest protein concentrations and dialyze with stirring against 500 mL PBS, overnight at 4 °C.
4. Regenerate the affinity column with 100 mL of PBS and store in 10 mL PBS containing 0.02% (w/v) sodium azide at 4 °C. Affinity columns can be kept for many years without losing their ability to purify antibodies.

3.4 Validation Method 1: hH_3R Isoform Selectivity Using Heterologous Expression Methods with Individual Isoforms Transiently Expressed in HEK 293 Cells

In order to confirm the selectivity of the antibodies generated, a series of three types of validation methods can be used.

3.4.1 Cell Culture and Transfection of HEK 293 Cells

Preparation of Dulbecco's Modified Eagle Medium/F12 (DMEM/F12, 1:1 ratio) Media.

All procedures should be performed under sterile conditions.

1. Mix powdered DMEM/F12 (15 g/L) and 15 mM HEPES with 800 mL of sterile water. Supplement the media with 40 mL of 10% (v/v) fetal calf serum (FCS), 7.5% (w/v) $NaHCO_3$ giving a final concentration of 3.0 g/L, and 20 mL of penicillin (500 μg/mL)/streptomycin (500 μg/mL) solution.
2. Adjust the pH of the media to pH 7.6 using 10 M NaOH and the final volume made up to 1 L using sterile dd.H_2O. Filter-sterilize the media using a 0.2 μm Sartorius Satolab-V150 filter unit, and then store at 4 °C.

Sub-culturing of HEK 293 Cells

Perform all procedures under sterile conditions. HEK 293 cells are grown in 250 mL Greiner flasks containing DMEM/F12. The flasks are incubated in an incubator (e.g., Sanyo) at 37 °C, humidified in 5% CO_2. The cells are sub-cultured every 3–4 days, at approx.80% confluence.

1. 30 min before, pre-warm sterile PBS, DMEM/F12 media and trypsin-EDTA to 37 °C.
2. Remove the old medium from the cells and wash the cells in 10 mL of pre-warmed PBS.
3. Remove the PBS and incubate the cells for 2 min in 2 mL of trypsin-EDTA, at 37 °C.
4. Resuspend the cells in 10 mL of fresh pre-warmed DMEM/F12 media by gentle pipetting up and down.
5. Add 2 mL of the cell suspension to a fresh sterile flask with a further 10 mL of fresh media and return back to the CO_2 incubator.

Polyethyleneimine (PEI) Transfection Method.

Mammalian cells can be transfected efficiently (up to 30%) using several different simple techniques, including calcium precipitation, and methods using PEI or lipofectamine (the former two being relatively inexpensive if finances are tight). Herein, the PEI method for the transfection of HEK 293 cells adapted from [11], for a 3 mL petri dish of cells (approximately 80% confluent), is described.

1. Dilute 1 μg cDNA (pC DNA Flag-tagged hH_3R isoform) (*see* **Note 5**) in 100 μL 0.9% (w/v) NaCl in a 1.5 mL eppendorf, then add 2 μL of 1 mg/mL PEI (linear MW ~25,000) and flick gently to mix the contents.
2. Incubate the cDNA/PEI mixture freestanding for 10 min at RT. During the incubation period, remove the old media from the HEK 293 cells and add 2 mL of fresh pre-warmed media.
3. Following the incubation period, add the 1 μg DNA/PEI mixture to the HEK 293 cells, gently mix, and incubate at 37 °C in a standard CO_2 incubator.

Harvesting Cells and Membrane Preparation of HEK 293 Cells

1. 48 h post-transfection, remove/aspirate the culture media and replace with 1 mL of homogenization buffer.
2. Scrape cells from the bottom of the petri dish using a Greiner cell scraper. Homogenize the resuspended cells using a dounce glass/glass homogenizer, kept ice cold.

3. Pellet the homogenate by centrifugation at 18,000 × *g* at 4 °C for 5 min.
4. Discard the supernatant and resuspend the pellet in 1 mL of ice-cold homogenization buffer.
5. Rehomogenize the membranes and divide in 100 μL aliquots and store at −20 °C.

3.4.2 Immunoblots

One of the standard methods to utilize the antibodies is immunoblotting. SDS polyacrylamide gel electrophoresis (SDS-PAGE) is commonly carried out using either 7.5 (v/v) or 10% (v/v) polyacrylamide slab gels [appropriate for analyzing monomeric (M_r 30–45 kDa) and dimeric species (M_r 75–90 kDa)] under reducing conditions. Lower percentage polyacrylamide can be used for higher molecular weight proteins. Immunoblots can then be probed either with anti-FLAG antibody (commercial; Sigma-Aldrich, UK) in the case of the FLAG tagged human H_3R clones, or with the appropriate rabbit anti-H_3R antibodies (untagged human H_3R clones).

Preparation of Resolving Gel

1. Prepare the resolving gel by mixing 6 mL of dd.H_2O with 3 mL of resolving gel buffer [50 mM Tris, 384 mM glycine, 1.8 mM EDTA, and 0.1% (w/v) SDS pH 8.8], 6 μL of TEMED, 3 mL of stock 30% acrylamide, and 60 μL 10% (w/v) APS. Immediately pour the polyacrylamide solution gently into a preassembled Hoefer SE 245 dual gel caster, using two gel plates of 10 × 8 cm and spacers of 1 mm width.
2. Layer 100 μL of saturated water/butanol solution over the top of each gel. Cover the gels with parafilm and allow to polymerize for 40–60 min at RT. The gels can be used immediately or stored by wrapping the gels individually in tissue paper and stored in electrode buffer [50 mM Tris, 384 mM glycine, 1.8 mM EDTA, and 0.1% (w/v) SDS pH 8.8] at 4 °C until required. These can be kept for up to 1 month.

Preparation of Protein Samples for SDS-PAGE.

Protein samples for SDS-PAGE are precipitated using the chloroform/methanol precipitation method.

1. To the protein sample (25–50 μg), add 4× volumes of ice-cold methanol and vortex-mix samples and centrifuge at RT at 18,000 × *g* for 1 min.
2. Add 1× volume of ice-cold chloroform to the samples, vortex-mix and centrifuge at RT at 18,000 × *g* for 1 min.
3. Add 3× volumes of ice-cold water to the samples, vortex-mix and centrifuge at RT at 18,000 × *g* for 1 min.

4. Carefully discard the upper layer and add 1× volume ice-cold methanol to the samples, vortex-mix and centrifuge at RT at 18,000 × *g* for 4 min.
5. Discard the supernatant and air-dry the pellet. Resuspend the dried protein pellet by vortex mixing in 5 μL of sample buffer [30 mM sodium hydrogen phosphate, pH 7.0, 30% (v/v) glycerol, 0.05% (v/v) bromophenol blue and 7.5% (w/v) SDS, 2 μL of 200 mM DL-Dithiothreitol (DTT)] and 8 μL of water to a final volume of 15 μL.
6. Boil the samples at 95 °C in the heat block for 5 min and then centrifuge at 18000 × *g* for 30 s at RT before analysis by SDS-PAGE.

SDS-PAGE

1. Carefully clamp the resolving mini-slab acrylamide gel into a Hoefer mini-vertical gel electrophoresis unit SE260.
2. Prepare the stacking gel by mixing 2.3 mL of water with 1 mL of stacking gel buffer [0.5 M Tris-glycine, pH 6.8, containing 8 mM EDTA and 0.4% (w/v) SDS, 650 μL of stock 30% acrylamide, 5 μL of TEMED, and 80 μL of 10% (w/v) APS].
3. Pour the stacking gel mixture immediately and gently (avoiding air bubbles) into the mini-slab gel on the top of the resolving gel and insert a welled comb into the stacking gel. Polymerization takes up to 10 min.
4. Check and carefully remove the comb and wash the wells with dd.H_2O.
5. Pour approximately 300 mL of electrode buffer (*see* above) into and behind the wells and into the base of the electrophoresis unit.
6. Load using a Hamilton syringe or pipette with gel-loading tip extension 15 μL of protein samples and prestained standards (protein molecular weight range of 200–6.5 kDa, Takara Bio Group, USA) into the ten wells of the stacking gel. Ensure all lanes are loaded.
7. Perform electrophoresis at a constant current 10 mA (per gel) initially and then increase the current by 5 mA or 10 mA (per gel) once the samples reach the resolving gel. Gel run time is approximately 2 h or until the appropriate prestained molecular weight marker (M_r 25 kDa) is at the bottom of the resolving gel.

Immunoblotting stage.

After SDS-PAGE is complete, the proteins from the gels are transferred to a nitrocellulose membrane.

1. In order to do this, construct a transfer cassette in the following order of components each of which has been pre-equilibrated in transfer buffer sponge, two sheets of blotting paper, nitrocellulose membrane, SDS-PAGE gel, two sheets of blotting paper, and finally a piece of sponge.
2. On the addition of each component to the transfer cassette, remove air bubbles carefully using a glass pipette or plastic tube. Transfer proteins at a constant voltage of 50 V for 2 h using a Hoefer TE 22 tank transfer unit containing transfer buffer kept cool with external ice packs.
3. Following the transfer of the proteins, briefly rinse the nitrocellulose and incubate with 15 mL of blocking buffer, which comprises of PBS, containing 5% (w/v) dried milk and 0.02% (v/v) Tween-20, for 1 h at RT with gentle agitation.
4. After blocking of the nonspecific antibody sites, wash the nitrocellulose membrane with 10 mL of PBS. Dilute the appropriate affinity-purified primary antibodies in incubation buffer, which comprises of PBS, containing 2.5% (w/v) dried milk to working concentrations of (0.25–5 μg purified antibody/mL).
5. Incubate the nitrocellulose membranes with 10 mL of the diluted primary antibody solution for 2 h at RT, or overnight at 4 °C with gentle agitation (petri dish or plate).
6. After incubation with the primary antibody, wash the nitrocellulose membranes four occasions in 10 mL of wash buffer, consisting of PBS, containing 2.5% (w/v) dried milk and 0.2% (v/v) Tween-20, for 10 min intervals with gentle agitation on a shaker at RT.
7. Incubate the nitrocellulose membranes for 1 h with gentle agitation with horseradish peroxidise (HRP) labeled secondary antibody, either anti-rabbit or anti-mouse depending on the host species for primary antibody, at a dilution of 1/2000 in 10 mL of incubation buffer.
8. Remove the unbound secondary antibody by washing the membrane as detailed above.
9. Drain the nitrocellulose and briefly rinse with PBS.
10. Develop the immunoreactive bands on the nitrocellulose membrane by processing in a solution containing 100 μL of 68 mM p-coumaric acid, 10 mL of 1.25 mM luminal, and 6 μL of 30% (v/v) H_2O_2, for 1 min at RT (*see* **Note 6**).
11. After incubation, wrap the immunoblot in cling film, and place in a film cassette.
12. Expose the immunoblots to Hyperfilm™ for various times between 1 and 5 min, and develop the film developed in Kodak D-19 Developer until the immunoreactive bands are visible and fix in Kodak Unifix for 5 min at RT.

3.5 Validation Method 2–Omission of the Primary Antibody and a Peptide Block

Controls for immunoblots should include the omission of the primary antibody and a peptide block where the primary antibody is pre-incubated with the relevant peptide immunogen (100-fold excess) to confirm antibody specificity.

3.5.1 Peptide Block to Confirm Antibody Specificity for Individual Immunogen

In order to confirm that immunoreactivity detected either in the immunoblots or in immunohistochemical analysis is specific to the amino acid sequence of the immunizing peptide, a peptide block can be carried out.

1. Pre-incubate the antibody overnight at 4 °C with an equal volume of the relevant peptide. The peptide is used in molar excess (500 μg/mL) to ensure complete blockade of antibody binding. Control irrelevant peptides (same concentration) can be used to confirm the sequence specificity.
2. Adjust the final antibody dilution to take into account the initial 1:2 dilution with the peptide.

Any immunoreactive bands or staining that persists after the antibody block is considered to be due to nonspecific antibody binding. Anti-human H_3R isoform-specific antibodies have been validated against HEK 293 cells transfected with the respective H_3R isoform cDNA.

3.6 Representative Examples of Results for Specificity Demonstration and Control Experiments

Figure 3 shows the peptide sequences selected from the overall sequences in Fig. 2, to produce the H_3R isoform-specific antibodies.

3.6.1 Isoform Specificity of the Anti-$rH_{3A/C}/hH_3R_{(445/453)}$ (268–277) Antibody

The sequence chosen is specific to the third intracellular loop region of the $rH3_{C\,(397)}$ isoform. The antibody is shown to be selective for the $rH3_{A\,(445)}$ and $rH3_{C\,(397)}$, but not rat $rH3_{B\,(413)}$ (not shown). Herein, it is shown that the antibody in terms of human isoform also detects both the full-length $hH_{3\,(445)}$ and $hH_{3\,(453)}$ isoforms (Fig. 4). The $hH_{3\,(453)}$ isoform is the result of an additional

Ab 1 Rat H_{3C} isoform rH_{3C}	(268 - 277)	EAMPLHRGSK-Cys
Ab 2 Human $H_3R_{(365)}$ peptide 1	(268 - 281)	EAMPLHRKVAKSLA-Cys
Ab 3 Human $H_3R_{(365)}$ peptide 2	(268 - 278)	Cys-EAMPLHRKVAK
Ab 4 Human $H_3R_{(329)}$ Δ/3	(222 - 231)	Cys-YLNIQSFTQR
Ab 5 Human $H_3R_{(200)}$	(191 - 200)	Cys-RRPRPRWRSA

Fig. 3 Anti-human H_3R isoform antibody panel

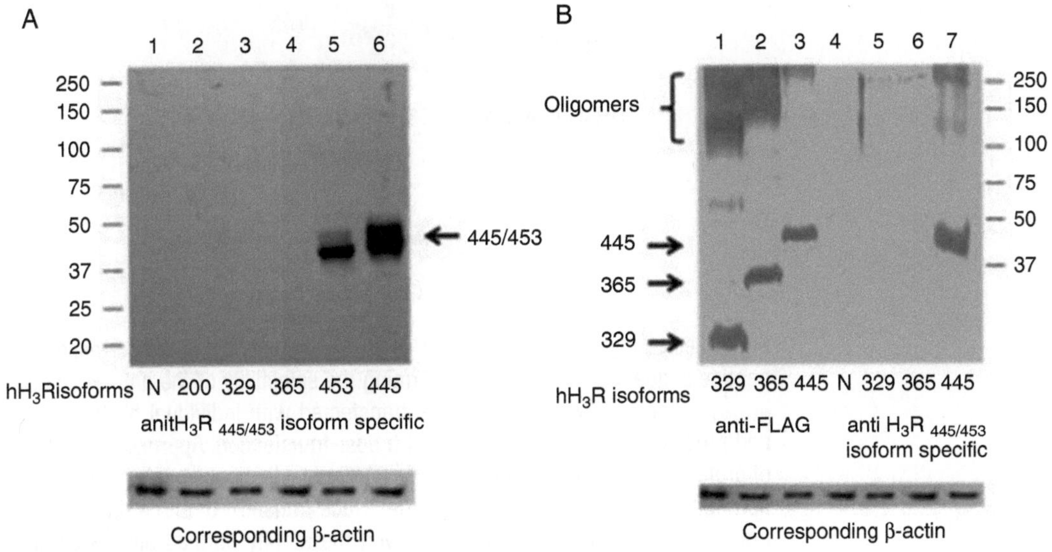

Fig. 4 (**a**) Immunoblot of five different human H_3R isoforms probed with anti-$rH_{3AC}/hH_3R_{(445/453)}$-specific antibody. HEK 293 cells were transfected with individual hH_3R isoforms and processed for immunoblotting 24 h-post-transfection. Approximately 25 μg of protein/well was loaded onto a 7.5% PAGE gel. Once transferred the membrane was probed with affinity purified anti-$rH_{3AC}/hH_3R_{(445/453)}$ antibody (1 μg/mL concentration). The antibody detects only the full-length $hH_3R_{(445)}$ and $hH_3R_{(453)}$ isoforms with no cross reactivity with the shorter isoforms. The lower panel shows the corresponding β-actin, probed with monoclonal mouse anti β-actin antibody (1:5000). *Lane 1*, HEK 293 cells untransfected but still contain PEI; *Lane 2*, HEK 293 cells expressing $hH_3R_{(200)}$; *Lane 3*, HEK 293 cells expressing $hH_3R_{(329)}$; *Lane 4*, HEK 293 cells expressing $hH_3R_{(365)}$; *Lane 5*, HEK 293 cells expressing $hH_3R_{(453)}$; *Lane 6*, HEK 293 cells expressing $hH_3R_{(445)}$. (**b**) Immunoblot of three different FLAG tagged human H_3R isoforms probed with anti-FLAG (*lanes 1–3*) and the anti-$rH_{3AC}/hH_3R_{(445/453)}$ specific antibody (*lanes 4–7*). Homogenates of HEK 293 cells transfected with three different human H_3R isoforms (329, 365, and 445), all epitope tagged with FLAG, were prepared. Approximately 25 μg of protein/well was loaded onto a 7.5% PAGE gel. Identical sample were run on both left and right-hand sides of the gel. Once transferred onto a nitrocellulose membrane, the left-side panel was probed with a monoclonal mouse anti-FLAG antibody (1:5000 dilution) while the right-side panel probed with affinity purified anti-$rH_{3AC}/hH_3R_{(445/453)}$ antibody (1 μg/mL concentration). The FLAG antibody reacts with all three isoforms with monomeric species migrating at approximately M_r 33, 36, 44 kDa. The anti-$rH_{3AC}/hH_3R_{(445/453)}$ antibody detects only the full-length 445 isoform with no cross reactivity with the two shorter isoforms. Lower panel shows corresponding β-actin signal, probed with monoclonal mouse anti β-actin antibody (1:5000). *Lanes 1* and *5*, HEK 293 cells expressing $hH_3R_{(329)}$; *Lanes 2* and *6*, HEK 293 cells expressing $hH_3R_{(365)}$; *Lanes 3* and *7*, HEK 293 cells expressing $hH_3R_{(445)}$; *Lanes 4*, HEK 293 cells untransfected but still contain PEI. All blots shown are representative blots from at least eight similar experiments

exon utilized resulting in an additional eight amino acids added at the C-terminus [9]. The significance of this very rare isoform is yet to be determined.

3.6.2 Immunoblot Showing Labeling of the Human $H_3R_{(445/453)}$ Isoforms Using the Anti-$rH_3R_{AC}/hH_3R_{(445/453)}$ Antibody

The sequence specific to the i3 region in the $rH3_{C(397)}$ isoform is selected. This antibody is shown to be selective for the rat H_{3A} and $rH3_{C(397)}$ isoforms and, surprisingly only the full-length human $H_{3(445/453)}$ isoform (Fig. 4a, b). Antibodies purified from this sequence in different rabbits and different bleeds consistently showed the same human $H_{3(445)}$ selectivity.

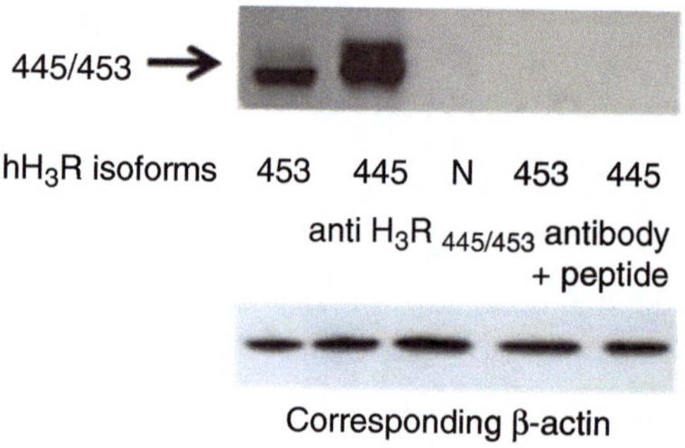

Fig. 5 Selectivity of the anti-rH$_{3AC}$/ hH$_3$R $_{(445/453)}$ antibody using the corresponding peptide sequence: Immunoblot confirming the selectivity of the anti-rH$_{3AC}$/ hH$_3$R $_{(445/453)}$ antibody. HEK 293 cells were transfected with individual hH$_3$R isoforms and processed for immunoblotting 24 h post-transfection. Approximately 25 μg of protein/well was loaded onto a 7.5% PAGE gel. Identical samples were run on both left and right-hand sides of the gel. Once transferred onto a nitrocellulose membrane, the left side was probed with the affinity purified anti-rH$_{3AC}$/ hH$_3$R $_{(445/453)}$ antibody (1 μg/mL concentration) while the right side was probed with affinity purified anti-rH$_{3AC}$/hH$_3$R $_{(445/453)}$ antibody pre-incubated with the antigen peptide (1 μg/mL concentration)

Once the reactivity of antibody against the human H$_3$R isoform transfected cells was determined, the selectivity of the antibody was determined using peptide blockade (Fig. 5). The major immunoreactive bands labeled in HEK 293 expressing the hH$_3$R $_{(453)}$ or hH$_3$R $_{(445)}$ (lanes 1 and 2, respectively) were greatly suppressed by pre-incubation with the antigen peptide (lanes 4 and 5), demonstrating the sequence selectivity of the antibody. Lane 3, HEK293 cells mock transfected. Lower panel shows corresponding β-actin signal, where the immunoblot is re-probed with monoclonal mouse anti β-actin antibody (1:5000). The anti-rH$_3$R$_{AC}$/hH$_3$R $_{(445/453)}$ antibody has been shown to detect only the full-length human and rat isoforms as well as a truncated rH3$_{A\,(445)}$ isoform. Therefore, this antibody is useful for looking at the full-length H$_3$R in both rodent and human tissue.

Occasionally, the peptide-directed antibody production approach yields unexpected results. One such example is the following where an attempt was made to generate an anti-hH$_3$R $_{(365)}$ selective antibody. However, when screened it was found to only selectively identify the hH$_3$R $_{(445)}$ isoform.

3.6.3 Isoform Specificity of the Anti-hH$_3$R $_{(365)}$ Peptide 2 (268–278) Antibody

The sequence chosen is specific to the third intracellular region in the human H$_3$R $_{(365)}$ isoform. This antibody was shown to be selective for the human H$_3$R $_{(445)}$ isoform only (Fig. 6).

In contrast, the following antibody was found to selectively label the isoform to which it was directed, namely the hH$_3$R $_{(329)}$ isoform (Fig. 7).

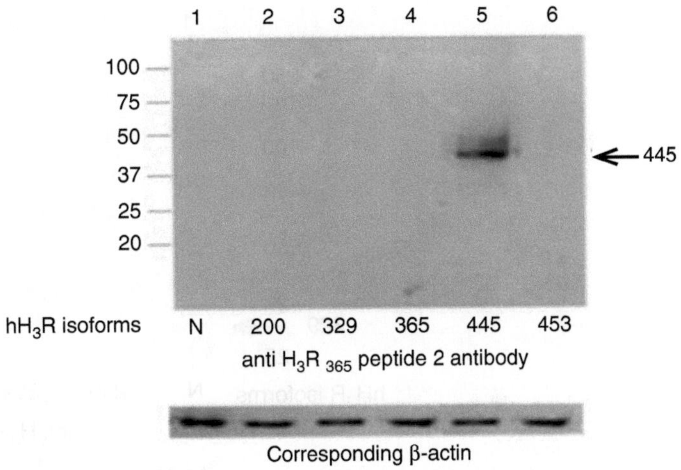

Fig. 6 Immunoblot of five different human H$_3$R isoforms probed with anti-hH$_3$R $_{(365)}$ peptide 2 specific antibody. HEK 293 cells were transfected with individual hH$_3$R isoforms and processed for immunoblotting 24 h post-transfection. Approximately 25 μg of protein/well was loaded onto a 7.5% PAGE gel. Once transferred the membrane was probed with affinity purified anti-hH$_3$R $_{(329)}$ antibody (3 μg/mL concentration). The anti-hH$_3$R $_{(329)}$ antibody detects only the H$_3$R $_{(329)}$ isoform. No cross reactivity with the other shorter or longer isoforms was detected. Lower panel shows the corresponding β-actin, probed with monoclonal mouse anti β-actin antibody (1:5000). *Lane 1*, HEK 293 cells mock transfected; *Lane 2*, HEK 293 cells expressing hH$_3$R $_{(200)}$; *Lane 3*, HEK 293 cells expressing hH$_3$R $_{(329)}$; *Lane 4*, HEK 293 cells expressing hH$_3$R $_{(365)}$; *Lane 5*, HEK 293 cells expressing hH$_3$R $_{(445)}$; *Lane 6*, HEK 293 cells expressing hH$_3$R $_{(453)}$

3.6.4 Isoform Specificity of the H$_3$R $_{(200)}$/Isoform 5 (191–200) Antibody

The sequence was generated to the C terminus of the human H$_3$R $_{(200)}$ because of its unique C terminal sequence. The antibody was shown to detect immunoreactivity in both human putamen (not shown) and recombinant HEK 293 cells expressing the H$_3$R $_{(200)}$ cDNA (Fig. 8).

3.7 Validation Method 3

3.7.1 Immunohistochemical Analysis

Immunohistochemical analysis is carried out as essentially described previously [7, 8].

Diaminobenzidine IHC

1. Perfusion-fix adult mouse brains with 4% (w/v) paraformaldehyde, 0.05% (v/v) glutaraldehyde in 0.1 M phosphate buffer, pH 7.4.
2. Remove brains, post-fix in 4% (w/v) paraformaldehyde (0.05% (v/v) glutaraldehyde in 0.1 M phosphate buffer, pH 7.4 overnight, and then cryoprotect the tissue by incubation in 10%, 20%, and 30% (w/v) sucrose in 0.01 M phosphate buffer, pH 7.4 at 4 °C for 48 h in an even step-wise-manner.
3. Freeze the tissue at −80 °C in isopentane for 1.5 min, and cut coronal sections (25 μm thick) on a cryostat set to −20 °C.

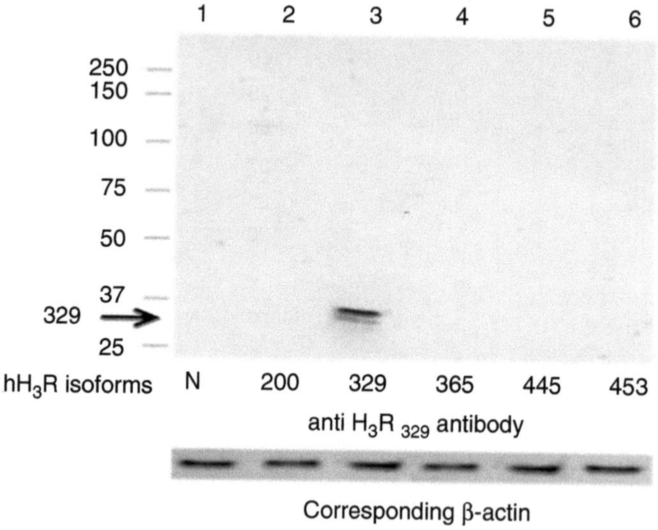

Fig. 7 Immunoblot of five different human H_3R isoforms probed with anti-hH_3R $_{(329)}$ specific antibody. HEK 293 cells were transfected with individual hH_3R isoforms and processed for immunoblotting 24 h post-transfection. Approximately 25 μg of protein/well was loaded onto a 7.5% PAGE gel. Once transferred the membrane was probed with affinity purified anti-hH_3R $_{(329)}$ antibody (3 μg/mL concentration). The anti-hH_3R $_{(329)}$ antibody detects only the H_3R $_{(329)}$ isoform. No cross reactivity with the other shorter or longer isoforms was detected. *Lower panel* shows the corresponding β-actin, probed with monoclonal mouse anti β-actin antibody (1:5000). *Lane 1*, HEK 293 cells mock transfected; *Lane 2*, HEK 293 cells expressing hH_3R $_{(200)}$; *Lane 3*, HEK 293 cells expressing hH_3R $_{(329)}$; *Lane 4*, HEK 293 cells expressing hH_3R $_{(365)}$; *Lane 5*, HEK 293 cells expressing hH_3R $_{(445)}$; *Lane 6*, HEK 293 cells expressing hH_3R $_{(453)}$

Pick up sections using a fine paintbrush and store in PBS (with 0.05% sodium azide) for not more than 2 weeks at 4 °C. Care should be taken to remove the sodium azide prior to completion of IHC methods as this can inactivate the peroxidase enzyme.

4. Treat free-floating sections initially with 10% (v/v) methanol and 3% (v/v) hydrogen peroxide in 50 mM TBS, pH 7.4, for 10 min to quench endogenous peroxidise activity.
5. Incubate sections in PBS, 0.2% (w/v) glycine and 0.2% (v/v) Tween-20, for 15 min to mop up residual un-reacted aldehyde groups from the fixative.
6. Block nonspecific antibody binding sites on the tissue by incubating with 2% (v/v) FCS in PBS, 0.02% (v/v) Tween-20 for 1 h.
7. Incubate sections overnight at 4 °C in the primary anti-H_3R antibody at a range of concentrations (0–5 μg/mL) in 1% (v/v) FCS/PBS.

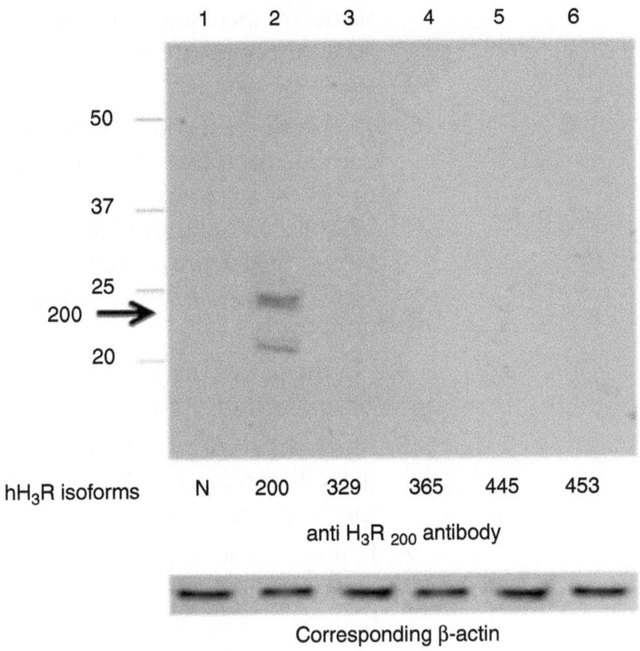

Fig. 8 Immunoblot of five different human H_3R isoforms probed with anti-$hH_3R_{(200)}$ specific antibody. HEK 293 cells were transfected with individual hH_3R isoforms and processed for immunoblotting 24 h post-transfection. Approximately 25 μg of protein/well was loaded onto a 10% PAGE gel. Once transferred the membrane was probed with affinity purified anti-$hH_3R_{(200)}$ antibody (3 μg/mL concentration). The anti-$hH_3R_{(200)}$ antibody detects only the $hH_3R_{(200)}$ isoform. No cross reactivity with the longer isoforms was detected. *Lower panel* shows the corresponding β-actin, probed with monoclonal mouse anti β-actin antibody (1:5000). *Lane 1*, HEK 293 cells mock transfected; *Lane 2*, HEK 293 cells expressing $hH_3R_{(200)}$; *Lane 3*, HEK 293 cells expressing $hH_3R_{(329)}$; *Lane 4*, HEK 293 cells expressing $hH_3R_{(365)}$; *Lane 5*, HEK 293 cells expressing $hH_3R_{(445)}$; *Lane 6*, HEK 293 cells expressing $hH_3R_{(453)}$

8. After washing the sections on three occasions in PBS/0.1% (v/v) Triton X 100, detect antibody binding using the Vectastain ABC Elite kit.
9. Incubate the sections with a biotin linked, anti-rabbit secondary antibody for 2 h followed by incubation for 1 h with streptavidin-horse radish peroxidase (HRP) complex.
10. Visualize the immune reaction using 3,3′-diaminobenzidine tetrahydrochloride as the HRP substrate.

Immunofluorescence Protocol

1. Perfuse-fix adult mouse brains (wild-type and H_3R KO) with 4% (w/v) paraformaldehyde in 0.1 M phosphate buffer, pH 7.4.
2. Remove brains, post-fix in 4% (w/v) paraformaldehyde in 0.1 M phosphate buffer, pH 7.4 overnight, and then cryoprotect the

tissue by incubation in 10%, 20% and 30% (w/v) sucrose in 0.01 M phosphate buffer, pH 7.4 at 4 °C for 48 h in an even step-wise-manner.

3. Freeze the tissue at −80 °C in isopentane for 1.5 min and cut coronal (or other appropriate orientation) sections (14 μm thick) on a cryostat set to −20 °C. Free-floating sections may be collected as above, alternatively if thinner sections are preferred (8–16 μm), they can be collected onto poly-l-lysine coated slides, air dried, and stored at −80 °C in air-tight boxes until use.
4. On the day of the assay remove the slides from the freezer and air dry again for 1 h.
5. Block the sections for 45 min at RT in PBS pH 7.4 containing 0.4% Triton X-100, 4% FCS or normal serum from the same species as the secondary antibodies are raised in, and 1% BSA.
6. Following the blocking stage, rinse the sections briefly in PBS and then incubate for 48 h at 4 °C with primary anti-H_3R antibody at a range of concentrations (0–5 μg/mL). The antibody diluent for both the primary and secondary antibodies is PBS pH 7.4 containing 0.1% Triton X-100, 1% FCS (or normal serum as before), and 1% BSA.
7. Rinse sections and wash in PBS (3 × 10 min), and then apply secondary antibodies: fluorophore linked anti-rabbit antibodies, e.g., Cy3 or Alexa 488, for 1 h.
8. Rinse sections and wash in PBS as before and mount in Citifluor AF4 or equivalent.

3.7.2 Demonstration of Selectivity Using H_3R KO Mice

Immunoblotting Studies in Mice.

As an illustration of this approach, the specificity of the anti-r$H_{3A/C}$/anti-h$H_{3\,(445)}$ antibody for murine H_3Rs was confirmed by using it to probe immunoblots of H_3R wild-type (WT) and H_3R KO mouse brain. Two bands at Mr 50,000 (±2000) and Mr 44,000 (±2000) are consistently detected in WT mouse brain but not in the KO material. Occasionally, a Mr 40,000 species is also selectively detected (Fig. 9).

IHC Studies in the Mouse.

IHC studies using anti-r$H_{3A/C}$/anti-h$H_{3\,(445)}$ antibody to compare immunoreactivity in H_3R KO mice with WT mice clearly demonstrate the specificity of this antibody. The anti-r$H_{3A/C}$/h$H_{3\,(445)}$ isoform-specific antibody is used to carry out a detailed mapping of the anatomical distribution of the H_3R in mouse brain. IHC is carried out in WT mouse brain slices alongside identical slices obtained from H_3R KO animals. Additional controls include the prior incubation of the anti-h$H_{3\,(445)}$ antibody

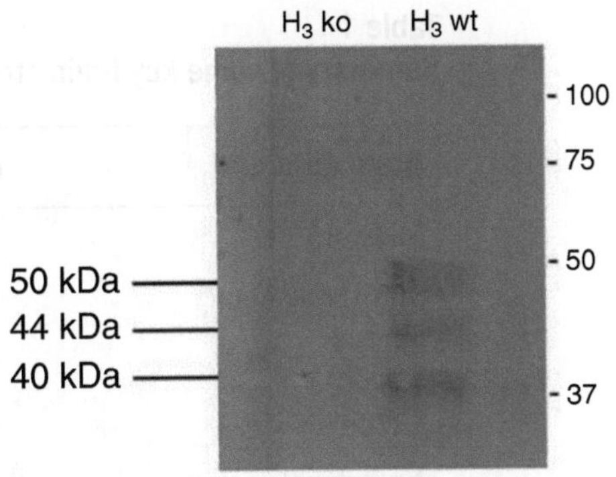

Fig. 9 Immunoblot using anti-rH$_{3A/C}$/anti-hH$_{3\,(445)}$ to compare H$_3$ receptor immunoreactivity in H$_3$R −/− knockout (KO) mice with H$_3$R +/+ wild-type (WT) mice. KO and WT mouse forebrain membranes (10 μg protein) were probed in parallel with anti-rH$_{3A/C}$/hH$_{3\,(445)}$ R used at 1 μg/mL. Two bands at Mr. 50,000 ± 2000 and 44,000 ± 2000 were consistently detected in WT but not in KO material (n = 3 separate mice). After each immunoblot the nitrocellulose sheet was stained with Ponceau S to confirm that the total protein loading was the same for both the KO and WT lanes

with its respective peptide such that specific immunoreactivity would be blocked. To achieve this, the primary antibody is incubated with the peptide at a final concentration of 500 μg/mL overnight at 4 °C. Before use the antibody/peptide mixture is diluted such that the final antibody concentration is the same as for the unblocked antibody. As a second control, IHC is carried out with the secondary antibody alone.

A descriptive summary of the immunoreactivity in selected brain regions is shown in Tables 1 and 2 for both wild-type (WT) and H$_3$R KO mice. Tables 1 and 2 show results using the pan anti-H$_3$R (346–358) antibody and the isoform-specific anti-rH$_{3A/C}$/anti-hH$_{3\,(445)}$ antibody, respectively. The data are from three different mice and the findings are in agreement with those from an independent laboratory using our antibodies to screen at least four further WT and KO animals (Dr Keri Cannon, Albany, USA). Intensity of staining is graded 0–4, with 0 being equivalent to background and 4 representing intense labeling. The strongest specific staining (that is not present in knockout animals) is seen in cortical laminae II, somatosensory cortex (Fig. 10), piriform cortex, and the amygdaloid complex (Fig. 10). Moderate reactivity is also noted in the stratum terminalis, str: caudate putamen, fimbria of the hippocampus, and the cingulum. Weak nonspecific reactivity is observed in some of the brain structures of knockout animals using the anti-rH$_{3A/C}$/anti-hH$_{3\,(445)}$ antibody (Fig. 10). This nonspecific staining was not seen with an immunofluorescence detection system using rhodamine linked anti-rabbit secondary antibodies.

Table 1
Summary of some key brain structures using pan-H_3 receptor antibody

Brain structure	H_3R wild-type mice	H_3R KO mice
Striatum	+3–4	0
Substantia nigra	+3	0
S1/S2 cortex	+3–4	+1
Cingulate cortex	+3	0
Entorhinal cortex	+3	0
Thalamus	+3	0
Amygdaloid complex	+3–4	0
Hippocampus CA1	0–1	0–1
Medial septal cortex	0	0

Wild-type (WT) and H_3R KO Mice produced by Janssens/J&J, USA on a C57Bl6 mouse background. 0 = no detectable labeling, +1 = weak labeling, +2 = moderate labeling, +3 strong labeling, +4 very strong labeling

Table 2
Summary of some key brain structures using anti- $rH_{3A/3C}/hH_{3\,(445)}$ antibody

Brain structure	H_3R wild-type mice	H_3R KO mice
Substantia nigra	+4	+1
Striatum	+3	+1
Cingulum	+3	+2
Somatosensory cortex	+3	0
Fimbria of the hippocampus	+3	+2
Hippocampus: CA1/CA2/CA3 subfields	0	0
Cortex layer II	+4	0
Piriform cortex	+4	0
Stratum terminalis	+4	+1
Amygdaloid complex	+4	0

Wild-type (WT) and H_3R KO Mice produced by Janssens/J&J, USA on a C57Bl6 mouse background. 0 = no detectable labeling, +1 = weak labeling, +2 = moderate labeling, +3 strong labeling, +4 very strong labeling

The background strain of the H_3R KO mice is C5731/6J (US Patent no. 7151200). In contrast to results using the pan anti-H_3 (346–358) in B6C3Fe mice [7], there is negligible immunostaining in the deeper cortical layers and little detectable signal above

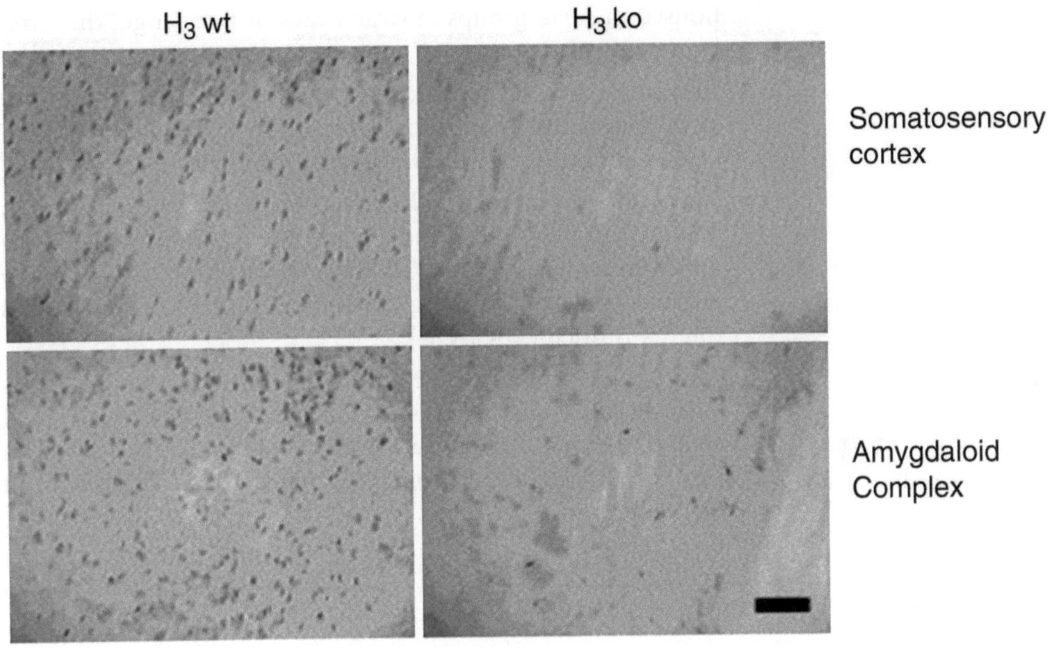

Fig. 10 Immunohistochemical detection of H$_3$R immunoreactivity in a couple of representative brain structures. Immunohistochemical analysis was performed using anti-rH$_{3A/C}$/anti-hH$_{3\,(445)}$ antibody to compare immunoreactivity in H$_3$R KO mice with wild-type (WT) mice to clearly demonstrate the specificity of this antibody. 10 μm brain cryoslices were probed with anti-H$_3$R antibody at 1 μg/mL for 16 h at 4 °C and developed using the DAB/peroxidase method. Scale bar is 100 μm

background in the CA1, CA2, and CA3 regions of the hippocampus. In B6C3Fe mouse brain slices pan anti-H$_3$ (346–358) immunoreactivity is detected in cortical layers II and V, and in the CA3 region of the hippocampus [7].

4 Notes

1. Synthetic peptides can be purchased commercially from various companies (e.g., Cambridge Research Biochemical, Billingham, UK), at >98% purity that is sufficient. Ideally at least 15 mg is required for all procedures.
2. Complete emulsification is very important for a successful protocol. Routinely, this is checked by leaving the sample to stand for at least 30 min at RT and ensuring that the adjuvant and conjugate do not separate into two layers. If this occurs further mixing is required and retested prior to inoculation.
3. In order to ensure that both inoculation and bleeding procedures are stress-free, rabbits are withstrained gently by an experienced handler in a dedicated clean lab coat with holes cut out for ears to protrude, and back legs supported to ensure the animals do not injure themselves. Rabbits are routinely

housed in small groups in large cages or free-range, the latter being more stress-free.

4. Retain the unbound fraction and store in case the affinity column is overloaded and does not retain all the available antibody. This is rare but does happen occasionally.
5. This CMV promoter cDNA construct, ideal for expression in mammalian cells, was a kind gift from [5], epitope tagged with a FLAG sequence (DYKDDDDK) which offers an alternative method of detection using commercial anti-FLAG antibodies (Sigma-Aldrich (UK), UK).
6. This is a homemade recipe developed in the laboratory. It has a drawback in that it lacks a stabilizer and has a use limit of approx. 10 min. There are a number of commercial products that can be used which contain stabilizers and can be utilized for longer.

5 Conclusions

This chapter describes the development and characterization of a selection of novel anti-human H_3R isoform selective immunoprobes. These probes can be used to investigate expression of three of the human H_3R isoforms 445, 365, and 329 in native human tissue. Different isoforms have been shown for the first time to be expressed at the protein level in the human CNS (e.g., [12; 13]). Future studies can now explore whether there are changes in human H_3R isoforms expression in ageing or disease.

5.1 The Rat $H_{3C}/H_{3\,(397)}$ Isoform Antibody is a Specific Human $H_{3\,(445)}$ Antibody

A peptide sequence unique to the rat $H_{3C\,(397)}$ isoform was chosen and used to immunize rabbits for the generation of sequence-specific antibodies. The antibody was affinity purified and screened against rat and human H_3R isoforms expressed in HEK 293 cells. Immunoblotting of cell homogenates revealed that in addition to detecting the $rH_{3C\,(397)}$ isoform it also labeled the full-length 445 isoforms of *both* the human and the rat H_3R. The peptide sequence EAMPLHRGSK is found within the third intracellular loop of the rat $rH_{3C\,(397)}$ isoform, aa 268–277. The sequence is present in both the human and rat full-length forms but in the $rH_{3C\,(397)}$ isoform it is split: EAMPLHR appearing on the 5′ side of the deletion site and GSK on the 3′ side. Presumably, the tertiary structure of the receptor is such that the two halves are brought together in a structural form that the antibody can recognize. One might have expected the antibody to react with $hH_{3\,(365)}$ (deletion 275–354) and $rH_{3B\,(413)}$ (deletion 275–306) since only the last two amino acids are missing from the EAMPLHRGSK sequence in these two isoforms. In addition in the full-length mouse H_3R the sequence is EAMPLHR**YGV**, with the last three amino acids being different from the immunizing peptide; nevertheless, specific anti-H_3R immunostaining was detected with both the pan anti-H_3 and the anti-$rH_{3A/3C}$/anti-$hH_3R_{(445)}$ in mouse brain slices (validated by H_3 KO mice). However, the tertiary structure of the $hH_{3\,(365)}$ and $rH_{3B\,(423)}$ may have been unfavorable, with the peptide sequence presumably not accessible to the antibody within these isoforms. The $hH_{3\,(329\,\Delta IC)}$ (deletion 227–342) does not possess any of this particular peptide sequence and, as expected, no reactivity was seen with this expressed clone.

5.2 Oligomerization of Human H_3R

Immunoblots of receptors expressed in HEK 293 cells revealed the presence of higher molecular weight species in addition to bands running at the expected molecular weight of the respective receptor. The receptor is not being expressed in its natural environment and expression levels are generally considerably higher than in native tissue. However, higher molecular weight species were also observed in immunoblots of native tissue, especially in the human material. Oligomerization of rat H_3R has been described by us and others [14, 15] and there is a growing consensus that many GPCRs, possibly all of them, function as dimers or higher molecular weight oligomers. With rat isoform, $rH_{3\,(397)}$ expressed in HEK 293 cells, higher molecular weight species were less apparent than with the full-length $rH_{3\,(445)}$ isoform.

5.3 Human H_3R Isoform-Specific Antibodies

5.3.1 Immunoblotting Methods Probing Heterologously Expressed Human H_3R Isoforms

Attempts were made to generate antibodies against three more human H_3R isoforms using an identical strategy. This strategy yielded in some cases unexpected results, for example Ab2 designed to be a selective $hH_{3\,(365)}$ antibody actually yielded a $H_{3\,(445/365)}$ specific antibody, Ab3 designed to produce a $hH_{3\,(365)}$ selective antibody surprisingly yielded a $H_{3\,(445)}$ selective antibody. In contrast, Ab4 designed to produce an anti-$H_{3\,(329)}$ antibody, proved successful in yielding such an antibody; finally, Ab5 directed to a unique sequence with the highly truncated $H_{3\,(200)}$ receptor again proved successful despite the limited available selective immunogen sequence. Therefore, to date, a panel of anti-$H_{3\,(200)}$, $H_{3\,(329)}$ and $H_{3\,(445)}$ antibodies have been successfully generated; the mixed specificity $H_{3\,(365)}$ /$H_{3\,(445)}$ antibody may have some utility using immunoblotting methods.

5.3.2 Immunohistochemical Techniques with KO Mice

Immunohistochemical (IHC) studies using wild-type and H_3R KO mice showed a marked ablation in immunoreactivity in the knockout animals compared to the wild-type, demonstrating the specificity of the antibodies. The immunoreactivity in wild-type animals was similar for both the original pan anti-hH_3 (346–358) antibody (not shown) and the new isoform selective antibody. The findings also confirmed those of a previous study using the pan anti-hH_3 (346–358) antibody [7] to map the anatomical distribution of the H_3R in mouse brain slices; with the exception of cortex layer V that showed moderate/strong staining in the first study but only light staining in the present investigation, and the hippocampus (regions CA1–CA3 and dentate gyrus) where there was some moderate reactivity, not found here (Table 1). It is possible that these differences might be accounted for by the fact that different mouse strains were used (B6C3Fe, [7]; C5731/6 J in the more recent study); however, further work is necessary to validate these observations and confirm their reproducibility. IHC using the anti-$rH_{3C}/hH_{3\,(445)}$ antibody demonstrated clear specific immunoreactivity in striatum, substantia nigra, cortical laminae II, somatosensory cortex, piriform cortex, and the amygdaloid complex. Moderate reactivity was also noted in the str terminalis, fimbria of the hippocampus, and the cingulum (Table 2). Background labeling was evident in some brain areas in knockout animals, notably the fimbria of the hippocampus and cingulum, and to a lesser degree in the striatum; nevertheless, it was at a significantly lower level than in equivalent areas from wild-type mice. This background labeling was not apparent using an immunofluorescent detection system, e.g., basal ganglia (not shown). A similar picture was observed in the pain circuits study with the pan-H_3R antibody; clear labeling was observed in wt mice for a subpopulation of A delta fibers, and was completely absent in H_3R KO mice; however, a small subset of A beta fibers were labeled nonspecifically as evidenced by maintenance of this immunoreactivity in H_3R KO mice [8]. Furthermore, in immunoblots comparing mouse brain homogenates from WT and KO the animals there was an indication of some immunoreactivity in the KO material [8]. Care should be taken with screening antibodies in KO mice. In the H_3R KO mice, the H_3R gene is disrupted by homologous recombination (US Patent no. 7151200). A 0.7 kb region covering part of the first intron and the 5′ end of the second exon is replaced. Although the gene is rendered nonfunctional by this disruption with no detectable [^{3}H] RAMH binding in KO animals [16] (US Patent no. 7151200), there could possibly be some low level expression of nonfunctional H_3R protein remaining. This was a significant issue in some of the early H_3R KO mice (personal communication). This is also unlikely to be due to the closely related H_4R; as the EAMPLHRGSK sequence is not found within the H_4R aa sequence and the anti-$rH_{3C}/hH_{3\,(445)}$ antibody does not detect recombinant H_4R expressed in HEK 293 cells. The high expression in the basal ganglia (Fig. 10), particularly in the striatum and substantia nigra, is consistent with recent double labeling confocal studies using these H_3 receptor antibodies. These have shown that the H_3 receptor is expressed on subpopulations of GABA-ergic neurons in the sustantia nigra and frontal cortex, and furthermore on subpopulations of histaminergic neurons in the tubermammilary nucleus, which suggests distinct control of output neurons to other brain regions by the H_3 receptor [17].

5.4 Overall Conclusion

In conclusion, generating human H_3R isoform-specific antibodies requires a high level of knowledge and expertise, plus a little bit of fortune. Thorough validation of the antibodies, as described herein, with multiple methods and in combination with in situ hybridizaton and ligand autoradiographical studies is essential before they can be used as reliable probes to investigate the physiological relevance of alternative splicing in the human H_3 receptor.

Dedication

P.L.C. would like to dedicate this chapter to the memory of Sheila Chazot for her love and support.

References

1. Lovenberg TW, Roland BL, Wilson SJ et al (1999) Cloning and functional expression of the human histamine H_3 receptor. Mol Pharmacol 55:1101–1107
2. Arrang JM, Garbarg M, Schwartz JC (1983) Auto-inhibition of brain histamine release mediated by a novel class (H3) of histamine receptor. Nature 302:832–837
3. Morisset S, Sasse A, Gbahou F et al (2001) The rat H_3 receptor: gene organization and multiple isoforms. Biochem Biophys Res Commun 280:75–80
4. Wiedemann P, Bönisch H, Oerters F et al (2002) Structure of the human histamine H_3 receptor gene (HRH3) and identification of naturally occurring variations. J Neural Transm (Vienna) 109:443–453
5. Cogé F, Guénin SP, Audinot V et al (2001) Genomic organization and characterization of splice variants of the human histamine H_3 receptor. Biochem J 355:279–288
6. Harper EA, Shankley NP, Black JW (1999) Evidence that histamine homologues discriminate between H_3-receptors in guinea-pig cerebral cortex and ileum longitudinal muscle myenteric plexus. Br J Pharmacol 128:751–759
7. Chazot PL, Hann V, Wilson C et al (2001) Immunological identification of the mammalian H3 histamine receptor in the mouse brain. Neuroreport. 12:259–262
8. Cannon KE, Chazot PL, Hann V et al (2007) Immunohistochemical localization of histamine H3 receptors in rodent skin, dorsal root ganglia, superior cervical ganglia, and spinal cord: potential antinociceptive targets. Pain 129:76–92
9. Wellendorph P, Goodman MW, Burstein ES et al (2002) Molecular cloning and pharmacology of functionally distinct isoforms of the human histamine H(3) receptor. Neuropharmacology 42:929–940
10. Chazot PL, Pollard, S, Stephenson FA (1999) Immunoprecipitation of Receptors 257–285 In Vitro Neurochemical Techniques. In: Boulton AA, Baker GB, Bateson AN (eds) Springer Publishing (USA)
11. van Rijn RM, van Marle A, Chazot PL et al (2008) Cloning and characterization of dominant negative splice variants of the human histamine H_4 receptor. Biochem J 414: 121–131
12. Shan L, Bossers K, Luchetti S et al (2012) Alterations in the histaminergic system in the substantia nigraand striatum of Parkinson's patients: a postmortem study. Neurobiol Aging 33:1488.e1–1488.13
13. Lethbridge N (2011) Histamine H_3 receptor hetrogeniety in the Central nervous system in ageing and dementia. PhD thesis
14. Shenton FC, Hann V, Chazot PL (2005) Evidence for native and cloned H_3 histamine receptor higher oligomers. Inflamm Res 54(S1):S48–S49
15. Bakker RA, Lozada AF, van Marle A et al (2006) Discovery of naturally occurring splice variants of the rat histamine H3 receptor that act as dominant-negative isoforms. Mol Pharmacol 69:1194–1206
16. Toyota H, Dugovic C, Koehl M et al (2002) Characterization of mice lacking histamine H(3) receptors. Mol Pharmacol 62: 389–397
17. Giannoni P, Passani MB, Nosi D et al (2009) Heterogeneity of histaminergic neurons in the tuberomammillary nucleus of the rat. Eur J Neurosci 29:2363–2374

Chapter 3

Approaches to Recombinant Histamine H_3/H_4 Receptor Expression in Mammalian Cells

Tadeusz Karcz, Urszula Cichoń, and Katarzyna Kieć-Kononowicz

Abstract

Recombinant receptor techniques are very commonly utilized in pharmacological studies nowadays. This state of affairs is a result of recent development of genetic engineering and DNA cloning methods, which made the expression of foreign genes in various cellular environments possible. The starting point for the application of recombinant proteins in studies on seven-transmembrane receptors (7TMRs) was marked by cloning of the first two 7TMRs-cholinergic and adrenergic receptors in the late 1980s. Resolving of gene sequences for successive receptors enabled the use of expression techniques for already well-characterized 7TMRs, but also for orphan receptors. Within the toolbox of available systems for expression of recombinant receptors, mammalian cells constitute the most frequently used model, since they offer a high probability for maintenance of full functional activity of artificially overexpressed receptors. Taking into consideration the importance of mammalian expression systems in relation to current challenges of molecular pharmacology, some of the available protocols for recombinant 7TMRs production in mammalian cells will be discussed in this chapter.

In the first part, details of transient transfection of CHO cells with genetic construct encoding for fusion protein of histamine H_3 receptor and fluorescent protein-mCherry using polyethylenimine as transfection reagent will be given. Then, methods for establishing a monoclonal cell lines stably expressing receptor protein following the lipofection procedure will be presented. Finally, the utility of retroviral expression systems for recombinant receptor production will be discussed using the histamine H_4 receptor as an example.

Key words Histamine H_3 and H_4 receptors, Mammalian expression systems, Polyethylenimine (PEI) transfection, Recombinant receptors, Retroviral transduction, Stable transfection

1 Introduction

In recent years, an increasing access to enlarging libraries of both natural and synthetic compounds determines a need for creating efficient and rapid screening methods to examine the pharmacological properties of novel chemical structures such as potential G protein-coupled receptors (GPCR, seven transmembrane receptors, 7TMRs) ligands.

Ekaterini Tiligada and Madeleine Ennis (eds.), *Histamine Receptors as Drug Targets*, Methods in Pharmacology and Toxicology, DOI 10.1007/978-1-4939-6843-5_3, © Springer Science+Business Media LLC 2017

Still in the late 1990s, preliminary pharmacological studies were mainly based on assays utilizing genetically unmodified material from primary cultures, animal tissues and preparation of membranes from native cells [1]. However, the advancement of knowledge about genome sequences of various organisms and development of genetic engineering techniques resulted in increasing use of models based on recombinant receptor expression [2–4].

Numerous expression systems can be used to obtain recombinant proteins. For the expression of GPCRs there are four types of host organisms available: yeast, bacteria, insect, and mammalian cells. Each of them has both advantages and important limitations.

The most common models used to investigate receptors interacting with G proteins are mammalian cell lines. They provide a sophisticated machinery of posttranslational modifications of proteins and give a possibility of obtaining membrane localization of recombinant receptors. Moreover, mammalian cells contain compatible set of intrinsic signalling mediators, which enables researchers to perform functional tests on 7TMRs. Another advantage of this system is the appropriate content of lipid bilayer, being essential for proper functioning of many G protein-coupled receptors. On the other hand, mammalian expression systems also have some disadvantages. Difficulties that may occur during the transfection of cells with foreign DNA and demanding conditions to maintain cell cultures appear as major limitations. Due to high overall cost and rather low yield in production of recombinant proteins, mammalian cell systems are not recommended for structural studies of 7TMRs. However, they can be useful for development of functional and binding assays resembling receptors in native conditions [5, 6].

Expression of recombinant proteins in mammalian cell lines can be either transient or stable. Development of stable cell lines is related to lower expression level of recombinant proteins in single cells, but there is no need to repeat the procedure of transfection before each particular pharmacological experiment. Moreover, it provides greater reproducibility of conducted studies. In the case of transient expression, higher expression level of the protein of interest can occur, but after a few days it is normally completely diminished due to loss of expression vector by cells, or because of their death. In this kind of expression, transcription of the introduced receptor gene is based on non-replicating material occurring in cytosol, which can be either viral or plasmid vector. Conversely, in stable expression an integration of introduced receptor's cDNA into the genome of host organism is the core of foreign gene maintenance in recombinant cells (episomally replicating plasmids, which are further discussed in the text, constitute an exception to this rule) [7]. However, the frequency of integration of recombinant gene into host genome is rather low. It is estimated to appear only in one per 10,000 cells [8]. The number of cDNA copies being incorporated as well as their localization within the chromosomes of modified cells determine the level of protein expression, which can be decreased, e.g., after integration into transcriptionally inactive region or as a result of genetic instability related to recombination [9]. With regard to low frequency of spontaneous recombination events, there is a need for proper selective pressure while preparing a cell line with stable expression of target protein. The most common way to fulfil this condition is to include a suitable antibiotic into cell culture medium after transfection or transduction. Resistance to a particular antibiotic occurs in response to the expression of the resistance gene, which is usually introduced to the cells with use of the same vector that also contains DNA encoding for recombinant protein of interest.

Introduction of foreign genetic material to mammalian cell lines can be performed using either methods of transfection or transduction. Transduction is a technique in which virus-based methods are used to transfer desired genes into cells. On the other hand, transfection is the term reserved for all of the other methods of introducing foreign DNA into mammalian cells.

1.1 Transfection

Transfection of mammalian cells can be performed using both physical and chemical methods. There are a few chemical components that can facilitate the process of transfection:

1. Inorganic salts, e.g., tricalcium phosphate in co-precipitation with DNA, where foreign genetic material is captured in the structure of crystals composed of calcium phosphate. In this form, DNA can be taken up by the cells in the process of endocytosis [10]. Transfection efficiency using the co-precipitation technique can yield up to 80% in case of HEK293 cell line, if the experiment is conducted under optimal conditions [11]. Unfortunately, the discussed method has some limitations. It is time-consuming and there is a need for strict control of the process of crystal formation, since they should not grow too large. Moreover, this technique can be inappropriate for some cell lines. For example, in case of CHO cells, additional procedures must be considered to ensure high performance of transfection, including the execution of osmotic shock to cells. Key parameters for high efficiency of co-precipitation method involve: proper pH of phosphate buffer, good quality of prepared crystals, which should be homogenous and relatively small, and also the addition of compounds that promote the pinocytosis, like DMSO, sucrose, glycerol, or sodium butyrate.
2. Cationic polymers, which include diethylaminoethyl-dextran (DEAE-dextran). Due to major disadvantage of DEAE-dextran, being its cytotoxicity, this transfection reagent is nowadays substituted with polyethylenimines (PEIs). PEI can

be used for transfection both in its linear and branched form. The average molecular mass of PEIs utilized for introduction of foreign genes to mammalian cells falls into ranges from 25 to 800 kDa. Each monomer of polyethylenimine contains nitrogen, which following its protonation can create ionic bonds with dissociated and negatively charged phosphate groups in DNA. The diameter of obtained DNA-PEI complexes varies from 50 to 1000 nm and depends on the form of used PEI and applied reaction conditions. Created complexes are transported into cells in the process of endocytosis and are further released into the cytosol, due to swelling and rupture of endosomes and lysosomes. This process is probably related to high ionic strength created by the abundant presence of amine residues [7, 12–14].

3. Cationic lipids, which are the major components of commercial transfection reagents, including FuGENE HD, TurboFect, and Lipofectamine2000. Most of them contain a mixture of cationic, mono- or polyvalent, and neutral lipids, for example cholesterol or dioleoyl-phosphatidylethanolamine (DOPE). They are either dissolved in water, where they can aggregate to form liposomes, or in ethanol, where they form micelles. Transfection with the use of cationic lipids is called lipofection. The technique can be characterized as the most efficient among all aforementioned chemical methods of transfection. Cationic lipids form complexes with negatively charged DNA similar to cationic polymers. An additional advantage of lipofection is the hydrophobic character of created complexes, which promotes direct diffusion through the cell membranes [7, 15].

Physical methods of transfection include biolistic particle delivery, microinjection, and electroporation. Only the last method is used in vitro for genetic modifications of eukaryotic cells on a larger scale.

The principle of electroporation is to apply an electric impulse of high voltage to a high-density suspension of cells (from 10^6 to 10^7 cells per mL) combined with foreign genetic material in special cuvettes. The electric pulse leads to a transient increase of cell membrane permeability, which enables the introduction of recombinant DNA into the cells. Usually, the voltage of applied electric impulse ranges from 100 to 1000 V and electric capacity ranges from 25 to 1000 μF. Pulse duration and amplitude can be the subject of further optimization. Electroporation is usually used for nonadherent cells. Adherent cells have to be first detached from the culture dishes. This technique is suitable for either stable or transient expression of the desired transgene. Electroporation experiments are normally performed at room temperature and, following the electric treatment, cells are placed on ice. This step is included to prolong the partial disintegration of cell membranes, which allows foreign genetic material to enter the cells. The major disadvantages of electroporation are: the requirement for higher numbers of cells and genetic materials in comparison to chemical methods of transfection and the need of individual optimization of experimental conditions for different cell lines [16, 17].

1.2 Transduction

Transduction of eukaryotic cells is a method of introduction of DNA into the cells with the use of viral vectors. Transduction can lead to a transient expression of transgene due to transduced cells death a few days post-infection, when recombinant alphaviruses (*Semliki Forest virus*) or Cowpox viruses (*Vaccinia virus*) are utilized. On the other hand, use of retroviral vectors enables cell survival and results in the integration of introduced gene into the host genome [5, 7, 18]. The application of retroviruses is restricted to cloning of DNA fragments smaller than 11 kilobase pair, since larger fragments cannot be closed into the virus capsid. Moreover, this technique can be used only with actively dividing cells.

The retroviral genome constitutes of a single-stranded RNA, which is located in protein capsid together with viral enzymes responsible for replication. The capsid is surrounded by the layer of lipids, which also contains specific viral glycoproteins.

Genetically unmodified, wild-type viruses enter cells by endocytosis, where specific receptors on the cell surface recognizing viral glycoproteins are engaged in the process. Immediately after endocytosis, the virus genome is amplified, based on the activity of host cell and viral components, including reverse transcriptase encoded by one of *pol* genes. Later, the transcribed viral DNA integrates into host chromosome, with the use of integrase, another protein product of *pol* genes. Virus genome integrated into the DNA of host cell is called provirus and undergoes replication together with the genetic material of the infected cell. The genome of wild-type viruses consists of all of genes, which are essential for production of complete virions: *gag*, *pol*, and *env*. Each of these genes is responsible for synthesis of distinct viral proteins. Capsid proteins are encoded by *gag* gene (*group-specific antigen*), reverse transcriptase, protease, and integrase are coded by *pol* genes, whereas *env* gene (*envelope proteins*) is responsible for production of glycoproteins from the outer lipid layer of virion, which are recognized by specific receptors on the host cell. Retrovirus genome also contains a signalling sequence ψ, which is recognized by proteins responsible for assembling of viral particles and leads to packaging of RNA molecules possessing packaging signal into maturing virions. Wild-type retroviruses, budding from the cells are fully virulent and can infect subsequent cells initiating the next viral life-cycle [19, 20].

Retroviruses adopted as vectors in genetic engineering experiments are modified to be no longer capable of self-replication. The genome of such viruses is devoid of sequences essential for

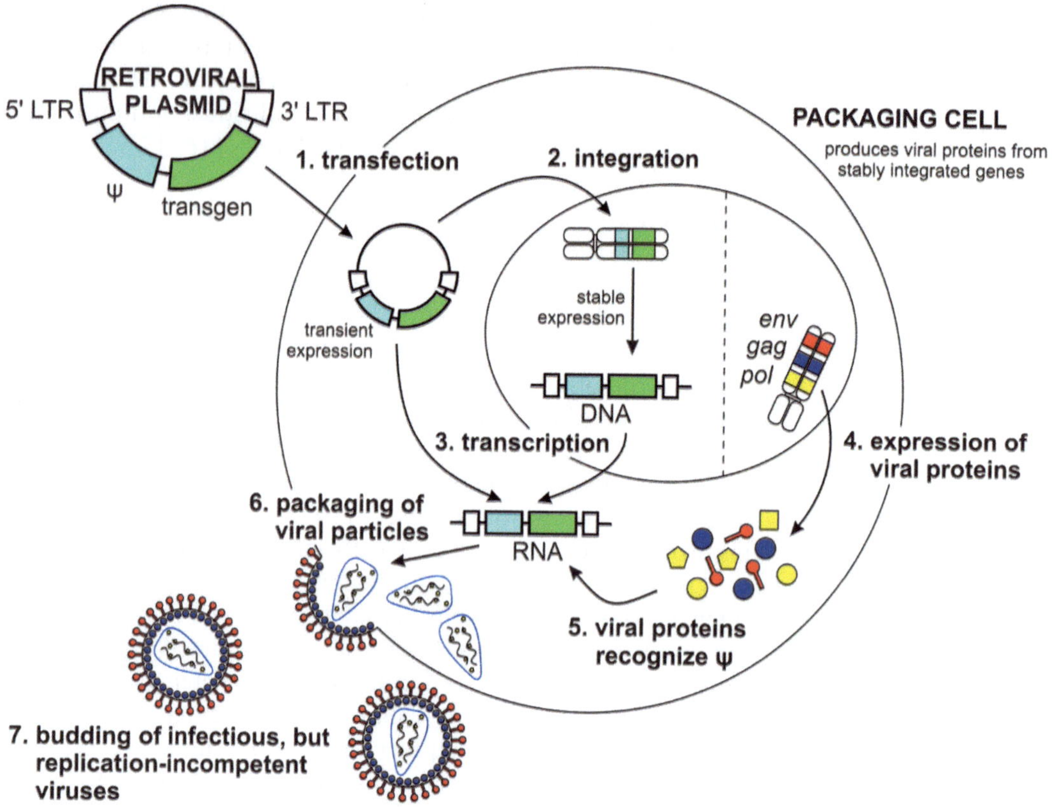

Fig. 1 Recombinant retroviruses production in packaging cells in response to transfection with retroviral plasmid (description in the text)

creation of viral particles. In order to obtain complete virions, special packaging cell lines have to be utilized. Packaging cells are stably transfected with *gag*, *pol*, and *env* genes and constitute a core element of retroviral expression system (Fig. 1). Another relevant component of this system is retroviral plasmid. It consists of eukaryotic promoter, signal sequence ψ, multi-cloning site, where the foreign gene is inserted, and selectable marker. These sequences are located between virus long terminal repeat sequences (LTR). These fragments contain viral promoter and also enhancing, polyadenylation and termination of transcription sequences [20, 21].

In the first step of retroviral transduction experiment, packaging cells are transfected with the retroviral plasmid. Subsequently, based on the promoter sequence present in the 5′ LTR region, the process of transcription of plasmid DNA into RNA takes place. At the same time, *gag*, *pol*, and *env* genes are expressed based on the sequences integrated into packaging cell chromosomes. Synthesized viral components, originating from retroviral plasmid and packaging cell sequences, are caught in protein capsid in response to packaging signal ψ and complete viruses are released into culture medium. It is important to emphasize that the genome of emerging viruses contains only sequences located between LTR fragments from utilized retroviral plasmid, and *gag*, *pol*, and *env* genes are not inserted into viral particles [20].

Obtained virions can be further transferred into the culture flask containing the desired target cell line. Later, recombinant viruses infect the cells and their genetic material undergoes the process of reverse transcription and is then stably integrated into the genome of target cells. Unlike the case with wild-type viruses, the life-cycle of genetically modified retroviruses finishes at that point, because they are not able to restore structure of viral particles, i.e., due to the lack of sequences encoding for capsid components. Based on transduced genetic material, only the expression of transgene and antibiotic resistance gene occurs in host cells [20]. That way, the construction of retroviral expression systems protects from uncontrolled spreading of genetically modified viruses into the environment and provides the sufficient safety level for investigators.

2 Materials

2.1 Cell Lines

2.1.1 Cell Lines Used for the Expression of GPCR

Most of the described attempts to achieve expression of GPCR in mammalian cells refer to cell lines derived from fibroblasts (CHO, HEK293, COS, A9, BHK-21, NIH/3T3, L-929, Rat-1) or cells derived from the nervous system (C6, PC-12, or SH-SY5Y) [16]. Among the above-mentioned lines the most commonly used are Chinese hamster ovary (CHO) and Human embryonic kidney (HEK293) cell lines, which is dictated by ease of transfection, simple culture conditions, short doubling time, safety, and a relatively small amount of endogenous receptors [16, 18].

The CHO cell line (#CCL-61; ATTC) was obtained in the 1950s from a Chinese hamster's ovary and was rapidly adapted for basic research in the field of metabolism and cell cycle. Currently, it is estimated that up to 70% of recombinant proteins for therapeutic use are produced using CHO cells [22].

The HEK293 line, the second mammalian line most frequently used for the production of recombinant proteins, was derived by Graham in 1977 [23]. The studies conducted in subsequent years allowed for its detailed characterization. mRNA levels for over 100 genes encoding GPCR were determined using microarray techniques, which allowed for a better understanding of the molecular context, in which the overexpression of recombinant receptors is performed [24]. Moreover, some additional genetic modifications of HEK293 cells were carried out to increase the intracellular copy number of plasmids containing viral origins of replication. Introduction of genes encoding Epstein-Barr virus nuclear antigen 1 or Simian virus 40 large T antigen into HEK293 cells and obtaining their stable expression led to HEK293EBNA and HEK293T

(#CRL-3216; ATCC) cell lines, respectively. Development of these lines enabled episomal replication of compatible plasmids in these cells. This leads to the increase in: the gene copy number in a transfected cell, the expression level of recombinant protein, as well as the likelihood of permanent integration of the transgene into the host genome [18, 25].

2.1.2 Retrovirus Packaging Cell Lines

Retrovirus packaging cells are obtained as a result of stable transfection with *pol*, *env*, and *gag* genes. The lines that are most often used for this purpose include: HEK293 and COS cells or mouse fibroblasts NIH/3T3 [20, 26]. An example might be a packaging cell line-GP+*env*AM-12 (#CRL-9641, ATCC) [27]. This was a result of transfection of the NIH/3T3 line with a plasmid containing *gag* and *pol* genes, derived from Moloney murine leukemia virus. Subsequently, a series of clones of the obtained cell line characterized by a high level of expression of *gag* and *pol* genes (including a reverse transcriptase that was used as a marker) was transfected again-this time with a plasmid containing the *env* gene of the 4070A amphotropic murine leukemia virus. This resulted in a cell line that efficiently produces structural and functional proteins of retroviruses. Sequences conditioning the formation of a fully active virus were spatially separated in the GP+*env*AM-12 line. Therefore, the risk of a triple recombination (between *gag/pol* and *env* sequences in the genome of packaging cells and a retroviral plasmid), which would lead to a formation of replication-competent viruses, is negligible [27].

2.2 Plasmids

Obtaining recombinant protein expression by transfection of mammalian cells requires the use of genetic vectors, which are carriers for a foreign DNA. For this purpose, the expression plasmid vectors are used, which should contain:

- a promoter sequence, binding endogenous transcription factors and controlling gene transcription-eukaryotic plasmids most frequently contain constitutive promoters derived from viral genomes, e.g., Cytomegalovirus (CMV) or Simian virus 40 (SV40) promoter, while the use of the CMV promoter gives generally better results [16].
- a polyadenylation site, conditioning the proper termination of transcription and stability of the resulting mRNA.
- a so-called prokaryotic cassette comprising prokaryotic sites of initiation of replication and an antibiotic resistance gene, enabling amplification of the plasmid in bacterial cells.
- a multi-cloning site (MCS) containing sequences recognized by restriction enzymes and allowing for the introduction of a foreign gene.

– an eukaryotic antibiotic resistance gene (geneticin, hygromycin B) allowing for the formation of a selective pressure necessary for obtaining of stable expression of the recombinant protein.

Optionally, the eukaryotic plasmid may contain Epstein-Barr virus (EBV) or SV40 origins of replication. Plasmids of this type may undergo episomal replication in mammalian cells characterized by expression of: Epstein-Barr nuclear antigen 1 or SV40 large T antigen, respectively. Episomal replication of the plasmid increases the efficiency of expression of recombinant proteins by increasing the gene copy number in the cell [18].

In order to obtain genetic vectors in the form of retroviral particles, plasmid DNA, used to introduce a foreign gene into the packaging cells, is also applied. Suitable retroviral plasmids differ in structure from the classic eukaryotic expression plasmids and contain (as described in Sect. 1.2) sequences allowing for the transcription of a transgene to viral RNA and its incorporation into emerging viral particles. Plasmids utilized in the following experimental protocols include:

- pmCherry-N1 plasmid (Clontech Laboratories Inc., Mountain View, CA, USA), containing histamine H_3 receptor cDNA devoid of TGA stop codon, obtained in PCR reaction from plasmid pcDNA3.1-*h*H_3R (Missouri S&T cDNA Resource Center, Rolla, MO, USA; #HRH0300000): fusion protein construct, with open reading frame covering receptor sequence and fluorescent mCherry protein fragment. Size: 6053 base pairs.
- pQCXIN retroviral plasmid (Clontech Laboratories Inc., Mountain View, CA, USA) with histamine H_4 receptor gene cloned by means of PCR reaction, using pcDNA3.1-*h*H_4R (Missouri S&T cDNA Resource Center, Rolla, MO, USA; #HRH0400000) as a template DNA. Size: 8526 base pairs.
- pcDNA3.1-VSV-G plasmid encoding the envelope glycoprotein (G) of vesicular stomatitis virus (VSV). Size: 6913 base pairs.

2.3 Reagents

- FuGENE HD transfection reagent; #E2311; Promega.
- DMEM medium, high-glucose, #11995; ThermoFisher Scientific.
- DMEM/F12 medium, with HEPES, #11330; ThermoFisher Scientific.
- Fetal bovine serum, heat inactivated, US origin; #16140 10500-064; ThermoFisher Scientific.
- geneticin sulfate (G418), cell culture tested; #345810; Merck Millipore.
- GlutaMAX supplement; #35050; ThermoFisher Scientific.
- Hygromycin B; #H3274; Sigma Aldrich.

- Hypoxanthine; #A1148; Alfa Aesar.
- Mycophenolic acid; #475913; Merck Millipore.
- Penicillin/Streptomycin solution; #15140; ThermoFisher Scientific.
- Polybrene solution; #TR-1003-G; Merck Millipore.
- Polyethylenimine, branched, average Mw ~25,000 by LS; #408727; Sigma-Aldrich.
- Sodium butyrate solution; #TR-1008-G; Merck Millipore.
- TurboFect transfection reagent; #R0533; ThermoFisher Scientific.
- Xanthine; #0210329005; MP Biomedicals.

3 Methods

3.1 Transient Transfection of CHO Cells Using PEI

1. This protocol enables cost-effective production of cellular material representing a high expression level of recombinant receptor that can be utilized, i.e., for membrane preparation to be used in radioligand-binding studies. Using a single 175 cm^2 culture dish allowed us to obtain specimens containing app. 1 mg protein, which were characterized by *Bmax* value of 2 pmol/mg in saturation-binding studies.
2. The assay protocol was optimized for the pmCherry-N1 vector containing cDNA of histamine H_3 receptor. The total size of the construct was 6053 bp. As a standard, large-scale preparations of DNA plasmids are obtained in our laboratory from bacterial lysates with the use of spin columns utilizing silica-based membrane technology (GeneJET Plasmid Maxiprep Kit; #K0491; ThermoFisher Scientific), guarantying appropriate quality of preparations (*see* **Note 1**).
3. All experimental steps should be performed in the laminar flow cabinet paying attention to aseptic techniques.
4. Maintain CHO (#CCL-61; ATTC) cells in good condition, keep the passage number as low as possible, and routinely check for mycoplasma contamination (*see* **Note 2**). Grow the cells in DMEM/F12 medium, supplemented with 10% FBS. Split the cells every 3–4 days in the ratio of 1:10 using standard procedures. Do not let the cells overgrow.
5. One day before the transfection, seed 5.4×10^6 cells in a total volume of 30 mL of standard medium per single 175 cm^2 culture dish, so that the cells achieve confluence of 80% on the following day.
6. On the day of experiment, in a 50 mL conical tube, combine 72 μg of plasmid containing receptor cDNA with 6 mL of DMEM/F12 medium without FBS.

7. Add 180 μL of polyethylenimine solution (1 mg/mL in water; branched; average molecular weight determined by static light scattering: 25 kDa) and incubate for 20 min at room temperature (*see* **Note 3**).
8. Transfer the suspension of obtained complexes dropwise to CHO cells in culture. Scale up the necessary amounts of reagents proportionally to the number of dishes you want to use in the experiments (e.g., 360 μg DNA and 900 μL PEI solution in 30 mL of medium for five 175 cm^2 dishes).
9. Check for receptor expression after 24 h post-transfection. Expression of fluorescent fusion constructs can be tested with fluorescent microscopy or FACS.

3.2 Stable Transfection of HEK293T Cells

1. HEK293T cells (#CRL-3216; ATCC) are grown in DMEM medium with the addition of 10% FBS in humidified CO_2 incubator at 37 °C. Cells are passaged every 6 days in a ratio of 1:10. Between the passages medium is changed every 2 days. All the culturing procedures and following transfection steps should be performed in a laminar flow hood.
2. Twenty four hours before the planned experiment plate 3×10^5 HEK293T cells (*see* **Note 4**) on 10 cm^2 Petri dish containing 2 mL of complete growth medium (DMEM, 10% FBS, without antibiotics).
3. On the next day, combine in 1.5 mL tube a solution containing 2 μg of circular plasmid p*h*H_3R-mCherry (*see* **Note 5**), diluted with DMEM medium without FBS to the volume of 100 μL and add 5 μL of FuGENE HD transfection reagent.
4. Mix thoroughly and incubate at room temperature for 15 min (*see* **Note 3**).
5. Add the transfection complexes to the cells in a dropwise manner or add below the surface of the medium. Swirl the dish to ensure even distribution over the entire cell surface.
6. After 48 h, inspect the cells for the possible cytotoxicity of transfection mixture and verify the expression of recombinant receptor with the use of fluorescent microscope (for critical aspects of transfection efficiency, *see* **Note 6**).
7. Next, collect the cells from 10 cm^2 dish by trypsinization and remove the medium by centrifugation (180 × *g*, 10 min, RT).
8. Resuspend the obtained cell pellet in fresh DMEM medium containing 800 μg/mL G418 (30 mL) and place the transfected cells in a 175 cm^2 culture flask (*see* **Note 7**). From this point on the selection of stably transfected cells is conducted.
9. Continue the culture of transfected HEK293T cells, changing the medium every 2 days to remove the cell debris. First necrotic cells occur after 4 days of culturing in medium con-

taining G418. Selection process should be finished in 2 weeks and well distinguishable cell colonies will be visible at that time.

10. In order to isolate the single clones of stably transfected cells conduct the subcloning procedure by seeding the cells at low cell densities into individual wells of 96-well plates (*see* **Note 8**).
11. Before proceeding, estimate the plating efficiency of desired cell line by seeding the non-transfected HEK293T cells into 96-well plates in a density of 1–10 cells/well. After 7 days of incubation verify which cell concentration resulted in growing of an average of a single colony per well. Choose that seeding density for further experiments. In our case plating efficiency was app. 30%, so for the purposes of subcloning procedure stably transfected cells were plated on 96-well plates in concentration of 3 cells/well.
12. Trypsinize the cells after selection, centrifuge and discard the disintegrating medium. Resuspend the pellet in DMEM/10% FBS medium with reduced concentration of G418 (200 μg/mL) and adjust the volume to obtain the cell density of 30 cells/mL.
13. Add PBS to all marginal wells of three 96-well plates to reduce the evaporation of medium from central part of plate.
14. Place 100 μL of the cell suspension in the remaining wells of prepared microplates and leave them in the humidified CO_2 incubator.
15. Following 1 week of incubation check wells for single cell-derived colonies. Inspect the cells under a fluorescence microscope to confirm the expression of fluorescently tagged receptors. Mark the positive wells (should have at least five marked wells).
16. Change media on marked wells.
17. Allow cells to continue growing until each colony is large enough to be transferred to a bigger dish (may take another 5–7 days).
18. Transfer homogenous, intensively fluorescent colonies to the 10 cm^2 Petri dishes containing 2 mL of culture media, by pipetting the content of well several times up and down.
19. When the cells reach confluence expand the culture to the 75 cm^2 flask that will be used to prepare backups and to obtain the material for desired downstream applications.

3.3 Retroviral Transduction of CHO Cells

1. Two separate CO_2 incubators are needed to conduct the retroviral transduction experiment.
2. CHO cells are cultured in DMEM/F12 medium with the addition of 10% FBS (Sect. 3.1).

3. After thawing frozen stock of GP+*env*AM-12 cells (#CRL-9641, ATCC) at 37 °C, cultures are grown in DMEM medium, supplemented with 10% FBS, 2 mM Glutamax, 100 U/mL penicillin, and 100 μg/mL streptomycin (medium without HXM). Following the first passage of packaging cells, growth medium is changed to HXM medium (DMEM, 10% FBS, 200 μg/mL hygromycin B, 250 μg/mL xanthine, 15 μg/mL hypoxanthine, 25 μg/mL mycophenolic acid, 2 mM Glutamax, 100 U/mL penicillin, and 100 μg/mL streptomycin). Cells are cultured in a humidified CO_2 incubator at 37 °C and should not be allowed to overgrow. Cultures should be passaged when 80% confluent, with the splitting ratio in a range of 1:3–1:6.
4. In order to prepare for the retroviral transduction experiment, set the temperature of one cell culture incubator to 32°C.
5. Then, seed GP+*env*AM-12 cells at a density of 1.0×10^6 cells in a 25 cm^2 culture flask in DMEM medium containing only 10% FBS and 2 mM Glutamax.
6. On the following day, transfect the packaging cells with retroviral plasmid containing the gene of interest using Turbofect reagent. Mix in a 1.5 mL tube: 11.25 μg of pQCXIN-*h*H_4R plasmid and 6.75 μg of pcDNA3.1-VSV-G plasmid (*see* **Note 9**) diluted to 600 μL with DMEM medium without FBS and add 24 μL of Turbofect reagent.
7. Incubate for 15 min at room temperature and add the mixture dropwise to the culture of GP+*env*AM-12 cells.
8. Fourteen hours post-transfection, replace the medium for packaging cells with 3 mL of DMEM medium containing 10% FBS, 2 mM Glutamax, 100 U/mL penicillin and 100 μg/mL streptomycin.
9. Next, add 30 μL of 500 mM aqueous solution of sodium butyrate (*see* **Note 10**) and transfer the culture flask to the incubator with a set temperature of 32 °C and CO_2 level of 5%.
10. Continue the culture for 48 h.
11. Meanwhile, i.e., 24 h post-transfection, seed CHO cells (cultured in parallel to GP+*env*AM-12 cells) at a density of 1.0×10^6 cells in a 25 cm^2 flask and culture them at 37 °C so that on the next day confluency would reach app. 80%.
12. At the end of 48-h-long period of incubation of transfected GP+*env*AM-12 cells, inspect the virus-producing cells microscopically. Cells should be significantly larger and contain multiple granules.
13. Collect 3 mL of culture medium containing viral particles. Pass it through the syringe filter with a 0.45 μm pore size and combine with 2.4 μL of 10 mg/mL aqueous solution of polybrene (*see* **Note 11**).

14. Discard the medium from a previously prepared CHO cell culture flask and replace it with the obtained suspension of viral particles.
15. Two hours later, change the medium at CHO cells for fresh one (DMEM/F12, 10% FBS) and move the culture flask back to the incubator (37 °C, 5% CO_2).
16. After further 48 h collect the transduced CHO cells by trypsinization, centrifuge, resuspend in selection medium containing G418 (800 μg/mL) and place in a 175 cm^2 culture flask.
17. Perform selection of transduced cells and isolation of single clones in accordance with procedures described before (Sect. 3.2).

4 Notes

1. Sufficient DNA purity is essential for the process of transfection. It has significant influence on the effectiveness of transgene delivery to the cells. Genetic material used to perform transfection should be devoid of various contaminations, like organic compounds (for instance phenol or chloroform), proteins, bacterial RNA, endotoxins, and high concentration of inorganic salts [7, 16, 18].
2. Overall condition of the utilized cells is a crucial parameter for transfection efficiency. Cells should be transfected in the logarithmic phase of growth, and should be free of contaminations, including mycoplasma [17]. Another aspect that can have negative effect on stable transfection is the passage number of the cell culture. Some publications suggest that cells cannot be efficiently transfected when their passage number exceeds 30 [17, 28, 29].
3. Optimization of the transfection protocol can include the changes in the ratio of transfection mixture components, time of pre-incubation before adding the transfection complexes to cells and volume of culture medium used for dilution of transfection mixture. Density of transfected cells can also be the subject of optimization. Various cell confluences should be checked to select the conditions that result in enhanced efficiency of transfection and at the same time are not significantly cytotoxic to cells. More information about the optimization of transfection protocols can be found in manuals provided by manufacturers of transfection reagents.
4. In presented protocol the T-variant of HEK293 cell line (#CRL-3216, ATCC) was used. One of its features is the expression of large T antigen from Simian virus number 40 (SV40) [25]. Presence of this protein determines episomal

replication of plasmids, which contain origin of replication from SV40. Plasmid pmCherry-N1, which was utilized in experiments, fulfils that requirement and can be therefore maintained inside the transfected HEK293T cells for a longer time.

5. According to some protocols, stable transfection can be performed with the use of a linear form of the plasmid. That approach may potentially increase the efficiency of transgene integration into the host genome. Linear plasmids can be obtained by cleavage with the use of the appropriate restriction enzyme. The location of restriction cut site should be beyond the fragment that encodes for the receptor protein. Moreover, cutting the plasmid with restriction enzyme should not destroy the promoter sequences nor the antibiotic resistance gene.
6. Crucial parameters of lipofection experiments are:
   - Simultaneous incubation of cationic lipids and DNA in medium without serum, because it contains sulfate proteoglycans and other proteins, which compete with DNA in the process of forming complexes with cationic lipids.
   - Using culture medium without antibiotics during experiment.
   - Prevention of forming of potentially cytotoxic lipofection polyplexes, by reduction of DNA and/or cationic lipids amounts in transfection samples [7, 15].
7. Geneticin (G418) is a selective antibiotic for eukaryotic cells. It belongs to the group aminoglycosides and has a similar structure to neomycin, gentamicin, and kanamycin. Its cytotoxic activity in eukaryotic cells arises from inhibition of protein biosynthesis, due to the interaction of G418 with ribosomes. Geneticin resistance results from the expression of a gene of a bacterial origin encoding for aminoglycoside phosphotransferase, which is responsible for deactivation of antibiotic culture medium [9]. Eukaryotic cells have varying sensitivities for G418 and because of that, survival curves for wild-type cells should be determined prior to the stable transfection experiment. As for the utilized cell lines (HEK293T and CHO), cellular death rate of 100% was observed in G418 concentrations equal to or higher than 800 μg/mL after 14 days of cell culture in a culture medium with antibiotic. Based on these observations, it was stated that for the selection of transfected cells geneticin should be used at a concentration of 800 μg/mL. Efficacy of G418 is decreased when penicillin and streptomycin are also present in a culture medium; therefore, the selection procedure should be conducted in medium without these antibiotics.
8. The experience of our group indicates that subcloning procedure is crucial for obtaining cell lines with stable expression of

recombinant 7TM receptors. Our previous experiments revealed that despite high efficiency of transient transfection (up to 80%), at the end of selection stage only 20–30% of clones exhibited expression of recombinant protein, even though the antibiotic resistance was observed for all clones. Moreover, it is well recognized that in heterogeneous cell culture, with clones showing different levels of transgene expression, cells without recombinant protein grow faster. This can lead to the decrease in number of cells overexpressing the recombinant receptor in subsequent passages. Therefore, to avoid the described circumstances, subcloning should be considered in every stable transfection experiment.

9. Retroviral genes *env* encode for glycoproteins of the viral envelope and determine virus ability to enter different cell types in the mechanism of receptor-driven endocytosis. In order to increase the efficiency of infection of Chinese hamster cells by viruses produced in amphotropic GP+*env*AM-12 cells, a virus pseudotyping procedure was conducted, by the replacement of the native *env* gene product with the glycoprotein G from lipid envelope of *Vesicular Stromatitis Virus* (VSV). This protein, unlike other products of *env* gene, interacts with cell membrane phospholipids in a receptor-independent manner during the virus entry into the cells [30, 31]. Stable expression of VSV-G protein in packaging cells is harmful for them; therefore, pseudotyping of viruses was obtained by means of transient transfection of virions-producing cells with the plasmid containing VSV-G cDNA sequence. No additional actions were necessary to attach the recombinant VSV-G protein to the envelope of produced retroviruses [30].
10. Sodium butyrate enhances the transient expression of plasmids containing the SV40 early promoter in transfected cells.
11. Polybrene (1,5-dimethyl-1,5-diazaundecamethylene polymethobromide, hexadimethrine bromide) is a cationic polymer that is a highly efficient enhancer of gene transfer into mammalian cells through infection with retroviral vectors. The efficiency of retroviral transduction can be increased significantly, 100 to 1000-fold in some cells, by including polybrene during the infection.

Acknowledgments

The authors acknowledge the financial support of Polish National Science Centre within the frame of Meastro grant No. 2011/02/A/NZ4/00031 and Preludium grant No. 2011/01/N/NZ4/01126, which enabled the development and optimization of protocols described in this manuscript.

References

1. Hill SJ (2006) G-protein-coupled receptors: past, present and future. Br J Pharmacol 147(Suppl 1):S27–S37
2. Bockaert J, Brand C, Journot L (1997) Do recombinant receptor assays provide affinity and potency estimates? Ann N Y Acad Sci 812:55–70
3. Kenakin T (1996) The classification of seven transmembrane receptors in recombinant expression systems. Pharmacol Rev 48: 413–463
4. Sautel M, Milligan G (2000) Molecular manipulation of G-protein-coupled receptors: a new avenue into drug discovery. Curr Med Chem 7:889–896
5. Sarramegna V, Talmont F, Demange P et al (2003) Heterologous expression of G-protein-coupled receptors: comparison of expression systems from the standpoint of large-scale production and purification. Cell Mol Life Sci 60:1529–1546
6. Tate CG, Grisshammer R (1996) Heterologous expression of G-protein-coupled receptors. Trends Biotechnol 14:426–430
7. Colosimo A, Goncz KK, Holmes AR et al (2000) Transfer and expression of foreign genes in mammalian cells. Biotechniques 29:314–318 320-312, 324
8. Mortensen RM, Kingston RE (2009) Selection of transfected mammalian cells. Curr Protoc Mol Biol 86:9.5.1–9.5.13
9. Makrides SC (1999) Components of vectors for gene transfer and expression in mammalian cells. Protein Expr Purif 17:183–202
10. Jordan M, Schallhorn A, Wurm FM (1996) Transfecting mammalian cells: optimization of critical parameters affecting calcium-phosphate precipitate formation. Nucleic Acids Res 24:596–601
11. Meissner P, Pick H, Kulangara A et al (2001) Transient gene expression: recombinant protein production with suspension-adapted HEK293-EBNA cells. Biotechnol Bioeng 75:197–203
12. Reed SE, Staley EM, Mayginnes JP et al (2006) Transfection of mammalian cells using linear polyethylenimine is a simple and effective means of producing recombinant adeno-associated virus vectors. J Virol Methods 138:85–98
13. Ehrhardt C, Schmolke M, Matzke A et al (2006) Polyethylenimine, a cost-effective transfection reagent. Signal Transduct 6:179–184
14. Benjaminsen RV, Mattebjerg MA, Henriksen JR et al (2013) The possible "proton sponge" effect of polyethylenimine (PEI) does not include change in lysosomal pH. Mol Ther 21:149–157
15. Hawley-Nelson P, Ciccarone V, Moore ML (2008) Transfection of cultured eukaryotic cells using cationic lipid reagents. Curr Protoc Mol Biol 81:9.4.1–9.4.17
16. Hermans E (2004) Generation of model cell lines expressing recombinant G-protein-coupled receptors. Methods Mol Biol 259: 137–153
17. Freshney RI (2005) Culture of animal cells: a manual of basic technique, 5th edn. Wiley-Liss, Hoboken, NJ
18. Baldi L, Hacker DL, Adam M et al (2007) Recombinant protein production by large-scale transient gene expression in mammalian cells: state of the art and future perspectives. Biotechnol Lett 29:677–684
19. Zaremba ML, Borowski J (2004) Mikrobiologia lekarska: podręcznik dla studentów medycyny, 3rd edn. Wydawnictwo Lekarskie PZWL, Warszawa
20. Cepko C, Pear W (2001) Overview of the retrovirus transduction system. Curr Protoc Mol Biol 36:9.9.1–9.9.16
21. Miller AD, Buttimore C (1986) Redesign of retrovirus packaging cell lines to avoid recombination leading to helper virus production. Mol Cell Biol 6:2895–2902
22. Jayapal KP, Wlaschin KF, Hu W-S et al (2007) Recombinant protein therapeutics from CHO cells—20 years and counting. Chem Eng Prog 103:40
23. Graham FL, Smiley J, Russell WC et al (1977) Characteristics of a human cell line transformed by DNA from human adenovirus type 5. J Gen Virol 36:59–74
24. Atwood BK, Lopez J, Wager-Miller J et al (2011) Expression of G protein-coupled receptors and related proteins in HEK293, AtT20, BV2, and N18 cell lines as revealed by microarray analysis. BMC Genomics 12:14
25. Thomas P, Smart TG (2005) HEK293 cell line: a vehicle for the expression of recombinant proteins. J Pharmacol Toxicol Methods 51:187–200
26. Witte DG, Yao BB, Miller TR et al (2006) Detection of multiple H_3 receptor affinity states utilizing [^{3}H]A-349821, a novel, selective, non-imidazole histamine H_3 receptor inverse agonist radioligand. Br J Pharmacol 148:657–670
27. Markowitz D, Goff S, Bank A (1988) Construction and use of a safe and efficient

amphotropic packaging cell line. Virology 167:400–406
28. Hughes P, Marshall D, Reid Y et al (2007) The costs of using unauthenticated, over-passaged cell lines: how much more data do we need? Biotechniques 43:575 577-578, 581-572
29. Jacobsen L, Hughes P (2007) Effects of passage number on cell line transfection. Biochemica 3:2
30. Emi N, Friedmann T, Yee JK (1991) Pseudotype formation of murine leukemia virus with the G protein of vesicular stomatitis virus. J Virol 65:1202–1207
31. Burns JC, Friedmann T, Driever W et al (1993) Vesicular stomatitis virus G glycoprotein pseudotyped retroviral vectors: concentration to very high titer and efficient gene transfer into mammalian and nonmammalian cells. Proc Natl Acad Sci U S A 90:8033–8037

Chapter 4

Histamine H_2 Receptor Biased Signaling Methods

Natalia C. Fernández, Carina Shayo, Carlos Davio, and Federico Monczor

Abstract

Advances in the study of G protein-coupled receptors (GPCRs) allow understanding of the existence of multiple possible receptor conformational states. Among the wide range of possible events that could be mediated by a receptor (second messenger modulation, dimerization, desensitization, internalization, G protein-dependent signaling, gene regulation, etc), the ligand–receptor complex governs the ultimate downstream signaling event and the final cellular response. To analyze the pluridimensional aspect of ligand efficacy, there is a need to employ a wide range of experimental tools that enable the study of receptor behaviors.

In an attempt to contribute to the study and comprehension of the biased behavior of histamine H_2 receptor (H2R) ligands, the aim of this chapter is to provide experimental tools that facilitate the exploration and analysis of the pluridimensional nature of H2R ligands. We hope that in the future it would be possible to develop ligands that take advantage of biased signaling by selectively activating the beneficial signaling events of the H2R and blocking the undesired ones.

Key words Biased agonism, Biased quantification, Functional selectivity, Pluridimensional efficacy, Receptor conformation

1 Introduction

1.1 The Receptor Concept

Pharmacological studies rely on the understanding of the effects of a given ligand on a biological system, which includes knowing structure activity relationships, molecular interactions, pharmacokinetics and therapeutic uses of compounds. The strong link that exists between advances in pharmacology and the evolution of receptor theory demonstrates the importance of elucidating the mechanisms of the actions of drugs to properly understand physiology and treat disease. The receptor concept represents one of the most important concepts in pharmacology, if not the most important. Advances in physics, biology, and chemistry have allowed the evolution of the receptor concept from the first studies in 1878 where Paul Ehrlich and John Langley proposed that there are chemical substances of the cells that are specific and "receptive" and more important, with therapeutic "utility" [1, 2], until to our

Ekaterini Tiligada and Madeleine Ennis (eds.), *Histamine Receptors as Drug Targets*, Methods in Pharmacology and Toxicology, DOI 10.1007/978-1-4939-6843-5_4, © Springer Science+Business Media LLC 2017

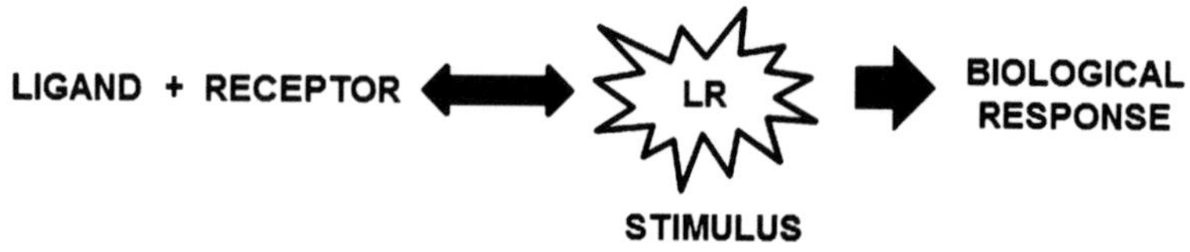

Fig. 1 Black and Leff operational model. In this model, formation of ligand receptor complex (stimulus) and eliciting of response are considered as separate events

current concept of receptors as macromolecules, of protein nature, that bind an active substance and elicit a response.

In an attempt to accurately quantify the key characteristics of receptor–ligand interaction and the consequences of such interaction on biological systems, several mathematical models have been designed that allow the estimation of ligand affinity and efficacy. Archibald Hill was a pioneer in applying mathematical models in order to quantify the relationship between ligand concentration and biological response [3].Since then, the increasing knowledge of receptor transduction mechanisms has led to the development of more sophisticated mathematical models of efficacy estimation. One of the most accepted is the two-step model of James Black and Paul Leff (Fig. 1) which considers as separated processes, the formation of ligand–receptor complex and the transduction of the stimulus into a biological response [4].

This model deals with the black-box issue of ligand-induced cell response considering that whole process consists in two steps, namely the binding of the ligand to the receptor molecule, and the triggering of the cell response by ligand–receptor complexes. In this scenario, both affinity and efficacy are determining factors for each step and should be considered to quantify the behavior of a drug.

The binding of a ligand to its receptor to form the ligand–receptor complex [LR] is a dynamic equilibrium that can be described with the equation of a rectangular hyperbola (Eq. 1):

$$[LR] = \frac{R_{tot} \cdot [L]}{[L] + K_{\mathrm{A}}} \quad (1)$$

where $[L]$ represents ligand concentration, R_{tot} is the membrane receptor density and K_A is the functional affinity of the ligand. The latter is not the affinity for the bare receptor (dissociation constant K_D) but it is the affinity for the receptor species that triggers the response, usually ternary complexes (i.e. ligand–receptor complex coupled to the G-protein or to β-arrestin). This is a crucial distinction and will be clarified below when quantification of bias will be specifically discussed.

The second step of signal transduction can also be accommodated considering a hyperbolic function (Eq. 2)

$$\text{Response} = \frac{S \cdot E_{\max}}{S + K_{\mathrm{E}}} \tag{2}$$

In this case, S is the stimulus able to initiate cell response, E_{max} is the maximum effect and K_E corresponds to the concentration of ligand–receptor complex that elicits half-maximal response.

Considering that ligand-bound receptor [LR] is the stimulus S, Eqs. (1) and (2) can be combined to obtain Eq. (3).

$$\text{Response} = \frac{[\mathrm{L}] \cdot \tau \cdot E_{\max}}{[\mathrm{L}] \cdot (1+\tau) + K_{\mathrm{A}}} \tag{3}$$

Equation (3) represents a hyperbolic relationship between ligand concentration and cell response, involving a term τ which comprises the intrinsic efficacy of the ligand and the sensitivity of the system to agonism and is defined as $\tau = R_{tot}/K_E$.

1.2 Affinity and Efficacy at GPCRs

In the particular case of GPCRs, transduction of the extracellular signal into an intracellular response comprises multiple and amplified events. It begins with the activation of heterotrimeric G protein, which exchanges guanosine diphosphate (GDP) for guanosine triphosphate (GTP) and dissociates into subunits Gα and Gβγ [5]. This dissociation then promotes the activation of effector proteins, namely adenylyl cyclase (AC) or phospholipase C (PLC). For that reason, GPCRs were originally thought to lead to the cytosolic increase of second messengers:cyclic adenosine monophosphate (cAMP) as a consequence of AC activation and inositol 1,4,5-trisphosphate (IP3) after PLC stimulation. However, it is currently well known that there are multiple classes of Gα subunits by means of which GPCRs can also activate other signaling pathways. In this way the Gs class of G proteins acts to stimulate AC; Gi/o inhibits AC and some members of this subfamily inhibit ion channels or activate phosphodiesterases that degrade cAMP; Gq and G11 types activate PLC; and finally, G12/13 class of G proteins modulates Rho/Rac/cdc42 small GTP binding family of protein [6]. In addition to the activation of signaling cascades by means of Gα subunit, the Gβγ dimer can also modulate the activity of some of the mentioned effector enzymes or even regulate the activity of ion channels. This dimer can also stimulate phosphoinositide 3-kinase (PI3K) and mitogen-activated protein kinases (MAPK) signaling pathways, which were generally associated to other types of membrane receptors, mainly of the tyrosine kinase membrane receptor type [7, 8].

As mentioned above, the two-step model of James Black and Paul Leff discriminates between the binding of the ligand to the receptor and the subsequent activation of the signaling pathway as separate processes [4]. With the aim of studying these processes two key conceptual tools associated with receptor pharmacology may be used, these are ligand *affinity* and ligand *efficacy*.

The *affinity* of a ligand characterizes the strength of the interaction between the ligand and the receptor but binding to the receptor is not enough to predict the biological effect of that ligand on cellular behavior. The property that accounts for the biological impact of the ligand is the *efficacy*, which indicates the ability of the ligand to evoke an observable response and can be quantified at different levels by measuring, for example, a physiological event such as muscle contraction or a molecular intracellular event such as signal transduction [9]. Biochemical assays in cellular or animal models are useful to evaluate the pharmacologic effect of ligands on the biological system, and measurement of receptor signaling is many times, the assay of choice.

If we consider the myriad of intracellular events that can occur after GPCR stimulation, it is not easy to choose an indicator of receptor response in order to quantify ligand efficacy [10]. However, in an attempt to understand the pharmacology of a ligand, the selection of any reasonable modification in the basal behavior of the system of study may represent, although arbitrary, a consistent response and may be measured to estimate the efficacy of that ligand. This can be determined by studying the effects of the compound on the selected biological end point in concentration/dose-response assays. The concentration–response plot, in a linear scale, results in a hyperbolic curve; but by plotting the effect of the ligand vs. its concentration in a semi-log fashion; we obtain a sigmoidal curve, often referred to as a dose-response curve, where it is easy to derive the ligand *potency* and *maximal response* of the ligand [11]. The International Union of Pharmacology defines potency as the concentration or amount needed to produce a defined biological response and is described in terms of the half-maximal effect or *EC50* obtained from a concentration–response curve [12] (Fig. 2). The maximal response of the ligand refers to the maximal effect elicited by the compound in the particular biological system where it is studied and was classically associated with ligand efficacy. However, in the present chapter we will not consider efficacy as the maximal response evoked by a ligand, instead of that we will refer to the general idea of *what drugs do*, or in other words, the ability of a compound to change target behavior.

Based on this, compounds that mimic the biological effect of the physiological ligand are defined as agonists or ligands with positive efficacy. Ligands that do not induce full activation of the receptor's signaling capacity are referred to as partial agonists, namely the response evoked by the partial agonist is lower than the maximal response of the physiological ligand in that system. Those compounds that after binding to the receptor block the effect of a

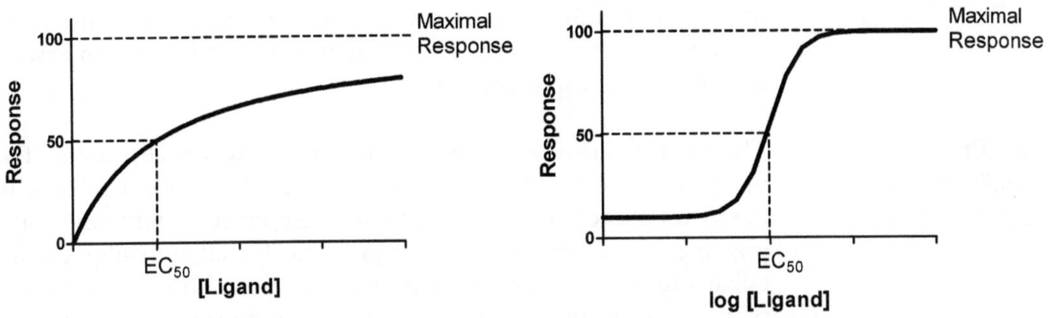

Fig. 2 Concentration response curves. Plotting of response vs agonist concentration in a linear plot produces a hyperbolic curve. Plotting the data in a semi-log plot reveals the typical sigmoidal curve. Shown are the effective concentration 50% (EC50) and the maximal response (Rmax). These values give information about potency and efficacy respectively

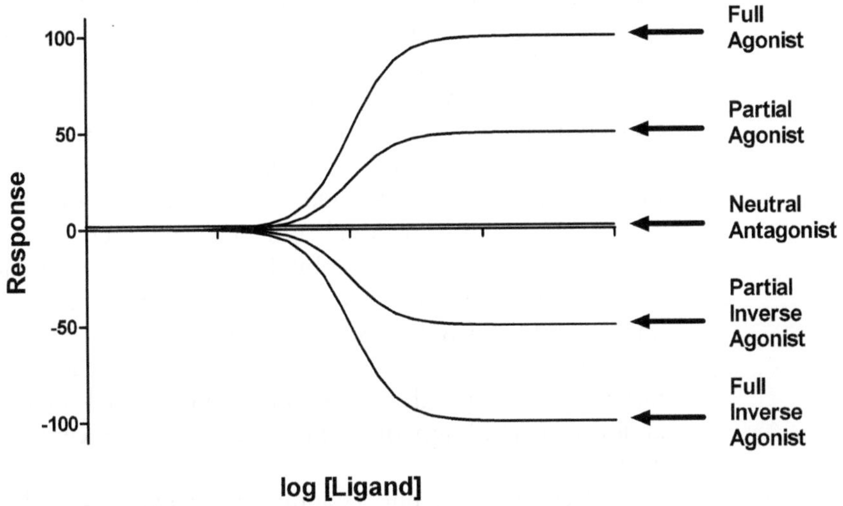

Fig. 3 Ligand efficacy. Concentration–response curves for ligands with positive (agonist and partial agonist) null (antagonist) or negative (inverse agonist and partial inverse agonist) efficacy

naturally occurring ligand but do not evoke a response per se, are classified as antagonists of the receptor, and considered ligands with null efficacy [12]. These ligands are usually studied by measuring the ability of increasing concentration of the antagonist to inhibit the effect of the agonist in competition assays, and their potency is often estimated as the concentration of antagonist that produces half-maximal inhibition of the response (*IC50*). Lastly, with the development of more sensitive methodologies that allow the detection of the spontaneous activity of GPCRs it was found that some compounds inhibit the basal constitutive activity of the receptors. These ligands are termed inverse agonists or ligands with negative efficacy and are responsible for the decrease in the basal response of a given system (Fig. 3). To evaluate the efficacy of inverse agonists it is necessary to assess receptors with high constitutive activity or in assays with enough sensitivity to measure a decrease in basal activity [13].

1.3 The Pluridimensional Aspect of Efficacy

The ligand classification mentioned above was really useful for many years; however, it presents a principal limitation in that it is based on the concept that receptors are entities with only one possible active conformation responsible for all signaling events occurring downstream of receptor stimulation. This vision implies that receptors are, in some way, passive conduits that transmit the message of the extracellular signaling molecule to an intracellular signaling event and by doing so they act as switches that alternate between an "on" active state and an "off" inactive one. In this context, GPCRs were thought to be inactivated by different mechanisms that involved receptor phosphorylation, principally mediated by G protein-coupled receptor kinases (GRKs) or second messengers-dependent kinases; β-arrestin binding to the phosphorylated receptor, which leads to uncoupling from heterotrimeric G protein and consequent receptor desensitization; and finally internalization of receptors by clathrin-coated vesicles [14].

Interestingly, all of the mechanisms of receptor switch off mentioned above were considered a consequence of the induction of the active conformational state achieved after ligand binding. This assumption was refuted by data showing that, antagonists of several GPCRs can cause receptor internalization with no concomitant receptor activation. Several antagonists for receptors for cholecystokinin, parathyroid hormone, serotonin, chemokines, and histamine among others have been shown to lead to receptor endocytosis although they fail to activate the receptor signaling cascades [15].

Advances in the understanding of proteins as fluid structures with inherent conformational dynamism, allow the understanding that receptors play an active role at transmitting the stimulus across the plasma membrane and that there are multiple possible conformational states distinct from the unique "active" or "inactive" ones. This conformational fluidity of proteins was hypothesized long ago by Changeux who postulated that "ligands shift the equilibrium of the protein structure between conformations, selectively stabilizing the one for which it has the highest affinity" [16].

All known GPCRs are able to bind multiple ligands and the conformation stabilized by a specific ligand may be different from the conformation stabilized by a different ligand. If the ligand–receptor complex is considered to act as a ligand for the intracellular partners of GPCRs, namely G proteins, GRKs and arrestins, it can be assumed that depending upon the receptor conformation that is stabilized by the ligand, the activated intracellular partners and the signaling output. In this way, the ligand–receptor complex is the one who governs the ultimate downstream signaling event and not the receptor itself [17]. Based on that, the efficacy for receptor internalization does not have to mirror the efficacy to produce receptor activation.

GPCRs are pleiotropic regarding their intracellular effects and ligand binding stabilizes specific conformations among the texture of conformational variants of receptor [18]. This process has been referred to as conformational selection and explains why only a part of receptor's signaling possibilities is selectively activated. A direct consequence of this is functional selectivity or biased agonism since the ligand causes differential activation of only some of the signaling events associated with a particular receptor [19]. Therefore, a ligand can stabilize a particular conformation that although fails to stimulate G-protein signaling, it may result in receptor desensitization, internalization or even G-protein independent signaling (Fig. 4).

This pluridimensional aspect of efficacy represents a revolutionary concept in pharmacology and was first described for adrenergic receptors by Galandrin and Bouvier in 2006 [20], to refer to the different behaviors modulated by a GPCR [21]. However, to see the whole picture of the action of a receptor ligand consideration of the molecular dynamic view of receptor multiple active states is not sufficient. To evaluate pluridimensional efficacy we also need a wide range of "experimental eyes" that make possible the study of those receptor behaviors [22, 23]. It is not surprising that the pluridimensional aspect of efficacy was not evident until more sensitive techniques, that improved the measurement of the ability of compounds to produce a biological response, were developed.

1.4 Pharmacological Advantages of the Pluridimensional Nature of Efficacy

Far from being a curiosity, functional selectivity provides the ability to fine-tune drug action in the context of multiple responses. From this pharmacological perspective, ligand bias allows to produce a wanted agonist activity over a specific signaling pathway while having null activity over other unwanted cellular responses. In the same way that in the past, the strategy to achieve therapeutic drug selectivity was through interaction with specific GPCR subtypes, the more recent introduction of molecular dynamics to receptor theory, offered the opportunity of considering bias signaling as a new dimension of selectivity. Therapeutically, by ligand stabilization of unique arrays of GPCRs conformations, different ligands of the same receptor can produce very different physiological outcomes [24, 25].

Although the identification of pluridimensional efficacy was several years ago, there is not much evidence regarding the therapeutic use of biased ligands and whether they actually lead to physiological relevant manifestations of the biased events. However, it is well known that many of the side effects of drugs are not a consequence of off-target interactions but of on-target signaling instead. Based on that, drug design could be oriented to the development of ligands that selectively activate the beneficial signaling events of a receptor and antagonize the undesired ones.

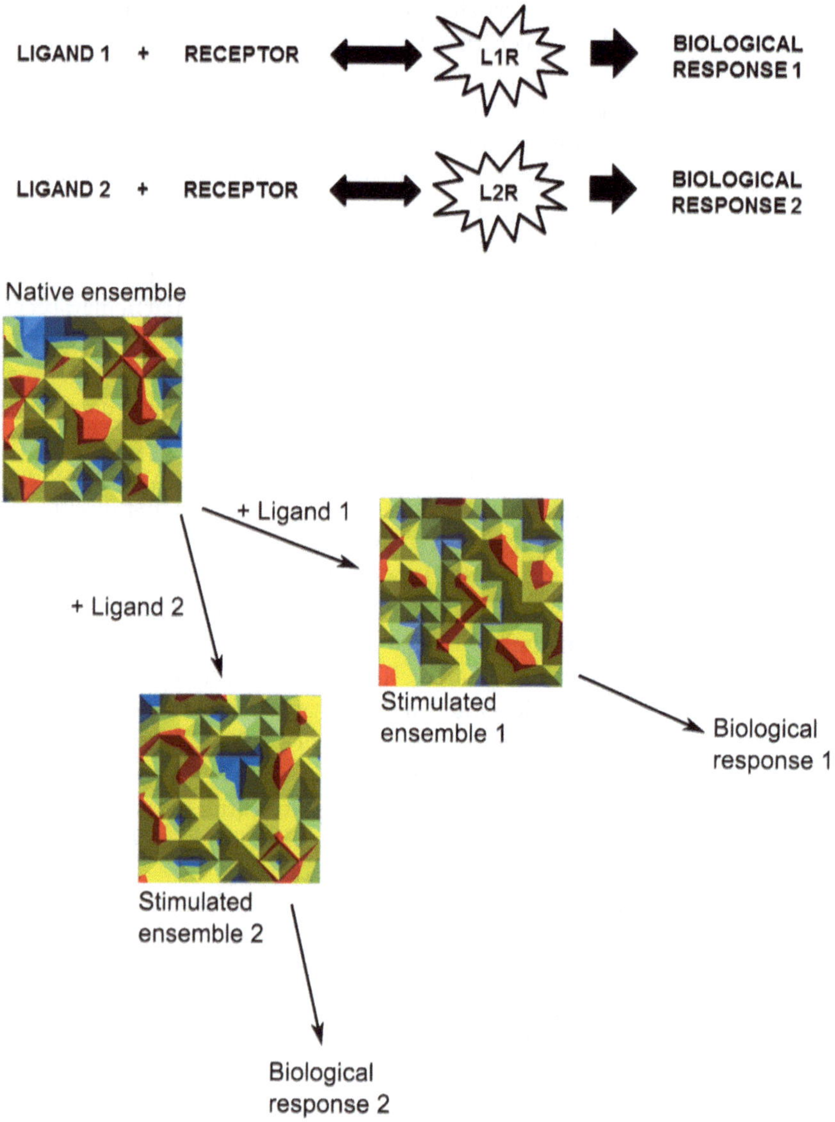

Fig. 4 Statistical interpretation of ligand efficacy. The receptor exists in multiple conformations in equilibrium that bind to ligand with different affinities. After binding to ligand, a particular set of receptor conformations is stabilized. This set has its own affinity for the available signal transducers (G proteins, arrestins, kinases, etc). Some ligand receptor conformations predominantly activate one signaling pathway, while others can activate different ones. *Top*: Adaptation of Black and Leff Operational model for biased signaling. *Bottom*: Schematic diagram of how conformational dynamics of receptors leads to biased signaling. The plot depicts the relative frequency for each conformation in a color scale from blue (less frequent) to red (more frequent). Each ligand enriches some populations at expenses of others

1.5 Histamine H_2 Receptor and Biased Agonism

The H2R is a GPCR coupled to Gαs protein so its activation by histamine stimulates adenylyl cyclase-mediated cAMP production [26]. It was discovered in the early 70s by Powell and Brody [27] four years after its pharmacological identification by Sir James Black [28]. It is highly expressed in parietal cells of the gastric mucosa and in various parts of the brain, including the basal ganglia, hippocampus, amygdala, and cerebral cortex [29] and, to a lower degree, in cerebellum and hypothalamus. In addition, there is a significant expression of H2R in neutrophils, eosinophils, monocytes, macrophages, dendritic cells, T and B cells, chondrocytes, and in smooth muscle, endothelial and epithelial cells [30]. It has been proved to present lower affinity for histamine than the receptor subtypes H_3 (H3R) and H_4 (H4R) and to present high constitutive activity towards cAMP production [31, 32].

In some H2R expressing cells, besides the classical signaling through Gs protein, it can also couple to Gq/11 proteins, leading to inositol phosphate formation and increases in cytosolic Ca^{2+} concentration [26, 33]. It has been described that H2R stimulation by histamine can also modulate the release of arachidonic acid by potently inhibiting the activity of phospholipase A2 [34]. Interestingly, H2R can also modulate other signaling pathways classically associated with tyrosine kinase receptors. In this context, some histamine actions mediated by the H2R such as modulation of cell proliferation, cell migration, cellular permeability, gene expression, and memory have been proved to involve the activation of extracellular signal-regulated kinases (ERK1/2) [35–37]. In homologous and heterologous H2R expression systems, it has been described that ERK activation by H2R ligands is achieved through a Gs protein, adenylyl cyclase and PKA-independent pathway [38–40].

There is also evidence that some typical histamine actions mediated by H2R, such as acid gastric secretion, involve the modulation of PI3K [41], a traditional mediator of growth factors and cytokines responses classically associated with cell survival and proliferation. In contrast, histamine and H2R ligands inhibit PI3K/Akt signaling in leukemic cell lines. Interestingly, in this cellular model as well as in myeloid cells of most patients with acute myeloid leukemia this signaling pathway is constitutively active resulting in malignant cells survival, chemoresistance, and, in consequence, poor survival prognosis [42–44].

In addition, it has been established that histamine or H2R agonists inhibit, in myeloid cells, the activity of nicotinamide adenine dinucleotide phosphate (NADPH) oxidase which is responsible of the generation of reactive oxygen species (ROS). By inhibiting NADPH action, histamine and H2R ligands were suggested to facilitate survival of antineoplastic lymphocytes and natural killer (NK) cells in acute myeloid leukemia (AML) [45, 46].

As with the rest of the GPCRs, the H2R loses responsiveness after long lasting or repetitive stimulation [47–49]. GRK2 and GRK3 are able to phosphorylate and desensitize the H2R in heterologous expression systems as COS-7 transfected cells [50, 51]. However, in cellular systems that endogenously expresses the H2R, only GRK2 was proved to be responsible for the desensitization of the receptor [52, 53]. The classical desensitization mechanism of GPCRs involves phosphorylation of receptor intracellular domains by GRKs, and recruitment of cytosolic arrestin proteins that uncouple the receptor from heterotrimeric G proteins. In the case of the H2R, after receptor activation, the regulator of G protein signaling (RGS) domain of GRK2 mediates the desensitization of the cAMP response while GRK2-mediated phosphorylation is only responsible for receptor internalization [54]. Although receptor phosphorylation by GRK2 recruits arrestin 3, the lack of receptor coupling to Gs is not due to steric hindrance mediated by arrestin 3 or GRK2 association to the receptor but due to the inactivating action of the RGS domain of GRK2 over Gs protein. After agonist evoked receptor phosphorylation and the recruitment of arrestin 3, the H2R is internalized in clathrin-coated vesicles by the action of dynamin (a GTPase, regulates the pinching off from the cell surface of clathrin-coated pits) dephosphorylated in endosomes and recycled back to the cell surface [55, 56] (Fig. 5).

Until now, some of the most clinically relevant uses of histamine receptor ligands were achieved through the regulation of H2R. The first clinically used H2R antagonist was cimetidine. After that, famotidine, ranitidine, and nizatidine also proved to be very active agents for the treatment of acid-related diseases such as

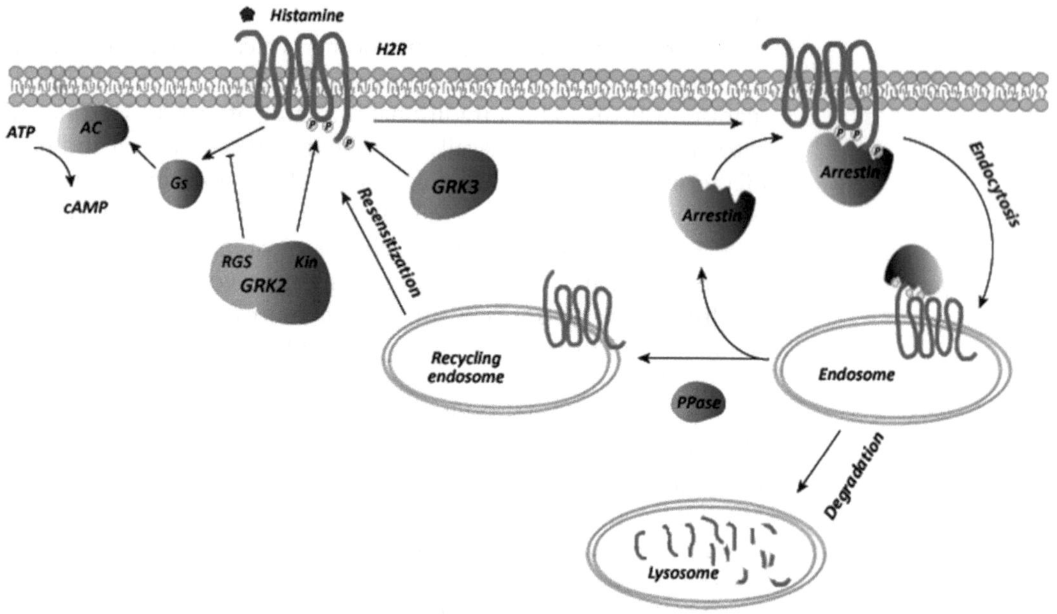

Fig. 5 Histamine H2 receptor (H2R) desensitization, phosphorylation, internalization, and recycling. Upon agonist binding, H2Rs are phosphorylated (P) by GRK2 and 3 leading to the recruitment of β2-arrestins (arrestin-3). β2-Arrestins, target the H2R to clathrin-coated pits-mediated endocytosis which also involves dynamin action. The H2R is then internalized into endosomes and dephosphorylated before returning to the cell surface. Some ligands of H2R lead to receptor degradation into lysosomes

Zollinger–Ellison syndrome, dyspepsia, duodenal and gastric ulcers, reflux and esophagitis. H2R antagonists have an excellent safety profile that supports their common use as over-the-counter medications [57, 58].

Although gastroesophageal reflux disease (GERD) is one of the most common gastrointestinal (GI) disorders and approximately 40% of adults in the USA complain of monthly, 20% of weekly, and approximately 7% of daily heartburn [59], the use of H2R antagonists diminished in the last years due to the launch of antibiotic therapies for Helicobacter infections [60, 61] and the discovery of proton pump inhibitors [62]. In spite of the preference for proton pump inhibitors for the treatment of GERD, current guide lines recommend prescribing H2R antagonists to prevent gastrointestinal ulcers for patients taking nonsteroidal anti-inflammatory drugs (NSAIDs). For example, a fixed-dose combination of NSAID, and the H2R antagonist, famotidine is available for the symptomatic treatment of arthritic symptoms and to reduce the risk of GI ulcers in patients requiring ibuprofen therapy. Interestingly, the use of the combination of these two drugs was shown to reduce the risk of ulcers by 50% when compared with ibuprofen alone [63].

Interestingly, H2R blockers currently used in the clinic, such as cimetidine, famotidine, and ranitidine, behave as inverse agonists regarding cAMP production [32, 64]. However, when other events of the H2R such as desensitization and internalization are evaluated, biased agonism towards these behaviors is observed [38, 39].Two of them, famotidine and ranitidine, even present a biased profile towards activation of the ERK signaling pathway. One of the agents that governs the expression of histidine decarboxylase (HDC), the enzyme responsible of histamine synthesis, is ERK [65, 66]. The positive efficacy displayed by ranitidine and famotidine towards ERK signaling, may lead to the induction of HDC resulting in increased levels of the enzyme and in turn, increased histamine synthesis [39]. This biased behavior of the most commonly used H2R ligands may explain why after withdrawal, these H2R blockers produce rebound acid hypersecretion.

In addition to the classical use of H2R antagonists, H2R ligands have been demonstrated to have therapeutic utility for treating disorders unrelated to acid gastric secretion based on the important role that H2R plays in inflammation and immune related diseases. In this context, H2R ligands have been proposed as promising drugs for the inhibition of neutrophil and eosinophil effector functions since they were proved to inhibit superoxide anion formation by these cell types [67]. Moreover, histamine dihydrochloride (Ceplene1) has been approved for the treatment of patients suffering from acute myeloid leukemia [68] and H2R agonists are being extensively studied as promising drug candidates for the treatment of acute myeloid leukemia and inflammatory diseases [69–73]. Histamine has been typically considered an effector molecule for chronic and immediate hypersensitivity [74]. However, growing evidence suggest that it is a potent modulator of the immune system. At low physiological concentrations histamine can act as an immune-stimulant exerting its action mainly through the H1 receptor (H1R). At higher concentrations, histamine released by basophils, mastocytes, or tumor cells acts as immune-suppressor through H2R, activating suppressor T cells and inhibiting T helper cytokine production [75]. As mentioned above, histamine also inhibits the production of reactive oxygen species (ROS) in isolated monocytes [76] and neutrophils [67, 77] which are known to create a reduced environment that impedes the activation of NK cells the first line defense against tumors [78, 79]. By inhibiting ROS production, H2R ligands allow NK activation having a great impact on clinical cancer immunotherapy [80].

Remarkably, it has been reported that the effect of histamine and H2R ligands on the oxidative burst of granulocytes is not mediated by cAMP accumulation. In contrast, there is substantial evidence for ligand specific conformations of the H2R, showing that dimaprit and impromidine are biased towards ROS inhibition in both neutrophils and eosinophils [67]. These results suggest that H2R biased signaling might be an important concept to consider for the design of clinical treatments. It can be envisaged that the advantages of ligands acting on H2Rs that are biased towards the inhibition of ROS production would allow the immune system to fight cancer.

Several worldwide marketed drugs have been identified in the last years as biased agonists. Although much has been speculated regarding the potential advantages of this pharmacological complexity in GPCRs signaling, until now there are no drugs marketed in base of unique biased therapeutic profiles. However, both wanted and undesired effects should also be interpreted in the light of understanding the pluridimensional efficacy of ligands. In general, biased ligands could surpass on-target undesirable events by avoiding signaling pathways, or increase their efficacy by avoiding or stimulating specific negative or positive feedback loops in their signaling pathways. Cumulative knowledge demonstrates that there is a need for physicians, pharmacists and researchers to understand and continue with the study of biased agonism in order to take advantage of the potential clinical relevance of this phenomenon. In an attempt to contribute in this direction, the aim of the following sections of this chapter is to provide some experimental tools that facilitate the exploration and analysis of the pluridimensional nature of H2R ligands.

2 Methods

2.1 Selection of the Model of Study

2.1.1 General Criteria to Evaluate Bias

The first step to identify agonist bias is to analyze two or more different responses of the receptor to a defined ligand. When one response is plotted as a function of the other, if the amount of signal produced in pathway 1 equals the amount of signal produced in pathway 2 in response to an equimolar concentration of the ligand, a straight line relation is obtained. However, if the ligand "prefers" one of the pathways instead of the other, a higher signal will be obtained for that response and a deviation from the straight line will be observed [24].

That is the general idea of the term "bias" and can be easily visualized in biased plots when response 1 is graphically express as a function of response 2 (Fig. 6). However, deviations from a straight line relationship can be due to different mechanisms where only one of them, referred to as agonist bias, actually reflects the ligand preference for one pathway over the other and can be therapeutically useful.

GPCRs function as multimeric signaling complexes where the stoichiometry of the different components, among other factors, determines the final cellular response after receptor stimulation. Since the composition, and expression levels of the signaling machinery varies among tissues and cellular types, knowledge of the proteomics of the chosen system is important. It is no surprise that the same receptor–ligand pair has a different bias profile if the

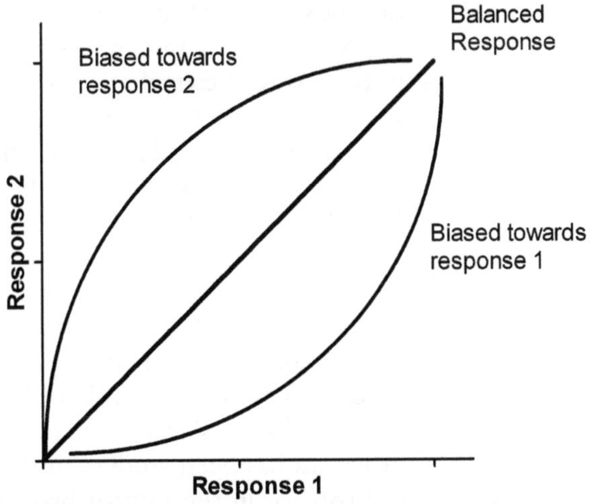

Fig. 6 Bias plot. Responses to ligands in two assay system. The plot shows the Response 1 as a function of the Response 2. The *straight line* indicates that both responses induced by the ligand are equally intense, hence the ligand is balanced. The *curved lines* indicate a bias towards a particular response depicting the bias of the ligand

cellular context is different depending upon the relative efficiency of each different pathways to signal in that context [81]. This type of bias that does not depend on the set of receptor conformations stabilized by the ligand but instead, on the cellular efficiency to signal can be thought as a *system-dependent bias* and can be easily misunderstood as ligand bias.

Another limitation arises when different methodologies are used to evaluate receptor responses. This *observational bias* is a consequence of the arbitrary differences in the potency of ligands due to the relative sensitivity between the assays carried out to quantify ligand responses. Observational bias not only depends on the experimental conditions but also on the temporal distance between the events that are being measured and the intrinsic amplification of the intracellular signals evaluated [20].

A way to remove system and observational bias is by comparing the activity of a set of ligands, for each one of the receptor responses. By expressing the relative activity of a ligand respect to a reference agonist, all the differences in the efficacy of the intracellular signaling as well as in assay sensitivities will be overcome. Based on that, the way to evaluate true ligand bias is in the context of another standard ligand that allows us to assert for example that ligand A is biased towards ERK signaling instead of cAMP in comparison to ligand B, both evaluated in the same system and by using the same methodology.

2.1.2 Homologous Expression Systems

Several cell lines that are commonly used for research studies present endogenous expression of the H2R. However, the selection of the most suitable cell line to evaluate the action of H2R ligands depends on the specific response to be measured.

Some of the more interesting models to study histamine action in the gastrointestinal tract are human gastric carcinoma AGS and KATO III cell lines [39, 82]. H2R expression has been also detected in Caco-2, HT29 and the mucus-producing HT29-MTX, intestinal epithelial cell models [83], as well as in LoVo and in HCT116 colorectal cells [84].

Several cellular systems have been used to evaluate H2R-mediated histamine action in allergy and inflammation related mechanisms. HaCaT keratinocytes and normal human keratinocites predominantly expressed H1R and H2R and can be used as models to evaluate the role of histaminergic ligands in the allergic response of the skin [85]. The action of histamine in lung related processes has been studied in the mice model of 3LL lung tumor cell [86] or in the human bronchial epithelial cell line BEAS-2B, both of which have been proven to express H2R [87].

In MA-10 Leydig tumor cells it has been described that H2R activation leads to both cAMP production and ERK phosphorylation [88]. This could be an interesting model to study the modulation of these two different signaling pathways mediated by H2R histaminergic ligands. MCF-10A and HBL-100 cells derived from nontumorigenic human breast epithelia and MDA-MB-231 and MCF-7 breast tumor cell lines express H2R and have been used to evaluate the protective effects of histamine over radiation treatment and its interaction with other currently approved antineoplastic treatments [33, 89, 90].

Human myeloid U937, THP-1 and HL-60 cells have been described to express significant levels of H2R [73, 91–93]. The action of H2R ligands on proliferation and differentiation processes has been extensively studied [52, 94, 95]. In these models, H2R stimulation increases the intracellular production of cAMP by means of Gs action and leads to rapid receptor desensitization and downregulation [47]. Some studies indicate that besides coupling to Gs, the H2R can signal through Gq-PLC-Ca^{2+} in HL-60 cells [73, 96]. H2R expression has also been described in mouse RAW 264.7 macrophage cells and monocyte J774A.1 cell line. In the latter, the H2R has been described to be downregulated after macrophage differentiation [97, 98].

In addition to these cellular models, interesting results have been obtained from studies carried out in neutrophils and eosinophils as well as in bone marrow-derived mast cells (BMMCs) that can be easily isolated and possess endogenous expression of the H2R [67, 99]. Those systems of the myeloid linage are often used to evaluate the effects of histamine on proliferation, differentiation, and apoptosis as well as to study inflammation related events as free radical formation [48, 67, 100].

Other options to evaluate the action of H2R histaminergic ligands in cells that endogenously express the receptor are: Rat phaeochromocytoma PC12 cells [101]; rat liver BRL-3A cell [102]; human umbilical-vein endothelial cells, HUVEC, and HUVEC derived human endothelial cell line EA.hy 926 [103, 104]; PANC-1 [105] and DU-145 human prostate cancer cells [106].

2.1.3 Heterologous Expression Systems

Human embryonic kidney HEK293 and HEK293T cells represent some of the most popular cell lines for heterologous expression of GPCRs. They are commonly used to express wild-type, truncated, or dominant negative variants of the different components of the transduction machinery of practically any known signaling pathway. They are easily transfected and offer high transfection efficiencies. However, these cells express many endogenous GPCRs, such as the β2-AR which has been described to interact with multiple GPCRs, including the α1B-AR, the adenosine A1R, the angiotensin II AT1R and the δ-opioid receptor, among others [107–109]. On that basis, functional analysis and screening assays performed in these cells will not necessarily yield the same results as tests done in other cellular models. For that reason, it is recommended to confirm the more physiologically relevant results in other cell models where the receptor is endogenously expressed.

As well as HEK293T cells, the COS-7 African green monkey kidney fibroblast-like cell line, is a suitable model for transfection by vectors requiring expression of SV40 T antigen. Both cell lines contain T antigen, and support high plasmid replication and protein expression levels. It has been suggested that COS-7 cells present lower endogenous levels of GRKs and arrestins than HEK293 cells. For this reason, they are not considered a suitable model to study dominant-negative proteins or RNAi but a good choice to study the effect of overexpressing these proteins. Therefore, cells expressing higher levels of these proteins, such as HEK293 or Chinese hamster ovary cells (CHO-K1 cells), are preferred to study the effect of RNAi or dominant negative variants over GRKs or arrestin proteins-mediated receptor internalization. In the case of H2R, both of COS-7 and HEK293 cells have proven to be useful models to evaluate receptor phosphorylation, desensitization, and internalization and the role of GRKs and arrestins in those mechanisms [32, 51, 55, 110].

2.2 Evaluation of G Protein-Dependent Signaling

The first event that occurs after ligand binding to a GPCR is activation of the G protein bound to the receptor and subsequent G protein-mediated signaling. For that reason, a straight forward way to evaluate H2R activation relies in measuring either G protein activation by, for example, GTPγs assays or second messenger production by kinetic or concentration–response assays respectively. Any of them allows discrimination of positive and negative efficacy as well as of neutral antagonism.

2.2.1 GTPγS Binding Assay

GTPγS binding assay allows direct determination of guanine nucleotide exchange (*see* **Note 1**). The replacement of GDP for GTP after G protein activation represents a well established step necessary to elicit downstream signal transduction by G proteins and can be monitored by measuring the amount of [^{35}S]-GTPγS accumulation on membrane fractions [111].

Although classical techniques were not easily applied to determine with good efficiency GDP-GTP exchange in other G proteins distinct from the more abundant Gi type, different strategies have been developed in the last years that allow working with non-Gi-coupled GPCRs. They are mainly based on the previous enrichment of samples by immunoprecipitation with antisera against the G protein of interest [111]. Recent strategies also allow utilization of nonhydrolysable analogs of GTP that are not radioactive such as the europium-labeled GTP analog which can be detected by time-resolved fluorescence (TRF) technology [112].

Beyond these variants, a classical approach involves following the next steps:

1. Prepare crude membrane fractions by harvesting PBS-rinsed monolayers of histamine H2R expressing cells from a 90–100%

confluent 10 cm plate. Lyse the cells with chilled hypotonic (50 mM Tris–HCl, pH 7.4) buffer. Centrifuge at 20,000 × *g* and decant the supernatant (this can be stored at −80 °C until use) and yields 24 wells.

2. Resuspend membrane fractions in assay buffer (50 mM HEPES, 5 mM $MgCl_2$, 150 mM NaCl, 0.2 mM EDTA, 100 mg/L ascorbic acid, pH 7.4) containing 20 μM GDP and [^{35}S] GTPγS (300 pM).
3. Distribute the suspension into 1.5 mL collecting tubes and add equal volumes of the ligand in 2× concentration. Incubate for 90 min at room temperature and then separate bound from free fraction by filtration through glass fiber filters.
4. Soak the filters in liquid scintillation cocktail and quantify beta emission in a liquid scintillation counter. Determine nonspecific binding at the maximum concentration of ligand in presence of 10 μM of a suitable antagonist. Background signal is determined in the presence of 10 μM unlabeled GTPγS.
5. Plot total [^{35}S]-GTP binding as a function of the logarithm of the molar concentration of the ligand. Perform a nonlinear regression curve in Prism (Graph Pad Software) or similar using a concentration response model.

2.2.2 Determination of cAMP Production

Since in the great majority of cellular systems the H2R is coupled to the Gs protein, the effect of H2R ligands can be easily evaluated by measuring cAMP production in kinetic or concentration–response assays. To avoid the natural degradation of cAMP to 5′AMP, phosphodiesterase (PDEs) activity should be blocked by pre-incubation of the cells with isobutyl methyl xanthine (IBMX) a general PDEs inhibitor previous to receptor stimulation. For PDE4 expressing cell lines, the more specific PDE4 inhibitor, rolipram, can also be used.

In some cases, relevant information can be obtained from measuring the amount of cAMP that results from the production–degradation balance which may account for the physiological downstream effects of cAMP. In those cases, kinetic experiments without IBMX may be preferred where the response to a fixed concentration of the ligand is measured after different end points. A theoretical example of kinetic experiment with and without IBMX and a concentration–response assay are shown in Fig. 7.

A general protocol to evaluate cAMP production in response to different concentrations of an H2R ligand, in adherent cells, is described below (*see* **Note 2**).

1. Receptor expressing cells are seeded in, at least 10 wells of a 48-well plate in 400 μL of culture medium to achieve 90–100% confluence the next day. Taking into account the number of parameters that are estimated in a sigmoidal curve, the minimum number of concentrations to be evaluated is five.

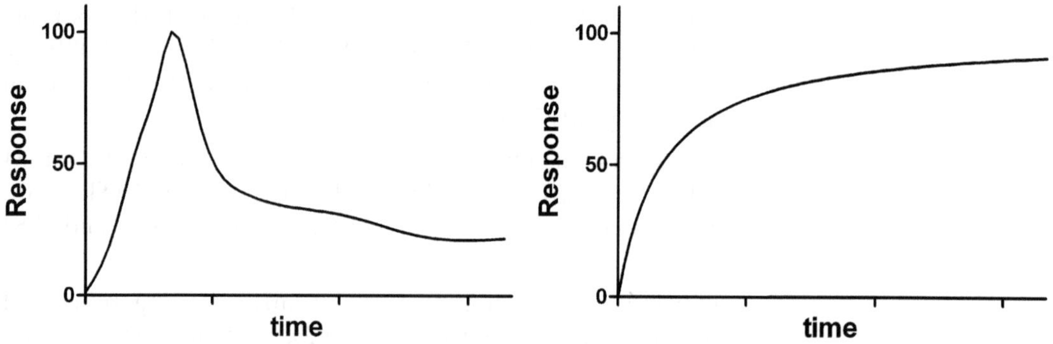

Fig. 7 cAMP production as a function of time. *Left panel* shows a kinetic experiment in the absence of PDEs inhibitor (for example IBMX) where cAMP levels reflect the balance between production and degradation. *Right panel* shows the same assay performed after pretreatment of cells with PDEs inhibitor. In this case the levels of cAMP quantified correspond to cAMP accumulation

2. On the day of the assay, media should be replaced by 100 μL of assay medium (minimal culture medium) and cells pre-incubated for 30 min at 37 °C.
3. Cells are pre-treated for 3 min with 50 μL of a 3× solution of IBMX prepared in the assay media.
4. Cells are then stimulated by addition of 150 μL of 1× dilution of IBMX and 2× solution of ligand (with a final concentration of ligand ranging from 0.1 nM to 10 or 100 μM in duplicate). It is also recommended to include as positive control a stimulus with 25–100 μM forskolin and a basal (vehicle without ligand) condition.
5. After 10–15 min, cAMP accumulation is stopped by removing the media and lysing the cells.

   At this point, the mechanism of lysis depends on the technique used for detection and quantification of cAMP. This is usually performed with competitive radiometric assays using [^{3}H] labeled cAMP [113] or [^{125}I] labeled cAMP (Perkin Elmer, USA) where the cellular cAMP present in the samples competes with the labeled form of cAMP for binding to an acceptor protein for instance an anti-cAMP antibody or purified PKA.

   More recently, these assays have been replaced with nonradioactive fluorescence or luminescence-based assays such as the HitHunter™ (DiscoveRx, USA) and AlphaScreen™ (Perkin Elmer, USA), CatchPoint cAMP assay (Molecular Devices, USA). Fluorescence polarization (FP)-based cAMP kits are also available from Molecular Devices (USA), GE Healthcare (USA) and Perkin Elmer (USA) [23].
6. Plot the amount of cAMP quantified for each concentration. This can be normalized to the basal cAMP amount as

appropriate and plotted as a function of the logarithmic molar concentration of the ligand.

Perform a nonlinear regression curve in Prism (GraphPad Software) or similar, using a concentration–response model and obtain the maximal response (*Top*) and the effective concentration 50% (*EC50*) values.

2.2.3 Determination of IPs and Ca^{2+} Released

The concept of functional selectivity can be applied to the specificity of coupling to G proteins. Evidence obtained from different systems has shown that the H2R can couple to Gs or Gq proteins [96]. Based on these observations, it may happen that two related ligands of the H2R exhibit different efficacies for these two downstream signaling pathways. For example, one agonist might preferentially activate Gs whereas the second might signal through Gq.

Activation of Gq pathway leads to PLC-mediated hydrolysis of phosphatidylinositol bisphosphate (PIP2) to form the second messengers, diacylglycerol (DAG) and IP3. IP3 activates calcium channels of the endoplasmic reticulum (ER) leading to efflux of Ca^{2+} to the cytoplasm and elevation of intracellular Ca^{2+} levels. By a series of enzymatic reactions, IP3 is rapidly hydrolyzed to IP2, IP1 and inositol. Both Ca^{2+} and DAG in turn activate protein kinase C (PKC) which phosphorylates downstream substrates [114]. To evaluate activation of this signaling cascade, IP3 accumulation (*see* **Note 3**) or intracellular Ca^{2+} increase (*see* **Note 4**) could be measured as follows.

Quantification of inositol phosphates

1. Receptor expressing cells are cultured in 24-well plates to 80% confluency.
2. To label the phosphatidylinositol of the cell membrane, the day before the assay, cells are incubated overnight in 400 μL culture medium without calf serum and supplemented with 2 μCi/mL myo-[^{3}H]-inositol.
3. Cells are washed and incubated for 20 min at 37 °C with 300 μL culture medium without calf serum, containing 20 mM LiCl to inhibit the degradation of IPs.
4. 50 μL of medium, containing 20 mM LiCl and the respective ligands in 7× concentration is added to the cells and incubation is carried out for 20 min at 37 °C. Each compound should be tested in duplicate. In addition to the tested ligand, points for determination of basal activity and maximal agonist stimulation as positive control should be included for activity calculations.
5. To stop the reaction, the medium is aspirated and IPs are extracted by the addition of 900 μL of cold chloroform, methanol, 0.12 M HCl (1:2:1 v/v, freshly prepared). Phases are

separated by the addition of 300 μL of water and 300 μL of chloroform.

6. The mixture is then centrifuged at 1500 × *g* for 15 min at 4 °C, and the aqueous phase is removed.
7. Total water-soluble inositol phosphate fraction is purified by anion exchange chromatography. Dowex AG-X8 column should be previously resuspended in 0.1 M formic acid solution and equilibrated with buffer Tris–Formic 10 mM, pH 7.4.
8. The elution scheme is as follows: 10 mL of myo-inositol 5 mM to elude the radioactive [^{3}H]-myo-inositol incorporated to cells but not to PIP2; 5 mL of water to wash the column and 10 mL of ammonium formate 1 M in formic acid 0.1 M, to elute total [^{3}H]-IPs, which are collected in 1 mL fractions in vials with scintillation cocktail.
9. The eluted fractions are collected and radioactivity measured in a liquid scintillation counter.
10. The activity of each ligand may be calculated as the percent of maximal activity (obtained with the maximal concentrations of the agonist control) and for antagonist as the percent of inhibition of receptor activity (in presence of an *EC50* concentration of the agonist). Alternatively, ligand activity may be normalized to total [^{3}H]-inositol radioactivity recovered from the initial water wash of the columns.

Ca2+ measurement

1. Cells are cultured in 96-well dishes to 100% confluence in culture medium.
2. The medium is aspirated and cells are loaded with 50 μL/well of calcium buffer (2 mM $CaCl_2$, 145 mM NaCl, 10 mM glucose, 5 mM KCl, 1 mM $MgSO_4$, and 10 mM HEPES, pH 7.4) containing 0.5 μL/well of the fluorescent Ca^{2+} indicator, fura-2 acetoxymethyl ester (fura-2 AM) and then incubated for 90 min at 37 °C to facilitate the uptake and hydrolysis of the ester to the acid form.
3. Excess dye is removed by aspiration and washing with calcium buffer without fura-2 AM. At this point it is recommended to incubate the cells with the fresh buffer for 10 min at 37 °C before replacement of the washing calcium buffer with 100 μL of fresh buffer for posterior fluorescence reading.
4. For measuring, excitation wavelengths are set at 340/380 nm and detection at 500 nm in a FlexStation 3 Multi-Mode Microplate Reader (Molecular Devices, USA). Basal fluorescence is measured for 10 s, then 25 μL of the test ligand or reference compound in 5× concentration are added to the wells and fluorescence recorded for 120 s (each ligand concentration is assayed in triplicate).

5. At the end of the time-course, $CaCl_2$ (20 mM) followed by Triton X-100 (0.25% v/v) is added to determine the maximal fluorescence (*Fmax*) followed by EGTA (6.25 mM, pH 8.6) to determine the minimal fluorescence (*Fmin*). Using these values intracellular Ca^{2+} concentrations are calculated as described by Grynkiewicz [115].
6. Results may be calculated as the percent of the maximal response of the system (considered as 100%), measured in the presence of 20 mM $CaCl_2$, 0.25% Triton X-100 where baseline or 0% is considered as the calcium levels determined in the first 20 s of recording. For concentration response assays, raw data (fluorescence units) for each concentration of ligand or reference agonist may be normalized to the baseline fluorescence (reported as fold increase over basal) and plotted as a function of the logarithm of the molar concentration of the ligand. A nonlinear regression curve may be plotted using Prism (GraphPad Software) or similar, using a concentration–response model and the maximal response and the *EC50* values are obtained.

2.3 Receptor Desensitization

The ability of ligands to induce receptor desensitization is a therapeutically relevant drug property that has been shown to be functionally heterogeneous and to closely depend on the ligand that binds to the receptor. Since receptor desensitization represents an adaptive mechanism of turning off receptor signaling to avoid system overstimulation, it was originally thought to only take place after treatment with receptor activating ligands (agonists). However, more recent findings proved that H2R desensitization can also occur as a consequence of antagonist or even inverse agonist treatment [38].

The more widely accepted definition of receptor desensitization is the loss of receptor responsiveness after repetitive or long term exposure to the ligand. Based on that, a useful way to measure receptor desensitization is to perform a desensitization kinetic assay. This consists of evaluating the remaining capability of the receptor to evoke second messenger accumulation in response to an agonist after being challenged for different periods of time with a ligand (which may be the same agonist or not). A general protocol is the following (*see* **Note 5**).

1. Receptor expressing cells are seeded in 48-well plate in 400 μL of culture medium the day before the assay. Four wells should be plated for each time point of pretreatment with the ligand. Two wells are used to evaluate basal cAMP levels and the other two to determine cAMP stimulated levels for each one of the specific pretreatment times. For example, if you are measuring the receptor response after 0; 0.5; 3; 10; 30; 60; 90; 120 min of pretreatment with a particular ligand, then 32 wells should be plated.

2. On the day of the assay, media should be replaced by 100 μL of assay medium (minimal culture medium) and cells pre-incubated for 30 min at 37 °C.
3. Cells are pretreated by addition of 50 μL of a 3× solution of the desensitizing stimulus beginning from the longer time periods to the shorter ones in order to wash all the wells of plate at the same time. For pretreatment of the cells IBMX should not be used.
4. Cells are then washed three times with room temperature PBS and resuspended in fresh medium containing 1 mM IBMX, incubated for 3 min, and exposed to 10 μM amthamine (or 100 μM histamine) for 10 min to determine whether the system is able to generate a cAMP response.
5. After 10–15 min, cAMP accumulation is stopped by removing the media and lysing of the cells depending upon the protocol of choice for determination of cAMP.
6. Stimulated and basal raw data can be plotted as a function of time. Alternatively, stimulated cAMP levels can be standardized over basal cAMP levels for each time of pretreatment or expressed as stimulus minus basal cAMP levels as a function of time. A representative plot is shown in Fig. 8.

If the ability of the system to recover the capability of response is going to be evaluated, after washing the desensitizing stimulus cells should be incubated in fresh medium for 60–90 min and then the cAMP response to the agonist should be evaluated at different time-points.

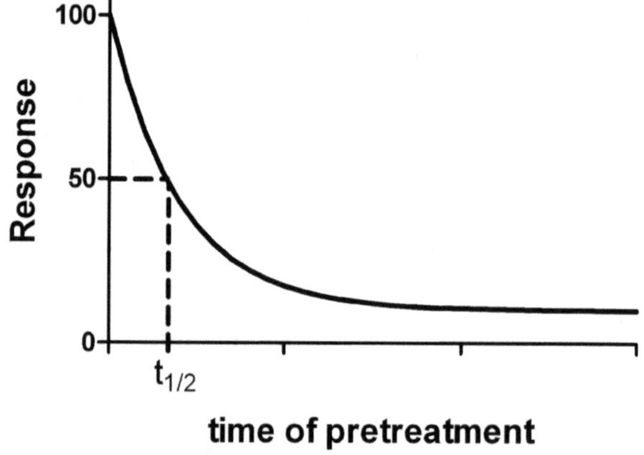

Fig. 8 Desensitization kinetic. The exponential decay curve reflects the fade in cAMP production after pretreatment of the cells with the H2R ligand. The desensitization phenomenon implies the loss of system responsiveness

2.4 Receptor Phosphorylation

In the canonical model of GPCR desensitization, agonist-induced activation leads to receptor phosphorylation by second messenger-dependent kinases and/or specific GRKs [116]. In turn, GRK-mediated phosphorylation facilitates the binding of the third intracellular loop and the carboxyl-terminal tail of the receptor to arrestins, which physically uncouple the receptor from the G protein.

It is well established that receptor phosphorylation by GRKs is dependent on the 3-dimensional shape of the receptor. GRKs recognize the ligand–bound conformation of GPCRs and solely phosphorylate those receptors that have been stimulated [117]. Where traditional agonists are thought to lead to the whole range of signaling events of a receptor, it is hypothesized for biased agonists that they stabilize a partial or limited regional shift in the shape of GPCRs. If this is the case, it is not difficult to imagine that a ligand, even a traditional antagonist, could stabilize a conformational state of the receptor that allows recognition by GRKs and subsequent phosphorylation, arrestins recruitment and receptor internalization without activation of signaling by G proteins. In this scenario, receptor phosphorylation, which was originally thought as part of the desensitization process, can be considered a biased response since it results in a change in the basal distribution of the receptor states. Moreover, advances in the research about other GPCRs demonstrate that different arrangements of GRKs may phosphorylate a receptor depending of the ligand that binds the receptor [118–120]. In addition, the conformation stabilized by different ligands may expose a particular array of serine and threonine residues that may be phosphorylated. These events could potentially lead to a unique pattern of phosphorylation that occurs depending on the ligand (even for an antagonist) where the phosphorylation barcode, encoded by the selective recruitment of kinases and the exposure of specific residues would yield unique downstream signaling consequences [121].

Evaluation of GPCR phosphorylation is not an easy task (*see* **Note 6**). This is mainly due to the lack of good commercial antibodies directed against GPCRs that allow specific and high yielding receptor immunoprecipitation. For that reason the following procedure outlines the use of receptors tagged with epitopes having good quality commercial antibodies for immunoprecipitation as myc, flag, hemagglutinin, 6-histidine, etc.

1. Receptor expressing cells are cultured in 100 mm dishes to 100% confluence.
2. On the day of the assay cells are pre-incubated forl h at 37 °C in phosphate-free medium, and labeled for 3 h with 100 μCi/mL of ^{32}Pi at 37 °C in fresh medium.
3. Cells are then treated with maximal concentration of the ligand for 5–30 min.

4. Stimulus is removed by two washings with ice cold PBS and cells lysed in ice with 0.5 mL immunoprecipitation buffer containing proteases and phosphatases inhibitors (150 mM NaCl, 50 mM Tris–HCl, pH 8, 1% Nonidet P-40, 0.1% SDS, 0.2 mM EDTA, 10 mM FNa, 1 mM sodium vanadate, 1 mM phenylmethylsulfonyl fluoride, 5 μM aprotinin, 10 μM leupeptin, and 5 μM pepstatin).
5. With the help of a scraper, cells are completely lysed and total volume is collected in 1.5 mL tubes.
6. Samples are incubated 30 min at 4 °C with rotation and then centrifuged at 12,000 × *g* during 30 min at 4 °C.
7. For preclearing, supernatants are incubated in rotation with A/G agarose beads during 1 h at 4 °C. After that samples are centrifuged for 3 min at 1000 × *g*.
8. Supernatants are incubated in rotation at 4 °C, overnight with 1 μg of specific antibody.
9. Protein A/G agarose beads are added to samples and incubated 3 h with rotation at 4 °C, then centrifuged at 12,000 × *g* for 30 min at 4 °C.
10. Pellets are washed three times with immunoprecipitation buffer and resuspended in approximately 40 μL of Laemmly sample buffer.
11. Complexes are dissociated by heating at 65 °C for 10 min in sample buffer and separated by 12% SDS-polyacrylamide gel electrophoresis. Gels are dried and ^{32}P label detected by autoradiography.

2.5 Receptor Internalization

It is well known that in addition to uncoupling from G proteins, arrestin binding to the receptor targets the phosphorylated GPCR to clathrin-coated pits and initiates receptor internalization. This process is mediated by the interaction of the carboxyl-terminal of arrestin with both the clathrin heavy chain and the 2-adaptin subunit of AP-2 complex [122]. After pinching off the vesicles from plasma membrane by dynamin [123], the receptors are sequestered into endosomes [124] where they may be dephosphorylated and recycled to the cell surface or retained in the endosomal compartment and targeted to lysosomes for degradation (down-regulation) [122, 125].

H2R internalization was first reported in HEK293 cells where the authors showed that histamine treatment induces loss of H2R membrane immunoreactivity [56]. Further studies in several cellular models showed that agonist promoted H2R internalization is crucial for the rapid recovery of H2R-mediated cAMP response, where β2-arrestin, dynamin, and clathrin are involved in both the internalization and resensitization of the H2R [55]. Surprisingly, treatment of H2R with cimetidine, famotidine, ranitidine, and tiotidine inverse agonists also leads to receptor endocytosis. However, the internalization promoted by these ligands differs from the internalization promoted by agonists. While amthamine-induced receptor internalization requires GRK2-mediated phosphorylation, inverse agonists promoted endocytosis is not inhibited in presence of kinase inactive dominant negative mutant of GRK2. Moreover, receptor endocytosis promoted by inverse agonists seems to lead to receptor downregulation instead of receptor recycling [38, 39].

There are several ways to evaluate the internalization of receptors. Fluorophore-labeled specific ligands as well as traditional radioligands can be used to visualize internalization of GPCRs. Other techniques involve the use of amino terminal tagged receptors or the use of specific antibodies against the extracellular loops or amino terminal portion of the receptor in order to follow cellular trafficking. Here, the traditional radioligand binding assay to quantify receptor internalization will be described (*see* **Note** 7).

1. Receptor expressing cells are seeded in 96-well plate in 200 μL of culture medium the day before the assay. For each time of internalization 24 wells should be plated. Six of them are used to evaluate nonspecific binding and the other 18 to determine, in duplicate, the specific binding for each one of the nine amounts of [^{3}H]-tiotidine radioligand used.
2. On the day of the assay, media should be replaced by 100 μL of assay medium (minimal culture medium) and cells preincubated for 30 min at 37 °C.
3. H2R expressing cells are pretreated for 1 h with maximal concentration (10–100 μM) of the ligand (agonists, antagonist or inverse agonists to be evaluated as promoters of receptor internalization).
4. Cells are then washed three times with room temperature PBS and 25 μL of binding buffer is added to each well. At this point, 25 μL of a 1 μM unlabeled tiotidine solution is added to the 6 wells for measuring unspecific binding.
5. 25 μL of each of the nine 2× solutions of [^{3}H]-tiotidine ranging from 0.4 to 240 nM is added to the rest of the wells. Cells are incubated at 4 °C for 40 min.
6. Incubation is stopped by washing three times with chilled 50 mM Tris/HCl (pH 7.4) and the bound fraction is collected in 200 μL of ethanol.
7. Ethanol fractions are transferred to vials containing liquid scintillation cocktail and beta emission is quantified in a liquid scintillation counter. Nonspecific binding curve is obtained from fitting of raw data from wells containing unlabeled tiotidine.

8. Plot specific bound [^{3}H]-tiotidine as a function of free [^{3}H]-tiotidine (this is obtained after subtraction of nonspecific binding). Perform a nonlinear regression fit in Prism (Graph Pad Software) or similar using a hyperbolic saturation binding model. Obtain *Bmax* and *Kd* values.

2.6 Receptor Dimerization

It has been described that many, if not all, GPCRs interact in the plasma membrane to form dimers or even higher order oligomers. However, the functional role of receptor self-association in most cases is unclear. While a single receptor molecule in active conformation is sufficient to activate G proteins, there is a wide range of other receptor functions (that are often overlooked) in which GPCR dimerization could play a role. In all cases, dimerization does not seem to be required for functional coupling of the GPCR to heterotrimeric G-protein [126, 127], but mainly for its intracellular trafficking (cell membrane targeting of newly synthesized receptors and processing of the activated receptors by arrestins and adaptor proteins prior to endocytosis [128, 129].

In the case of histamine receptors, it has been proven that H1R and H2R can exist as heterodimers, cross-desensitize and co-internalize upon ligand stimulation [100]. Although receptor dimerization is not detected at basal conditions, there is a strong interaction between these subtypes of histamine receptors when agonist-induced receptor co-internalization occurs. Based on that, H1R-H2R heterodimerization does not seem to be involved in receptor maturation or transport to the cell surface but it may play a role in the regulation of trafficking and/or signaling within the cells after receptors are activated and co-internalized [100].

GPCR high order organization may lead to distinct signaling properties and then, compounds that target receptor dimer/oligomers may have the potential to achieve specific therapeutic effects. This line of reasoning boosted techniques aiming to detect and confirm the existence and the functional relevance of receptor complexes. These include energy transfer approaches as fluorescence resonance energy transfer (FRET) and bioluminescence resonance energy transfer (BRET) and more conventional biochemical methodologies such as co-immunoprecipation followed by gel electrophoresis. A survey of these methods will be provided, with special emphasis on FRET methodology as this was used to identify histamine receptor heterodimerization [100].

2.6.1 Co-immunoprecipitation

With co-immunoprecipitation, it is intended to analyze the physical interaction between two receptors, or, more general, two proteins. This technique uses specific antibodies against one receptor, that are able to immunoprecipitate it, and then followed by probing for the other receptor. Cells are disrupted and the antibody-bound receptor is pulled out of the sample using affinity beads by centrifugation or magnetic attraction. The unbound proteins are washed away and the receptor–antibody complex is then resolved by SDS-PAGE for western blot analysis. Proteins are then transferred from the gel to a nitrocellulose membrane. An antibody against the second dimerizing receptor is used to visualize this receptor, supporting the hypothesis that this receptor is associated, and co-immunoprecipitated. Receptors can be native or differentially tagged if no available antibodies for native receptors are available.

Results can be questionable due to the required solubilization step with detergents which can result in artificial aggregation due to the highly hydrophobic nature of GPCRs. Different approaches have been utilized to overcome this issue. The demonstration that complexes are obtained only upon co-expression of receptors within the same cell and not merely upon mixing of cells individually expressing each receptor, or the use of an additional GPCR (as a negative control) to demonstrate the specificity of the receptor–receptor interaction. Also, the probability of artificial aggregation may be diminished by using different combinations of detergents or reducing conditions. Hence, under specific control of experimental conditions, co-immunoprecipitation is a valuable tool to study GPCR oligomerization (*see* **Note 8**).

2.6.2 FRET and BRET

In order to assess receptor–receptor interactions on the membrane of living or fixed cells, this microscopic technique is based on the principle that a chromophore can transfer energy to another chromophore by resonance (in a nonradiative manner) if they are close enough to each other. One chromophore (donor, e.g. cyan fluorescent protein, CFP) in its excitation state transfers energy when the second chromophore (acceptor, e.g. yellow fluorescent protein, YFP) is in its close proximity [130]. In case of BRET, the donor molecule can be an enzyme which causes energy to be released upon oxidation of a suitable substrate. The distance between the protomers must be 10–100 Å, which can be calculated by the energy transfer efficiency. Consequently, the donor's emission intensity reduces while the acceptor fluorescence increases. The excitation spectrum of the acceptor must overlap the emission spectrum of the donor [130].

Both FRET and BRET have several limitations (*see* **Note 9**). The efficiency of energy transfer depends on the relative orientation of the donor and acceptor moieties and the distance between them, so that absolute distances cannot be measured. Detection of an energy transfer signal indicates that the distance between fluorescent moieties is smaller than 50–60 Å. The size of 27 kDa fluorescent proteins and 34 kDa luciferase is comparable to that of the transmembrane core of GPCRs, possessing a diameter of approximately 40 Å. These proteins are usually attached to the receptor C-terminus, which in different GPCR subtypes varies in length from 25 to 150 amino acids, and then, polypeptides of this length in extended conformation can cover 80–480 Å. Thus, a FRET or BRET signal indicates that two fluorescent tags are within 60 Å of each other, which may occur when receptors form a true dimer or when they are >500 Å apart. Moreover, quantitative FRET and BRET measurements are limited by the quality of the signal and noise level. However, BRET techniques do not require a conventional light source to initiate energy transfer, thus having an improved signal-to-noise ratio. Fluorescent proteins yield background signals arising from incompletely processed proteins inside the cell and high cell autofluorescence in the spectral region used. Proper interpretation of energy transfer data requires quantitative analysis of signal dependence on the donor:acceptor ratio at different levels of receptor expression, estimation of labeling efficiency and possible contribution of unlabeled receptors, including endogenously expressed GPCRs with which labeled receptors may heterodimerize [131].

Below, a typical FRET assay to quantify receptor–receptor interaction by confocal microscopy is described.

1. HEK293T cells, grown to 80–90% confluency in p35 glass-bottom dishes (MatTek, Ashland, USA), are transfected with plasmids coding to H2R-yellow fluorescent protein (-YFP) and H1R-cyan fluorescent protein (-CFP) using LipofectAmine 2000 reagent (Invitrogen™) or similar according to manufacturer's instructions.
2. 48 h later, cells are serum-starved for 2 h and then stimulated with 10 μM of the H1R or H2R ligands.
3. Live cell imaging can be performed using a LSM 700 Zeiss confocal laser-scanning microscope with a Plan-Apochromat 63 Å 1.40 NA oil immersion objective (or similar) and incubation at 37 °C and 5% CO_2.
4. Images are acquired every 1–2 min over a period of 30 min. Excitation and filters should be set according to the donor and acceptor spectra (typically as follows: for CFP, 445 nm excitation, band-pass (BP) 460–500 nm emission; for YFP, 488 nm excitation, BP 520–600 nm emission.
5. The image and statistical analysis can be performed with the ImageJ software Colocalization Analysis plugin (NIH, Bethesda, MD, USA). To normalize FRET, the background given by the images from nontransfected cells is subtracted from the images from transfected cells, and the resulting images were processed. The plugin calculates the bleed-through of the pair of fluorophores as constant values and subtracts them from the raw FRET channel image [132]. This method reduces the interference of the user to a minimum by analyzing the entire image, pixel by pixel, and displays FRET images as a function of the colocalization of the two fluorescent partners.

2.7 Evaluation of G Protein-Independent Signaling

Increasing evidence indicates that GPCRs can transmit information to cells by mechanisms that do not require activation of heterotrimeric G proteins. β-arrestin proteins play a crucial role not only for desensitizing and internalizing GPCRs but also as mediator of GPCRs signaling within the cell. Since β-arrestin-mediated signaling has different physiological consequences from signaling mediated by G proteins, these processes are being extensively investigated and they promise to yield therapeutically relevant applications [133]. G protein-independent signaling is mainly focused on co-localization assays of GPCRs and β-arrestin or translocation studies as well as on the analysis of G protein-independent signaling cascades.

2.7.1 β-Arrestin Recruitment

β-Arrestin binding to the receptor has the capacity to function as an adaptor protein and signal through multiple mediators, in addition to mediating GPCR uncoupling from heterotrimeric G protein and receptor desensitization and internalization. However, it is still unclear whether the receptor conformation that leads to receptor desensitization is the same to that which mediates β-arrestin recruitment and signaling (*see* **Note 10**).

Although there is evidence supporting β-arrestin participation in H2R internalization and recycling there is no direct evidence of β-arrestin recruitment by the H2R. Recruitment of β-arrestin can be studied by evaluating the intracellular redistribution of diffused GFP-tagged β-arrestin from the cytosol to the plasma membrane or to coated vesicles by imaging techniques. For this purpose, many imaging-based β-arrestin recruitment assays have been commercialized [134]. As for any other imaging-based assays, it is advisable to use a cell type that presents good adherence properties and a large cytoplasm-to-nucleus ratio (for example HeLa cells). This will ensure high quality images suitable for further analysis.

Alternatively, β-arrestin recruitment can be studied by BRET. This kind of study attempts to evaluate interaction between two proteins and relies on the same theoretical basis as FRET studies. The receptor contains a C-terminus fluorescent protein tag (such as eGFP2, GFP10, or YFP) and β-arrestin is tagged with a Renilla luciferase (RLuc) or vice versa. When the two proteins come into close proximity the light emitted from the RLuc reaction excites the GFP, which then emits a detectable signal at a higher wavelength. BRET signal is then calculated as the ratio of the two emissions (GFP/RLuc) and gives information about the interaction between the tagged molecules [135]. Similar non-image based assays, as PathHunter™ technology (DiscoveRx) and the TangoTM assay (Invitrogen), are commercially available [136–138].

2.7.2 Activation of G Protein-Independent Signaling Cascades

As mentioned before, β-arrestins have been shown to act as scaffolds for numerous signaling pathways such as MAPK, Src, NF-κB, and PI3K or even for EGFR transactivation [139]. The signaling cascades mediated by G proteins and β-arrestins proved to be independent for many receptors, including the histamine H2R, and may be selectively modulated. β-Arrestin-mediated signaling represents one of the most relevant events to analyze biased agonism. An understanding of this may help to eliminate undesired side effects of histamine receptor modulation by selectively activating some signaling pathways and not others.

In this context, H2R inverse agonists that are widely used as blockers of histamine stimulated gastric acid secretion have the surprising effect of mimicking some histamine effects. In addition to leading to receptor desensitization and internalization, these ligands also increase ERK phosphorylation. In gastric cell lines, there is a strong link between ERK activation and induction of HDC, the enzyme responsible of histamine synthesis. Several agents that increase ERK phosphorylation cause upregulation of HDC [65, 66]. Interestingly, famotidine and ranitidine are more efficacious than the H2R agonist, amthamine, at activating ERK [38, 39]. These observations, as well as the H2R upregulation after prolonged H2R blockade [64] may explain some of the undesired effects that are commonly observed after withdrawal of H2R blockers as rebound gastric acid hypersecretion [140].

The easier way to study the activation of these signaling pathways is to evaluate the amount of phosphorylated versions of the components of G protein-independent signaling cascades, for instance, ERK, p38, JUNK, Akt, among others. This can be done by western blot analysis following standard protocols (*see* **Note 11**).

2.8 Evaluation of Gene Expression

Modulation of second messenger levels after GPCRs activation may alter gene transcription or cellular events coupled to gene expression. Several lines of evidence demonstrate that some of the effects of histamine that are mediated by the H2R involve regulation at the transcriptional level.

One of the first pieces of evidence regarding H2R-mediated regulation of gene expression was obtained from peripheral blood mononuclear cells where histamine treatment, through activation of the H2R, suppressed the expression of the tumor necrosis factor α (TNF-α). It has also been described that histamine and the H2R agonist, dimaprit, increase c-fos expression at the transcriptional and translational levels in the human promonocytic U937 cell line [95]. Lectin-like oxidized low-density lipoprotein receptor-1 (LOX-1) is a member of the scavenger receptor family that is expressed in monocytes/macrophages and its expression is via the H2R in human monocytic THP-1 cells [93]. The expression levels of several cytokines are also modulated by histamine acting, at least partially, through the H2R [141, 142]. Most of the modulations of gene expression exerted by histamine in these cellular models of the myeloid lineage were proved to depend on the stimulation of cAMP production after H2R activation.

In melanoma cell lines, by means of H2R activation, histamine and related ligands modulate the expression of proteins involved in melanogenesis. It has been described that histamine stimulates v-ets erythroblastosis virus E26 oncogene homolog 1 (Ets-1) synthesis which is involved in the regulation of melanoma growth [143]. In the same way, the expression of growth-differentiation factor-15, a protein belonging to transforming growth factor beta which has a relevant role in melanogenesis is induced by histamine-mediated activation of the H2R. Interestingly, through induction of growth-differentiation factor-15, the H2R also modulates the expression of other proteins as melanin, tyrosinase, tyrosinase-related protein 1, and tyrosinase-related protein 2 [144].

Based on these observations, analysis of the regulation of gene expression allows the elucidation of long term effects of H2R signaling. In this scenario, reporter gene assays or quantitative PCR provide popular and cost-effective platforms to evaluate the action of histamine H2R ligands.

2.8.1 Gene Reporter Assays

The histamine H2R ligands, by modulating cAMP production and MAPK pathways may regulate the cAMP response element (CRE), the nuclear factor of activated T-cells response element (NFAT-RE), the serum response element (SRE) and the serum response factor response element (SRF-RE) among others. Therefore, cell-base gene reporter assay, using some of these regulatory sequences, will provide an interesting tool to measure the histamine H2R response (*see* **Note 12**). Gene reporter constructs usually contain a reporter enzyme that is under the control of the responsive element of interest cloned upstream a minimal promoter. Reporter enzymes commonly used are luciferase, β-galactosidase, β-lactamase, alkaline phosphatase, among others. The response to ligand treatment could be easily measured by evaluating the activity of these enzymes by luminescent, colorimetric or fluorescent detection.

One of the most commonly used reporter genes is the luciferase gene from the firefly *Photinus pyralis*. This gene encodes a 61 kDa enzyme that oxidizes D-luciferin in the presence of ATP, oxygen, and Mg^{2+} to a product that can be easily quantified by measuring the emitted light. A general luciferase reporter assay is described below.

1. Cells seeded on 12-well plates are transfected following the manufacturer's instructions with the reporter plasmid containing luciferase coding sequence under the transcriptional control of the responsive element of interest (for example CRE, SRE) and, if necessary, a plasmid coding for the H2R.
2. 24 h later, transfected cells are harvested and seeded in 96-well plates. Cells are starved for 2 h and stimulated with the ligands of interest.

3. After 6–48 h part of the medium is removed and cells are lysed by adding equal amount of the luciferase reagent (a detergent-containing buffer plus the luciferase substrate) to the remaining culture medium (typically 50 μl).
4. Luminescence should be measured within a certain time-range, depending on the commercial kit used. For this purpose the content of the well is transferred to a white plate and luminescence determined in a single point or kinetic measurement.
5. Reporter activity is normalized to control activity. The accuracy of the data obtained is improved by using a second constitutively expressed Renilla luciferase, which removes false positives due to cell death from compound toxicity and normalizes well-to-well variations differentiating genetic responses of interest from nonrelevant influences in the experimental system. The Dual-Luciferase® Reporter (DLR™) Assay and Dual-Glo™ Assay from Promega Biosciences Inc. enable the sequential measurement of both firefly and Renilla luciferases from one sample.
6. Raw data is expressed as Relative Light Units (RLUs) which do not represent an absolute value. This is because the current output by the photomultiplier tube measured by typical luminometers cannot be translated into photons, unlike photon-counter instruments. Results can be normalized to total protein content, total ATP content, total cell content or to a control vector reporter. The most used normalization methods are the first and the last one, with the total protein content typically used to remove variability due to cell number in stable transfected cells and the control vector reporter for transfection efficiency variations in transiently transfected cells. Each sample is normalized to the control reporter value and triplicates are then averaged. Comparison between test groups could be done by relativizing normalized values to basal/control samples.

2.8.2 Quantitative PCR

Quantitative polymerase chain reaction (qPCR) enables the measurement of the number of DNA molecules containing a specific sequence in a sample of interest (*see* **Note 13**). It is useful to quantify gene expression by converting messenger RNA (mRNA) to its complementary sequence of DNA (cDNA) by reverse transcription. The sample obtained in this way is subjected to fluorescence-based PCR amplification where, theoretically, during each cycle, two new duplex DNA molecules are produced for each duplex DNA molecule present in the sample. Properly carried out, this valuable technique allows measuring the relative change of the sequence of interest compared to a reference sequence and the determination of molecule number in the starting sample.

1. Cells are seeded in 6-well dishes, and when 100% confluence is reached, starved and treated for 6–48 h with the ligand of

interest (performing initial kinetic studies is very useful in identifying the optimal expression window of the target gene).

2. Total RNA can be isolated from cells by acidphenol-guanidinium thiocyanate-chloroform extraction. The quality of the RNA obtained can be verified by 2% agarose gel electrophoresis where two defined bands corresponding to ribosomal RNA should be observed.
3. For the first-strand cDNA synthesis, 1 μg of total RNA may be reverse-transcribed using random primers and commercial reverse transcriptase. At this point, cDNA sample could be stored for several months give temperature until qPCR performance.
4. Design primers complementary to the ends of opposite strands of the target sequence and located between 100 and 300 bp apart (short amplicon are advisable to avoid incomplete products amplification). Ideally, primer set should be of approximately 17–22 nucleotides in length with a Tm between 56 and 66 °C (preferentially 60 °C). If published primers pairs for a target exist, it may be advisable to use the published sequences. The specificity of the chosen pair of primers could be evaluated using blast programs and verified using standard PCR to ensure that a single product of the expected size is obtained. Commercial primers coding for β-Actin, GAPDH, or Ciclophilin-A are commonly use to standardize the content of the cDNA of interest.
5. Plan the quantitative real-time PCR (qPCR) to perform at least triplicates of each sample and sample dilutions (if necessary). A standard curve ranging from 100-fold above and below the number of expected molecules of the template should be done in order to estimate the absolute numbers of mRNA in the sample.
6. Add the experiment reagents into a microtiter plate. A general reaction may contain:
   - Master mix (Buffer, DNA polymerase, fluorescent dye or probe).
   - Target DNA.
   - Primer Fw (10 pmol).
   - Primer Rv (10 pmol).
   - H_2O (in enough quantity to the final volume of reaction)
7. After the plate reactions are assembled, seal the plate and start the run. A general amplification program would involve the following steps: a denaturing step of 4 min at 94 °C followed by 40–45 cycles of denaturing (15 s at 94 °C), annealing (20 s at melting temperature, 60 °C), and extension (30 s at 72 °C)

steps. Then, a melt or dissociation curve should be performed in order to verify the production of only one product.

8. The amplification plot shows the fluorescence signal for each cycle of the run. The Ct is defined as the PCR cycle at which the fluorescent signal cross an arbitrary placed threshold. It inversely correlates with the initial template amount. Absolute quantitation provides the exact copy number following transformation of the data via a standard curve. Relative quantitation calculates the ratio between the amount of target template and a reference template in the sample. In this case, the quantification of the target mRNA sequence could be performed using the comparative $\Delta\Delta Ct$ method relative to the housekeeping gene of choice.
9. Determine the PCR efficiency of gene of interest and control gene. Make tenfold serial dilutions of cDNA and perform qPCR for both primers. Plot the *Ct* vs. cDNA dilutions. PCR efficiency is then calculated by the equation $m = (1/\log E)$, where m is the slope of the line and E is the efficiency. PCR efficiency should be 2. Use this curve also to determine working range.
10. Analyze the melting curve. The product formed in each well should present a homogeneous, unique melting peak at its characteristic temperature. Lowering the primer concentrations will often reduce the amount of nonspecific products.

2.9 Quantification of Ligand Bias

Receptor pharmacology deals with numbers as result of experiments and interprets experimental data to simple mathematical models, thus concluding about ligand behavior related to the molecular properties of drugs. From this standpoint, quantifying ligand bias is an extremely useful way to obtain a single number that represents how biased a ligand is and applies statistics to assess true differences in ligand behavior. The goal is to obtain a unique numerical parameter accompanied by its statistical uncertainty that allows the researcher to evaluate a feature that relies only on the ligand and that can be extrapolated among different experimental systems.

Since ligand bias was recognized as a true property of drug molecules and it was realized that this feature could have an enormous impact in pharmacology, several methods were developed and used in order to measure the degree of bias that can be assigned to a ligand [24]. However, as mentioned above, there can be at least three sources of signal bias. The system bias, which is characteristic of the specific pathways to be considered, (i.e. differential amplifications steps); the observational bias, which is related to the methodology used to measure drug responses (i.e. differential sensitivity of techniques employed); and the ligand bias, which can be ascribed specifically to the differential efficacy of the ligand to activate different pathways. The first two origins of bias should be discriminated from true ligand bias if we want to extrapolate the observations made at the bench to therapy.

The strategy to distinguish and dissect the ligand bias from the methodological and system-dependent biases is to establish a comparative parameter relative to a reference ligand. The responses of the reference ligand acting on the same system as the assayed ligand will be affected by equivalent system bias; hence the ratio of efficacies of both ligands would overcome undesired sources of bias. All the methods proposed to quantify bias would then allow the measurement of how biased the test ligand is compared to the reference ligand.

Usually, the reference ligand chosen is the natural ligand of the receptor, and by definition it would be considered as a balanced ligand. It is worth noting that this property is arbitrarily assigned to the reference ligand, since there is no way to know the absolute magnitude of system and methodological biases.

Comparing only *EC50s* of the ligands fails to consider the efficacy of the ligand, and comparing maximal responses cannot differentiate between full agonists whose response is limited by the ability of the system to generate a response.

However, if both ligands are full agonists (e.g. they have the same observed maximal response) simple comparison of *EC50s* ($\Delta pEC50$) is sufficient to determine bias. Nevertheless, if at least one of the ligands is a partial agonist, this simplification cannot be made, and more considerations should be taken into account. In fact, the comparison should include the differences in the efficacy by contrasting *equiactive concentrations*. This was originally developed to estimate relative affinity of partial agonists and compares concentrations of full and partial agonists needed to achieve the same response [145].

Certainly, the attempt to measure the differential efficacies of a ligand to trigger different responses relies on the model chosen to interpret the mechanisms by which a ligand acts on a cell system. Most methods explicitly involve the assumptions made by Black and Leff in their operational model of ligand action as described above [4].

Hence, the comprehensive ability of a ligand to elicit a response can be obtained by fitting experimental data to Eq. (3) in order to find its τ value, which comprises the intrinsic efficacy of the ligand and the sensitivity of the system to agonism and has been previously defined as $\tau = R_{tot}/K_E$, and then the ratio of τs for test and reference ligands $\sigma_{lig} = \log(\tau_{lig}/\tau_{ref})$ [146].

Employing this approach, τ values are fitted assuming a constant independent value for the functional constant K_A that is usually determined in binding experiments under conditions that prevent formation of a ternary complex. In other words, the K_A value in Eq. (3) is supposed to be equivalent to the affinity of ligand for the bare receptor, K_D. This is not entirely true in most cases. Considering an allosteric point of view, only those receptor species coupled to transducers (e.g. G-proteins or β-arrestins) are the functional entities accountable for the generation of cell response. The ligand-receptor-transducer ternary complex and not the ligand–receptor complex is the minimal biological unit needed to elicit a response. As in any allosteric model, the affinity of the ligand depends on the property and amounts of the partner proteins or receptor state. This was clearly discussed by David Colquhoun [147]. The assumption that the agonist binds with the same affinity to all receptor species, whether they are coupled to transducer partners or not, may drive to error since it is expected that agonists possess differential affinities for different receptor species [32, 148–150]. In fact, in modern ligand–receptor interaction models, this differential affinity is considered the ultimate cause of ligand efficacy [151].

Regarding this, a value of K_A fitted from concentration–response curves would better represent the actual scenario where the ligand binds with different affinities to the different receptor species. Within this frame, the ratio τ/K_A, namely the transduction ratio, is a unique proportion that can characterize the behavior of a specific ligand. A new parameter $\Delta\log(\tau/K_A) = \log(\tau/K_A)_{lig} - \log(\tau/K_A)_{ref}$ can be calculated. This parameter represents the ratio of power of each ligand to induce a response using a reference agonist that will cancel the effects of system and observational bias [152]. Remarkably, signaling bias can be assessed if a response can be measured in both pathways. In general, bias can only be evaluated when a response is observed (*see* **Note 14**).

After calculating the relative efficacies of test and reference ligands (e.g. $\Delta pEC50$, σ_{lig} or $\Delta\log(\tau/K_A)$) for a given path, ratios for the relative efficacy of each ligand throughout different paths can be determined as a degree of agonist bias ($\Delta\Delta pEC50$, $\Delta\sigma_{lig}$ or $\Delta\Delta\log(\tau/K_A)$). The detailed procedure to determine the different parameters mentioned will be described below.

1. As a first step, a reference ligand should be chosen. It is irrelevant which compound is chosen as the reference, although the natural ligand is the usual choice. It is important to point out that the same ligand should be used as the reference for all the paths studied to allow comparison between pathways.
2. Raw data obtained from concentration response assays for all ligands should be expressed as a fraction of the maximal response of the system E_{max}. These fractional values are comparable between ligands and are scaled to the assay since they are referenced to a system constant. The E_{max} value may be determined independently (e.g. using forskolin to achieve the maximal adenylyl cyclase activation) or may be inferred if several different agonists possess the same maximal response levels, making reasonable to assume that they actually achieve the maximal response of the system.

3. With the data from concentration–response curves a nonlinear fitting procedure should be done fitting the data to the Hill equation (Eq. 4):

$$\text{Response} = \frac{[L]^n \cdot R_{\text{max}}}{[L]^n + EC_{50}} \tag{4}$$

4. The slope value n obtained from the analysis should be evaluated. If the fitted value for the slope n is not significantly different from unity, a simple comparison of Rmax/EC50 can be done. It can be demonstrated that when the Hill coefficient factor n is not different from unity, log(Rmax/EC50) is equal to log(τ/KA). Hence, for some systems, a more simple comparison of parameters can be used to quantify agonist bias.

   On the other hand, if the slope factor n is significantly different from unity, τ or τ/K_A values ought to be calculated from fitting the operational model of Black and Leff using Eq. (5), a modified version of original Eq. (3).

$$\text{Response} = \frac{[L]^n \cdot \tau^n \cdot E_{\text{max}}}{[L]^n \cdot \tau^n + ([L] + K_A)^n} \tag{5}$$

   As before, τ is the efficacy of the ligand, and the maximal response capability of the assay is given by E_{max}, hence the maximal response for partial agonists will be less than E_{max}.

   For high efficacy agonists, nonlinear fitting procedures can encounter local minimums, and therefore the whole process will not converge properly. Usually, these problems can be solved using suitable starting values for the parameters to be fit, τ and K_A. If it is not the case, a more manageable form of the Eq. (5) can be used (Eq. 6):

$$\text{Response} = \frac{E_{\text{max}}}{1 + \exp[n \ln[1 + \exp\frac{(\ln(K_A))}{[L]}] - n \ln(\tau)]} \tag{6}$$

   Please note that the slope factor n and E_{max} are values defined by the system and must be common for all ligands tested in a certain assay.

5. Once values of τ or τ/K_A were obtained for each ligand, the ratio between the tested ligands and the reference ligand should be found as follows: $\sigma_{lig} = \log(\tau_{lig}/\tau_{ref})$ or $\Delta\log(\tau/K_A) = \log(\tau/K_A)_{lig} - \log(\tau/K_A)_{ref}$ respectively. The quotient between tested and reference ligands cancel the effects that are not strictly due to the drug, and these are the parameters that should be considered for further analysis.

   The values of σ_{lig} and $\Delta\log(\tau/K_A)$ denote the ratio of ligands for a given pathway. A value of zero indicates that the ligand has the same degree of activity than the reference for the pathway considered. One relative value should be found for each pathway studied.

6. Next step implies obtaining a ratio of efficacy for both pathways (path1 and path2) to effectively quantify the degree of bias of a ligand relative to the reference. A parameter β_{lig} can be found using Eq. (7):

$$\beta_{lig} = \frac{\sigma_{lig}{}^{\text{path 1}} - \sigma_{lig}{}^{\text{path 2}}}{\sqrt{2}} \quad (7)$$

As previously stated, it would be expected that for a balanced agonist, the signaling would be equal for both pathways, and then on a graph that compares these two values balanced agonists would be located on a line of unity. Therefore, Eq. (7) represents the distance between the pair of σ_{lig} factors for both pathways and the line of unity.

In turn, it can be calculated $\Delta\Delta log(\tau/K_A)$ using Eq. (8) as an index of ligand bias

$$\Delta\Delta\log(\tau / K_A) = \Delta\log(\tau / K_A)^{\text{path1}} - \Delta\log(\tau / K_A)^{\text{path2}} \quad (8)$$

The order of subtraction is not relevant; however this will orientate the bias vector. Values obtained using Eq. (8), are the logarithms of the bias towards pathway 2 given an amount of signal in pathway 1, always compared to the reference ligand.

The distance between β_{lig} or $\Delta\Delta\log(\tau/K_A)$ and zero is the log of the magnitude of the bias towards a given pathway. Whether the value is positive or negative and statistically different from zero indicates that the ligand possesses bias towards path1 or path2 respectively.

To obtain a bias factor the antilog of the parameters can be calculated. If so, conclusions can be drawn by evaluating their differences from unity.

7. If several ligands are going to be evaluated assessing different responses, graphical representation can be very useful to interpret results. For instance, when ligand bias is considered for drug development process, therapeutic combinations of ligands and receptors transformed in therapeutic combinations of ligands, receptors and signaling proteins. Hence the concept of target validation is replaced by pathway validation. Individual readouts for efficacy became a considerable collection of efficacies, which represents large amounts of data difficult to interpret.

Different graphical solutions have been proposed to tackle the issue of the interpretation of the amounts of data. For instance, webs of efficacy have been developed to show graphs with multiple axes depicting ligand efficacy at various paths. In these schemes, each ligand possesses a differential plot that is very useful to visualize the tendency to activate particular responses [39, 67].

In turn, hierarchical clustering analysis was proposed using *pEC50* data using GeneCluster software where the different responses and drugs represent the two axes. Then a similarity matrix is produced via the correlation method and a complete linkage clustering is performed [153]. With this approach, patterns of functional selectivity can be found and used for the discovery of novel compounds with the desired features.

Final Considerations for Bias Quantification

The difference in the conclusions that can be drawn using β_{lig} or $\Delta\Delta\log(\tau/K_{\text{A}})$ lies in how different are K_{A} and K_{D}. As their difference approaches to zero, β_{lig} and $\Delta\Delta\log(\tau/K_{\text{A}})$ become equivalent. It can be demonstrated that [24]

$$\sqrt{(2)}\beta_{lig} = \Delta\Delta\log(\tau / K_{\text{A}})_{lig\ ref} + \log(K_{\text{A}\ ref} / K_{\text{A}\ lig})^{\text{path2}} - \log(K_{\text{A}\ ref} / K_{\text{A}\ lig})^{\text{path1}} \quad (9)$$

Equation (9) shows the relationship between both parameters. It illustrates that β_{lig} and $\Delta\Delta\log(\tau/K_{\text{A}})$ differ in the possible difference of affinity of the agonists when they bind to receptor and subsequently bind to signaling partners in pathways 1 and 2 (second and third terms of the right side).

If the affinity of both ligands is identical when both pathways are activated, those terms become zero and Eq. (9) reduces to Eq. (10).

$$\sqrt{(2)}\beta_{lig} = \Delta\Delta\log(\tau / K_{\text{A}})_{lig\ ref} \quad (10)$$

The effect of signaling proteins on ligand affinity determines whether there will be an error in bias estimates using β_{lig} or $\Delta\Delta\log(\tau/K_{\text{A}})$. It cannot be discarded beforehand that in some instances a single binding affinity (K_{D}) seems to model the functional affinity of agonists (K_{A}), and therefore both β_{lig} and $\Delta\Delta\log(\tau/K_{\text{A}})$ will give an accurate estimate of ligand bias.

3 Notes

1. **GTPγS Binding Assay**. *Advantages*: Since GDP-GTP exchange is an early event in GPCRs signal transduction, it is less subjected to regulation by other cellular processes. *Disadvantages*: Classical techniques involve the use of radioactive [^{35}S]-GTP and titration steps. There is also a poor signal to background window for GPCRs that do not signal through to Gi protein.

2. **Determination of cAMP production** . *Advantages*: since the production of cAMP is an amplified step in the signal transduction cascade of GPCRs, this response should be detected with good sensitivity. *Disadvantages*: cAMP production is subject to regulation by other cellular processes as heterologous desensitization or receptor internalization among others.
3. **Quantification of inositol phosphates** . *Advantages*: A functional assay that can be used for low binding ligands. *Disadvantages*: Difficult, tedious, and time-consuming to perform for a large amount of compounds.
4. **Ca2+ measurement** . *Advantages*: Ca^{2+} assays are robust and can be used to rapidly test a large amount of compounds in live cells. *Disadvantages*: Some compounds may interfere with fluorescence. Since calcium mobilization is rapid and transient it cannot be used to detect slow binding agonists. In addition, it cannot be used to evaluate inverse agonists because increases in basal Ca^{2+} levels are not observed after expression of constitutive active forms of GPCRs. For these cases, IP accumulation assays are preferred.
5. **Receptor desensitization** . *Advantages*: since the rate of desensitization limits G protein signaling, desensitization studies bring important information regarding the differential duration of G protein action. *Disadvantages*: cAMP production may be subjected to regulation by other cellular processes such as heterologous desensitization or receptor turnover among others.
6. **Receptor phosphorylation**. *Advantages*: the selective recruitment of various kinases yields a phosphorylation "barcode" that may determine the fate of the receptor (recycling-degradation or arrestin-mediated signaling) [154]. *Disadvantages*: In general, antibodies directed against GPCRs are of poor quality. Classical techniques involve immunoprecipitation of GPCRs, which is a tricky task, and the use of radioactive reagents. Despite the typical disadvantages that are associated with the use of radioactive substances such as availability and generation of radioactive waste, phosphorylation studies imply the use of ^{32}P a high energy, beta emitter.
7. **Receptor internalization**. *Advantages*: the study of receptor trafficking can be done in living cells. Receptor binding assay is a very robust technique and can be used to quantitatively evaluate receptor internalization and recovery of membrane sites. *Disadvantages*: Binding assays involve the use of radioactive compounds with their concomitant disadvantages in availability and generation of radioactive waste. However, the study of receptor trafficking by image-based techniques often implies the use of not naïve, artificial tagged receptors.

8. **Receptor dimerization by co-immunoprecipitation.** *Advantages*: Can be done in native systems expressing native receptors. *Disadvantages*: Specific controls should be carried out to discard artifacts concerning protein aggregation in denaturing conditions.
9. **FRET and BRET**. *Advantages*: Very sensitive and reliable method. *Disadvantages*: It cannot be performed in native tissues. Recombinant systems expressing tagged receptors must be used. Interpretation of experimental data may be complex.
10. **β -Arrestin recruitment**. *Advantages*: It can be performed by imaging techniques in living cells. The identification of the recruitment of *β*-arrestin opens a new range of possibilities for G protein-independent signaling. *Disadvantages*: To discriminate whether *β*-arrestin binding is going to lead to receptor internalization or to G protein-independent signaling, further pathway analysis is required.
11. **Activation of G protein-independent signaling cascades.** *Advantages*: It is easy to evaluate for example, MAPKs signaling pathway in western blot assays by using anti-phosphorylated MAPKs antibodies. *Disadvantages*: Need to know the signaling pathway that is regulated.
12. **Evaluation of gene expression by gene reporter assays.** *Advantages*: High sensitivity, low cost, simple, and fast. There is usually a large signal-to-background ratio. It allows detection of gene expression modulation even for weak agonists. It brings biologically relevant information since it involves a genomic ligand effect. *Disadvantages*: It cannot be done in unmodified naïve systems. Ligand effects could be missed by evaluating such a downstream response. Gene expression may be modulated by multiple converging pathways which could lead to false positive measure. Relative values are obtained which can be difficult to standardize. For absolute values, a standard curve with purified luciferase must be obtained.
13. **Evaluation of gene expression by quantitative PCR** . *Advantages*: It brings biologically relevant information since it involves a genomic ligand effect. It can be done in unmodified naïve systems. qPCR is exceptionally sensitive; in theory, it can detect a single molecule of RNA. *Disadvantages*: Previous information about target genes is needed. The quantified increase in the levels of a transcript does not always represent a physiologically significant one. Special equipment is needed.
14. **Quantification of ligand bias.** If no response can be observed for a given pathway, that not necessarily means that the ligand possesses no efficacy for that cell response. In some cases, assays can have a poor sensitivity to show a response. It is tempting to assume that the ligand is totally biased towards the more sensitive assay. However, this conclusion is attained based on a technical artifact.

4 Conclusions

The study of functional selectivity profoundly relies on using correct and accurate methodologies to screen GPCR responses. In order to have the whole picture of histaminergic ligands' action, currently studies in pharmacology need to consider not just the receptor molecule, but the myriad of behaviors of the histamine receptors as well, even of those going beyond the strict concept of signaling pathways since they may also account for biased agonism. This wider vision will surely result in a successful identification of drugs' mechanisms of action and their biological effects.

References

1. Langley JN (1905) On the reaction of cells and of nerve-endings to certain poisons, chiefly as regards the reaction of striated muscle to nicotine and to curari. J Physiol 33:374–413
2. Prull CR (2003) Part of a scientific master plan? Paul Ehrlich and the origins of his receptor concept. Med Hist 47:332–356
3. Hill A (1910) The possible effects of the aggregation of the molecules of haemoglobin on its dissociation curves. J Physiol 40:4–7
4. Black JW, Leff P (1983) Operational models of pharmacological agonism. Proc R Soc Lond B Biol Sci 220:141–162
5. Johnston CA, Siderovski DP (2007) Receptor-mediated activation of heterotrimeric G-proteins: current structural insights. Mol Pharmacol 72:219–230
6. Wettschureck N, Offermanns S (2005) Mammalian G proteins and their cell type specific functions. Physiol Rev 85:1159–1204
7. Luttrell LM, van Biesen T, Hawes BE et al (1997) G-protein-coupled receptors and their regulation: activation of the MAP kinase signaling pathway by G-protein-coupled receptors. Adv Second Messenger Phosphoprotein Res 31:263–277
8. Lefkowitz RJ, Shenoy SK (2005) Transduction of receptor signals by beta-arrestins. Science 308:512–517
9. Stephenson RP (1997) A modification of receptor theory. 1956. Br J Pharmacol 120: 106–120
10. Perez DM, Karnik SS (2005) Multiple signaling states of G-protein-coupled receptors. Pharmacol Rev 57:147–161
11. Kenakin T (2009) Pharmacology primer: theory, applications and methods, 3rd edn. Elsevier Inc United Kindom
12. Neubig RR, Spedding M, Kenakin T et al (2003) International union of pharmacology committee on receptor nomenclature and drug classification. XXXVIII. Update on terms and symbols in quantitative pharmacology. Pharmacol Rev 55:597–606
13. Strange PG (2002) Mechanisms of inverse agonism at G-protein-coupled receptors. Trends Pharmacol Sci 23:89–95
14. Ligeti E, Csepanyi-Komi R, Hunyady L (2012) Physiological mechanisms of signal termination in biological systems. Acta Physiol (Oxf) 204:469–478
15. Kenakin T (2007) Collateral efficacy in drug discovery: taking advantage of the good (allosteric) nature of 7TM receptors. Trends Pharmacol Sci 28:407–415
16. Changeux JP (1964) Allosteric Interactions interpreted in terms of quaternary structure. Brookhaven Symp Biol 17:232–249
17. Kenakin T, Miller LJ (2010) Seven transmembrane receptors as shapeshifting proteins: the impact of allosteric modulation and functional selectivity on new drug discovery. Pharmacol Rev 62:265–304
18. Kenakin T (2004) Principles: receptor theory in pharmacology. Trends Pharmacol Sci 25:186–192
19. Ghanouni P, Gryczynski Z, Steenhuis JJ et al (2001) Functionally different agonists induce distinct conformations in the G protein coupling domain of the beta 2 adrenergic receptor. J Biol Chem 276:24433–24436
20. Galandrin S, Bouvier M (2006) Distinct signaling profiles of beta1 and beta2 adrenergic receptor ligands toward adenylyl cyclase and mitogen-activated protein kinase reveals the pluridimensionality of efficacy. Mol Pharmacol 70:1575–1584
21. Luttrell LM, Kenakin TP (2011) Refining efficacy: allosterism and bias in G protein-coupled receptor signaling. Methods Mol Biol 756:3–35

22. Kenakin TP (2009) Cellular assays as portals to seven-transmembrane receptor-based drug discovery. Nat Rev Drug Discov 8:617–626
23. Zhang R, Xie X (2012) Tools for GPCR drug discovery. Acta Pharmacol Sin 33:372–384
24. Kenakin T, Christopoulos A (2013) Signalling bias in new drug discovery: detection, quantification and therapeutic impact. Nat Rev Drug Discov 12:205–216
25. Whalen EJ, Rajagopal S, Lefkowitz RJ (2011) Therapeutic potential of beta-arrestin- and G protein-biased agonists. Trends Mol Med 17:126–139
26. Hill SJ, Ganellin CR, Timmerman H, Schwartz JC et al (1997) International union of pharmacology. XIII. Classification of histamine receptors. Pharmacol Rev 49:253–278
27. Powell JR, Brody MJ (1976) Identification and specific blockade of two receptors for histamine in the cardiovascular system. J Pharmacol Exp Ther 196:1–14
28. Black JW, Duncan WA, Durant CJ et al (1972) Definition and antagonism of histamine H2 -receptors. Nature 236:385–390
29. Traiffort E, Pollard H, Moreau J et al (1992) Pharmacological characterization and autoradiographic localization of histamine H2 receptors in human brain identified with [125I]iodoaminopotentidine. J Neurochem 59:290–299
30. Panula P, Chazot PL, Cowart M et al (2015) International union of basic and clinical pharmacology. XCVIII. Histamine receptors. Pharmacol Rev 67:601–655
31. Alewijnse AE, Timmerman H, Jacobs EH et al (2000) The effect of mutations in the DRY motif on the constitutive activity and structural instability of the histamine H(2) receptor. Mol Pharmacol 57:890–898
32. Monczor F, Fernandez N, Legnazzi BL et al (2003) Tiotidine, a histamine H2 receptor inverse agonist that binds with high affinity to an inactive G-protein-coupled form of the receptor. Experimental support for the cubic ternary complex model. Mol Pharmacol 64:512–520
33. Davio C, Mladovan A, Lemos B et al (2002) H1 and H2 histamine receptors mediate the production of inositol phosphates but not cAMP in human breast epithelial cells. Inflamm Res 51:1–7
34. Traiffort E, Ruat M, Arrang JM et al (1992) Expression of a cloned rat histamine H2 receptor mediating inhibition of arachidonate release and activation of cAMP accumulation. Proc Natl Acad Sci U S A 89:2649–2653
35. Bonini JS, Da Silva WC, Da Silveira CK et al (2011) Histamine facilitates consolidation of fear extinction. Int J Neuropsychopharmacol 14:1209–1217
36. Kim NH, Lee AY (2010) Histamine effect on melanocyte proliferation and vitiliginous keratinocyte survival. Exp Dermatol 19:1073–1079
37. Luo T, Chen B, Zhao Z et al (2013) Histamine H2 receptor activation exacerbates myocardial ischemia/reperfusion injury by disturbing mitochondrial and endothelial function. Basic Res Cardiol 108:342
38. Alonso N, Monczor F, Echeverria E et al (2014) Signal transduction mechanism of biased ligands at histamine H2 receptors. Biochem J 459:117–126
39. Alonso N, Zappia CD, Cabrera M et al (2015) Physiological implications of biased signaling at histamine H2 receptors. Front Pharmacol 6:45
40. Xu AJ, Kuramasu A, Maeda K et al (2008) Agonist-induced internalization of histamine H2 receptor and activation of extracellular signal-regulated kinases are dynamin-dependent. J Neurochem 107:208–217
41. Mettler SE, Ghayouri S, Christensen GP et al (2007) Modulatory role of phosphoinositide 3-kinase in gastric acid secretion. Am J Physiol Gastrointest Liver Physiol 293:G532–G543
42. Grandage VL, Gale RE, Linch DC et al (2005) PI3-kinase/Akt is constitutively active in primary acute myeloid leukaemia cells and regulates survival and chemoresistance via NF-kappaB, Mapkinase and p53 pathways. Leukemia 19:586–594
43. Min YH, Eom JI, Cheong JW et al (2003) Constitutive phosphorylation of Akt/PKB protein in acute myeloid leukemia: its significance as a prognostic variable. Leukemia 17:995–997
44. Werner K, Neumann D, Seifert R (2016) High constitutive Akt2 activity in U937 promonocytes: effective reduction of Akt2 phosphorylation by the histamine H-receptor and the beta-adrenergic receptor. Naunyn Schmiedebergs Arch Pharmacol 389:87–101
45. Aurelius J, Martner A, Brune M et al (2012) Remission maintenance in acute myeloid leukemia: impact of functional histamine H2 receptors expressed by leukemic cells. Haematologica 97:1904–1908
46. Thoren FB, Romero AI, Brune M et al (2009) Histamine dihydrochloride and low-dose interleukin-2 as post-consolidation immunotherapy in acute myeloid leukemia. Expert Opin Biol Ther 9:1217–1223

47. Lemos Legnazzi B, Shayo C, Monczor F et al (2000) Rapid desensitization and slow recovery of the cyclic AMP response mediated by histamine H(2) receptors in the U937 cell line. Biochem Pharmacol 60:159–166
48. Monczor F, Fernandez N, Riveiro E et al (2006) Histamine H2 receptor overexpression induces U937 cell differentiation despite triggered mechanisms to attenuate cAMP signalling. Biochem Pharmacol 71:1219–1228
49. Shayo C, Legnazzi BL, Monczor F et al (2004) The time-course of cyclic AMP signaling is critical for leukemia U-937 cell differentiation. Biochem Biophys Res Commun 314:798–804
50. Rodriguez-Pena MS, Timmerman H, Leurs R (2000) Modulation of histamine H(2) receptor signalling by G-protein-coupled receptor kinase 2 and 3. Br J Pharmacol 131:1707–1715
51. Shayo C, Fernandez N, Legnazzi BL et al (2001) Histamine H2 receptor desensitization: involvement of a select array of G protein-coupled receptor kinases. Mol Pharmacol 60:1049–1056
52. Fernandez N, Monczor F, Lemos B et al (2002) Reduction of G protein-coupled receptor kinase 2 expression in U-937 cells attenuates H2 histamine receptor desensitization and induces cell maturation. Mol Pharmacol 62:1506–1514
53. Fernandez N, Monczor F, Tubio MR et al (2007) Regulatory mechanisms underlying GKR2 levels in U937 cells: evidence for GRK3 involvement. Biochem Pharmacol 73:1758–1767
54. Fernandez N, Gottardo FL, Alonso MN et al (2011) Roles of phosphorylation-dependent and -independent mechanisms in the regulation of histamine H2 receptor by G protein-coupled receptor kinase 2. J Biol Chem 286:28697–28706
55. Fernandez N, Monczor F, Baldi A et al (2008) Histamine H2 receptor trafficking: role of arrestin, dynamin, and clathrin in histamine H2 receptor internalization. Mol Pharmacol 74:1109–1118
56. Smit MJ, Timmerman H, Alewijnse AE et al (1995) Visualization of agonist-induced internalization of histamine H2 receptors. Biochem Biophys Res Commun 214: 1138–1145
57. Hershcovici T, Fass R (2011) Gastro-oesophageal reflux disease: beyond proton pump inhibitor therapy. Drugs 71:2381–2389
58. Sigterman KE, van Pinxteren B, Bonis PA et al (2013) Short-term treatment with proton pump inhibitors, H2-receptor antagonists and prokinetics for gastro-oesophageal reflux disease-like symptoms and endoscopy negative reflux disease. Cochrane Database Syst Rev 5:CD002095
59. Sandler RS, Everhart JE, Donowitz M et al (2002) The burden of selected digestive diseases in the United States. Gastroenterology 122:1500–1511
60. Marshall BJ, Goodwin CS, Warren JR et al (1988) Prospective double-blind trial of duodenal ulcer relapse after eradication of *Campylobacter pylori*. Lancet 2:1437–1442
61. Marshall BJ, Warren JR (1984) Unidentified curved bacilli in the stomach of patients with gastritis and peptic ulceration. Lancet 1:1311–1315
62. Olbe L, Carlsson E, Lindberg P (2003) A proton-pump inhibitor expedition: the case histories of omeprazole and esomeprazole. Nat Rev Drug Discov 2:132–139
63. Laine L, Kivitz AJ, Bello AE et al (2012) Double-blind randomized trials of single-tablet ibuprofen/high-dose famotidine vs. ibuprofen alone for reduction of gastric and duodenal ulcers. Am J Gastroenterol 107:379–386
64. Smit MJ, Leurs R, Alewijnse AE et al (1996) Inverse agonism of histamine H2 antagonist accounts for upregulation of spontaneously active histamine H2 receptors. Proc Natl Acad Sci U S A 93:6802–6807
65. Colucci R, Fleming JV, Xavier R et al (2001) L-histidine decarboxylase decreases its own transcription through downregulation of ERK activity. Am J Physiol Gastrointest Liver Physiol 281:G1081–G1091
66. Wessler S, Hocker M, Fischer W et al (2000) Helicobacter pylori activates the histidine decarboxylase promoter through a mitogen-activated protein kinase pathway independent of pathogenicity island-encoded virulence factors. J Biol Chem 275:3629–3636
67. Reher TM, Brunskole I, Neumann D et al (2012) Evidence for ligand-specific conformations of the histamine H(2)-receptor in human eosinophils and neutrophils. Biochem Pharmacol 84:1174–1185
68. Martner A, Thoren FB, Aurelius J et al (2010) Immunotherapy with histamine dihydrochloride for the prevention of relapse in acute myeloid leukemia. Expert Rev Hematol 3:381–391
69. Burde R, Buschauer A, Seifert R (1990) Characterization of histamine H2-receptors in human neutrophils with a series of guanidine analogues of impromidine. Are cell type-

specific H2-receptors involved in the regulation of NADPH oxidase? Naunyn Schmiedebergs Arch Pharmacol 341: 455–461

70. Burde R, Seifert R, Buschauer A et al (1989) Histamine inhibits activation of human neutrophils and HL-60 leukemic cells via H2-receptors. Naunyn Schmiedebergs Arch Pharmacol 340:671–678
71. Copsel S, Garcia C, Diez F et al (2011) Multidrug resistance protein 4 (MRP4/ABCC4) regulates cAMP cellular levels and controls human leukemia cell proliferation and differentiation. J Biol Chem 286: 6979–6988
72. Jutel M, Akdis M, Akdis CA (2009) Histamine, histamine receptors and their role in immune pathology. Clin Exp Allergy 39:1786–1800
73. Seifert R, Hoer A, Schwaner I et al (1992) Histamine increases cytosolic Ca^{2+} in HL-60 promyelocytes predominantly via H2 receptors with an unique agonist/antagonist profile and induces functional differentiation. Mol Pharmacol 42:235–241
74. Pearce FL (1991) Biological effects of histamine: an overview. Agents Actions 33:4–7
75. Jutel M, Blaser K, Akdis CA (2006) The role of histamine in regulation of immune responses. Chem Immunol Allergy 91:174–187
76. Hellstrand K, Asea A, Dahlgren C et al (1994) Histaminergic regulation of NK cells. Role of monocyte-derived reactive oxygen metabolites. J Immunol 153:4940–4947
77. Ching TL, Koelemij JG, Bast A (1995) The effect of histamine on the oxidative burst of HL60 cells before and after exposure to reactive oxygen species. Inflamm Res 44:99–104
78. Malmberg KJ (2004) Effective immunotherapy against cancer: a question of overcoming immune suppression and immune escape? Cancer Immunol Immunother 53:879–892
79. Murdoch C, Giannoudis A, Lewis CE (2004) Mechanisms regulating the recruitment of macrophages into hypoxic areas of tumors and other ischemic tissues. Blood 104: 2224–2234
80. Hellstrand K (2002) Histamine in cancer immunotherapy: a preclinical background. Semin Oncol 29:35–40
81. Kenakin TP, Ambrose JR, Irving PE (1991) The relative efficiency of beta adrenoceptor coupling to myocardial inotropy and diastolic relaxation: organ-selective treatment for diastolic dysfunction. J Pharmacol Exp Ther 257:1189–1197
82. Hahm KB, Park IS, Kim HC et al (1996) Comparison of antiproliferative effects of 1-histamine-2 receptor antagonists, cimetidine, ranitidine, and famotidine, in gastric cancer cells. Int J Immunopharmacol 18:393–399
83. Diebel LN, Liberati DM, Hall-Zimmerman L (2011) H2 blockers decrease gut mucus production and lead to barrier dysfunction in vitro. Surgery 150:736–743
84. Cianchi F, Cortesini C, Schiavone N et al (2005) The role of cyclooxygenase-2 in mediating the effects of histamine on cell proliferation and vascular endothelial growth factor production in colorectal cancer. Clin Cancer Res 11:6807–6815
85. Fujimoto S, Komine M, Karakawa M et al (2011) Histamine differentially regulates the production of Th1 and Th2 chemokines by keratinocytes through histamine H1 receptor. Cytokine 54:191–199
86. de Lera RM, Zheng J, Berlin MY et al (2013) Bicyclic and tricyclic heterocycle derivatives as histamine H3 receptor antagonists for the treatment of obesity. Bioorg Med Chem Lett 23:6004–6009
87. Muller T, Myrtek D, Bayer H et al (2006) Functional characterization of histamine receptor subtypes in a human bronchial epithelial cell line. Int J Mol Med 18:925–931
88. Pagotto RM, Monzon C, Moreno MB et al (2012) Proliferative effect of histamine on MA-10 Leydig tumor cells mediated through HRH2 activation, transient elevation in cAMP production, and increased extracellular signal-regulated kinase phosphorylation levels. Biol Reprod 87:150
89. Martinel Lamas DJ, Cortina JE, Ventura C et al (2015) Enhancement of ionizing radiation response by histamine in vitro and in vivo in human breast cancer. Cancer Biol Ther 16:137–148
90. Porretti JC, Mohamad NA, Martin GA et al (2014) Fibroblasts induce epithelial to mesenchymal transition in breast tumor cells which is prevented by fibroblasts treatment with histamine in high concentration. Int J Biochem Cell Biol 51:29–38
91. Davio C, Baldi A, Shayo C et al (1995) H1 and H2 histamine receptors in histiocytic lymphoma cell line U-937. Inflamm Res 44(S1):S72–S73
92. Nagai Y, Tanaka Y, Kuroishi et al (2012) Histamine reduces susceptibility to natural killer cells via down-regulation of NKG2D ligands on human monocytic leukaemia THP-1 cells. Immunology 136:103-114

93. Tanimoto A, Murata Y, Nomaguchi M et al (2001) Histamine increases the expression of LOX-1 via H2 receptor in human monocytic THP-1 cells. FEBS Lett 508:345–349
94. Brodsky A, Davio C, Shayo C et al (1998) Forskolin induces U937 cell line differentiation as a result of a sustained cAMP elevation. Eur J Pharmacol 350:121–127
95. Shayo C, Davio C, Brodsky A et al (1997) Histamine modulates the expression of c-fos through cyclic AMP production via the H2 receptor in the human promonocytic cell line U937. Mol Pharmacol 51:983–990
96. Mitsuhashi M, Payan DG (1991) Multiple signaling pathways of histamine H2 receptors. Agents Actions 33:289–294
97. Cho EJ, An HJ, Shin JS et al (2011) Roxatidine suppresses inflammatory responses via inhibition of NF-kappaB and p38 MAPK activation in LPS-induced RAW 264.7 macrophages. J Cell Biochem 112:3648–3659
98. Kimura S, Wang KY, Yamada S et al (2015) CCL22/Macrophage-derived chemokine expression in apolipoprotein e-deficient mice and effects of histamine in the setting of atherosclerosis. J Atheroscler Thromb 22: 599–609
99. Mirzahosseini A, Kovacs M, Kanai K et al (2015) BODIPY((R)) FL histamine as a new modality for quantitative detection of histamine receptor upregulation upon IgE sensitization in murine bone marrow-derived mast cells. Cytometry A 87:23–31
100. Alonso N, Fernandez N, Notcovich C et al (2013) Cross-desensitization and cointernalization of H1 and H2 histamine receptors reveal new insights into histamine signal integration. Mol Pharmacol 83:1087–1098
101. Shen Y, Hu WW, Fan YY et al (2007) Carnosine protects against NMDA-induced neurotoxicity in differentiated rat PC12 cells through carnosine-histidine-histamine pathway and H(1)/H(3) receptors. Biochem Pharmacol 73:709–717
102. Wu T, Gan X, Zhou S et al (2013) Histamine at low concentrations aggravates rat liver BRL-3A cell injury induced by hypoxia/reoxygenation through histamine H2 receptor in vitro. Toxicol In Vitro 27:378–386
103. Hadri L, Pavoine C, Lipskaia L et al (2006) Transcription of the sarcoplasmic/endoplasmic reticulum Ca2+-ATPase type 3 gene, ATP2A3, is regulated by the calcineurin/NFAT pathway in endothelial cells. Biochem J 394:27–33
104. Huwiler A, Doll F, Ren S et al (2006) Histamine increases sphingosine kinase-1 expression and activity in the human arterial endothelial cell line EA.hy 926 by a PKC-alpha-dependent mechanism. Biochim Biophys Acta 1761:367–376
105. Cricco G, Martin G, Medina V et al (2006) Histamine inhibits cell proliferation and modulates the expression of Bcl-2 family proteins via the H2 receptor in human pancreatic cancer cells. Anticancer Res 26:4443–4450
106. Ramos-Jimenez J, Soria-Jasso LE, Lopez-Colombo A et al (2007) Histamine augments beta2-adrenoceptor-induced cyclic AMP accumulation in human prostate cancer cells DU-145 independently of known histamine receptors. Biochem Pharmacol 73:814–823
107. Hiller C, Kuhhorn J, Gmeiner P (2013) Class A G-protein-coupled receptor (GPCR) dimers and bivalent ligands. J Med Chem 56:6542–6559
108. Schmitt JM, Stork PJ (2000) beta 2-adrenergic receptor activates extracellular signal-regulated kinases (ERKs) via the small G protein rap1 and the serine/threonine kinase B-Raf. J Biol Chem 275:25342–25350
109. Shaw G, Morse S, Ararat M et al (2002) Preferential transformation of human neuronal cells by human adenoviruses and the origin of HEK 293 cells. FASEB J 16:869–871
110. Smit MJ, Timmerman H, Blauw J et al (1996) The C terminal tail of the histamine H2 receptor contains positive and negative signals important for signal transduction and receptor down-regulation. J Neurochem 67:1791–1800
111. Milligan G (2003) Principles: extending the utility of [35S]GTP gamma S binding assays. Trends Pharmacol Sci 24:87–90
112. Labrecque J, Wong RS, Fricker SP (2009) A time-resolved fluorescent lanthanide (Eu)-GTP binding assay for chemokine receptors as targets in drug discovery. Methods Mol Biol 552:153–169
113. Davio CA, Cricco GP, Bergoc RM et al (1995) H1 and H2 histamine receptors in N-nitroso-N-methylurea (NMU)-induced carcinomas with atypical coupling to signal transducers. Biochem Pharmacol 50:91–96
114. Berridge MJ (1993) Inositol trisphosphate and calcium signalling. Nature 361:315–325
115. Grynkiewicz G, Poenie M, Tsien RY (1985) A new generation of Ca2+ indicators with greatly improved fluorescence properties. J Biol Chem 260:3440–3450
116. Pitcher J, Lohse MJ, Codina J et al (1992) Desensitization of the isolated beta 2-adrenergic receptor by beta-adrenergic receptor kinase, cAMP-dependent protein

kinase, and protein kinase C occurs via distinct molecular mechanisms. Biochemistry 31:3193–3197
117. Lohse MJ, Andexinger S, Pitcher J et al (1992) Receptor-specific desensitization with purified proteins. Kinase dependence and receptor specificity of beta-arrestin and arrestin in the beta 2-adrenergic receptor and rhodopsin systems. J Biol Chem 267: 8558–8564
118. Kim J, Ahn S, Ren XR et al (2005) Functional antagonism of different G protein-coupled receptor kinases for beta-arrestin-mediated angiotensin II receptor signaling. Proc Natl Acad Sci U S A 102:1442–1447
119. Ren XR, Reiter E, Ahn S et al (2005) Different G protein-coupled receptor kinases govern G protein and beta-arrestin-mediated signaling of V2 vasopressin receptor. Proc Natl Acad Sci U S A 102:1448–1453
120. Zidar DA, Violin JD, Whalen EJ et al (2009) Selective engagement of G protein coupled receptor kinases (GRKs) encodes distinct functions of biased ligands. Proc Natl Acad Sci U S A 106:9649–9654
121. Liggett SB (2011) Phosphorylation barcoding as a mechanism of directing GPCR signaling. Sci Signal 4:pe36
122. Oakley RH, Laporte SA, Holt JA et al (1999) Association of beta-arrestin with G protein-coupled receptors during clathrin-mediated endocytosis dictates the profile of receptor resensitization. J Biol Chem 274:32248–32257
123. Sever S (2002) Dynamin and endocytosis. Curr Opin Cell Biol 14:463–467
124. Tsao P, Cao T, von Zastrow M (2001) Role of endocytosis in mediating downregulation of G-protein-coupled receptors. Trends Pharmacol Sci 22:91–96
125. Prossnitz ER (2004) Novel roles for arrestins in the post-endocytic trafficking of G protein-coupled receptors. Life Sci 75:893–899
126. Chabre M, le Maire M (2005) Monomeric G-protein-coupled receptor as a functional unit. Biochemistry 44:9395–9403
127. Gurevich VV, Gurevich EV (2008) GPCR monomers and oligomers: it takes all kinds. Trends Neurosci 31:74–81
128. Bulenger S, Marullo S, Bouvier M (2005) Emerging role of homo- and heterodimerization in G-protein-coupled receptor biosynthesis and maturation. Trends Pharmacol Sci 26:131–137
129. Terrillon S, Bouvier M (2004) Roles of G-protein-coupled receptor dimerization. EMBO Rep 5:30–34
130. Lohse MJ, Nuber S, Hoffmann C (2012) Fluorescence/bioluminescence resonance energy transfer techniques to study G-protein-coupled receptor activation and signaling. Pharmacol Rev 64:299–336
131. Milligan G, Ramsay D, Pascal G et al (2003) GPCR dimerisation. Life Sci 74:181–188
132. Youvan DC, Silva CM, Bylina EJ, Coleman WJ et al (1997) Calibration of fluorescence resonance energy transfer in microscopy using genetically engineered GFP derivatives on nickel chelating beads. Biotechnol Alia 3:1–18
133. Luttrell LM (2014) Minireview: more than just a hammer: ligand "bias" and pharmaceutical discovery. Mol Endocrinol 28:281–294
134. Haasen D, Wolff M, Valler MJ et al (2006) Comparison of G-protein coupled receptor desensitization-related beta-arrestin redistribution using confocal and non-confocal imaging. Comb Chem High Throughput Screen 9:37–47
135. Kamal M, Marquez M, Vauthier V et al (2009) Improved donor/acceptor BRET couples for monitoring beta-arrestin recruitment to G protein-coupled receptors. Biotechnol J 4:1337–1344
136. Barnea G, Strapps W, Herrada G et al (2008) The genetic design of signaling cascades to record receptor activation. Proc Natl Acad Sci U S A 105:64–69
137. Wetter JA, Revankar C, Hanson BJ (2009) Utilization of the Tango beta-arrestin recruitment technology for cell-based EDG receptor assay development and interrogation. J Biomol Screen 14:1134–1141
138. Yin H, Chu A, Li W et al (2009) Lipid G protein-coupled receptor ligand identification using beta-arrestin PathHunter assay. J Biol Chem 284:12328–12338
139. Rajagopal S, Rajagopal K, Lefkowitz RJ (2010) Teaching old receptors new tricks: biasing seven-transmembrane receptors. Nat Rev Drug Discov 9:373–386
140. Chen D, Aihara T, Zhao CM et al (2006) Differentiation of the gastric mucosa. I. Role of histamine in control of function and integrity of oxyntic mucosa: understanding gastric physiology through disruption of targeted genes. Am J Physiol 291:G539–G544
141. Gschwandtner M, Bunk H, Kother B et al (2012) Histamine down-regulates IL-27 production in antigen-presenting cells. J Leukoc Biol 92:21–29
142. Gutzmer R, Langer K, Lisewski M et al (2002) Expression and function of histamine receptors 1 and 2 on human monocyte-

derived dendritic cells. J Allergy Clin Immunol 109:524–531

143. Hegyesi H, Horvath B, Pallinger E et al (2005) Histamine elevates the expression of Ets-1, a protooncogen in human melanoma cell lines through H2 receptor. FEBS Lett 579:2475–2479
144. Lee CL, Hsu SH, Jong YJ et al (2013) Inhibition of histamine H1 receptor activity modulates proinflammatory cytokine production of dendritic cells through c-Rel activity. Int Arch Allergy Immunol 160:265–274
145. Barlow RB, Scott KA, Stephenson RP (1963) An attempt to study the effects of chemical structure on the affinity and efficacy of compounds related to acetylcholine. Br J Pharmacol Chemother 21:509–522
146. Rajagopal S, Ahn S, Rominger DH et al (2011) Quantifying ligand bias at seven-transmembrane receptors. Mol Pharmacol 80:367–377
147. Colquhoun D (1985) Imprecision in presentation of binding studies. Trends Pharmacol Sci 6:197
148. McLoughlin DJ, Strange PG (2000) Mechanisms of agonism and inverse agonism at serotonin 5-HT1A receptors. J Neurochem 74:347–357
149. McPherson J, Rivero G, Baptist M et al (2010) mu-opioid receptors: correlation of agonist efficacy for signalling with ability to activate internalization. Mol Pharmacol 78:756–766
150. Rasmussen SG, DeVree BT, Zou Y et al (2011) Crystal structure of the beta2 adrenergic receptor-Gs protein complex. Nature 477:549–555
151. Clarke WP, Bond RA (1998) The elusive nature of intrinsic efficacy. Trends Pharmacol Sci 19:270–276
152. Kenakin T, Watson C, Muniz-Medina V et al (2012) A simple method for quantifying functional selectivity and agonist bias. ACS Chem Nerosci 3:193–203
153. Thompson GL, Lane JR, Coudrat T et al (2015) Biased agonism of endogenous opioid peptides at the mu-opioid receptor. Mol Pharmacol 88:335–346
154. Shenoy SK, Lefkowitz RJ (2011) beta-Arrestin-mediated receptor trafficking and signal transduction. Trends Pharmacol Sci 32:521–533

Chapter 5

Ligand-Binding Kinetics on Histamine Receptors

Reggie Bosma, Tamara A.M. Mocking, Rob Leurs, and Henry F. Vischer

Abstract

Equilibrium-binding affinities of ligands for a drug target do not always accurately reflect the success of drug candidates in the clinic. Affinity-based predictions concerning competitive antagonism on the target will only be accurate if equilibrium binding of both ligands is allowed. Unless equilibrium for ligand binding is obtained really quickly, it is unlikely that equilibrium is established in vivo. Instead, concentrations of (endogenous) ligands rapidly fluctuate over time. Hence, the velocity in which binding equilibrium is reached and the duration of target occupancy by the ligand (also known as residence time) are thought to be more important predictors of drug in vivo efficacy. This chapter provides the theoretical background on ligand-binding kinetics and several experimental approaches to determine the target residence time of antihistamines on histamine receptors.

Key words Antihistamines, Drug optimization, Histamine receptors, Insurmountable antagonism, Kinetic-binding rate constant, Ligand dissociation, Radioligand binding, Residence time

1 Introduction

In life, timing is everything. Correct spatio-temporal regulation of signaling molecules (ligands) determines the physiological response. In allergies for example, mast cells are triggered by allergens to release histamine [1, 2]. Histamine subsequently induces a variety of different responses such as the recruitment of immune cells, cytokine production, and vascular permeability [3–6]. Yet, high concentrations of histamine will only be present for a limited amount of time before returning to basal levels [7]. This means that if cells are not activated in a timely fashion by histamine, they have to wait for the next histamine surge. Here lies a possibility of optimizing antihistamines based on their dissociation rate, which predicts how fast blocked histamine receptors become available again to respond to histamine. In contrast, optimization of binding affinity during drug development only predicts the displacement of the antagonist by histamine under the assumption that there is ample time for ligands to have fully associated with, and fully dissociated

Ekaterini Tiligada and Madeleine Ennis (eds.), *Histamine Receptors as Drug Targets*, Methods in Pharmacology and Toxicology, DOI 10.1007/978-1-4939-6843-5_5,

from the receptor. However, this assumption is likely unfit for a dynamic system such as the human body. This notion has been getting considerable attention from the last decade for its implications in drug discovery [8–12]. In this review, we will discuss the therapeutic relevance of ligand-binding kinetics, the way to measure the ligand-binding kinetics, and the way to incorporate the information in the optimization of antihistamines.

1.1 Histamine and Antihistamines

Histamine is found throughout the body and is involved in the paracrine and autocrine regulation of numerous physiological processes based on the receptor subtype that is activated. Four human G protein-coupled receptors (GPCRs) are responsive to histamine, named the histamine 1–4 receptor (H_1R–H_4R). H_1R is successfully targeted for the treatment of allergic rhinitis, allergic conjunctivitis, urticaria, motion sickness, whereas H_2R is targeted to treat increased gastric acid secretion [13, 14]. The H_3R and H_4R have been implicated as promising targets for the treatment of narcolepsy, Alzheimer's disease, depression, obesity (H_3R), pruritus, asthma, allergic rhinitis, and dermatitis (H_4R) [15, 16].

Ligand-binding kinetics currently receive increased attention to predict the functional efficacy of a drug, since binding affinity might not always accurately predict this in vivo as exemplified by the non-equilibrium situation above [8]. Lack of drug efficacy is an important reason for failure in clinical phase II studies [17, 18]. Incorporating ligand-binding kinetics early in the drug discovery process might address some of these efficacy problems and is therefore thought to potentially reduce attrition rates [8–11]. In Fig. 1, the ligand-binding reaction is schematically depicted. As can be seen, binding is assumed to be a one-step reaction with a single ligand (L) binding a receptor (R) forming a ligand-receptor complex (RL). Derived models interpret this reaction according to the law of mass action that states that the reaction rate is proportional to the products of the concentration reactants (i.e., ligand, receptor, and ligand-receptor complex) multiplied by a kinetic-binding rate constant. This means that the forward rate and reverse rate of the binding reaction can be described as $[L]\cdot[R]\cdot k_{on}$ (binding rate) and $[RL]\cdot k_{off}$ (dissociation rate). Upon addition of a ligand concentration [L] to a receptor population [R], rate of formation will cause [RL] to increase until the rate of binding is the same as the rate of dissociation. At this state of *equilibrium*, the ratio between bound and free ligand can be predicted by the ratio of k_{off} over k_{on}, which is a new constant called the dissociation constant (K_d). Figure 1 shows how the association and dissociation of a ligand to and from the receptor are dependent on the binding rate constants k_{on} and k_{off}.

A commonly used ligand-binding parameter is the *residence time*, which reflects the time a ligand is bound to the receptor and is defined as the reciprocal of the dissociation rate ($1/k_{off}$) and is therefore analogous to the dissociation half-life ($t_{1/2} = \ln 2/k_{off}$) (Fig. 1).

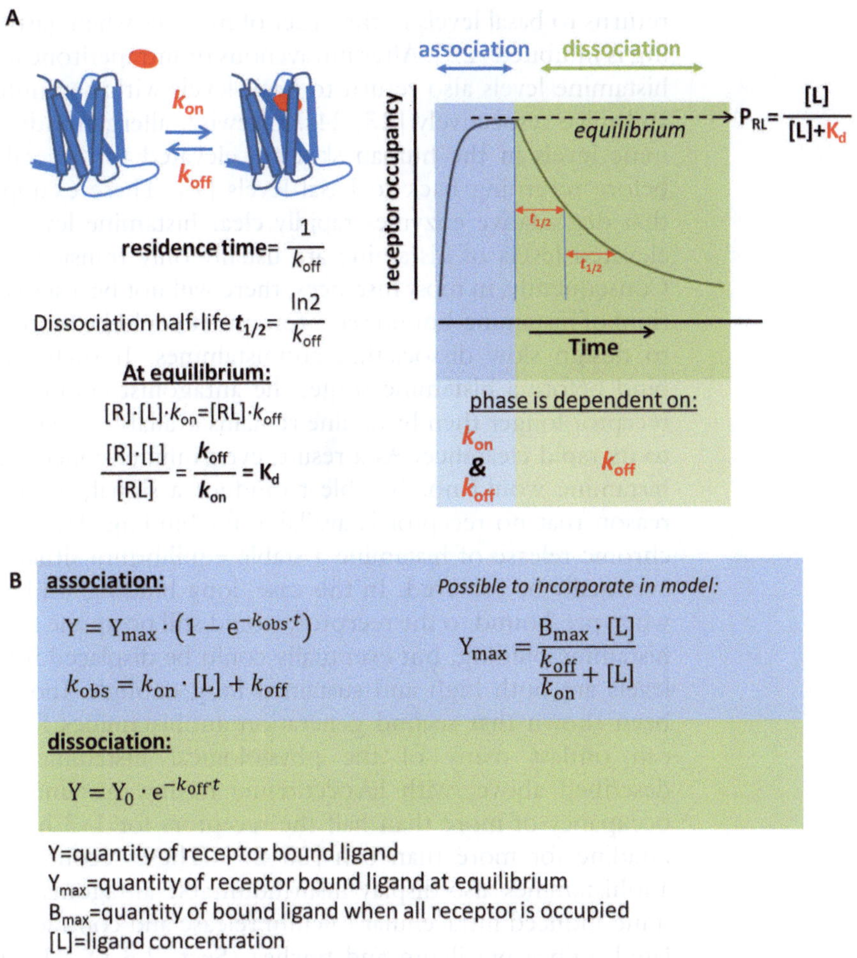

Fig. 1 Ligand binding to the receptor over time. (**a**) Ligand binding to the receptor is a reversible reaction. At equilibrium, the forward rate and reverse rate are equally fast. According to the law of mass-action this would mean that the rate of the complex association (product of receptor concentration [R], ligand concentration [L], and association rate constant k_{on}: $[R]\cdot[L]\cdot k_{on}$), equals the rate of dissociation (product of ligand-bound receptor concentration [RL] and dissociation rate constant k_{off}: $[RL]\cdot k_{off}$). The ratio of k_{off} over k_{on} is equal to the equilibrium dissociation contant (K_d), which reflects binding affinity of the ligand for the receptor. One concentration of ligand associates in time with the receptor until binding equilibrium is reached (**a**, *blue panel*). As can be seen in the *blue panel* of **b**, the time to reach equilibrium is dictated by k_{obs}, which can be described as a function of k_{on}, k_{off}, and [L]. Proportional receptor occupancy (P_{RL}) at equilibrium is dependent on ligand concentration and K_d (**a**). When free ligand is then continuously removed, there are no free ligands to form complexes with receptors and only dissociation of ligand-receptor complex will be possible (**a**, *green panel*). The time needed for ligands to dissociate from the receptor is only dependent on the k_{off} (**b**, *green panel*). Alternatively, the k_{off} can be expressed as the residence time or dissociation half-life (**a**). The latter corresponds to the time that is necessary for half of the ligands to dissociate as depicted in the *green panel* of (**a**)

Local histamine levels vary over time. Neuronal histamine release (in vitro) and breakdown in rat brain seem to occur in the order of minutes [19–21]. Moreover, histamine release in the rat stomach can be elevated for hours in response to gastrin, but returns to basal levels in the order of minutes when gastrin signaling is inhibited [22]. After intravenous or intraperitoneal injection histamine levels also return to basal levels within minutes in rats and mice respectively [23, 24]. Likewise, allergen-induced histamine levels in the human skin are elevated for several minutes before returning back to basal levels [7]. These examples show that degradative enzymes rapidly clear histamine levels and that elevated levels of histamine are usually only transiently present. Consequently, in most instances, there will not be a stable equilibrium of histamine-bound receptors and it could be more attractive to design slow dissociating antihistamines. If such antagonists bind before a histamine surge, the antagonist could occupy the receptor longer then histamine remains available in the tissue due to its rapid clearance. As a result, even infinite concentrations of histamine would not be able to induce a signal, for the simple reason that no receptor is available for binding. However, upon chronic release of histamine a stable equilibrium situation could eventually be achieved. In this case, long binding antihistamines, when pre-bound to the receptor, would still postpone the onset of histamine binding, but eventually could be displaced if histamine levels are both high and sustained long enough. Indeed, it has been shown that second generation antihistamines for the H_1R can outlast many of the physiological histamine responses described above, with levocetirizine having sustained receptor occupancy of more than half the receptors for 1–3 h and desloratadine for more than 6 h [25–27]. These second generation antihistamines also display insurmountable antagonism on histamine-induced intracellular calcium release and contraction of isolated guinea pig ileum and trachea (Sect. 2.3.1). This indicates that in controlled settings effective H_1R inhibition can be predicted based on a slow dissociation rate (k_{off} value) and not a high affinity (Fig. 2) [28, 29].

One important argument to optimize the residence time of drugs is that receptor occupancy in vivo will decrease at a slower rate than their clearance from the circulation, consequently increasing their therapeutic efficacy (Fig. 3). Such effects have also been described for H_1R antihistamines like levocetirizine and fexofenadine, referred to as "hysteresis" in the literature (delay between available concentration and biological activity) [30]. Moreover, it has also been suggested that long residence times of ligands can lead to accumulation of drugs in tissues expressing the target receptor rather than in plasma [9]. However, chronic treatment with the long residence time H_2R (insurmountable) antagonist loxitidine resulted gastric tumors in rats, which was not the case for high doses of the short residence time H_2R (surmountable) antagonist ranitidine, indicating that the long-lasting inhibitory effect on H_2R might lead to on target toxicity [31, 32]. This hypothesis is supported by the fact that an hypoacidic environ-

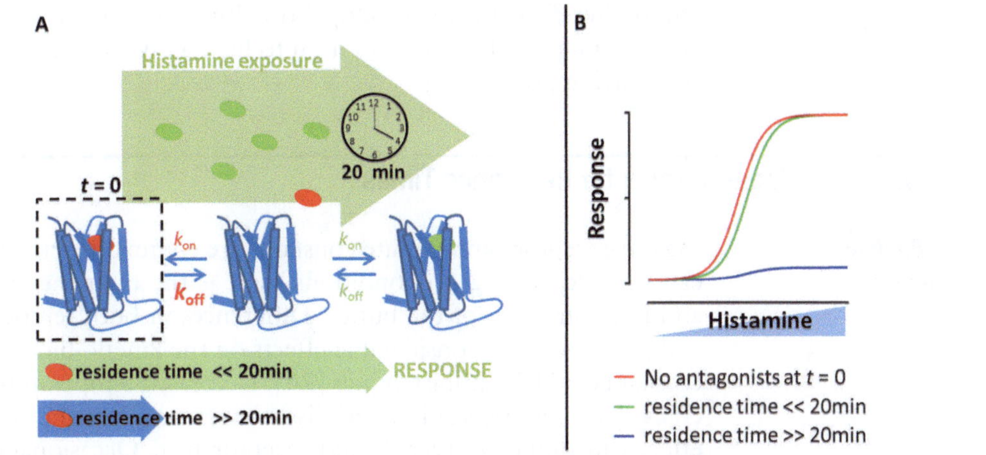

Fig. 2 Insurmountable antagonism based on dissociation rate of antihistamines. (**a**) Upon allergy stimulation, histamine (*green*) levels are increased for approximately 20 min [7]. This histamine surge (*green arrow*) can only activate the receptor within this timeframe. If pre-bound antihistamine (in *red*) at $t = 0$ does not dissociate from the receptor within this 20 min, then the receptor cannot be activated. If antihistamines dissociate readily within this 20 min, then histamine can bind the receptor based on the concentration and affinity. Since histamine competes with the antihistamine for the same receptor, higher histamine concentrations are necessary to obtain the same effect. This is reflected by a right shift of the histamine concentration response curve (**b**, *green*). If there is hardly antihistamine dissociation in 20 min, then a small number of receptors become available to respond to histamine (**b**, *blue*)

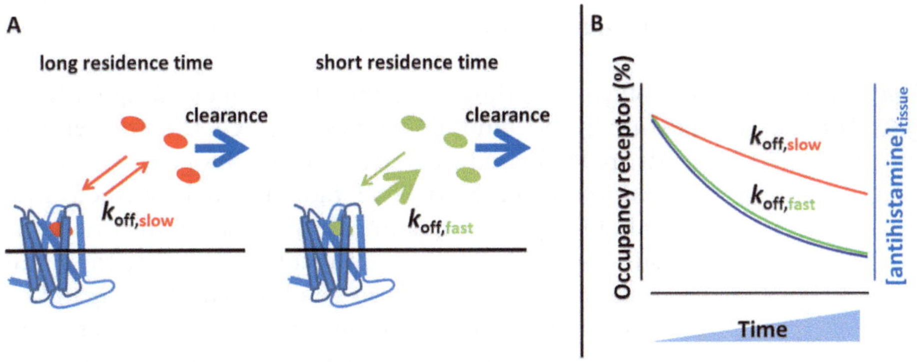

Fig. 3 Prolonged receptor occupancy based on the ligand dissociation rate. In vivo, drug concentrations can decrease rapidly due to metabolism and excretion, this clearance of the drug (**a**, *blue arrow*) can be much faster than the rate in which drugs dissociate from the target receptor. If dissociation from the receptor is rapid (**a**, *green*), receptor occupancy (**b**, *green line*) decreases in line with drug concentration (**b**, *blue line*). Hence, receptor occupancy is a function of ligand concentration and affinity (K_d). In contrast, slow dissociating drugs (**a**, *red*) will occupy the receptor (**b**, *red line*) beyond the decrease in drug concentration

ment of the stomach, a direct result of H_2R antagonism, indeed seems to increase the development of gastric tumors [33–35].

To summarize, ligand-binding kinetics can have a profound effect on the therapeutic efficacy of drug molecules. It will depend on the specific drug target whether long or short residence time ligands have a clinical advantage. A valid drug discovery strategy could therefore be to develop both long and short residence antihistamines in lead optimization to have a diverse set of ligands as a starting point.

2 Quantifying Ligand-Receptor Residence Times

2.1 Binding Conditions

Ligand-receptor-binding rate constants are context dependent and can vary depending on conditions such as the temperature, pH, and ionic strength of the buffer. Differences in both temperature and pH have, e.g., considerable effects on the kinetic-binding rate constants of H_1R antihistamines [26]. Decreased temperature generally decreases association and dissociation rate, but the absolute effect can differ between ligand-receptor pair. Occasionally, low temperatures are used to slow down binding, when kinetic-binding rates are too fast to determine experimentally [36]. Mixed effects of the pH on the kinetic-binding rate constants are known being receptor and ligand specific [26]. Moreover, the ionic strength can affect the association rate constant of charged ligands [37–39]. Interestingly, many binding studies, including studies that measure the kinetic-binding rate constants, use low ionic strength buffers based on Tris or HEPES which have much lower ionic strengths than observed in vivo (50–250 mM [40]). Since ligands targeting aminergic GPCRs typically require a positive charge to make an ionic interaction with the D3.32 in the transmembrane pocket, they might be susceptible to ionic strength effects.

2.2 Radioligand-Binding Studies

Radioligand-binding experiments are most frequently used to measure ligand-binding kinetics to GPCRs. To this end, radioligands are incubated with cells or cell homogenate expressing the desired receptor. Next, free radioligand is washed away and bound radioligand is quantified. By isolating the bound fraction of radioligands after different incubation times, the binding of the radioligand over time can be obtained. Radioligand binding can also be used in competition with an unlabeled ligand to indirectly determine the binding rate constants of the latter. An important benefit of radioligand binding is that receptors can be used in their native membrane bound state. A downside of conventional radioligand-binding methods is a low throughput, since receptor bound radioligand has to be separated from free radioligand. Limitations of this *stop-flow*-based determination of binding are discussed and alternatives are suggested to tackle throughput issues.

2.2.1 Production of Cell Homogenate from Transiently Transfected Cells

Originally, radioligand-binding assays were performed on homogenized native tissues expressing the relevant receptor [41, 42]. Nowadays, it is more common to use (homogenized) immortalized cell lines expressing the receptor of interest either endogenously (often lower expression) or upon stable/transient transfection (often higher expression). Highly expressing transfected cells are often first choice for kinetic-binding studies, because it is crucial to have a good signal-to-noise ratio, since differences in curvature that shape the fitted k_{on} and k_{off} rates are often quite subtle. However, it has to be realized that receptor overexpression might increase the number of receptor dimers that might display positive or negative-binding cooperativity between their ligand-binding sites [43, 44]. Moreover, receptor densities could possibly also affect rebinding when ligands diffusion rates are limited [45]. Preferably, experiments are designed in such a way that rebinding does not affect the measured kinetic-binding rate constants (dissociation experiments, Sects. 2.2.3 and 2.2.5).

Method

1. Human embryonic kidney (HEK)293T cells are cultured in culture medium (i.e., Dulbecco's modified eagle medium (DMEM) containing 10% fetal bovine serum and 1% penicillin/streptomycin) in a humidified incubator at 37 °C and 5% CO_2.
2. One day before transfection 2×10^6 HEK293T cells are seeded in 7 mL culture medium in a 10 cm dish.
3. The next day, 5 μg DNA encoding the target receptor in 250 μL sterile NaCl solution (150 mM) is mixed with 30 μg 25-kDa linear polyethylenimine in 250 μL sterile NaCl solution (150 mM). The mixture is vortexed and incubated for 15 min. In the meantime, culture medium is refreshed with 7 mL new medium. After gentle resuspension (i.e., no vortexing), the transfection mixture is added dropwise to the cells.
4. 48 h later, cells are washed with PBS, collected and stored as dry pellets at ≤−20 °C before further experimentation.
5. To prepare cell homogenate, the pellets are thawed on ice and resuspended in ice-cold-binding buffer (e.g., 50 mM Na_2HPO_4/KH_2PO_4, pH 7.4). Cells are subsequently homogenized into fragments by an ultrasonic cell disruptor.
6. All models that describe a relation of the ligand concentration in the buffer assume that this concentration remains constant over time. In reality, however, binding of ligand to the receptor will decrease ligand concentration in solution. This *ligand depletion* is often assumed to be neglectable when bound ligand is less than 10% of the added radioligand concentration [46]. For radioligands, this can be easily determined by quantifying the concentration of the added ligand compared to the receptor-bound ligand. As a general rule for experiments with increasing concentrations of radioligand, the total receptor concentration should be less than 0.1 times the K_d value [47].

2.2.2 Terminating Binding Reactions and Quantifying Activity

Bound radioligand is often quantified using a radioactivity scintillation detector. If free radioligand is not separated from bound radioligand, it is normally impossible to quantify the latter. Since kinetic experiments require rapid termination and washing it is advisable to use filtration with ice-cold wash buffer to minimize undesired dissociation. Alternatively, scintillation proximity assays detect bound radioligand more efficiently than free radioligand, and consequently do not require a separation step (Sect. 2.2.9).

Method

1. Half an hour before the binding reaction is terminated, 96-well GF/C filter plates are presoaked in 0.5% 750 kDa branched polyethylenimine.
2. At the desired time point (see the specific assay format below) terminate the binding reactions over the 96-well filter plate using vacuum filtration, trapping the cell homogenate on the filter.
3. Residual free radioligand is removed by three rapid wash steps using ice-cold wash buffer (e.g., Tris–HCl, pH 7.4).
4. Filterplates are then dried in a stove at 52 °C for >45 min.
5. Next, scintillation liquid is added 25 μL per well, and bound radioligand is quantified using a radioactivity scintillation detector after a delay of >200 min to reduce variability in data.

2.2.3 Radioligand-Binding Kinetics

Kinetic-binding rate constants of radioligands can be directly quantified by measuring receptor occupancy in time. Ligand binding to a single site on the receptor with a one-step binding mechanism (Fig. 1) can be described as a function of time by Eq. (1):

$$Y = Y_{\max} \cdot \left(1 - e^{-k_{obs} \cdot t}\right) \tag{1}$$

Here, Y is the receptor-bound radioligand, $Y_{\max}$ is the radioligand binding at equilibrium, and k_{obs} is the rate in which equilibrium is approached (time^{-1}). The k_{obs} is dependent on the k_{on}, k_{off}, and ligand concentration [L]. This relationship is defined by Eq. (2):

$$k_{obs} = k_{on} \cdot [L] + k_{off} \tag{2}$$

To measure ***radioligand association***, cell homogenate expressing the receptor is incubated with radioligand for various time periods. The time required to reach 50% equilibrium binding equals $\ln 2/k_{obs}$ (Fig. 4a). Since k_{obs} encompasses both k_{on} and k_{off}, one cannot extract these binding rate constants from a single association curve. One way to determine k_{on} and k_{off} is to use multiple radioligand concentrations, leading to multiple k_{obs} values (Fig. 4a). The k_{obs} increases linearly as a function of radioligand concentration with k_{on} and k_{off} being the slope and intersection with Y-axis, respectively (Fig. 4b). Alternatively, kinetic-binding rate constants can be

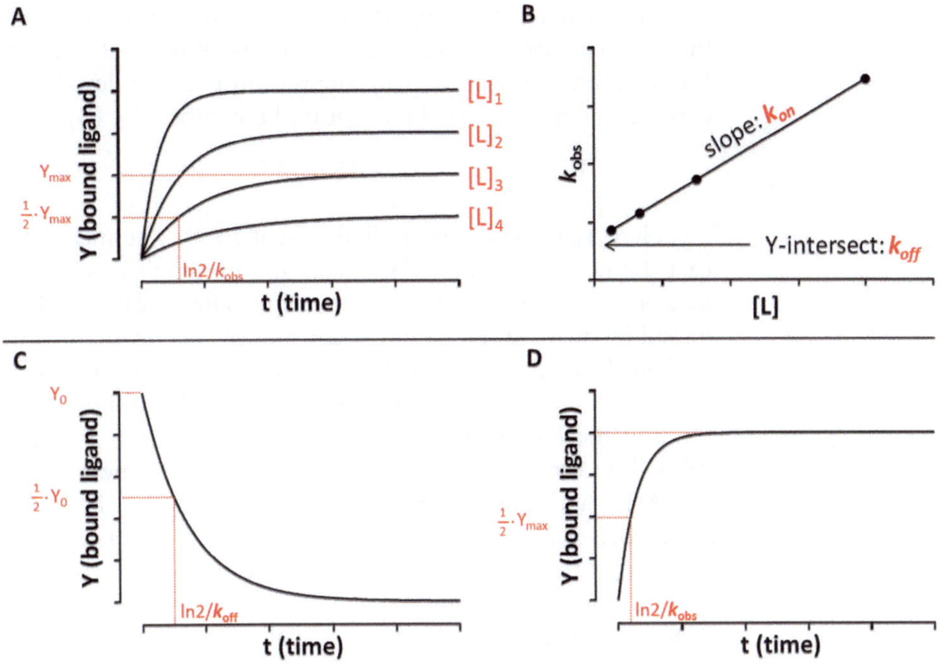

Fig. 4 Dissecting association and dissociation rates from radioligand-binding experiments. There are two common methods to dissect the binding rate constants of radioligands. The first (**a** + **b**) uses the fact that the speed in which equilibrium is obtained (k_{obs}) is dependent on the ligand concentration used. The k_{obs} can be measured by obtaining the maximal binding for a concentration of ligand and then to determine how long it takes to reach half maximal binding. This time correlates to the ratio of ln2 over the k_{obs}. (**a**) Measuring multiple k_{obs} can be used to distil the association and dissociation rates of the radioligand (**b**). Another way to obtain the binding rate constants (**c** + **d**) is to measure both the time to obtain half maximal dissociation (**c**) and to obtain the time to reach half maximal association (**d**). The time to reach half maximal dissociation is the ratio of ln2 over the k_{off}. Using Eq. (2) and the determined k_{obs} and k_{off}, the k_{on} can be calculated

determined from an association binding with one concentration radioligand in combination with a dissociation experiment (Fig. 4c–d). In the association curve the k_{obs} is obtained and from the dissociation curve the k_{off} is obtained (see below) so that k_{on} can be calculated using Eq. (2).

The *radioligand dissociation* from the receptor depends only on k_{off} (Fig. 1). Usually, cell homogenate is first incubated with radioligand for a certain amount of time before dissociation is initiated. To this end, either free radioligand is removed or excess unlabeled ligand is added so that radioligand rebinding is impossible. In the first method, the radioligand is often diluted to an amount that equilibrium switches entirely to the unbound state of the receptor ("infinite dilution"). Diluting the ligand concentration below 1% of its respective K_d value, it should be ensured that almost all ligands (≥99%) should have dissociated at equilibrium. The second method is probably best equipped to deal with rebinding, since wash steps and infinite dilution strategies might allow rebinding in the case that micro compartments near the receptor (like membrane structures) retain high concentrations of ligand [9]. Radioligand dissociation from the receptor can be described by an exponential decrease of ligand-bound receptor (Eq. (3)):

$$Y = Y_0 \cdot e^{-k_{off} \cdot t} \tag{3}$$

Here Y_0 is the bound radioligand at $t = 0$. The model assumes that the radioligand fully dissociates and binding (Y) should therefore be corrected for nonspecific binding. The k_{off} can then be determined by dividing the natural logarithm of two by the time needed for half the receptor-bound radioligand to dissociate (Fig. 4c).

However, the assumption that the ligand has a simple one-step binding mechanism to a single site of the receptor is not always valid. For example, the H_3R agonists [^{3}H]N-α-methylhistamine (NAMH) and [^{3}H]R-α-methylhistamine (RAMH) showed biphasic dissociation and biphasic association (for NAMH) curves, indicating that their binding mechanism might be more complex than the aforementioned one-step binding mechanism to a single site (Table 1) [51, 53]. This can be visualized by plotting the natural logarithm of specific binding over time, from either a radioligand association or dissociation experiment. Normally, this would lead to a straight line unless there is biphasic binding. Indeed, agonists might display more complicated binding mechanisms involving receptor isomerization to distinct conformational states and coupling to G proteins. If ligand binding is dependent on isomerization of the receptor (e.g., induced fit mechanism and conformational selection), it is expected that a nonlinear relation exists between k_{obs} and the ligand concentration [60, 61]. In these cases, where the binding does not comply with the presumed one-step binding mechanism to a single site of the receptor, it might be best to estimate a global k_{off} in a dissociation experiment, since this is the parameter that is thought to drive the functional efficacy of a drug in vivo. Moreover, dissociation is less complex for interpretation than the multifactorial association.

Association Binding: Method

1. Prepare the desired radioligand concentration(s) in binding buffer and dispense 25 μL per well. When using one concentration, prepare triplicate rows on a 96-well plate (4 times K_d as final concentration in the assay, *see* **Note 1**), when using multiple concentrations radioligand use duplicate rows with four different concentrations (0.25, 0.66, 1.5, and 4 times K_d as final concentrations in the assay, *see* **Note 1**).
2. Add 25 μL competitive unlabeled ligand (~4000 times K_i as final concentration in the assay, *see* **Note 1**) to the first column to quantify nonspecific radioligand binding, and 25 μL binding buffer to all remaining wells.

Table 1
Ligand-binding kinetics of radiolabeled antihistamines

Radioligand	K_d (k_{off}/k_{on}) (nM)	k_{on} (1/M min × 10)	k_{off} (1/min)	Notes	Refs.
[^{125}I] iodoaminopotentidine	0.43	30	0.013	gpH$_2$R (25 °C)	[48]
[^{3}H]tiotidine	10.6	11.6	0.123	gpH$_2$R (20 °C)	[49]
[^{125}I]iodoproxyfan	0.04	8380	0.332	rH$_3$R (25 °C)	[50]
[^{3}H]mepyramine	4	220	0.13	hH$_1$R (25 °C)	[26]
[^{3}H]levocetirizine	1.2	1.7	0.0020	hH$_1$R (25 °C)	[26]
[^{3}H]N-α-methylhistamine	1.1; 0.8	34; 660	0.036; 0.5	mfH$_3$R[a]; biphasic (30 °C)	[51]
[^{3}H]doxepin	0.96; 0.13	280; 600	0.27; 0.08	hH$_1$R; biphasic (37 °C)	[52]
[^{3}H]R-α-methylhistamine	3.9; 3.2	460; 24	1.8; 0.077	rH$_3$R; biphasic (30 °C)	[53]
[^{3}H]desloratadine	1.4	11	0.015[b]	hH$_1$R; aberrant dissociation[b] (RT)	[27]
[^{3}H]GSK189254	0.13	5600	0.72	hH$_3$R (37 °C)	[54]
[^{3}H]clobenpropit	0.05	700	0.044	gpH$_3$R (21 °C)	[55]
[^{3}H]A-349821	0.02	3500	0.07	hH$_3$R (RT)	[56]
[^{3}H]UR-PI294	1.5	140	0.21	hH$_3$R (22 °C)	[57]
[^{3}H]UR-PI294	12	2.7	0.033	hH$_4$R (22 °C)	[57]
[^{3}H]UR-DE257	20	0.86	0.024[c]	hH$_2$R; biphasic[c] (22 °C)	[58]
[^{3}H]histamine	10.7	7.8	0.08	hH$_4$R (25 °C)	[59]

Various radioligands for which association and or dissociation-binding experiments were performed were evaluated for their kinetic binding rate constants. Moreover, many examples of radioligands were found for which biphasic binding was observed, implying a more complicated binding mechanism. This means that obtained kinetic binding rate constants do probably not accurately reflect the binding of the ligand.

[a] *Macaca fascicularis*

[b] [^{3}H]desloratadine had much slower dissociation than expected based on the association-binding experiment. In a 6 h time frame hardly any dissociation was observed in a dissociation experiment

[c] Slow phase of dissociation much slower than depicted in table

3. After preheating all components to 25 °C, start binding reactions at different time points by adding 50 μL receptor-expressing cell homogenate to the wells (Sect. 2.2.1), and incubate under temperature-controlled conditions (25 °C) and gentle agitation (Fig. 5).
   - Use a different column for each time point with in total 11 time points (columns 2–12). The required incubation time

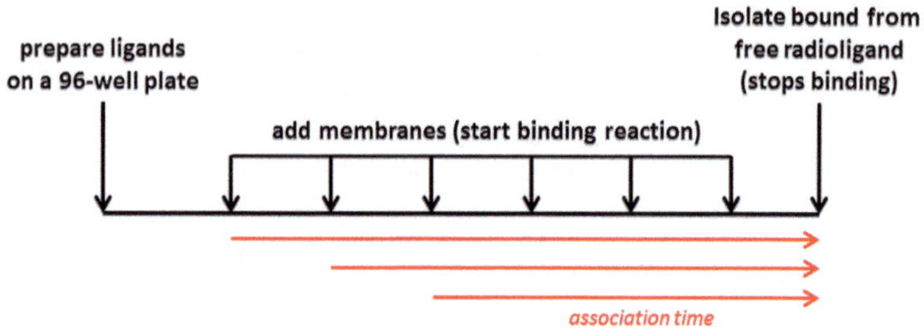

Fig. 5 (Competitive) ligand association-binding logistics

is dependent on the respective radioligand (Sect. 4.1). For [^{3}H]mepyramine the following time points in minutes could be used: 1, 2, 3, 4, 6, 9, 12, 16, 20, 25, 30. Incubations are started in the inverse order with all incubation times coming to an end simultaneously.

- Cell homogenate can be added at any time to the first column if nonspecific binding does not increase over time (*see* **Note 2**).

4. After the completion of the desired incubation times, all incubations are simultaneously terminated and bound ligand is quantified (Sect. 2.2.2).
5. Determined binding levels are baseline corrected for nonspecific binding determined in the first column determined for each concentration. Binding over time is analyzed by nonlinear regression using equation of Fig. 1b (blue panel) to obtain k_{on} and k_{off} (e.g., using Prism 6.0). Since the linear relationship between k_{obs} and $[L]$ is incorporated in the model, it is no longer required to extract the k_{on} and k_{off} from this straight line as in Fig. 4b. This can be done with the model that describes binding as a function of the bound ligand at equilibrium (Y_{max}), or a model in which equilibrium-bound radioligand is furthermore expressed as the B_{max}, ligand concentration, and the ratio between k_{off} and k_{on} (which reflects the K_d). The latter is recommended. If this experiment is performed in combination with a dissociation experiment, analysis is the same but the k_{off} should be constrained to the predetermined value of the radioligand.

Dissociation Binding: Method

1. Prepare 50 μL of the desired radioligand concentration (e.g., 4 times K_d as final concentration in the assay, *see* **Note 3**) in triplicate rows of a 96-well plate.
2. All components are preheated all to 25 °C before binding reaction is started. 50 μL receptor-expressing cell homogenate is added to the wells (Sect. 2.2.1) and incubated until equilibrium is obtained for radioligand association, as was established with association binding (>3.5/k_{obs}) (Fig. 6a). Alternatively, all

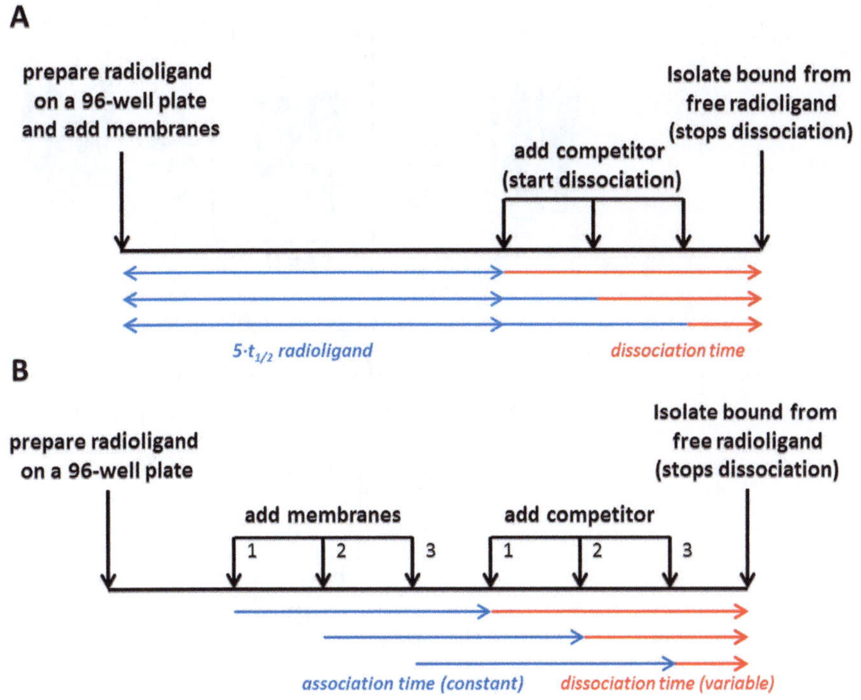

Fig. 6 Dissociation-binding logistics

samples are pre-incubated for exactly the same time before dissociation is initiated in the next step (Fig. 6b).

3. Dissociation is initiated at different time points, by adding an excess of competitive unlabeled ligand (~4000 times K_i as final concentration).
   - Use a different column for each time point.
   - To determine the binding at Y_0, the first column should not be supplemented with unlabeled competitor.
   - Added volume should be ≤10% of total volume to prevent dilution of the radioligand. In this case, use 11 μL with a concentration that is ten times the final concentration.
4. After approximately five times radioligand dissociation half-life, dissociation reactions are simultaneously terminated and bound ligand is quantified (Sect. 2.2.2). Binding over time is analyzed with the model in Fig. 1b (green panel) using nonlinear regression. To accommodate nonspecific binding, the model can be adjusted as in Eq. (4):

$$Y = (Y_0 - NS) \cdot e^{-k_{off} \cdot t} + NS \tag{4}$$

2.2.4 Competitive Ligand-Binding Kinetics

Kinetic-binding rate constants of unlabeled ligands can be indirectly determined using a competitive radioligand. Motulsky and Mahan have developed a mathematical model to describe radioligand association binding to the receptor in the presence of a

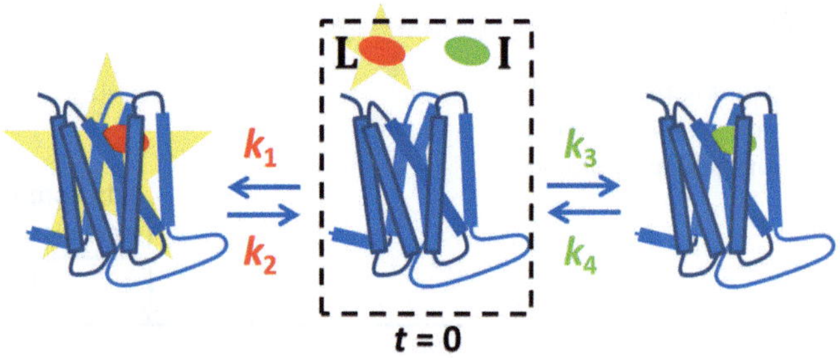

$$KA = k_1 \cdot [L] + k_2$$
$$KB = k_3 \cdot [I] + k_4$$
$$S = \sqrt{(KA - KB)^2 + 4 \cdot k_1 \cdot k_3 \cdot [L] \cdot [I]}$$
$$KF = \frac{1}{2} \cdot (KA + KB + S)$$
$$KS = \frac{1}{2} \cdot (KA + KB - S)$$
$$Q = \frac{B_{max} * k_1 \cdot [L]}{KF - KS}$$
$$Y = Q \cdot \left(\frac{k_4 \cdot (KF - KS)}{KF \cdot KS} + \frac{k_4 - KF}{KF} \cdot e^{-KF \cdot t} - \frac{k_4 - KS}{KS} \cdot e^{-KS \cdot t} \right)$$

Fig. 7 Competitive binding of two ligands to a receptor. Receptor is simultaneously subjected to the labeled ligand L and unlabeled ligand I. Binding of the labeled ligand can be measured and is described by the depicted mathematical model. In this model k_1 (k_{on}) and k_2 (k_{off}) are the association and dissociation rate constants of the radioligand, respectively, whereas the k_3 (k_{on}) and k_4 (k_{off}) are the association and dissociation rate constants of the unlabeled ligand. [L] and [I] are the concentrations of the labeled and unlabeled ligands, respectively. *Y* is the amount of receptor bound by the radioligand over time (*t*). B_{max} is the signal of *Y* when all receptors are occupied. When using this model, [L], [I], k_1, and k_2 are constrained to constant values

competitive unlabeled ligand [62]. This model assumes that both ligands are binding the receptor according to the law of mass action in a one-step binding reaction to the same site (i.e., no more than one ligand is bound at the same time), as depicted in Fig. 7. The k_{on} (k_1) and k_{off} (k_2) of the radioligand should be known, in order to determine the k_{on} ($k3$) and k_{off} (k_4) of the unlabeled ligand.

To initiate the experiment, both radioligand and one or more concentrations unlabeled ligand are simultaneously incubated with receptor-expressing cell homogenate for various incubation times. The use of multiple concentrations of unlabeled ligand results in a more robust estimation of k_3 and k_4 [54, 63]. A frequently used method to validate how well the model predicts the ligand-binding kinetics is to calculate the K_d from the obtained k_{on} and k_{off} values and compare it to predetermined K_i values derived from competition binding at equilibrium using the Cheng-Prusoff conversion

[64] (see Chap. 6). Another internal control would be to compare the k_1 and k_2 values of the radioligand to the k_3 and k_4 of the unlabeled analogue [25, 26].

Method

1. Prepare duplicate rows on a 96-well plate with 25 μL radioligand (e.g., 3 times K_d as final concentration, *see* **Note 1**) (Sect. 2.2.1) without and with three different concentrations unlabeled ligand (1, 3, and 10 times K_i as final concentrations in assay, *see* **Note 1**).
2. Add 25 μL competitive unlabeled ligand (~4000 times K_i as final concentration in the assay, *see* **Note 1**) to the first column to quantify nonspecific radioligand binding, and 25 μL binding buffer to all remaining wells.
3. After preheating all components to 25 °C, start the binding reaction at different time points by adding 50 μL receptor-expressing cell homogenate to the wells (Fig. 5).
   - Use a different column for each time point with in total 11 time points (columns 2–12). Required incubation time is dependent on the respective radioligand and unlabeled ligand (Sect. 4.1). For [^{3}H]mepyramine binding to the H_1R in competition with its unlabeled analogue, the following time points in minutes could be used: 1, 2, 3, 4, 6, 9, 12, 16, 20, 25, 30. Incubations are started in the inverse order with all incubation times coming to an end simultaneously.
   - Cell homogenate can be added at any time to the first column if nonspecific binding does not increase over time (*see* **Note 2**).
4. After the desired incubation times, reactions are simultaneously terminated and bound ligand is quantified (Sect. 2.2.2). Binding as a function of time is analyzed with the Motulsky-Mahan model using nonlinear regression with k_1, k_2, [L], and [I] as constraint values to obtain k_3 and k_4 (Fig. 7).

2.2.5 Dissociation of Unlabeled Ligands

If a complex binding mechanism for the unlabeled ligand is expected (e.g., Motulsky and Mahan model discussed in Sect. 2.2.4 does not fit the empirical data), the discussed method to determine the kinetic-binding rate constants is likely to be unfit for purpose. In order to still be able to measure a global dissociation rate, it would be easiest to specifically measure the dissociation of the unlabeled ligand. This can be done indirectly using a radioligand. It is required to know the equilibrium dissociation constants of unlabeled ligand and radioligands, since equipotent concentrations unlabeled ligand (as discussed in Sect. 4.1) are used in this assay. First, the receptor is pre-equilibrated with a 3 times K_i concentration unlabeled ligand to yield 75% receptor occupancy. Subsequent dilution with high concentration radioligand results in a new equilibrium in which almost all unlabeled ligand is displaced. For example diluting 10 μL of the pre-incubated unlabeled ligand/cell homogenate solution with 190 μL of a 20 times K_d concentration radioligand would lead to a situation in which <1% of the receptors are still occupied with unlabeled ligand, whereas the radioligand will occupy >94% of the receptors. Since radioligand binding requires first dissociation of the unlabeled ligand from the receptor, the association of radioligand over time reflects the dissociation rate of the unlabeled ligand [65]. It is important that the radioligand is binding sufficiently fast so that almost all binding sites are instantly occupied between interspacing time points. Furthermore, the radioligand should have a high concentration (relative to its K_d) to ensure that rebinding of the unlabeled ligand is impossible. As a final note, caution should be taken with interpreting the initial "dissociation," since the association of radioligand might be more rapid for early time points considering that not all receptors were occupied by unlabeled ligand during pre-equilibration. This is often inevitable, since radioligand concentrations can often not be used at concentrations that would fully displace saturating concentrations unlabeled ligand.

Method (for prerequisites *see* **Note 4**)

1. 20 μL suspensions cell homogenate are prepared in tubes with a single tube for each unlabeled ligand and time point. *Exactly* 60 min (*see* **Note 5**) before dissociation of the unlabeled ligand is planned (Fig. 8), 20 μL binding buffer or unlabeled ligand (3 times K_d as final concentration) is added to the respective tubes. The tubes are sealed, mixed, and incubated at 25 °C. These mixtures are then divided into triplicates of 10 μL per well on a 96-well plate, with one column for each desired dissociation time.
2. Dissociation of unlabeled ligand is started by adding 190 μL volume containing a 20 times K_d concentration radioligand. Initiate dissociation separately for each column at the desired time points.

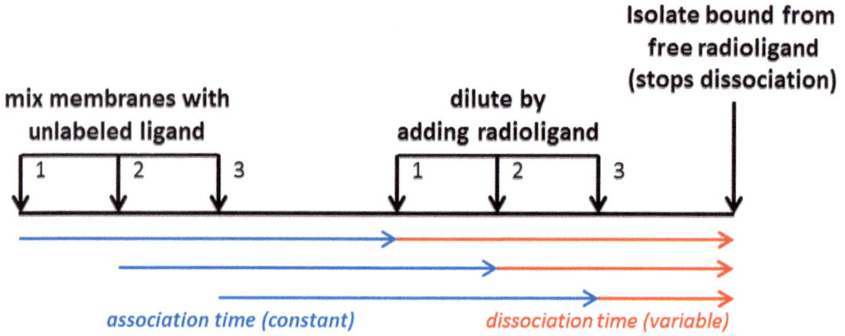

Fig. 8 Dissociation of unlabeled ligands logistics

3. Reactions are simultaneously terminated and bound ligand is quantified (Sect. 2.2.2). The radioligand association rate to full (>94%) receptor occupancy determines the temporal resolution in which dissociation of the unlabeled ligand can be followed. As a control, the amount of bound radioligand in the absence of unlabeled ligand should therefore approximate binding at equilibrium already at the first time point. Higher radioligand concentrations can be used to increase the k_{obs} and consequently the temporal resolution. To quantify the dissociation of the unlabeled ligand, the data can again be fitted by nonlinear regression to Eq. (4) (Sect. 2.2.3).

2.2.6 Dual-Point Competition Assay to Determine Relative-Binding Kinetics of Unlabeled Ligands

Association competition-binding experiments to determine the binding kinetic rate constants for unlabeled ligands are quite laborious considering all required time points and concentrations. To quickly distinguish whether unlabeled ligands dissociate faster or slower from the receptor as compared to the radioligand, a dual-point competition assay was designed [66]. This method requires only two time points and a single concentration of unlabeled ligand and works on the observation that unlabeled ligands that dissociate slower than the radioligand cause a typical overshoot pattern in radioligand binding (Fig. 9, purple), whereas unlabeled ligands with faster dissociation rates than the radioligand will delay the association of the latter to the receptor (Fig. 9, green). Two time points are then taken to calculate whether there is an overshoot pattern, or delayed association for the radioligand. The first time point is taken as the time needed for the radioligand, in the absence of unlabeled ligand, to reach ~90% binding of the binding at equilibrium (i.e., $t_1 \sim 2.3/k_{obs}$). This time point would lead to a good discrimination in binding levels as exemplified in Fig. 9. The second time point (t_2) should be taken as the point where equilibrium of all ligands is expected. An equipotent concentration (see Sect. 4.1) for all tested unlabeled ligands is used in competition with a constant concentration radioligand. The kinetic rate index (KRI) is then calculated by dividing the amount of bound radioligand at t_1 by the amount of radioligand bound at t_2. A drawback of this dual-point competition method is that it only allows an approximation of the dissociation rate and is therefore not reliable when ranking multiple slow dissociating ligands.

Method (for prerequisites *see* **Note 6**)

1. Add 25 μL unlabeled ligand (10 times K_d as final concentration, *see* **Note 1**) to six wells of a 96-well plate.
2. Add 25 μL radioligand (3 times K_d as final concentration, *see* **Note 1**) to all wells.
3. After preheating all components to 25 °C, start binding reaction by adding 50 μL receptor-expressing cell homogenate to

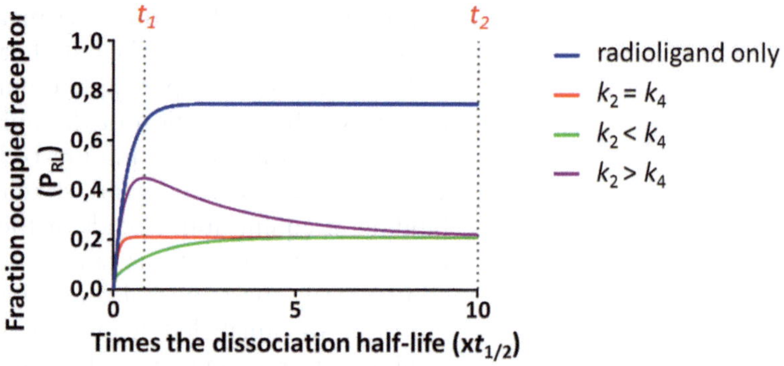

Fig. 9 Dual-point competition binding. Radioligand-binding curves at a 3 times K_d concentration ligand, depicted as a function of time (depicted as dissociation half-life's of the radioligand) in the absence (*blue*) or presence of equipotent concentration unlabeled ligands. If both radioligand and unlabeled ligand have similar dissociation rates, binding of the radioligand will be described by the *red curve*. An unlabeled ligand dissociating five times faster than the radioligand will delay binding of the radioligand (*green*), whereas unlabeled ligands that dissociate slower than the radioligand result in an overshoot for binding of the radioligand at early time points (*purple*). Binding of the radioligand will be measured after two incubation times: t_1, after which 90% of radioligand in the absence of competitor has bound the receptor, and t_2, after which all ligands are expected to have reached equilibrium. As can be seen, fast dissociating (*green*) and slow dissociating (*purple*) ligands will have a different level of binding at t_1, but not t_2 (since equipotent concentrations are used). By taking the ratio of measured radioligand binding at t_1 and t_2, the kinetic rate index (KRI) of unlabeled ligands can be determined

the first three wells of each unlabeled ligand. Do this with enough time before the planned termination of the binding reaction to allow equilibrium for each ligand (t_2 in Fig. 10).

4. Add 50 μL cell homogenate to the three remaining wells for each unlabeled ligand corresponding to a ~$2.3/k_{obs}$ incubation time (t_1 in Fig. 10).
5. After the desired incubation times, reactions are simultaneously terminated and bound ligand is quantified (Sect. 2.2.2). Estimate relative dissociation rate of unlabeled ligands by dividing the amount of bound radioligand at t_1 by the amount of bound radioligand at t_2 (KRI). KRI > 1 indicates slower dissociation of unlabeled ligand as compared to radioligand, whereas KRI < 1 indicates the opposite.

2.2.7 Two-Step Binding to Determine Relative Binding Kinetics of Unlabeled Ligands

Another efficient method compared to conventional analysis (Sect. 2.2.4) estimates the relative dissociation rates for unlabeled competitive ligands. For this method it is first required to determine IC_{50} values of the unlabeled ligands in equilibrium radioligand

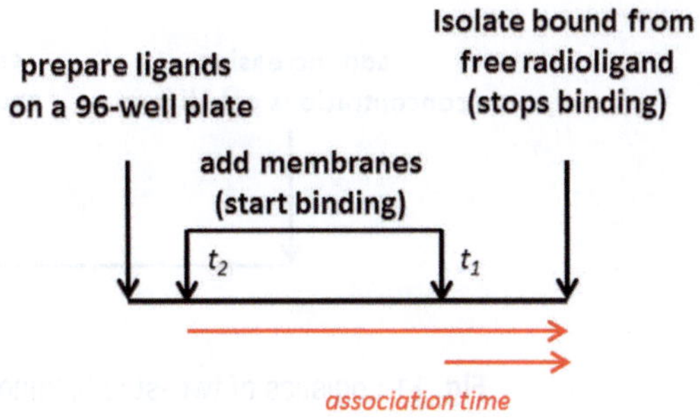

Fig. 10 Dual-point competition logistics

competition-binding experiments [67]. Next, receptor-expressing cell homogenate is pre-incubated with four to eight times IC_{50} concentrations of unlabeled ligand (step 1), followed by a filtration step in which the free ligand is removed and cell homogenate is incubated with the radioligand for a period of ~$2.3/k_{obs}$ (step 2). The k_{obs} can be adjusted by varying the concentration of radioligand (Eq. (2)). Rapid dissociating unlabeled ligands will hardly delay radioligand association, whereas slow dissociating competitors will make it impossible for the radioligand to bind and consequently delay its association. Although a very useful technique in terms of the throughput, only relative estimates of the dissociation rates can be obtained. This method is unable to discriminate unlabeled ligands that have a k_{off} that greatly exceeds the k_{obs} of radioligand association. In this limiting case, the association of the radioligand would be completely independent of the unlabeled ligand. An additional concern would be that not all free unlabeled ligand is removed leading to overestimation of the residence time; therefore, follow-up validation of selected hits is advisable.

Method (for prerequisites *see* **Notes 6** and 7)

1. 50 μL receptor-expressing cell homogenate (Sect. 2.2.1) is incubated with and without 50 μL of a solution containing a 4 times IC_{50} final concentration (*see* **Note 3**) unlabeled ligand in triplicate at 25 °C. Free unlabeled ligand is removed by filtration over a glass filter. Next, the filter is immediately soaked with 50 μL of a 3 K_d concentration radioligand.
2. Radioligand binding is terminated after an incubation time of ~$2.3/k_{obs}$ (Fig. 11) by vacuum filtration and subsequent wash steps with ice-cold wash buffer to remove free radioligand (Sect. 2.2.2).
3. Bound radioligand is quantified by scintillation counting. Binding levels are inversely proportional to the residence time of the unlabeled ligand.

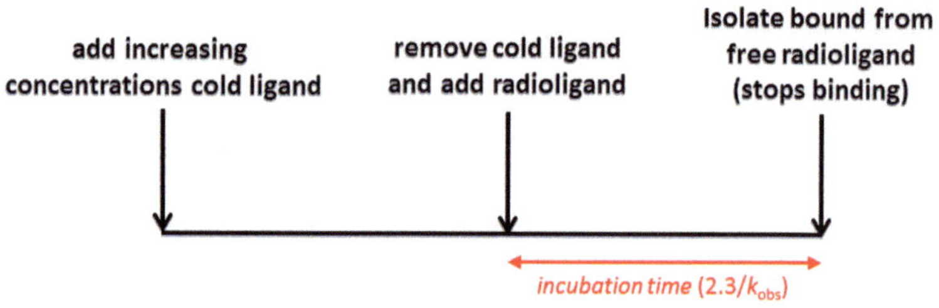

Fig. 11 Logistics of two-step binding experiments for fast ligands

2.2.8 Two-Step Binding (Unbiased) to Determine Dissociation Rate Constants of Unlabeled Ligands

The dissociation rate of a pre-incubated unlabeled competitive ligand can also be measured without prior knowledge of the unlabeled ligand using an alternative two-step binding approach [68]. However, this approach does require the association and dissociation rate constants (k_1 and k_2, respectively) of the radioligand. In Fig. 12, it is shown how this method can be used to calculate the dissociation rate constant of the unlabeled ligand (k_4). A concentration series of unlabeled ligand is pre-incubated with receptor-expressing cell homogenate in duplicate (step 1). Next, one of the duplicates is washed after an equilibration step (~30 min) to remove free ligand. Radioligand is subsequently added to all samples (step 2) and incubated for "t" minutes before the reaction is terminated. Depending on how fast the unlabeled ligand dissociates, the radioligand will not be able to bind the receptor to the same extent as in the absence of pre-incubated competitor. By increasing the incubation time "t," the more unlabeled ligand will dissociate and the less radioligand binding is affected.

The concentration unlabeled ligand corresponding to 25 times the IC_{50} value of the competition-binding curve in which free unlabeled ligand was not washed away (i.e., blue curve in Fig. 12b), will occupy >95% of the receptors after pre-incubation. The amount of radioligand bound to the receptor, after washing away this saturating concentration unlabeled ligand, is $[RL]_{I,\ max\ displacement}$ (i.e., "2" in Fig. 12b), whereas radioligand-bound receptor in the absence of unlabeled ligand is $[RL]_{no\ competitor}$. The dissociation rate constant (k_4) of the unlabeled ligand can then be calculated using the equation in Fig. 12a and known values [L], k_1 and k_2, of the radioligand. Moreover, it is assumed that all free unlabeled ligand is removed after the wash step, if not this will lead to an overestimation of the residence time (experiments with adherent cells are easier to wash than cell homogenates).

When pre-incubated unlabeled ligand dissociates completely within the time frame of the experiment or does not dissociate enough, the dissociation rate constant (k_4) cannot be determined. Between 20 and 80% dissociation of the initially bound unlabeled ligand should allow robust fitting of its k_{off}. This might be adjusted for by changing the incubation time. Advantage of using this two-step model compared to the Motulsky and Mahan model (Sect. 2.2.4) is that there are only two different time-points where

A

$$\frac{[RL]_{I,\text{max displacement}}}{[RL]_{\text{no antagonist}}} = \frac{(a+b)}{a}$$

$$a = \frac{k_1 \cdot [L] \cdot (1 - e^{-(k_1 \cdot [L] + k_2) \cdot t})}{k_1 \cdot [L] + k_2}$$

$$b = \frac{k_1 \cdot [L] \cdot (e^{-(k_1 \cdot [L] + k_2) \cdot t} - e^{-k_4 \cdot t})}{k_1 \cdot [L] + k_2 - k_4}$$

B

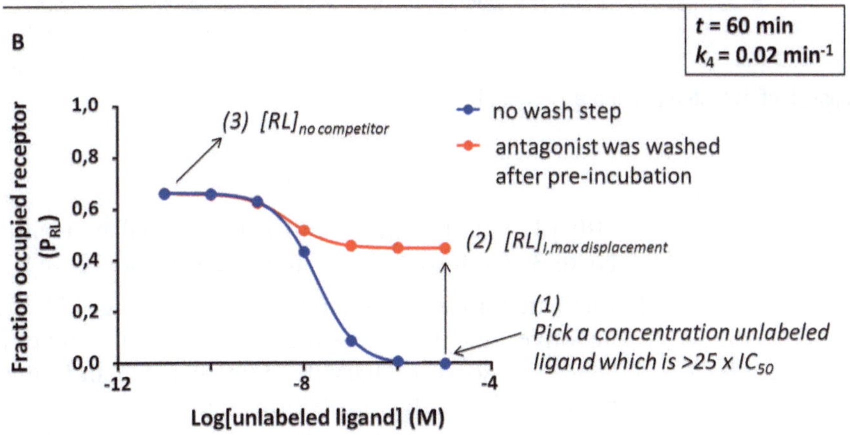

Fig. 12 Measuring dissociation rate using a two-step binding approach. In (**a**), a model is depicted which can be used to determine the dissociation rate of unlabeled ligands. This is done by an experiment (**b**) in which receptors are incubated with an increasing concentration unlabeled competitor. Receptors are subsequently incubated with a radioligand, either immediately (*blue curve*) or after washing away all free unlabeled ligands (*red curve*). From the radioligand displacement curve, depicted in *blue*, a concentration antagonist can be taken which displaces all radioligand (*1*). For the same concentration antagonist, the bound radioligand after washing away unlabeled ligand (*red curve*) can be determined (*2*; $[RL]_{I,\text{max displacement}}$). Bound radioligand in the absence of unlabeled ligand (*3*, $[RL]_{\text{no antagonist}}$) is determined from the concentration unlabeled ligand, in which no inhibition of the radioligand is observed. To calculate k_4, both k_1 and k_2 have to be known values

hands-on work is required. Additionally, both affinity (K_i) and residence time of the unlabeled ligand can be determined simultaneously. However, affinity can only be accurately determined if dissociation rate of unlabeled ligand is fast enough to reach equilibrium during the pre-incubation step for all concentrations unlabeled ligand (see also Sect. 4.1).

Method (*see* **Note 8**)

1. Seed receptor-expressing cells in a 96-well plate with a total volume of 100 μL fresh culture medium (cells should preferentially adhere better than HEK293T cells).
2. The next day, replace culture medium with 100 μL Hank's balanced salt solution (HBSS) containing increasing concentrations of unlabeled ligand with six wells per concentration. Also include a buffer only condition for six wells.
3. Remove free unlabeled ligand from three wells per used concentration of antagonist, after 1 h (Fig. 13), by several wash steps and reconstitute in 100 μL HBSS. Immediately after, add

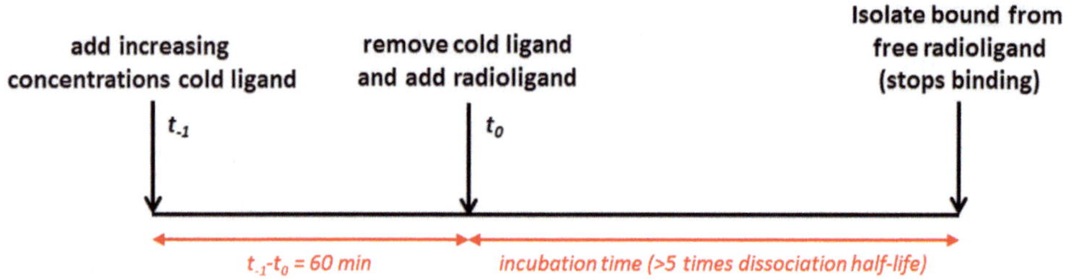

Fig. 13 Logistics of two-step binding experiments

100 μL radioligand (3 times K_d as final concentration, *see* **Note 3**) to all wells preheated to 25 °C (*see* **Note 9**).

4. Incubate for the desired incubation time (Fig. 13). This should be longer than five times the dissociation half-life of the radioligand. Dissociation half-life of unlabeled ligand can eventually be quantified if this incubation time corresponds to a time of ~0.32 to ~2.32 times the dissociation half-life of the respective unlabeled ligands (corresponding to approximately 20% to 80% dissociation of the unlabeled ligand).
5. Terminate all reactions simultaneously, by washing the cells three times with ice-cold wash buffer (e.g., Tris–HCl, pH 7.4) to remove unbound ligand. Cells are then lysed using lysis buffer (e.g., 1% NP-40, 0.5% sodium deoxycholate, 0.1% SDS) and mixed with water permissive scintillation liquid. Bound radioligand is then quantified using a radioactivity scintillation detector.
6. The IC_{50} value is determined from the competition-binding curve for which unlabeled ligand was not washed away using nonlinear regression. Select a concentration unlabeled ligand ≥25 times the IC_{50} value (concentration I,max displacement), and determine for this concentration the amount of bound radioligand after washing away free unlabeled ligand ($[RL]_{I,\text{ max displacement}}$). Determine the amount of bound radioligand in the absence of unlabeled ligand during pre-incubation ($[RL]_{\text{no antagonist}}$). Use these values together with k_1 and k_2 of the radioligand and the radioligand concentration to calculate the k_4 of the unlabeled ligand (Fig. 12a).

Notes

1. Concentration of ligands should be four times the final concentration to correct for dilution.
2. Verify that nonspecific binding does not increase over time. If it does increase over time, total binding should be corrected by the nonspecific binding determined for each individual time-point.

3. Concentration should be two times concentrated to compensate for dilution.
4. Equilibrium dissociation constants of unlabeled ligands (K_i) and radioligand (K_d), and k_1 and k_2 should be determined before the experiment.
5. Since for unlabeled ligands it will be unclear whether equilibrium has been reached within the pre-incubation, having a fixed pre-incubation time will ensure that binding levels unlabeled ligands upon dissociation is always the same.
6. The k_{obs} of association for a 3 times K_d concentration radioligand is determined prior to the experiment.
7. The IC_{50} of all antagonists is determined for inhibition of a 3 times K_d concentration radioligand.
8. Unlike conventional endpoint competition binding, this assay will at least indicate whether binding was indeed at equilibrium, since from the determined dissociation rate it can be calculated whether enough equilibration time was taken into account (>5 times the dissociation half-life of the slowest unlabeled ligand). Both the k_1 and k_2 of the radioligand should be determined before starting the experiment. However, no prior knowledge is required for binding affinity and kinetic-binding rate constants of unlabeled ligands.
9. Instead of using whole cells this experiment can also be performed with cell homogenates, as in Sect. 2.2.7. However, after washing away pre-incubated unlabeled ligand, half of the filtered samples should be reconstituted in buffer containing radioligand with the different concentrations unlabeled ligand, and half should be reconstituted in buffer with only radioligand.

2.3 Real-Time Readouts of Ligand-Binding Kinetics

Stop flow experiments are less useful when ligands reach equilibrium very fast due to the logistics of the experiment. However, if binding could be measured continuously it would be easier to have a well-defined association binding for fast compounds, especially when incubations can be started and measured simultaneously. Moreover, a big advantage of measuring binding continuously is that all required incubation times can be measured within the same incubation mixture. The same models as discussed for radioligand-binding studies (Sects. 2.2.3–2.2.8) can be used to analyze the data obtained with these real-time techniques.

2.3.1 Scintillation Proximity Assay (SPA)

Scintillation proximity assays use solid scintillation beads on which the target receptor is coupled, for example by linking the cell homogenate expressing the receptor to these beads. Since isotope disintegrations only convert into light when in very close proximity to these SPA beads, the enrichment of radioligands near the beads as a consequence of receptor binding can be specifically measured. Hence, this assay does not require separation of bound from free ligand and as such it can be measured continuously in a homogenous format [65]. However, temporal resolution might be limited by the specific activity of the radioligand, which determines the counting time per data point. Hitherto, SPA has only been used for equilibrium radioligand binding to histamine receptors [25, 69].

Method

1. Cell homogenates (Sect. 2.2.1) expressing the target receptor are incubated with PVT-PEI-WGA SPA, type A beads for 4 h at room temperature. For cell homogenates expressing the H_1R this is done by combining 1 mg of PVT-PEI-WGA SPA beads per 15 μg protein of cell homogenate in 50 μL total volume. For each well, 50 μL of this suspension is added to the respective ligands analogous to the fraction cell homogenate, as described in Sects. 2.2.3 and 2.2.4. The difference is that time points are no longer required as separate incubation conditions. After adding the cell homogenate/beads mixture, luminescence is immediately determined at various time points. Temporal resolution is limited by the speed of data acquisition (probably >10 s/well) and the number of samples.
2. Depending on the experiment, data are analyzed according to the respective models as discussed in Sects. 2.2.3 and 2.2.4.

2.3.2 Fluorescence Resonance Energy Transfer (FRET) and Bioluminescence Resonance Energy Transfer (BRET)-Based Ligand-Binding Assays

Binding of a fluorescent ligand to an N-terminally SNAP-tagged H_1R was measured in homogenous format using time-resolved fluorescence resonance energy transfer (TR-FRET) [70]. Fluorescent ligands are available for H_1R, H_2R, and H_3R [71–74]. This method allows continuous measurement of bound ligand by its FRET signal (Fig. 14); however, photobleaching of fluorescent ligands should be considered. Nevertheless, reasonable kinetic-binding rate constants for H_1R anthistamines were obtained as compared to radioligand-binding assays [70]. Another promising technique has also been recently published in which bound fluorescent ligand (acceptor) was not excited by a fluorescent donor but by bioluminescence [75]. In this case, the receptor N-terminus was fused to NanoLuc, a luciferase that yields bright luminescence upon conversion of the substrate furimazine. Upon binding of the fluorescent ligand this led to a high BRET signal over noise. The advantage of this BRET technique is that photobleaching is prevented; however, substrate availability might be limiting for prolonged incubation times. The SNAP-tag and NanoLuc methods are described below.

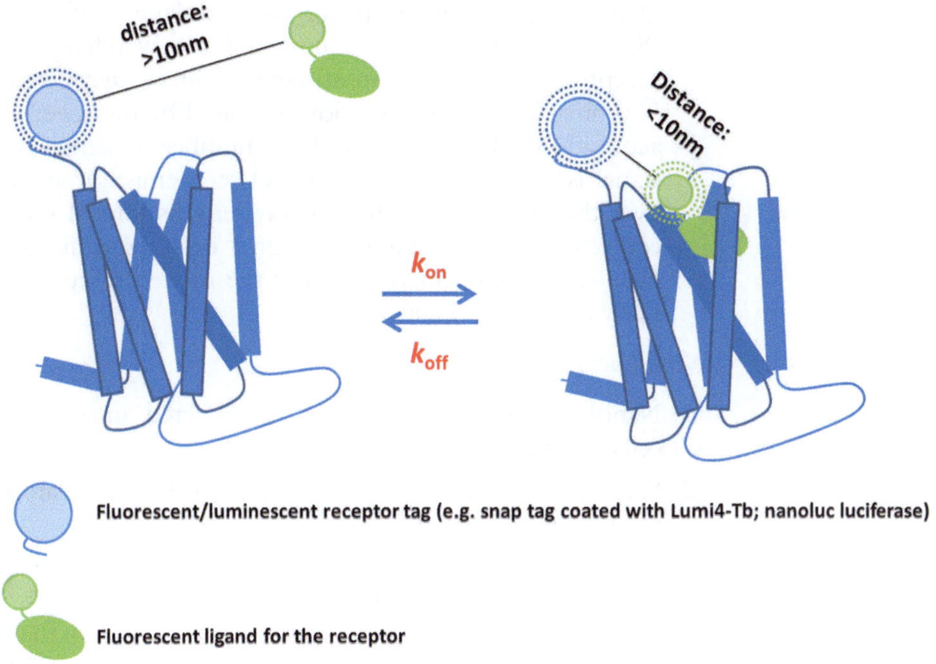

Fig. 14 Resonance energy transfer as a tool to study ligand binding. As an alternative to radioligands, fluorescent ligands can also be used to study binding. To do so, a fluorescent or luminescent energy donor is fused to the receptor, which emits light after excitation or by converting a substrate respectively. However, when a fluorescent ligand gets in close proximity to this energy donor, part of the energy will excite the fluorescent moiety of the ligand (acceptor) which will partially be emitted as light at a less energetic wavelength. Light emission of the ligand correlates therefore with a close proximity between ligand and receptor. This will be predominantly receptor-bound ligands

SNAP-tag: Method (for prerequisites *see* **Note 10**)

1. SNAP-tagged receptors are transfected into HEK293T cells (see Sect. 2.2.1).
2. The next day, cells are incubated with 6 mL 100 nM SNAP-Lumi4-Tb in taglite labeling medium for 1 h at 37 °C and 5% CO_2. Consecutively cells are detached from the plate using 5 mL enzyme free cell dissociation buffer. Using centrifugation and wash steps (5 min, 500 × *g*), the cells were washed three times in taglite labeling medium.
3. Ligands are dissolved in taglite labeling buffer and dispensed in a black 384-well plate in a total volume of 5 μL with a two times final concentration. Binding reactions are then started by adding 5 μL containing 5×10^4 labeled cells/mL. For dissociation experiments, dissociation is started by adding a small volume competitor (<10% final volume). It is best when binding can be started by machine injection so that signal can be immediately registered.
4. Signal is measured by exciting the SNAP-Lumi4-Tb with a wavelength of 337 nm. TR-FRET signal is then measured by

quantifying light intensity for the wavelength of the donor (SNAP-Lumi4-Tb; λ: 490 nm) and the wavelength of the acceptor (e.g., H_1R antihistamine *green mepyramine* λ: 520 nm). Temporal resolution is limited by the speed of data acquisition (>0.3 s/well) and the number of samples. FRET signal is expressed as the ratio between emission at 520 nm over the emission at 490 nm wavelengths. Signal should be corrected by subtracting the signal of nonspecific binding. Data can then be analyzed using the models discussed previously (Sects. 2.2.3 and 2.2.4).

NanoLuc: Method

1. NanoLuc-tagged receptors are transfected into HEK293T cells (see Sect. 2.2.1).
2. Seed receptor-expressing cells in a black 96-well plate with a total volume of 100 μL fresh culture medium.
3. Upon addition of 10 μM substrate (furimazine), BRET is measured by quantifying light intensity for the wavelength of the donor (NanoLuc; λ: 460 nm) and the wavelength of the acceptor (e.g., H_1R antihistamine *green mepyramine* λ: 520 nm). Temporal resolution is limited by the speed of data acquisition (>0.3 s/well) and the number of samples. BRET signal is expressed as the ratio between emission at 520 nm over the emission at 460 nm wavelengths. Signal should be corrected by subtracting the signal of nonspecific binding. Data can then be analyzed using the models discussed previously (Sects. 2.2.3 and 2.2.4).

2.3.3 Surface Plasmon Resonance (SPR)

Surface plasmon resonance is a technique that can measure the mass increase on a gold-layered glass chip. When a receptor is caught on this chip it can be used for binding studies, since the additional mass increase of a ligand binding the receptor can be registered by the SPR signal. Ligand is administrated as a continuous flow during which ligand binding will be detected. Protein stability remains a big challenge for using this technique in binding studies against GPCRs. Moreover, coupling strategies for GPCRs to the chip usually require purifying engineered protein, which was found to lead to discrepancies in ligand-binding data. New coupling methods have been developed and some successes were reported, though use of SPR for GPCRs has so far been limited [76, 77].

Notes

Fluorescent ligand for the target receptor is required and the receptor should be fused at the N-terminus with an SNAP-tag or NanoLuc. The used fluorescent ligand should be compatible with the used donor emission.

2.4 Functional Experiments to Determine Ligand-Binding Kinetics

Although functional experiments are harder to interpret for quantifying the kinetic-binding rate constants of ligands, they might give a better representation of their functional consequence under more relevant conditions. The possibilities of using functional experiments as handle in exploring the ligand-binding kinetics are therefore discussed.

2.4.1 Re-Equilibration Experiments (Insurmountable Antagonism)

A ligand bound to a receptor can only be displaced by another competitive ligand if there is sufficient time for the initially bound ligand to dissociate. This is the basis of insurmountable antagonism, which is frequently observed for different cellular responses. For example in the context of contraction of the guinea pig ileum (H_1R), cellular calcium response (H_1R), positive chronotropic response (H_2R), and stomach acid secretion (H_2R) insurmountable antagonism is observed for several histamine receptor antagonists [29, 31, 78, 79]. Fundamental for this effect is that receptor is preoccupied by the antagonist ($t = 0$ in Fig. 15), after which the cells are stimulated with agonist. For competitive orthosteric ligands it is expected that histamine dose-response curves shift limitless to the right without diminished maximal effect (E_{max}) in the presence of increasing concentrations antagonist since higher concentrations agonist are needed to initiate the same response. In contrast, if the antagonist does not have the chance to fully dissociate from the receptor in the incubation time of the experiment (incubation "t"), then at least part of the receptors will be unavailable for histamine-induced signaling. This can be seen as a depression of the maximal effect, because even high concentrations of histamine are unable to compete with an antagonist that will not dissociate from the receptor. Besides a depression of the E_{max} it is also possible to observe an initial shift to the right if there is a high receptor reserve, however for higher concentrations antagonist the E_{max} should eventually start to decrease [80]. A model was developed by Kenakin et al. in 2006 that predicts how the depression of the E_{max} is related to the dissociation rate of the antagonist and the time between agonist stimulation and quantification of the receptor response [81]. By pre-incubating with different concentrations of antagonist and subsequent stimulating with increasing concentrations of agonist, dose-response curves are obtained that shift to the right and/or show a depression in the E_{max} for high concentrations of antagonist (Fig. 15). There are three cases that can be distinguished: There is no E_{max} depression (fully competitive), there is an E_{max} depression that saturates for high concentration antagonists (hemi-equilibrium) and there is an E_{max} depression that abolishes all signal for high concentration antagonist (fully insurmountable). For the case in which hemi-equilibrium is obtained, the depicted model (Fig. 15) can be used to fit the dissociation rate constant of the antagonist, provided that equilibrium dissociation constant (K_A) of the agonist for the receptor is known [82, 83].

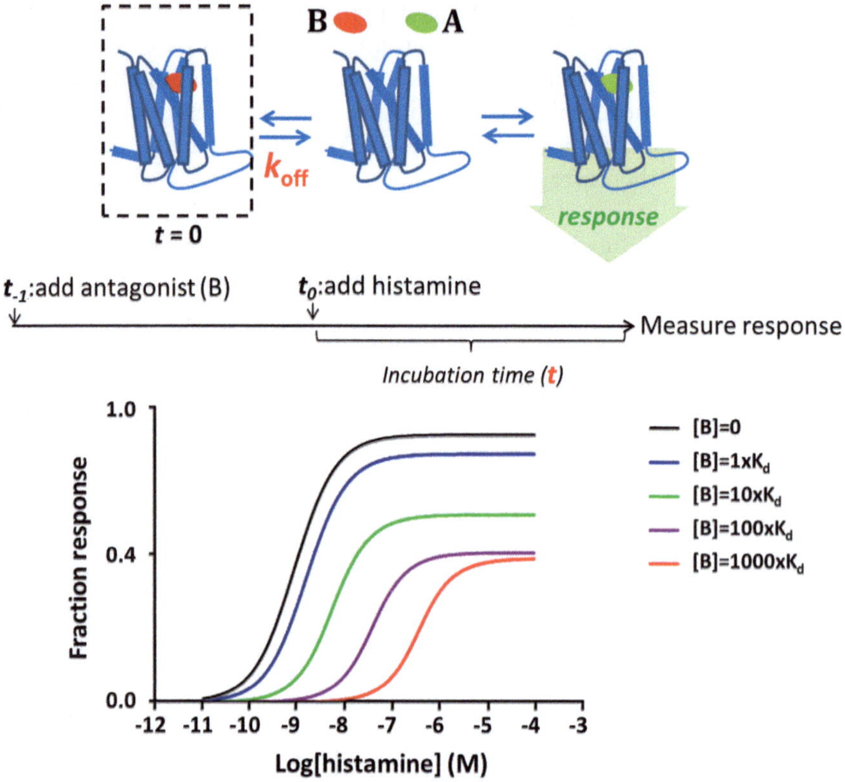

$$\alpha = \frac{\frac{[B]}{K_B}}{\frac{[B]}{K_B} + \frac{[A]}{K_A} + 1} \qquad \beta = \frac{\frac{[B]}{K_B}}{\frac{[B]}{K_B} + 1} \qquad \gamma = \frac{\frac{[B]}{K_B} + \frac{[A]}{K_A} + 1}{\frac{[A]}{K_A} + 1}$$

$$Y = \frac{\frac{[A]}{K_A} \cdot \left(1 - \left(\alpha \cdot \left(1 - e^{-k_{off} \cdot \gamma \cdot t}\right) + \beta \cdot e^{-k_{off} \cdot \gamma \cdot t}\right)\right) \cdot \tau \cdot E_{max}}{\frac{[A]}{K_A} \cdot \left(\left(1 - \left(\alpha \cdot \left(1 - e^{-k_{off} \cdot \gamma \cdot t}\right) + \beta \cdot e^{-k_{off} \cdot \gamma \cdot t}\right)\right) \cdot \tau + 1\right) + 1}$$

Fig. 15 Receptor activation after a pre-incubation with antagonist. Receptor is pre-incubated with antagonist. Consecutively, receptors are stimulated by increasing concentrations histamine and response is measured. A model is depicted that described the resulting response levels as a function of the antagonist concentration [B], agonist concentration [A], dissociation constants of the respective ligands (K_B and K_A) , the dissociation rate constant of the antagonist (k_{off}), the incubation time (t), and the efficacy and sensitivity of the system to induce a response (τ). This model can be used to obtain the k_{off} rate of antagonists

Furthermore, the incubation time (t) should be constrained as well. For the situation in which agonist and antagonist dissociate well within the incubation time and equilibrium is therefore obtained, the kinetic dissociation rate cannot be determined. It can only be said that full dissociation from the receptor is possible within the incubation time. Finally, in the case that antagonist is fully insurmountable by the agonist, then dissociation of the antagonist in the incubation time is close to zero and estimation of the dissociation rate is therefore impossible. However, it can be observed that the residence time must be much longer than the incubation time (t).

The incubation time is an interesting parameter in this experiment since it will determine what range of antagonist dissociation rates can be evaluated. For example, peak responses in intracellular calcium mobilization (see method below) and ERK1/2 phosphorylation were obtained after 15–75 s and 5 min, respectively [83]. This indicates that in many cases the specific cell response will often determine what incubation time will be applicable to an experiment.

Method (for prerequisites *see* **Note 11**)

1. Cells expressing the H_1R are seeded 3×10^4 cells/well in a black, clear-bottom 96-well plate.
2. Duplicate columns are incubated with 100 μL HBSS supplemented with 20 mM HEPES, containing increasing concentrations antagonist, corresponding to 0 to ~1000 times the K_i of the ligand, in the presence of Fluo4 NW and 4 mM probenecid. This is incubated for 30 min at 37 °C, in which substrate is enzymatically converted intracellularly into a calcium-sensitive fluorophore (Fig. 16).
3. After 30 min cells are stimulated with 10 μL, containing increasing concentrations (*see* **Note 12**) histamine and fluorescence is simultaneously recorded for approximately 1 min/well (Fig. 16). All components are preheated to 37 °C. To allow injection and detection at the same time, signal is acquired from the bottom of the plate using excitation at 494 nm and detection at 516 nm wavelengths.
4. Next, triton-X-100 is injected to a final concentration of 1.5% and signal is measured after cells are lysed.
5. Signal is normalized to baseline (before histamine injection) and saturated response after cell lysis. The normalized response is then plotted against log concentration agonist in the presence and absence of antagonist. This is analyzed with the discussed model (Fig. 15) by nonlinear regression in which affinity and ligand concentrations are constrained.

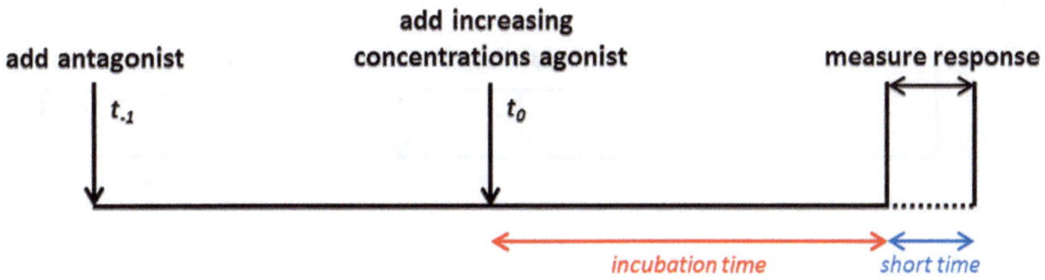

Fig. 16 Logistics of functional re-equilibration experiments

2.4.2 Recovery of Receptor Signaling After Washout

Another way to explore how long an antihistamine remains bound to the receptor is by observing the receptor response at different time points after removing the antagonist from solution. Receptor responsiveness should then return back to the level it had before it was inhibited. For H_1R and H_2R such experiments were performed for example using the chronotropic response of the guinea pig atria (H_2R), guinea pig ileum contraction (H_1R), or human lung contraction (H_1R) [28, 54, 79]. In these experiments, receptor response was measured at various times after washout of antihistamine or continuously in the presence of histamine. In the washout experiments in the context of the H_1R, recovery of receptor signaling did not seem completely dependent on the dissociation half-life, which was reported to be long (~100 min), but not nearly as long as suggested by the washout data (multiple hours-days) [28, 54].

Method (*see* **Note 13**)

1. 96-well plates with CHO cells expressing the target receptor are prepared as in Sect. 2.3.1.
2. When cells are strongly adherent to the plate, N wells are pre-incubated with a 3 times K_i concentration antagonist until equilibrium is expected for all used ligands. N represents the amount of time points for which antagonist is allowed to dissociate. Remove free antagonist by a few rapid wash steps, add buffer and stimulate at different time points after which response is immediately quantified (Fig. 17). All used components and incubation steps are performed at 37 °C.
3. Qualitative information about the recovery speed of receptor signaling is obtained.

Notes

1. Information is required about the kinetics of the cells' response to determine when the response should be quantified. Moreover, the approximate affinity of antagonist should be known.
2. Concentration should be 11 times concentrated to compensate for dilution.
3. Information is required about the kinetics of the cells' response to determine how response should be quantified over time.

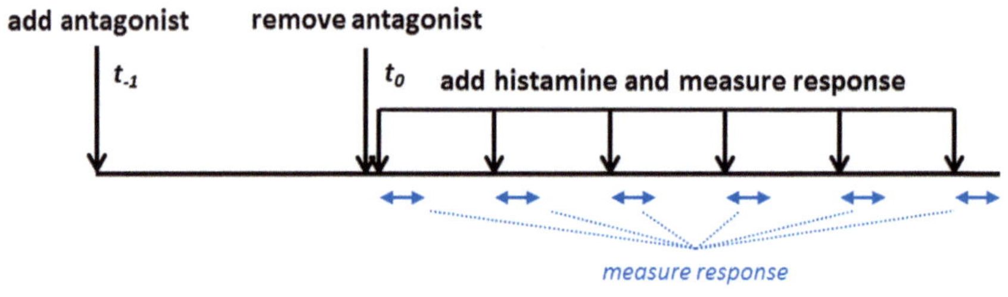

Fig. 17 Logistics of receptor signaling after washout

3 Choosing the Right Experiment

Choosing an experiment is very much dependent on the required information and desired throughput. For fragment-based drug discovery for example, it is likely that the dissociation rate of the ligands is relatively fast, as molecular size is an important determinant in shaping the ligand-binding kinetics [67, 84]. In stop flow experiments, the temporal resolution is limited (interspacing time points >30 s) making this a poor choice for very fast ligands. In this case, it might be better to go for a continuous readout such as the FRET-based ligand-binding experiment (Sect. 2.2.10) which can have a temporal resolution of ~0.3 s when measured in an individual well over time. Moreover, when evaluating the kinetic-binding rates in competition with the endogenous ligand it will be evaluated whether the antagonists have the desired kinetic-binding rates observed in a physiologically relevant competition for the receptor. Additionally, functional re-equilibration experiments (Sect. 2.3.1) could help in evaluating whether the respective dissociation rates of a set antagonist could have the potential to inhibit the respective cell response in an insurmountable manner. Table 2 shows a summary of the discussed techniques.

4 Experimental Design When Addressing Ligand-Binding Kinetics

In this section, some specific issues are discussed that should help in designing experiments meant to interrogate ligand-binding kinetics. Although mostly discussed in the context of radioligand-binding experiments, concepts will be more broadly applicable and therefore might warrant a careful read.

4.1 Equilibration Time and Equipotent Concentrations

For equilibrium saturation-binding and competition-binding experiments (see Chap. 6), it is very important that reactions have indeed reached equilibrium, since this is required for using the receptor occupancy models to analyze these data. In the mentioned experiments, a wide range of ligand concentrations is used (from very low concentrations to very high concentrations). In the case of low concentrations the product $k_{on}\cdot[L]$ will be neglectable compared to the k_{off} (see Eq. (2)). Experiments that use wide concentration ranges of a ligand will therefore be limited in its approach to equilibrium solely by the k_{off}. A rule of thumb was proposed by Motulsky and Mahan 1984, to wait five times the dissociation half-life ($3.5/k_{off}$) to ensure an approximation of equilibrium at all used concentrations. This is the case for both the binding of one ligand separately but also for two ligands binding competitively at the same time. In the latter case, the slowest k_{off} of the two ligands determines the required equilibration time [62].

Table 2
Experimental formats for quantifying/estimating ligand-binding kinetics

		Section	Temporal resolution	Notes
Stop flow	*radioligand*	2.2	>20 s[a]	Radioligand is required
Continuous	*SPA*	2.3.1	>10 s[b]	Less sensitive compared to stop flow-based radioligand binding
	FRET/BRET	2.3.2	>0.3 s	Modified receptor and fluorescent ligand are required

Format	Section	Quantitative/qualitative interpretation of binding rate constants	Throughput: Stop flow	Throughput: Continuous	Probe requirement	Notes
Association binding	2.2.3	Quantitative information	–	–[c]	Radioligand[d] for all ligands	Information about binding mechanism
Dissociation binding	2.2.3	Quantitative information	–	–[c]	Radioligand[d] for all ligands	Information about binding mechanism
Competitive association	2.2.4	Quantitative	–	+	Radioligand[d] required	
Competitive dissociation	2.2.5	Quantitative. For slow dissociating ligands compared to radioligand association (k_{obs})	–	+	Radioligand[d] required	Determines global k_{off}
Dual-point competition	2.2.6	Qualitative. Relative dissociation rate constants compared to radioligand	++	+	Radioligand[d] required	

Two step binding (fast compounds)	2.2.7	Qualitative. Relative dissociation rate dependent on incubation time	++	+	Radioligand[d] required	
Two step binding (unbiased)	2.2.8	Quantitative/qualitative. Dependent on incubation time	+/–	NA	Radioligand[d] required	Determines both affinity and ligand-binding kinetics
Re-equilibration experiments	2.4.1	Quantitative/qualitative. Dependent on incubation time until signal is, and can be, measured	–	NA	Agonist required	Information about mechanism of inhibition

An overview is depicted of the discussed different techniques and experimental formats that can assess the kinetic-binding rate constants of ligands

[a]Based on how fast the experimenter can start and stop incubations. Moreover, the amount of time points is limited, so temporal resolution can only be maintained for very short total incubation times.

[b]Depends on how high the signal is (available receptors, specific activity of the radioligand). The higher the signal, the faster the wells can be measured.

[c]Throughput still limited, since most ligands will not be labeled. Moreover, fluorescently labeled ligands will likely affect the kinetic-binding rate constants and therefore cannot be used to characterize the non-fluorescent ligands.

[d]Instead of radioligand, a fluorescent ligand could also be used in the context of BRET/FRET-based binding experiments.

In experiments interrogating the effects of ligand-binding kinetics it is often hard to make a fair comparison between ligands. One way to make sure that ligands only differ based on the dissociation rate and do not differ in their propensity to compete with another ligand is to use equipotent concentrations. This means that for each tested ligand the same ratio between concentration and affinity ($[L]/K_d$) is used. The effect of using equipotent concentration on receptor occupancy at equilibrium (in blue) and equilibration time (green) can be seen in Fig. 18. When taking x times the K_d as the ligand concentration, it can be observed that the fractional occupancy at equilibrium will be described by x, independent of the K_d of the ligand (Fig. 18a). However, the rate in which equilibrium is obtained (k_{obs}) will be dependent on both x and the k_{off} rate, which will differ between ligands (Fig. 18b). Note that for equipotent concentration the difference in k_{obs} between ligands does not depend on the k_{on} rate. Moreover, in the case of two ligands binding at the same time to a receptor, it can be seen that the fractional occupancy at equilibrium is again dependent on the relative concentrations to their individual K_d values (Fig. 18c). Based on the Motulsky and Mahan model, when substituting equipotent concentrations in the formula, it can be seen that binding (Y) becomes independent of the association rates of either ligand. Moreover, when comparing different ligands with equipotent concentrations, the exponential rate constants (KF and KS) only differ between ligands based on the dissociation rate (Fig. 18d). Therefore, fractional occupancies of the receptor at equilibrium should be the same when using equipotent concentrations of ligands, and differences observed in the onset of equilibrium are dependent solely on the dissociation rate of the used ligands.

4.2 Choosing Concentrations and Time Points

When measuring the binding kinetics of ligands it is most practical to not use too many concentrations of ligand or different incubation times, because all concentrations will also have to be measured on all chosen time points. In stop-flow-based experiments this could easily lead to a high number of conditions that need to be tested. It is therefore important to wisely choose concentrations and time points. In order to choose the required *time points* it helps if an educated guess can be made concerning the dissociation rate of the ligand. When information concerning the dissociation rate is known, then it can be calculated what would be a useful timeframe for the experiment. Probably 0 up to five times the $t_{1/2}$ would be a good pick for both association and dissociation experiments (Fig. 19a, b), as this will allow a close approximation of equilibrium for all relevant concentrations within the time frame of the experiment (see also Sect. 4.1). Moreover, it is useful to have more time points in the early phase binding/dissociation, since for this phase there are the biggest differences in binding.

Use an equipotent concentration ligand (x times the affinity value):

$$[L] = x \cdot K_{d,L} = x \cdot \frac{k_{off}(or\ k_2)}{k_{on}(or\ k_1)} \qquad [I] = y \cdot K_{d,I} = y \cdot \frac{k_{off}(or\ k_4)}{k_{on}(or\ k_3)}$$

(substitute in formula's below)

A Fractional occupancy at equilibrium

$$P_{RL} = \frac{[L]}{[L] + K_{d,L}}$$

$$P_{RL} = \frac{x \cdot K_{d,L}}{x \cdot K_{d,L} + K_{d,L}} = \frac{x}{x+1}$$

B Equilibration speed

$$k_{obs} = k_{on} \cdot [L] + k_{off}$$

$$k_{obs} = k_{on} \cdot x \cdot \frac{k_{off}}{k_{on}} + k_{off} = (x+1) \cdot k_{off}$$

C

$$P_{RL,I} = \frac{\frac{[L]}{K_{d,L}}}{1 + \frac{[L]}{K_{d,L}} + \frac{[I]}{K_{d,I}}}$$

$$P_{RL,I} = \frac{\frac{x \cdot K_{d,L}}{K_{d,L}}}{1 + \frac{x \cdot K_{d,L}}{K_{d,L}} + \frac{y \cdot K_{d,I}}{K_{d,I}}} = \frac{x}{1+x+y}$$

D

$$KA = (x+1) \cdot k_2$$

$$KB = (y+1) \cdot k_4$$

$$S = \sqrt{(KA - KB)^2 + 4 \cdot x \cdot y \cdot k_2 \cdot k_4}$$

$$KF = \frac{1}{2} \cdot (KA + KB + S)$$

$$KS = \frac{1}{2} \cdot (KA + KB - S)$$

$$Q = \frac{B_{max} \cdot x \cdot k_2}{KF - KS}$$

$$Y = Q \cdot \frac{k_4 - KF}{KF} \cdot e^{-KF \cdot t} - Q \cdot \frac{k_4 - KS}{KS} \cdot e^{-KS \cdot t} + Q \cdot \frac{k_4 \cdot (KF - KS)}{KF \cdot KS}$$

Fig. 18 The use of equipotent concentrations. When using equipotent concentrations ligand concentrations are chosen relative to the ligand affinity. Therefore, ligand concentrations are expressed as *x* (or *y*) times the K_d of the ligand (*gray square*). As can been seen in equilibrium (*blue square*), fractional occupancy of the receptor by a ligand (P_{RL}) can be expressed using the equations depicted in (**a**) as a function of ligand concentration ([L]) and the affinity (K_d) of L. Moreover, the same fractional occupancy of that ligand in competition with another ligand (I) for the receptor can be described by the equation in (**c**) as a function of ligand concentrations [L] and [I] and the affinity of those ligands. The ligand-bound ligand (Y) over time (*green square*) can be described for a single ligand to the receptor (**b**) or in competition with another ligand (**d**). In both cases, Y depends on the equipotent concentrations and on the kinetic dissociation rate constants of the respective ligand. However, binding over time is completely independent of the association rate constants when comparing equipotent concentrations

In order to choose the right *concentrations* of radioligand it is helpful to know the affinity of the radioligand. When association binding is performed to determine the k_{on} and k_{off} kinetic rate constants (Sect. 2.2.3), it is important to ensure that there is enough difference between the measured k_{obs} values to get a reliable fit of the k_{on} and k_{off}. This can be done by choosing sufficient differences in ligand concentrations that will result in variances in the k_{obs} (see Eqs. 1 and 2). Moreover by varying the Y_{max} sufficiently there is a more stringent fitting for the ratio between the k_{off}/k_{on} (i.e., the

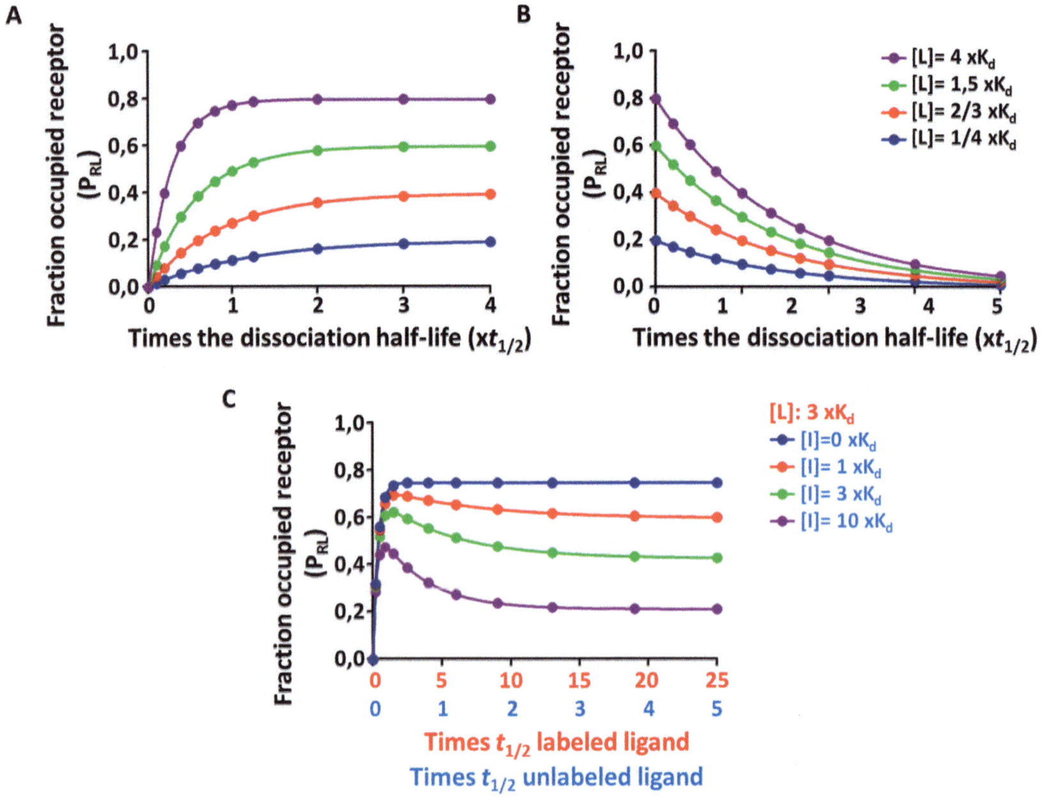

Fig. 19 Time points and concentrations in stop-flow-based experiments. *Lines* represent the theoretical models describing the association and dissociation of ligands to the receptor. (**a**) Depicts the association of ligand to its target receptor. It can be seen that equipotent concentrations will always lead to the same curves when binding is expressed as a function of the dissociation half-life. To best describe the theoretical curves, most data points should describe the early phase of binding where the biggest differences in binding are observed. Late phase time points are important to describe the amount of binding at equilibrium. (**b**) Depicts the dissociation of a ligand from the receptor. The curve will be completely dependent on the dissociation half-life and can be best described by measuring mostly early time points. Most ligands should have been dissociated after five times the dissociation half-life. (**c**) Describes the association of a ligand in the presence of another ligand. It can be seen that binding of L is dependent on the presence of a concentration [I]. Equilibrium will be reached based on the slowest dissociation half-life. In this case this is the unlabeled ligand I. Since the labeled ligand binds much faster, an increase in binding of the labeled ligand can be seen for early time points. Therefore, the measured early time points should be adjusted to the labeled ligand and the measured late time points should be adjusted to the slowest of the two ligands

K_d) when this is incorporated in the mathematical model (Fig. 1b, blue). Therefore, it is probably good to aim for a diversity in Y_{max} values to obtain well-separated curves (Fig. 19a).

For competitive association-binding experiments, both concentrations and time points are dependent on both ligands. Again, the equilibrium situation for applied ligand concentrations can be predicted using the affinities of both ligands. In Fig. 19c, an example of concentrations is shown (expressed as equipotent concentrations). It is important that antagonist displaces a substantial amount (but not fully) of the radioligand binding at equilibrium compared to radioligand binding in the absence of antagonist. When multiple concentrations of unlabeled ligands are used, clear differences between the different curves should be attained (e.g., 25, 50, and 75% inhibition of the radioligand at equilibrium). As for the chosen time points, the slowest ligand should be detrimental for how long the experiment lasts. Moreover, enough data points in the early phase of binding are also important and are dependent mostly on the dissociation half-life of the radioligand (time points between 0 and 3 times the $t_{1/2}$). An example for possible concentrations and time points are depicted in Fig. 19c.

5 Conclusion

Ligand-binding kinetic constants have been implicated to be an important drug parameter and would be valuable information for discriminating potential drug candidates. Due to the transient nature of histamine signaling, it was suggested that for the histamine receptors, the residence time is important in ligand optimization. It was therefore discussed what experiments would be appropriate for discriminating ligands based on their residence time. Discussed experimental formats were advantages in either their level of accuracy, throughput or physiological relevance. This overview should be a tool for researchers to design their experiments in a way that appropriate information is obtained. Additionally, it could provide insight and help in the design of new experimental formats.

Acknowledgments

The work was supported by the Innovative Medicines Initiative Joint Undertaking under grant agreement 115366, resources of which are composed of financial contribution from the European Union's Seventh Framework Programme (FP7/2007-2013) and European Federation of Pharmaceutical Industries and Associations (EFPIA) companies' in-kind contribution. This work was additionally supported by the TOPPUNT grant of the Netherlands Organization of Scientific Research.

References

1. Lowman M, Rees PH, Benyon RC et al (1988) Human mast cell heterogeneity: histamine release from mast cells dispersed from skin, lung, adenoids, tonsils, and colon in response to IgE-dependent and nonimmunologic stimuli. J Allergy Clin Immunol 81:590–597
2. Kinet JP (1999) The high-affinity IgE receptor (Fc epsilon RI): from physiology to pathology. Annu Rev Immunol 17:931–972

3. Hofstra CL, Desai PJ, Thurmond RL et al (2003) Histamine H4 receptor mediates chemotaxis and calcium mobilization of mast cells. J Pharmacol Exp Ther 305:1212–1221
4. Bäumer W, Wendorff S, Gutzmer R et al (2008) Histamine H4 receptors modulate dendritic cell migration through skin—immunomodulatory role of histamine. Allergy 63:1387–1394
5. Majno G, Palade GE (1961) Studies on inflammation. 1. The effect of histamine and serotonin on vascular permeability: an electron microscopic study. J Biophys Biochem Cytol 11:571–605
6. Wu L, Feng B-S, He S-H et al (2007) Bacterial peptidoglycan breaks down intestinal tolerance via mast cell activation: the role of TLR2 and NOD2. Immunol Cell Biol 85:538–545
7. Petersen LJ, Mosbech H, Skov PS (1996) Allergen-induced histamine release in intact human skin in vivo assessed by skin microdialysis technique: characterization of factors influencing histamine releasability. J Allergy Clin Immunol 97:672–679
8. Swinney DC (2004) Biochemical mechanisms of drug action: what does it take for success? Nat Rev Drug Discov 3:801–808
9. Vauquelin G, Charlton SJ (2010) Long-lasting target binding and rebinding as mechanisms to prolong in vivo drug action. Br J Pharmacol 161:488–508
10. Copeland R, Pompliano DL, Meek TD (2006) Drug-target residence time and its implications for lead optimization. Nat Rev Drug Discov 5:730–739
11. Lu H, Tonge PJ (2010) Drug-target residence time: critical information for lead optimization. Curr Opin Chem Biol 14:467–474
12. Hoffmann C, Castro M, Rinken A et al (2015) Ligand residence time at g-protein-coupled receptors—why we should take our time to study it. Mol Pharmacol 88:552–560
13. Simons FER, Simons KJ (2011) Histamine and H1-antihistamines: celebrating a century of progress. J Allergy Clin Immunol 128:1139–1150.e4
14. Feldman M, Burton ME (1990) Histamine2-receptor antagonists. Standard therapy for acid-peptic diseases. N Engl J Med 323: 1672–1680
15. Sander K, Kottke T, Stark H (2008) Histamine H3 receptor antagonists go to clinics. Biol Pharm Bull 31:2163–2181
16. Thurmond RL (2015) The histamine H4 receptor: from orphan to the clinic. Front Pharmacol 6:1–11
17. Cook D, Brown D, Alexander R et al (2014) Lessons learned from the fate of AstraZeneca's drug pipeline: a five-dimensional framework. Nat Rev Drug Discov 13:419–431
18. Waring MJ, Arrowsmith J, Leach AR et al (2015) An analysis of the attrition of drug candidates from four major pharmaceutical companies. Nat Rev Drug Discov 14:475–486
19. Hough LB, Khandelwal JK, Green JP (1984) Histamine turnover in regions of rat brain. Brain Res 291:103–109
20. Dismukes K, Snyder SH (1974) Histamine turnover in rat brain. Brain Res 78:467–481
21. Pollard H, Bischoff S, Schwartz JC (1974) Turnover of histamine in rat brain and its decrease under barbiturate anesthesia. J Pharmacol Exp Ther 190:88–99
22. Kitano M, Norlén P, Håkanson R (2000) Gastric submucosal microdialysis: a method to study gastrin- and food-evoked mobilization of ECL-cell histamine in conscious rats. Regul Pept 86:113–123
23. Irman-Florjanc T, Erjavec F (1993) Kinetics of histamine and tele-methylhistamine elimination from rat plasma. Agents Actions 38:C304–C306
24. Cash KJ, Clark H (2013) Phosphorescent nanosensors for in vivo tracking of histamine levels. Anal Chem 85:6312–6318
25. Gillard M, Van Der Perren C, Moguilevsky N et al (2002) Binding characteristics of cetirizine and levocetirizine to human H(1) histamine receptors: contribution of Lys(191) and Thr(194). Mol Pharmacol 61:391–399
26. Gillard M, Chatelain P (2006) Changes in pH differently affect the binding properties of histamine H1 receptor antagonists. Eur J Pharmacol 530:205–214
27. Anthes JC, Gilchrest H, Richard C et al (2002) Biochemical characterization of desloratadine, a potent antagonist of the human histamine H(1) receptor. Eur J Pharmacol 449:229–237
28. Christophe B, Carlier B, Gillard M et al (2003) Histamine H1 receptor antagonism by cetirizine in isolated guinea pig tissues: influence of receptor reserve and dissociation kinetics. Eur J Pharmacol 470:87–94
29. Matsumoto Y, Funahashi J, Mori K et al (2008) The noncompetitive antagonism of histamine H1 receptors expressed in chinese hamster ovary cells by olopatadine hydrochloride: its potency and molecular mechanism. Pharmacology 81:266–274
30. Schoepke N, Church M, Maurer M (2013) The inhibition by levocetirizine and fexofenadine of the histamine-induced wheal and flare response in healthy caucasian and japanese volunteers. Acta Derm Venereol 93:286–293
31. Brittain RT, Jack D, Reeves JJ et al (1985) Pharmacological basis for the induction of gas-

tric carcinoid tumours in the rat by loxtidine, an insurmountable histamine H2-receptor blocking drug. Br J Pharmacol 85:843–847
32. Poynter D, Pick CR, Harcourt RA et al (1985) Association of long lasting unsurmountable histamine H2 blockade and gastric carcinoid tumours in the rat. Gut 26:1284–1295
33. Fossmark R, Qvigstad G, Waldum HL (2008) Gastric cancer: animal studies on the risk of hypoacidity and hypergastrinemia. World J Gastroenterol 14:1646–1651
34. Fossmark R, Zhao CM, Martinsen TC et al (2005) Dedifferentiation of enterochromaffin-like cells in gastric cancer of hypergastrinemic cotton rats. APMIS 113:436–449
35. Waldum HL, Gustafsson B, Fossmark R et al (2005) Antiulcer drugs and gastric cancer. Dig Dis Sci 50:39–44
36. Guo D, Mulder-Krieger T, IJzerman AP et al (2012) Functional efficacy of adenosine A2A receptor agonists is positively correlated to their receptor residence time. Br J Pharmacol 166:1846–1859
37. Nolte HJ, Rosenberry TL, Neumann E (1980) Effective charge on acetylcholinesterase active sites determined from the ionic strength dependence of association rate constants with cationic ligands. Biochemistry 19:3705–3711
38. Radić Z, Kirchhoff PD, Quinn DM et al (1997) Electrostatic influence on the kinetics of ligand binding to acetylcholinesterase. Distinctions between active center ligands and fasciculin. J Biol Chem 272:23265–23277
39. Darling RJ, Kuchibhotla U, Glaesner W et al (2002) Glycosylation of erythropoietin affects receptor binding kinetics: role of electrostatic interactions. Biochemistry 41:14524–14531
40. Haraldsdottir HS, Thiele I, Fleming RM (2012) Quantitative assignment of reaction directionality in a multicompartmental human metabolic reconstruction. Biophys J 102: 1703–1711
41. Wallace RM, Young JM (1983) Temperature dependence of the binding of [3H]mepyramine and related compounds to the histamine H1 receptor. Mol Pharmacol 23:60–66
42. Rising TJ, Norris DB, Warrander SE et al (1980) High affinity 3H-cimetidine binding in guinea-pig tissues. Life Sci 27:199–206
43. May LT, Bridge LJ, Stoddart L et al (2011) Allosteric interactions across native adenosine-A3 receptor homodimers: quantification using single-cell ligand-binding kinetics. FASEB J 25:3465–3476
44. Corriden R, Kilpatrick LE, Kellam B et al (2014) Kinetic analysis of antagonist-occupied adenosine-A3 receptors within membrane microdomains of individual cells provides evidence of receptor dimerization and allosterism. FASEB J 28:4211–4222
45. Charlton SJ, Vauquelin G (2010) Elusive equilibrium: the challenge of interpreting receptor pharmacology using calcium assays. Br J Pharmacol 161:1250–1265
46. Hulme EC, Trevethick M (2010) Ligand binding assays at equilibrium: validation and interpretation. Br J Pharmacol 161:1219–1237
47. Chang K-J, Jacobs S, Cuatrecasas P (1975) Quantitative aspects of hormone-receptor interactions of high affinity. Biochim Biophys Acta 406:294–303
48. Ruat M, Traiffort E, Bouthenet ML et al (1990) Reversible and irreversible labeling and autoradiographic localization of the cerebral histamine H2 receptor using [^{125}I]iodinated probes. Proc Natl Acad Sci USA 87: 1658–1662
49. Gajtkowski GA, Norris DB, Rising TJ et al (1983) Specific binding of 3H-tiotidine to histamine H2 receptors in guinea pig cerebral cortex. Nature 304:65–67
50. Ligneau X, Garbarg M, Vizuete ML et al (1994) [125I]iodoproxyfan, a new antagonist to label and visualize cerebral histamine H3 receptors. J Pharmacol Exp Ther 271: 452–459
51. West RE, Wu RL, Billah MM et al (1999) The profiles of human and primate [3H]Nalpha-methylhistamine binding differ from that of rodents. Eur J Pharmacol 377:233–239
52. Kanba S, Richelson E (1984) Histamine H1 receptors in human brain labelled with [3H] doxepin. Brain Res 304:1–7
53. West RE, Zweig A, Granzow RT et al (1990) Biexponential kinetics of (R)-alpha-[3H]methylhistamine binding to the rat brain H3 histamine receptor. J Neurochem 55:1612–1616
54. Slack RJ, Russell LJ, Hall D et al (2011) Pharmacological characterization of GSK1004723, a novel, long-acting antagonist at histamine H1 and H3 receptors. Br J Pharmacol 164:1627–1641
55. Harper E, Shankley NP, Black JW (1999) Characterization of the binding of [3H]-clobenpropit to histamine H3-receptors in guinea-pig cerebral cortex membranes. Br J Pharmacol 128:881–890
56. Witte DG, Yao BB, Miller TR et al (2006) Detection of multiple H3 receptor affinity states utilizing [3H]A-349821, a novel, selective, non-imidazole histamine H3 receptor inverse agonist radioligand. Br J Pharmacol 148:657–670

57. Igel P, Schnell D, Bernhardt G et al (2009) Tritium-labeled N1-[3-(1H-imidazol-4-yl) propyl]-N2-propionylguanidine ([3H] UR-PI294), a high-affinity histamine H3 and H4 receptor radioligand. ChemMedChem 4: 225–231
58. Baumeister P, Erdmann D, Biselli S et al (2015) [3H]UR-DE257: development of a tritium-labeled squaramide-type selective histamine H2 receptor antagonist. ChemMedChem 10: 83–93
59. Smits R, Lim HD, van der Meer T et al (2012) Ligand based design of novel histamine H4 receptor antagonists; fragment optimization and analysis of binding kinetics. Bioorg Med Chem Lett 22:461–467
60. Tummino PJ, Copeland R (2008) Residence time of receptor-ligand complexes and its effect on biological function. Biochemistry 47:5481–5492
61. Vogt AD, Di Cera E (2012) Conformational selection or induced fit? A critical appraisal of the kinetic mechanism. Biochemistry 51: 5894–5902
62. Motulsky HJ, Mahan LC (1984) The kinetics of competitive radioligand binding predicted by the law of mass action. Mol Pharmacol 25:1–9
63. Andaloussi M, Lim HD, van der Meer T et al (2013) A novel series of histamine H4 receptor antagonists based on the pyrido[3,2-d]pyrimidine scaffold: comparison of hERG binding and target residence time with PF-3893787. Bioorg Med Chem Lett 23:2663–2670
64. Cheng Y, Prusoff WH (1973) Relationship between the inhibition constant (KI) and the concentration of inhibitor which causes 50 per cent inhibition (I50) of an enzymatic reaction. Biochem Pharmacol 22:3099–3108
65. Swinney DC, Beavis P, Chuang K-T et al (2014) A study of the molecular mechanism of binding kinetics and long residence times of human CCR5 receptor small molecule allosteric ligands. Br J Pharmacol 171:3364–3375
66. Guo D, van Dorp EJH, Mulder-Krieger T et al (2013) Dual-point competition association assay: a fast and high-throughput kinetic screening method for assessing ligand-receptor binding kinetics. J Biomol Screen 18:309–320
67. Tresadern G, Bartolome JM, Macdonald GJ et al (2011) Molecular properties affecting fast dissociation from the D2 receptor. Bioorg Med Chem 19:2231–2241
68. Packeu A, Wennerberg M, Balendran A et al (2010) Estimation of the dissociation rate of unlabelled ligand-receptor complexes by a “two-step” competition binding approach. Br J Pharmacol 161:1311–1328
69. Crane K, Shih DT (2004) Development of a homogeneous binding assay for histamine receptors. Anal Biochem 335:42–49
70. Schiele F, Ayaz P, Fernández-Montalván A (2015) A universal homogeneous assay for high-throughput determination of binding kinetics. Anal Biochem 468:42–49
71. Vernall AJ, Hill SJ, Kellam B (2014) The evolving small-molecule fluorescent-conjugate toolbox for Class A GPCRs. Br J Pharmacol 171:1073–1084
72. Rose RH, Briddon SJ, Hill SJ (2012) A novel fluorescent histamine H(1) receptor antagonist demonstrates the advantage of using fluorescence correlation spectroscopy to study the binding of lipophilic ligands. Br J Pharmacol 165:1789–1800
73. Malan SF, van Marle A, Menge WM et al (2004) Fluorescent ligands for the histamine H2 receptor: synthesis and preliminary characterization. Bioorg Med Chem 12:6495–6503
74. Amon M, Ligneau X, Camelin J-C, Berrebi-Bertrand I et al (2007) Highly potent fluorescence-tagged nonimidazole histamine H3 receptor ligands. ChemMedChem 2:708–716
75. Stoddart LA, Johnstone EKM, Wheal AJ et al (2015) Application of BRET to monitor ligand binding to GPCRs. Nat Methods 12:661–663
76. Bocquet N, Kohler J, Hug MN et al (2015) Real-time monitoring of binding events on a thermostabilized human A2A receptor embedded in a lipid bilayer by surface plasmon resonance. Biochim Biophys Acta 1848:1224–1233
77. Heym RG, Hornberger WB, Lakics V et al (2015) Label-free detection of small-molecule binding to a GPCR in the membrane environment. Biochim Biophys Acta 1854:979–986
78. Chand N, Diamantis W, Sofia RD (1986) Antagonism of histamine and leukotrienes by azelastine in isolated guinea pig ileum. Agents Actions 19:164–168
79. Arai H, Nakagawa M, Tanada K et al (1994) Histamine H2-receptor antagonism of T-593: studies on positive chronotropic responses in guinea pig atria. Jpn J Pharmacol 64:251–256
80. Kenakin TP (2009) Orthosteric drug antagonism. In: A Pharmacology primer. Elsevier Academic Press, London, 101–127
81. Kenakin T, Jenkinson S, Watson C (2006) Determining the potency and molecular mechanism of action of insurmountable antagonists. J Pharmacol Exp Ther 319:710–723
82. Mould R, Brown J, Marshall FH et al (2014) Binding kinetics differentiates functional antagonism of orexin-2 receptor ligands. Br J Pharmacol 171:351–363

83. Riddy DM, Valant C, Rueda P et al (2015) Label-free kinetics: exploiting functional hemi-equilibrium to derive rate constants for muscarinic receptor antagonists. Mol Pharmacol 88:779–790
84. Pan AC, Borhani DW, Dror RO et al (2013) Molecular determinants of drug-receptor binding kinetics. Drug Discov Today 18: 667–673

Chapter 6

Methods to Study the Molecular Pharmacology of the Histamine H_4 Receptor

Eléonore W.E. Verweij, Rob Leurs, and Henry F. Vischer

Abstract

The H_4R is the latest addition of the histamine receptor family. This GPCR was found to be involved in a multitude of allergic and inflammatory diseases. Antagonizing H_4Rs results in profound anti-inflammatory effects in various animal disease models, and a first phase 2a clinical trial in patients suffering from atopic dermatitis has already been conducted.

In order to accelerate and expand current drug discovery at H_4R, in-depth understanding of its molecular mechanisms and signaling pathways are key. Complexity of H_4R signaling pathways was highlighted by the discovery of so-called biased ligands, which can initiate differential efficacies in various GPCR responses. This chapter will provide an overview of commonly applied methods used to elucidate the molecular pharmacological aspects of the H_4R from receptor-ligand-binding interactions to downstream gene transcription.

Key words H_4R, $G\alpha_i$ protein signaling, Radioligand binding, β-arrestin2 recruitment, CAMYEL, CRE-luc

1 Introduction

1.1 Discovery of H_4R

The biogenic amine histamine is involved in many physiological and pathological processes in the human body. Histamine-induced responses are mediated by four receptor subtypes that all belong to class A G protein-coupled receptors (GPCR) [1]. The H_1, H_2, and H_3 receptor subtypes (H_1R, H_2R, and H_3R, respectively) were discovered by distinguished pharmacology of developed ligands [2–4], whereas the H_4 receptor (H_4R) gene was initially identified as an orphan GPCR gene lacking functional or pharmacological information. The H_4R gene was identified based on a sequence similarity search using a genomic database. An amino acid sequence alignment of the H_4R protein showed up to 35% homology with the H_3R [5–10]. Heterologous expression of human H_4R (hH_4R) in the human neuroblastoma cell line SK-N-MC revealed high affinity for histamine (5 nM) [5]. Most H_1R and H_2R compounds

Ekaterini Tiligada and Madeleine Ennis (eds.), *Histamine Receptors as Drug Targets*, Methods in Pharmacology and Toxicology, DOI 10.1007/978-1-4939-6843-5_6, © Springer Science+Business Media LLC 2017

showed only modest or no affinity at the H_4R, whereas H_3R ligands displayed divergent affinity/efficacy rankings on H_4R [5]. For example, hH_3R inverse agonist clobenpropit acts as a partial agonist at the hH_4R with nM affinity for both histamine receptor subtypes [5, 11].

Since its discovery, a quest to unravel the functional effects of the H_4R has been ongoing as other histamine receptor subtypes have proven to be designated targets for blockbuster drugs. H_1R antagonists are extensively used for treatment of allergic reactions [12], H_2R antagonists are crucial for treatment of ulcers by reducing gastric acid production [13], and H_3R antagonists show great potential in treatment of neurological diseases due to their modulatory role in neurotransmitter release in the brain [14]. A major milestone was reached in 2015 with the approval of the first H_3R inverse agonist, pitolisant (Wakix®), for treatment of narcolepsy [15].

The H_4R is suggested as a promising target in inflammatory diseases as indicated by its expression on hematopoietic cells [5–7, 16–22]. Therefore, in-depth understanding of its molecular mechanisms and signaling pathways is the key for drug discovery. Chemically distinctive ligands can display differential activation or efficacy patterns of receptor-induced responses. These so-called biased ligands might have therapeutical advantages as activation of one pathway might relieve symptoms, whereas another might cause adverse side effects. Indeed, for the angiotensin II type 1 (AT1R) receptor development of a biased ligand was demonstrated to be successful in the treatment of acute heart failure conditions [23, 24]. Recently, H_4R-biased ligands were reported that could initiate G protein-independent signaling pathways via β-arrestin2 recruitment [25–27]. This highlights the complexity of H_4R signaling mechanisms and gives opportunities for specific therapeutic intervention.

The aim of this chapter is to provide an overview of some of the main methods used to elucidate molecular aspects of the H_4R, describing the complete process of ligand binding till downstream signaling in a heterologous cell system. First, an overview of the currently known functional properties and the signaling pathways of the H_4R is provided.

1.2 H_4R Function

The H_4R is predominantly expressed on bone marrow and cells of hematopoietic origin, like mast cells, monocytes, dendritic cells, eosinophils, basophils, neutrophils, and T cells [5–7, 16–22], and was found to be involved in allergic and inflammatory processes [28]. Antagonizing the H_4R demonstrated profound anti-inflammatory effects in multiple preclinical disease models, like asthma, chronic pruritus, dermatitis, rheumatoid arthritis, gastric ulcerogenesis, and colitis [29–34]. Moreover, recently, the potent and selective H_4R antagonist JNJ39758979 has been evaluated for the treatment of atopic dermatitis (AD) in a Phase 2a clinical trial [35]. Although the study was preliminary terminated due to two patients suffering from neutropenia, the overall findings suggested beneficial effects of blocking the H_4R in the treatment of dermatitis. H_4R has also been mentioned as a possible target in neurological and psychiatric diseases [36], although conflicting data on both H_4R transcript and protein expression in the brain has been reported [36–40].

1.3 H_4R Signaling Pathways

1.3.1 G Protein Activation

Histamine inhibits forskolin-induced cAMP response element (CRE) driven transcription in H_4R expressing cells (Fig. 1) in a pertussis toxin (PTx)-sensitive manner, suggesting that H_4R signals via heterotrimeric $G\alpha_{i/o}$ proteins [6]. $G\alpha_{i/o}$ protein activation inhibits adenylyl cyclase (AC) activity resulting in reduced cAMP levels, and consequently reduced protein kinase A (PKA) and CRE-binding protein (CREB) activation (Fig. 1). Moreover, mitogen-activated protein kinase (MAPK) phosphorylation was increased in HEK293 cells upon H_4R-mediated $G\alpha_i$ activation [7].

1.3.2 Ca^{2+} Release and Chemotaxis

The $G\beta\gamma$ subunits of the heterotrimeric G protein complex activate phospholipase Cβ (PLCβ) to hydrolyze phosphatidylinositol 4,5,biphosphate (PIP_2) into diacylglycerol (DAG) and inositol 1,4,5-triphosphate (IP_3). Subsequently, IP_3 stimulates the release

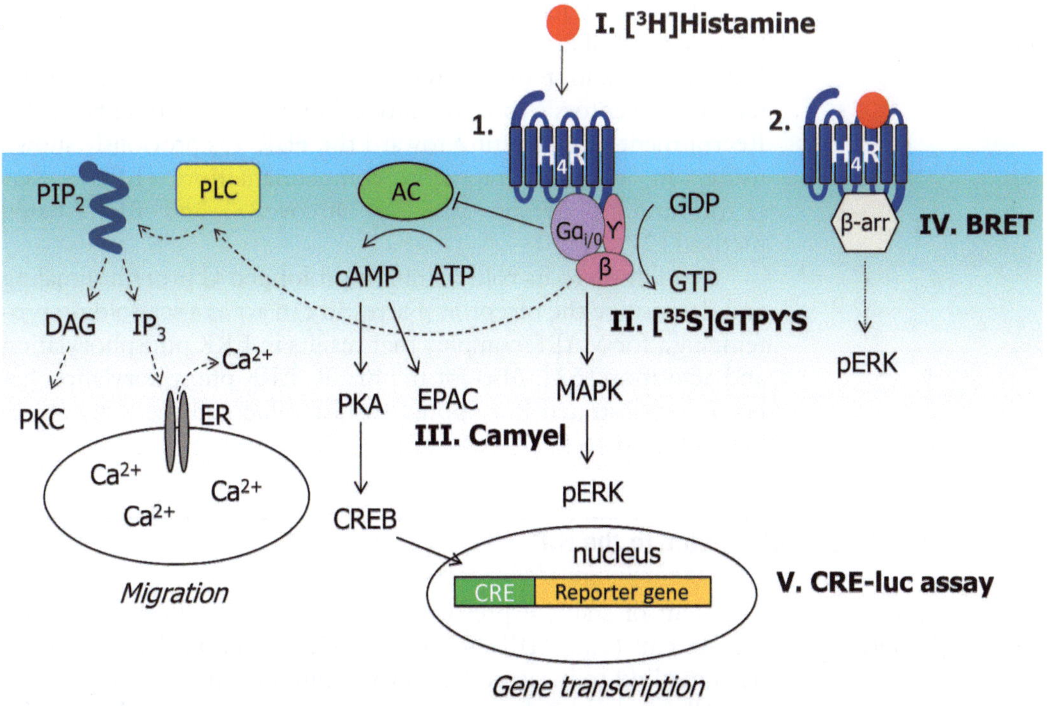

Fig. 1 Overview of H_4R signaling pathways described in in vivo or in vitro systems. *Solid arrows* indicate signaling induced by the $G\alpha_{i/o}$ subunit, *dashed arrows* represent signaling initiated by the $G\beta\gamma$ subunit, *dotted arrows* indicate signaling initiated by β-arrestin2. (*1*) H_4R interacting with its G protein, (*2*) H_4R interaction with β-arrestin2 which can occur in a G protein independent manner. Indicated experiments (*I–V*) are discussed in this review

of Ca^{2+} from intracellular stores as it binds to its receptor located at the endoplasmic reticulum (ER). Released Ca^{2+} induces chemotaxis of mouse-derived mast cell toward histamine [20]. The dual H_3R/H_4R antagonist thioperamide blocked the chemotactic response to histamine. Furthermore, mast cells from H_4R-deficient mice did not show this chemotactic response, while cells derived from H_3R-deficient mice still showed chemotaxis in response to histamine [20]. Induced chemotaxis has also been demonstrated in eosinophils, macrophages, and dendritic cells [19, 20, 41–44].

1.3.3 Constitutive H_4R Activity

GPCRs can also signal in the absence of an agonist, a phenomenon known as constitutive activity, which can be inhibited by inverse agonists [45]. Reduced basal signaling of the hH_4R was observed in $[^{35}S]GTP\gamma S$ assays in response to thioperamide, which was previously reported as an H_3R antagonist, implying that the hH_4R is constitutively active [7, 46]. Receptor number and G protein expression levels are determinants of constitutive activity as higher expression levels are often associated with more basal signaling [47, 48]. This indicates that in heterologous cell systems, in which receptor numbers are overexpressed compared to endogenous cell systems, the occurrence of constitutive activity is more easily observed.

1.3.4 β-Arrestin2 Recruitment

After G protein activation, GPCRs are rapidly phosphorylated by kinases to facilitate β-arrestin recruitment and activation [49]. Bound β-arrestin sterically prevents further G protein coupling and targets receptors toward intracellular compartments [50]. Recruitment of β-arrestin2 toward the H_4R was previously shown using an enzyme fragment complementation (EFC) assay (PathHunter β-arrestin assay of DiscoveRx) and BRET-based method [27, 51].

In addition to its role to inhibit prolonged G protein signaling and desensitize the receptor, β-arrestin can act as a scaffolding protein, e.g., for MAPK complex that results in ERK phosphorylation and activation [52]. Also for the hH_4R, ERK phosphorylation has been demonstrated in response to histamine and the β-arrestin2-biased ligand JNJ7777120 [27].

2 Methods Used to Characterize the H_4R

2.1 Cell Culture and Transfections

Transient or stable expression of H_4R (mutants) in heterologous cell systems (e.g., HEK293(T), COS7, or CHO cells) is a widely used method to measure H_4R ligand binding and signaling.

All protocols described in this review are applicable for HEK293T cells transiently expressing H_4R. Use of other cell lines or ex vivo samples should therefore be optimized and validated. Histamine receptor subtype specific antagonists can be used to validate whether observed binding and/or signaling is indeed mediated via the H_4R [21]. Alternatively, subtype-selective agonists such as, for example, 4-methylhistamine and VUF8430 can be used to favor H_4R-mediated signaling [11, 53].

Required materials, reagents, and plasmid DNA

- HEK293T cells.
- DNA constructs in mammalian expression vector (e.g., pcDNA3 and pcDEF3).
  - H_4R.
  - CAMYEL BRET sensor pcDNA3L-His-CAMYEL plasmid (ATCC, ATCC® MBA-277™).
  - Donor and acceptor BRET constructs; hH_4R-5Rluc8 and β-arrestin2-5mVenus.
  - Reporter gene construct; C21xCRE-luc.
- Culture medium: Dulbecco's modified Eagle medium (DMEM) containing 4 nM L-glutamine and 4.5 g/L glucose and 10% fetal bovine serum (FBS), 1% antibiotics (50 IU/mL penicillin, and 50 μg/mL streptomycin).
- Phosphate buffered saline (PBS).
- Trypsin ethylenediaminetetraacetic acid (EDTA) solution.
- Filter sterilized 25 kDa linear polyethyleneimine (PEI) in dH_2O (1 μg/μL), pH 7.4.
- Filter sterilized 150 mM NaCl in dH_2O.

Method

HEK293T cells are maintained in culture medium in a humidified incubator at 37 °C and 5% CO_2. DMEM without serum is only applied on HEK293T cells during stimulation conditions if not longer than 6 h. In all other conditions, serum is required as HEK293T cells will otherwise not survive. Refreshment of the culture medium should occur at least every 3–4 days depending on the growth rate of the cells. At 80% confluence, cells should be 10–20-fold diluted to keep them in the growth phase.

One day before transfection, 2×10^6 HEK293T cells are seeded in a 10 cm culture dish. Next day, cells are transiently transfected with cDNA using 25 kDa linear PEI. To this end, 5 μg cDNA in 250 μL NaCl (150 mM) is mixed by vortexing (>4 s) with 250 μL NaCl (150 mM) containing 20 μg of linear PEI (1:4 ratio) and incubated for 20–30 min at 22 °C. If less than 5 μg protein-encoding expression plasmid is used, supplement DNA with empty plasmid. Meanwhile, culture medium is aspirated from the cells and fresh medium is added (6 mL). The transfection mix is gently resuspended and dropwise added to the cells (Fig. 2).

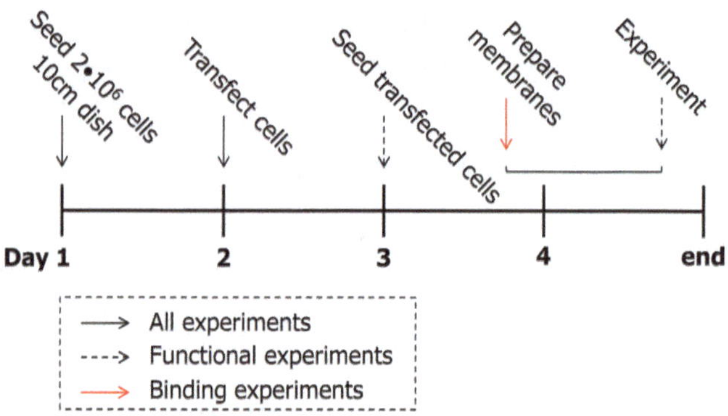

Fig. 2 Cell culture and transient transfection schedule

2.2 H_4R Radioligand-Binding Experiments

Receptor-ligand binding can be directly measured with various concentrations of radiolabeled ligands (saturation binding, Sect. 2.2.3.1) or indirectly with unlabeled ligands competing with a fixed concentration of radiolabeled ligand (competition binding, Sect. 2.2.3.2).

2.2.1 Theory: Receptor-Ligand Binding

For ligand-receptor binding a reversible two-state binding model is adopted (Eq. (1)).

$$[A]+[R] \underset{k_{off}}{\overset{k_{on}}{\rightleftarrows}} [AR] \tag{1}$$

According to this model, ligand $[A]$ and receptor $[R]$ can either occur in an unbound state $[A] + [R]$ or as a complex $[AR]$. A stable amount of $[AR]$ is obtained (i.e., equilibrium) once the rate of formation and deformation is the same (Eq. (2)).

$$k_{on}[A]*[R] = k_{off}[AR] \tag{2}$$

The rate of formation depends on the concentration of $[A]$, $[R]$, and association rate constant k_{on}. Deformation of $[AR]$ depends on the concentration of the formed complex and dissociation rate constant k_{off}. Based on k_{on} and k_{off} rate constants the equilibrium dissociation constant (K_d) of a ligand can be calculated (Eq. (3)).

$$K_d = \frac{k_{off}}{k_{on}} = \frac{[A]*[R]}{[AR]} \tag{3}$$

This value provides a measurement of strength for the interaction between the ligand and the receptor, known as the affinity. K_d (unity in M) equals the concentration of ligand that occupies 50% of the receptors.

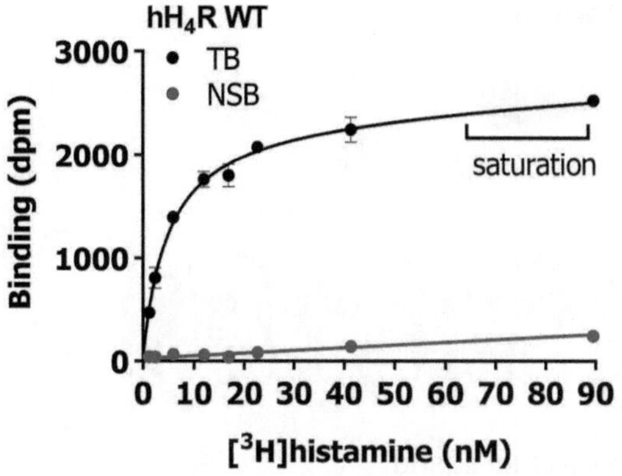

Fig. 3 HEK293T cells transiently expressing hH_4R show saturable binding of [^{3}H]histamine. Nonspecific binding was determined with 50 μM JNJ7777120 (10,000 × K_d). A K_d value of 4.9 nM was determined. *TB* Total binding, *NSB* nonspecific binding, *dpm* disintegrations per minute

In saturation-binding experiments, increasing concentrations of radiolabeled ligand are added to a constant amount of receptors. Saturation is obtained when all receptors are occupied (Fig. 3). This so-called B_{max} value is usually expressed as a number of receptor molecules per amount of tissue sample in the assay (e.g., pmol/mg protein).

The binding affinity of unlabeled ligands can be estimated in competition-binding assays with a radiolabeled ligand. In this case, increasing concentrations of unlabeled ligand are competing with a fixed concentration of radiolabeled ligand for binding on a constant number of receptors (Fig. 4). Usually, the concentration of radiolabeled ligand used in this assay is equivalent to its K_d value (*see* **Note 1**). Plotting radiolabeled ligand binding as a function of logarithmic concentration unlabeled ligand results in sigmoidal inhibitory curves from which the IC_{50} value can be obtained. The IC_{50} value represents the concentration of unlabeled ligand that displaces 50% of bound radiolabeled ligand from the receptor, and is dependent on both concentration (A^*) and affinity of the radiolabeled ligand. To calculate the equilibrium dissociation constant (K_i) of unlabeled ligands for the receptor, the Cheng-Prusoff equation is used (Eq. (4)) (*see* **Note 2**).

$$\text{Cheng-Prusoff equation } K_i = \frac{IC_{50}}{1 + \frac{[A*]}{K_d}} \tag{4}$$

Agonists have generally higher affinity for active G protein-(pre)coupled GPCR conformation(s) as compared to inactive G protein-uncoupled receptor conformation(s), and might consequently be sensitive to G protein availability [54]. In contrast,

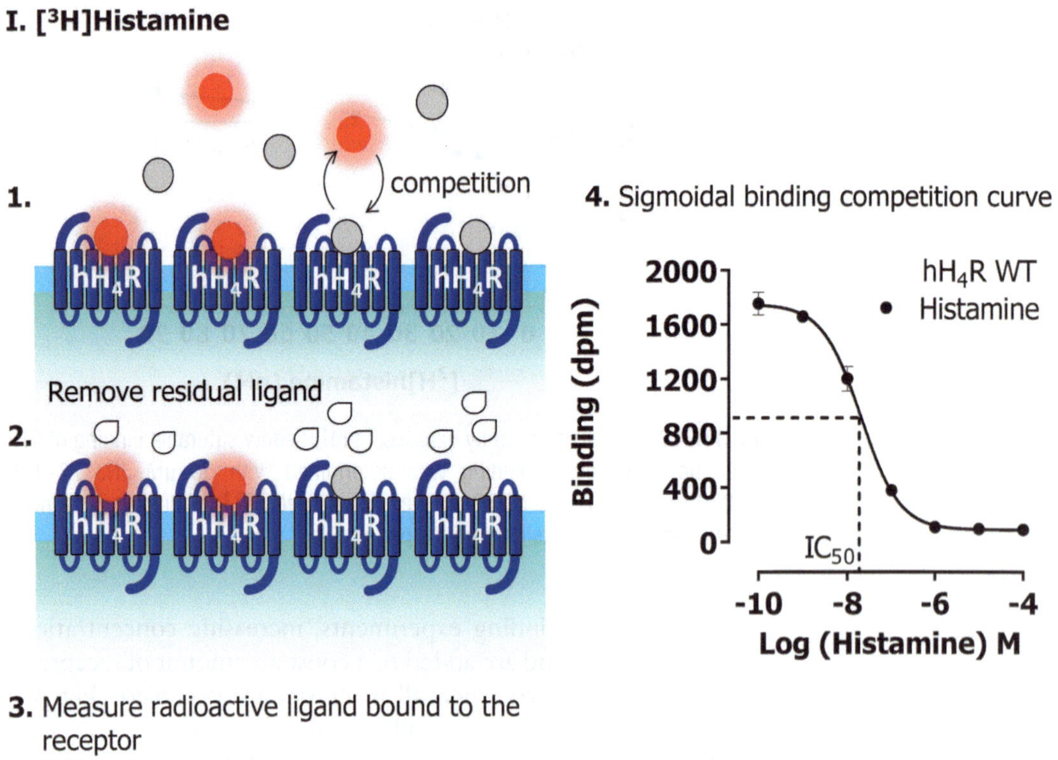

Fig. 4 Principle of a radioligand-binding competition assay. (*1*) Membranes expressing the hH_4R are incubated with a fixed concentration of radiolabeled ligand ([3H]histamine, *red dot*) and increasing concentrations of unlabeled ligand (*gray dot*). (*2*) Residual unlabeled- and radiolabeled ligand is removed from the membranes. (*3*) Radioactive ligand still bound to the receptor is measured. (*4*) Homogenates of HEK293T cells transiently transfected with 1 μg hH_4R cDNA. Membranes were incubated with 2 nM [3H]histamine and increasing concentrations of unlabeled histamine (100 pM–100 μM)

antagonists bind equally well to both G protein coupled and uncoupled GPCR conformations and are preferably used as radioligands to obtain single-site-binding curves. Home-made radiolabeled H_4R antagonists [^{125}I]iodophenpropit and [^{125}I]JNJ7777120 yielded comparable K_i values for unlabeled ligands in competition-binding experiments as full agonist [^{3}H]UR-PI294 and the commercially available full agonist [^{3}H]-histamine [11, 55]. Indeed, agonist binding at the hH_4R seems to be G protein independent [46, 56].

2.2.2 Preparation of H_4R Transfected Cell Homogenates for Binding Experiments

Required materials and reagents

- HEK293T cells transiently expressing H_4R.
- PBS, pH 7.4.
- Bicinchoninic acid (BCA) assay kit.
- Temperature-controlled centrifuge.

Method

1. HEK293T cells are transiently transfected with 0.1–1 μg H_4R cDNA and 4–4.9 μg empty plasmid (see Sect. 2.1) and incubated at 37 °C and 5% CO_2. Two days after transfections, cells are washed (2 mL) and resuspended in ice-cold PBS (2 mL), pH 7.4. Confluence of the cells should be around 95% (subconfluent). During the entire procedure cells are kept on ice to prevent protease activation.
2. Next, cells are centrifuged for 10 min at ~2000 × *g* and 4 °C. Supernatant is discarded and pellet resuspended in ice-cold PBS (1 mL/10 cm dish).
3. Cell suspension is divided into aliquots and centrifuged at 4 °C, ~2000 × *g* for 10 min, supernatant is discarded, and pellets stored at −20 °C until further use. Protein levels are determined using a BCA assay kit.

2.2.3 [^{3}H]Histamine-Binding Assays

Required materials and reagents

- Frozen (−20 °C) transfected cell homogenates (described in Sect. 2.2.2).
- Binding buffer: 50 mM Tris–HCl, pH 7.4.
- U-shaped 96-well plates.
- Ultrasonic homogenizer (Branson sonifier 250 set to a constant duty cycle and a microtip limit of 2).
- Radioactive ligand ([^{3}H]histamine, specific activity: 10–20 Ci/mmol).
- Unlabeled ligands.
- Specific H_4R ligand for nonspecific binding.
- Whatman GF/C filterplates, 96-well (Perkin Elmer).
- 0.5% polyethyleneimine (PEI) solution dissolved in dH_2O from 50% PEI stock solution (Sigma-Aldrich).
- Unifilter-96 harvester (Perkin Elmer).
- Scintillation fluid (MicroScint^{TM}-O, Perkin Elmer).

Method for [^{3}H]Histamine Saturation Binding

1. Homogenates prepared from HEK293T cells expressing the H_4R (Sect. 2.2.2) are resuspended in 5.5 mL binding buffer. Subsequently, cell homogenates are sonicated for 3–5 s to obtain a homogeneous suspension. Homogenates should be kept on ice until further use.
2. Homogenates (10–20 μg in 50 μL) are incubated with increasing concentrations (0.5–80 nM) of radiolabeled ligand (25 μL) and vehicle (25 μL binding buffer) or a high concentration of H_4R specific ligand (25 μL) (*see* **Note 3**) in U-shaped, clear 96-well plates until equilibrium is reached at 22 °C under

gently agitation (*see* **Note 4**). Radiolabeled ligand (25 μL) should also be spotted on a separate glass microfiber filter (GF/C, 96-well) to quantify added concentrations in the assay.

3. Incubation is terminated by rapid filtration under vacuum over a GF/C filter (96-well plate) followed by three additional wash steps of ice-cold-binding buffer. Excess free ligand is separated from the receptor-ligand complexes on cell homogenates. GF/C filters are presoaked in 0.5% PEI for at least 30 min to prevent free ligand to bind. The positively charged PEI neutralizes the negatively charged GF/C filters. To remove excess PEI, soaked GF/C filters are washed with ice-cold-binding buffer just before rapid filtration of cell homogenates.
4. Filters are dried at 52 °C for at least 30 min before 25 μL of MicroScintTM-O scintillation fluid is added to the wells. Sufficient drying of filters is required as MicroScintTM-O is not suitable for aqueous conditions.
5. Radioactivity of receptor-bound radiolabeled ligand is measured using a scintillation counter (Microbeta liquid scintillation counter), after a delay of at least 300 min to reduce variation in the data.
6. Data are analyzed using GraphPad Prism 6.0 software. Two methods can be applied, (1) manually subtract nonspecific binding from total binding to obtain specific binding. Specific binding is fitted by nonlinear regression using one site fit specific binding. (2) Directly fit total and nonspecific binding in nonlinear regression, one-site total and nonspecific binding (Fig. 3) (*see* **Note 5**).

Method for [^{3}H]Histamine Competition Binding

1. Cell homogenates (10–20 μg in 50 μL) (Sect. 2.2.2) are incubated with a fixed concentration of (25 μL) radiolabeled ligand and variable concentrations of unlabeled ligand (10 pM–100 μM), binding buffer or a high concentration of H_4R specific ligand (25 μL) in U-shaped, clear 96-well plates until equilibrium is reached at 22 °C under gently agitation (*see* **Note 4**). Radioligand (25 μL) should also be spotted on a separate glass microfiber filter (GF/C) to quantify added concentration in the assay.
2. Steps 3–5 are similar to saturation-binding assays (Sect. Method for [^{3}H]Histamine Saturation Binding).
3. Raw data are analyzed using GraphPad Prism 6.0 software, nonlinear regression, one site fit log *IC50* (Fig. 4).

Notes

1. A concentration equivalent to the radiolabeled ligand K_d value is usually selected in competition-binding assays to have sufficient measurement window. Higher concentrations of radiolabeled ligand will obviously increase the window, yet

require higher concentrations of competing ligand to be displaced, resulting in a right shift of the IC_{50} values.

2. The Cheng-Prusoff equation is only applicable to ligands competing for the same binding site on the receptor, and cannot be used for ligands that allosterically modulate each other's binding by acting at distinct sites on the receptor (Fig. 5). However, to our knowledge, allosteric ligands have not yet been identified for the H_4R.
3. Determination of nonspecific binding in radioligand binding assays is critical. This can be achieved by the addition of a high concentration (at least $1000 \times K_d$) of H_4R specific ligand to occupy all H_4R (e.g., JNJ7777120), which blocks binding of radiolabeled ligand to the receptor. Nonspecific binding is linearly correlated to radiolabeled ligand concentration (Fig. 3).
4. Acquiring equilibrium conditions is an essential step in saturation or competition-binding assays as non-equilibrium conditions can lead to inaccurate estimations of the ligand-binding affinity (K_d, K_i). As a general rule, use of an incubation time greater than five times the radioligand dissociation half-life ($t_{½}$) is sufficient to obtain equilibrium [57]. In this case, dissociation rates of the radioligand should first be determined (Eq. (5)).

$$t_{½} = \frac{ln2}{k_{off}} \tag{5}$$

For [^{3}H]histamine k_{off} of 0.083 ± 0.01/min was previously determined in H_4R-expressing HEK293T cell homogenates, corresponding to $t_{½}$ of 11.21 min [58]. An incubation time of at least 1 h should therefore be sufficient to reach equilibrium.

In the case of competition binding, the chosen incubation time is five times $t_{½}$ of the slowest compound in the assay. If this is unknown pilot assays should be performed using variable incubation times. If K_i values are constant between incubation times, equilibrium was reached.

5. To determine H_4R expression levels (B_{max}) on cell homogenates, binding with one concentration of radiolabeled ligand may be performed if its K_d value is known in that specific cell line. In different cell lines, K_d values might differ for the same radiolabeled ligand. The occupancy equation, based on the Langmuir isotherm (Eq. (6)), is used to determine the B_{max} value of cell homogenates.

$$\text{Langmuir's isotherm } \rho_A = \frac{[A]}{[A]+K_d} \tag{6}$$

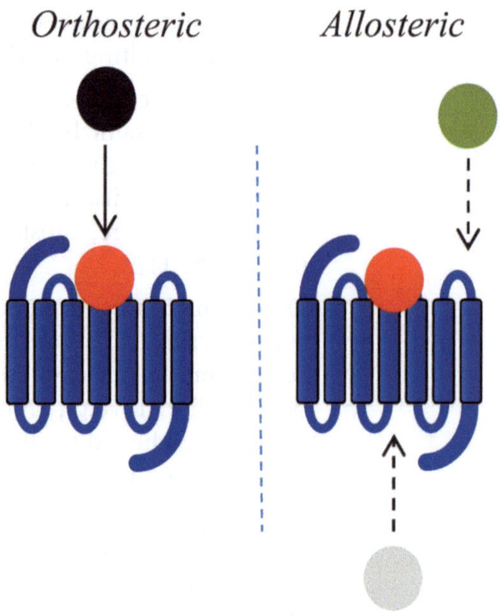

Fig. 5 Illustration of orthosteric and allosteric binding of ligands to a GPCR. *Red ligand* binds to the orthosteric-binding site of the receptor and can be replaced by the *black ligand* in a competition assay. Both the *green* and *gray ligand* bind to allosteric-binding sites at the receptor and will therefore be unable to directly compete with the *red ligand*

2.3 H_4R-Mediated $G\alpha_{i/o}$ Protein Activation—[^{35}S] GTPγS Accumulation Assay

Heterotrimeric G protein activation by GPCRs results in the exchange of guanosine diphosphate (GDP) with guanosine triphosphate (GTP) at the Gα subunit and the dissociation of Gα and Gβγ subunits. Association of GTP to the α-subunit leads to regulation of downstream effectors, like modulation of AC in case of the H_4R. The activity of the Gα is terminated by intrinsic GTPase activity resulting in hydrolysis of GTP into GDP and reconstitution with Gβγ.

[^{35}S]GTPγS is a radiolabeled non-hydrolyzable analogue of GTP, which binds irreversibly to activated heterotrimeric G proteins and leads to accumulation of the radiolabeled [^{35}S]GTPγS in cell homogenates upon receptor activation (Fig. 6). An advantage of this assay is that it is less subjective to signal amplification compared to second messenger assays (CAMYEL, 2.4.1) and reporter gene assays (CRE-luc, 2.5) since measurements are made upstream in the G protein-signaling cascade.

H_4R-mediated [^{35}S]GTPγS binding has been observed in, e.g., HEK293T, U2OS, and Sf9 insect cells in response to agonist stimulation [27, 46, 51] (*see* **Note 1**).

2.3.1 Preparation of H_4R Transfected Cell Homogenates for [^{35}S] GTPγS Assays

Required materials and reagents

- HEK293T cells transiently expressing H_4R.
- GTPγS membrane buffer: 15 mM Tris, 1 mM EGTA, 0.3 mM EDTA and 2 mM $MgCl_2$, pH 7.4 at 4 °C.

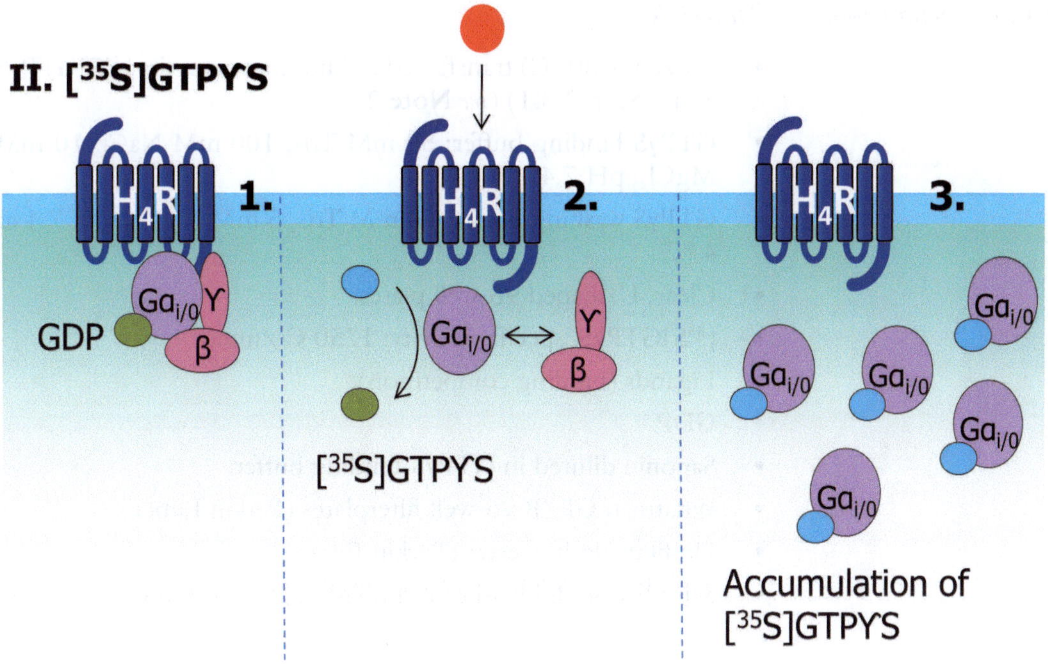

Fig. 6 Principle of a $[^{35}S]GTP\gamma S$ assay. (*1*) In its inactive conformation the heterotrimeric G protein is coupled to GDP. (*2*) When the receptor is bound by an agonist, its conformation changes toward the active state leading to dissociation of GDP and association of $[^{35}S]GTP\gamma S$. (*3*) The amount of radioactivity measured indicates activation of the receptor

- Tris-sucrose solution: 20 mM Tris, 250 mM sucrose, pH 7.4 at 4 °C.
- Ultrasonic homogenizer (Branson sonifier 250 set to a constant duty cycle and a microtip limit of 2).
- Temperature-controlled centrifuge.
- Bicinchoninic acid (BCA) assay kit.

Method

1. Cells are transiently transfected with 2.5–5 μg of H_4R cDNA and supplemented to 5 μg total DNA with empty expression plasmid in 10 cm dishes (Sect. 2.1).
2. Two days after transfection, cells are washed with 2 mL PBS and collected in 2.5 mL ice-cold GTPγS membrane buffer.
3. Cell suspension is sonicated for 20 s and centrifuged for 30 min, ~2000 × *g* at 4 °C. Supernatant is discarded and pellet is resuspended in 250 μL Tris-sucrose solution at 4 °C per 10 cm dish. To prevent degradation, cell homogenates are stored at −80 °C until further use. Protein levels are determined using a BCA assay kit.

2.3.2 [^{35}S]GTPγS Assay

Materials

- Frozen (−80 °C) transfected cell homogenates for [^{35}S]GTPγS assay (Sect. 2.3.1) (*see* **Note 2**).
- GTPγS-binding buffer: 50 mM Tris, 100 mM NaCl, 10 mM $MgCl_2$, pH 7.4.
- GTPγS washing buffer: 50 mM Tris, 5 mM $MgCl_2$, pH 7.4 at 4 °C.
- Clear, U-shaped 96-well plates.
- [^{35}S]GTPγS, specific activity: 1250 Ci/mmol.
- Ligands (binding competition).
- GDP.
- Saponin diluted in GTPγS-binding buffer.
- Whatman GF/B 96-well filterplates (Perkin Elmer).
- Unifilter-96 harvester (Perkin Elmer).
- Scintillation fluid (MicroScintTM-O, Perkin Elmer).

Method for [^{35}S]GTPγS accumulation assay

1. Receptor containing cell homogenates (*see* **Note 3**) are diluted in GTPγS-binding buffer till a concentration of 10 μg/100 μL.
2. GDP is diluted in GTPγS-binding buffer till a final concentration of 1–10 μM (optimization is required) supplemented with 0.2 μg/μL saponin. [^{35}S]GTPγS is added to this solution with a final concentration of 0.5–1 nM ([^{35}S]GTPγS mix).
3. 10 μg of membranes per well (100 μL) is added to 50 μL of ligand diluted in GTPγS-binding buffer and 50 μL of the [^{35}S]GTPγS mix (a total volume of 200 μL) in a clear, U-shaped bottom 96-well plate.
4. Samples are incubated for 1 h at 22 °C under gentle agitation.
5. Incubation is stopped by rapid filtration under vacuum over glass microfiber GF/B filters (96-well plate) followed by three additional flushes of ice-cold GTPγS washing buffer.
6. Perform steps 4 and 5 of radioligand binding (Sect. Method for [^{3}H]Histamine Saturation Binding).
7. Raw data are analyzed using GraphPad Prism 6.0 software, nonlinear regression, log(agonist) vs. response (three parameters).

Notes

1. This method is widely used for GPCRs coupling to $G\alpha_i$, since in general this protein is more abundant in cells compared to other G protein families [59]. In addition, a higher nucleotide exchange rate is observed for $G\alpha_i$, which results in a higher signal-to-noise ratio [59].

2. Cell homogenates prepared for [^{35}S]GTPγS assays are applicable for radioligand competition and saturation-binding assays. However, cell homogenates prepared for radioligand-binding assays cannot be used for [^{35}S]GTPγS assays.
3. [^{35}S]GTPγS is unable to cross cell membranes and can consequently only be used on membrane isolates.

2.4 BRET-Based Assay

Bioluminescence resonance energy transfer (BRET) is a widely used technique to measure protein-protein interactions or intramolecular conformational changes in living cells. BRET is based on the transfer of energy between luminescent enzyme (donor) in the presence of a substrate, and a fluorescent molecule/protein (acceptor) if their distance is less than 100 Å and their orientation allows dipole-dipole coupling (Fig. 7). By calculating the BRET ratios (i.e., luminescence at acceptor wavelength/luminescence at donor wavelength) the proximity between donor and acceptor can be determined. Real-time detection of BRET and luminescence makes this technique highly suitable for analysis of dynamic protein-protein interactions or conformational changes in a protein [60, 61].

2.4.1 CAMYEL Assay

The biosensor CAMYEL (cAMP sensor using YFP-EPAC-RLuc) is based on a truncated form of EPAC (exchange protein directly activated by cAMP) and consists of its cAMP-binding domain fused to *Renilla* luciferase (Rluc) at the N terminus and citrine (yellow fluorescent protein variant) at the C terminus [62]. In the absence of cAMP, CAMYEL adopts a closed conformation with donor and acceptor in close proximity, which results in a high BRET ratio. Binding of cAMP to the CAMYEL biosensor induces

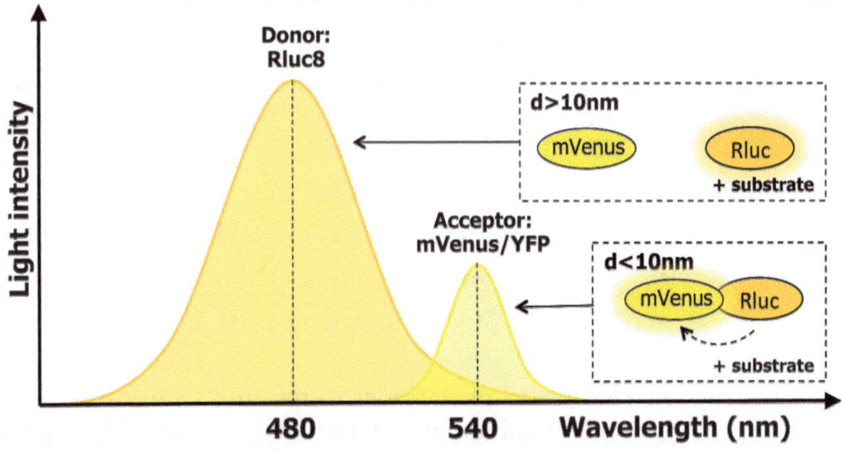

Fig. 7 Principle of a BRET assay. Emission spectra of donor (luminescent enzyme) must overlap with excitation spectra of acceptor (fluorophore) to facilitate energy transfer. Only if donor and acceptor are within 10 nm distance, excitation of acceptor is observed (BRET signal). Donor and acceptor can be tagged to the same protein (intramolecular BRET) or at different proteins (protein-protein interactions)

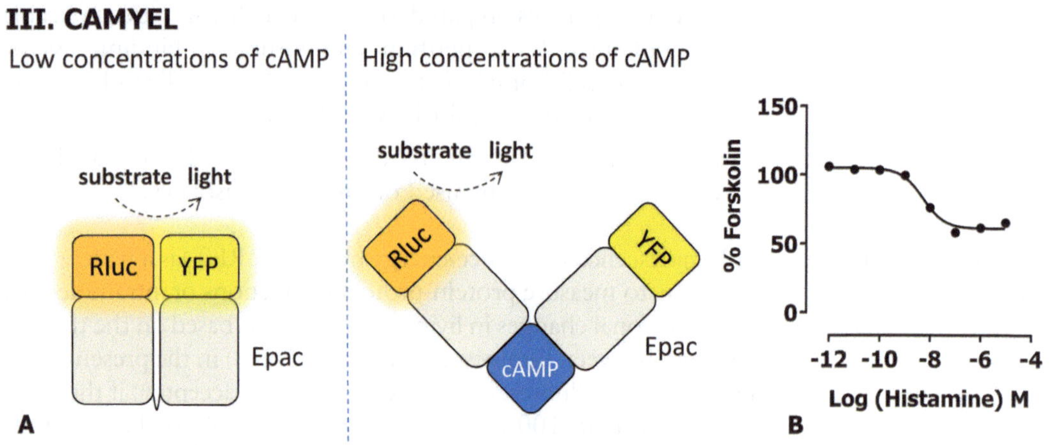

Fig. 8 (**a**) Principle of CAMYEL assay. Low levels of cAMP result in high BRET ratios, while high levels of cAMP result in low BRET ratios. (**b**) HEK293T cells transiently co-transfected with 1 μg of hH_4R and 4 μg CAMYEL cDNA. Cells were stimulated with increasing concentrations of histamine (1 pM–10 μM) in the presence of 10 μM forskolin

a conformational change resulting in decreased BRET ratio (Fig. 8a). For receptors that couple to $G\alpha_i$ proteins, like the H_4R, addition of forskolin is needed to directly activate AC and subsequent increase cAMP levels to observe the inhibitory $G\alpha_i$-mediated response upon receptor activation.

Materials

- HEK293T cells transiently transfected with the 1 μg of CAMYEL BRET sensor and 0.1–1 μg H_4R cDNA (Sect. 2.1).
- White, flat-bottomed 96-well tissue culture plates.
- Culture medium (Sect. 2.1).
- Coelenterazine-H (Promega), stock concentration of 1 mM in 0.1 mM HCl in methanol. Substrate is light sensitive and should be kept in the dark.
- Hanks' Balanced Salt Solution (HBSS).
- Poly-L-lysine (PLL) (Sigma-Aldrich, St. Louis, MO, USA).
- 3-isobuty-1-methylxanthine (IBMX).
- Forskolin, stock concentration 10 mM in dimethyl sulfoxide (DMSO).
- Multilabel plate reader to measure sequentially or simultaneously luminescence at 480 nm (Rluc) and 540 nm (BRET).

Method

1. 24 h post-transfection, HEK293T cells transiently transfected with 1 μg CAMYEL and 0.1–1 μg H_4R cDNA are seeded in white, flat-bottom shaped 96-well plates coated with 10% PLL

(*see* **Notes 1–3**). Each well contains 50,000 cells in 100 μL culture medium and cells are left to grow overnight at 37 °C and 5% CO_2.

2. The following day, medium is aspirated and cells are washed with 100 μL HBSS preheated at 37 °C to remove residual medium (*see* **Note 4**). Next 40 or 60 μL HBSS is added to the wells depending on whether cells will be treated with or without forskolin. If antagonists also need to be added 20 μL HBSS is used.
3. Add 20 μL coelenterazine-H (a final concentration of 5 μM) supplemented with IBMX (a final concentration 40 μM) to each well and incubate for 5 min at 37 °C in the dark. IBMX is a competitive, nonselective phosphodiesterase (PDE) inhibitor, thereby preventing the breakdown of cAMP. Assays should be performed in the absence of IBMX if BRET is measured in real time (study dynamics of cAMP levels).

   If pre-incubation of antagonists is required, this should occur prior to coelenterazine-H incubation. Incubation times are dependent on antagonist-binding kinetics. Viability of cells in HBSS is maintained for several hours.
4. Add 20 μL/well of ligand or vehicle (HBSS) and incubate cells in the dark at 37 °C. Incubation time of agonists and/or antagonists is dependent on their binding kinetics and needs optimization per ligand. For incubation times longer than 30 min, it is advised to pre-incubate cells with ligand before coelenterazine-H addition.
5. Add 20 μL forskolin (3 μM final concentration) to each well and incubate for 5 min at 37 °C in the dark (*see* **Notes 5** and **6**). As a control, a trio of wells should be treated with buffer instead of forskolin to determine the basal level of cAMP signaling in the cells (0% forskolin response).

   Cells treated with forskolin and vehicle instead of ligand serve as the maximal response induced by forskolin (100% forskolin response).
6. Measure sequentially or simultaneously luminescence at 480 nm (Rluc) and 540 nm (BRET) in a microplate reader.
7. BRET ratios are calculated by dividing the BRET signal by the Rluc signal (540/480 nm). Following, BRET ratios are normalized according to the 0 and 100% forskolin response. Graphs are plotted with GraphPad Prism 6.0 software using the nonlinear regression, dose response stimulatory fit (three independent parameters) (Fig. 8b).

2.4.2 β-Arrestin2 Recruitment Assay

Recruitment of β-arrestin2 to hH_4R in response to agonist stimulation can be detected using BRET [51]. To this end, hH_4R and β-arrestin2 were C-terminally fused to Rluc8 and mVenus, respectively (*see* **Note 7**).

Required materials and reagents

- HEK293T cells transiently transfected with 1 μg H_4R-5Rluc8 and 4 μg β-arrestin2-5mVenus (Sect. 2.1) (*see* **Note 8**).
- Culture medium (Sect. 2.1).
- White, flat-bottomed 96-well tissue culture plates.
- PLL (Sigma-Aldrich, St. Louis, MO, USA).
- Coelenterazine-H (Promega), stock concentration 1 mM in 0.1 mM HCl in methanol.
- HBSS.
- Multilabel plate reader to measure sequentially or simultaneously luminescence at 480 nm (Rluc) and 540 nm (BRET).

Method

1. 24 h post-transfection, HEK293T cells transiently co-transfected with 1 μg H_4R-Rluc8 and 4 μg β-arrestin2-mVenus cDNA are seeded in white 96-well plates (see Sect. 2.4.1, step 1).
2. 48 h after transfection, medium is aspirated for the cells and replaced by 50 μL HBSS.
3. Expression of β-arrestin2-mVenus is measured on a multilabel plate reader suitable for 96-well plates (excitation 485 nm; emission 535 nm).
4. 50 μL coelenterazine-H (final concentration 5 μM in HBSS) (Promega, Madison, WI, USA) is added to the cells and incubated for 5 min at 37 °C in the dark. Subsequently, Rluc8 luminescence (emission 480 nm) is measured using a BRET multiplate reader to monitor expression of H_4R-Rluc8.
5. Add 10 μL ligands in HBSS or vehicle (HBSS) and incubate at 37 °C (incubation times depend on ligand-binding kinetics) or directly measure luminescence at 480 and 540 nm in the microplate reader at 37 °C.
6. BRET ratios are calculated as described in Sect. 2.4.1, step 7. If measurements are made in real time, BRET ratios increase over time and should be corrected for the BRET ratios obtained from vehicle conditions (Fig. 9).

Notes

1. Coating 96-well plates with poly-L-lysine is recommended to reduce cell loss during washing.
2. White plates are recommended for BRET to avoid light absorption.
3. To monitor cell growth, cell viability, and transfection efficiency of fluorescently labeled proteins (light microscopy), cells are also plated in clear, flat-bottom shaped 96-well plates coated with PLL.

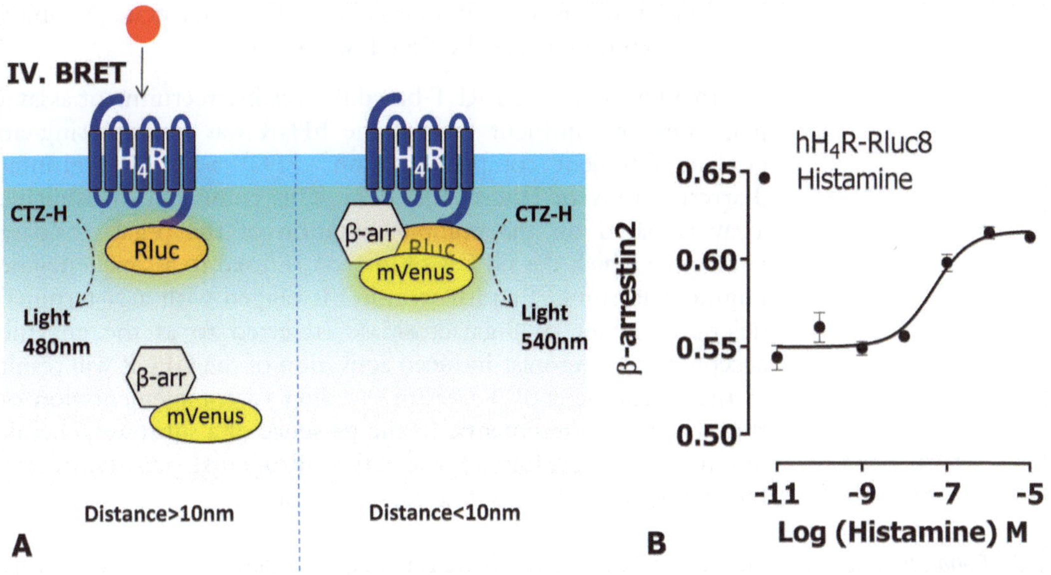

Fig. 9 (**a**) Principle of β-arrestin2 recruitment assay. (**b**) HEK293T cells transiently co-transfected with 1 μg of hH_4R-Rluc8 and 4 μg β-arrestin2-mVenus cDNA. Cells were stimulated with increasing concentrations of histamine (10 pM–10 μM)

4. Phenol red in the medium interferes with bioluminescence and should therefore be avoided.
5. Forskolin is added after receptor stimulation with ligands. Since cAMP is not degraded by PDE in the presence of IBMX, accumulation of cAMP will occur in cells stimulated with forskolin. To allow the ligand to bind to the receptor and induce an inhibitory effect on the production of cAMP, it is important to add the ligand before forskolin.
6. Forskolin concentration needs optimization to obtain highest window as the foskolin response is cell line dependent [63]. The optimal concentration can be determined with a forskolin concentration response curve in which the chosen concentration should correspond to the EC_{50} value of forskolin in the experimental system [64, 65].
7. The number of amino acids (linker) between the receptor/interacting protein and donor/acceptor can affect BRET. In most cases, a linker length of about 5–10 amino acids is used [60]. hH_4R-Rluc8 and β-arrestin2-mVenus both contained a linker length of five amino acids.
8. Optimization of acceptor/donor ratio might be required to obtain an optimal response window. Increasing concentrations of acceptor/donor proteins will eventually lead to nonspecific BRET signals as random collision between these proteins becomes more visible. On the other hand, low concentrations of acceptor/

donor proteins might not be sufficient to demonstrate proximity between proteins as the BRET signal is too low.

In addition to the BRET-based β-arrestin2 recruitment assays, β-arrestin2 recruitment toward the hH_4R was shown using an enzyme fragment complementation (EFC) assay (PathHunter β-arrestin assay of DiscoveRx) [27]. This commercially available assay is based on the complementation of the β-galactosidase enzyme in which the GPCR of interest is fused to a small enzyme fragment ProLink™ and β-arrestin2 is tagged with a N-terminal deletion mutant of β-galactosidase (referred to as the enzyme acceptor; EA). Agonist-induced activation of the GPCR will result in the recruitment of β-arrestin2 leading to complementation of the two enzyme fragments. In the presence of a substrate, chemiluminescent PathHunter® Detection Reagents, activity of the reconstituted β-galactosidase can be measured.

2.5 Reporter Gene Assay

GPCR signaling can activate transcription factors that subsequently bind to DNA response elements to regulate gene transcription. Reporter gene constructs consist of a promoter region with defined response elements regulating the expression of an easily detectable bioluminescent or enzymatic protein (e.g., luciferase, β-galactosidase, or β-lactamase). Numerous reporter gene constructs are (commercially) available for detection of various signaling pathways [66]. Key advantages of reporter gene assay are the relative ease by which the assay is performed, low cost of required chemicals, and ability to use a high-throughput format. Agonist-induced H_4R signaling decreases cAMP-dependent CREB activity, which can be measured using a CRE reporter gene (Fig. 10) (*see* **Notes 1** and **2**) [11, 25].

Required materials and reagents

- HEK293T cells transiently transfected with the 2.5 μg CRE-luc reporter gene and the 1 μg hH_4R (Sect. 2.1).
- Culture medium (Sect. 2.1).
- DMEM.
- White, flat-bottomed 96-well tissue culture plates.
- PLL (Sigma-Aldrich, St. Louis, MO, USA).
- Luciferase assay reagent (0.83 mM ATP, 0.83 mM D-luciferin, 18.7 mM $MgCl_2$, 0.78 μM Na_2HPO_4, 38.9 mM Tris/H_3PO_4 (pH 7.8), 0.39% glycerol, 0.03% Triton X-100 and 2.6 μM dithiothreitol (DTT)).
- Forskolin, stock concentration 10 mM in DMSO.
- Multilabel plate reader to measure luminescence.

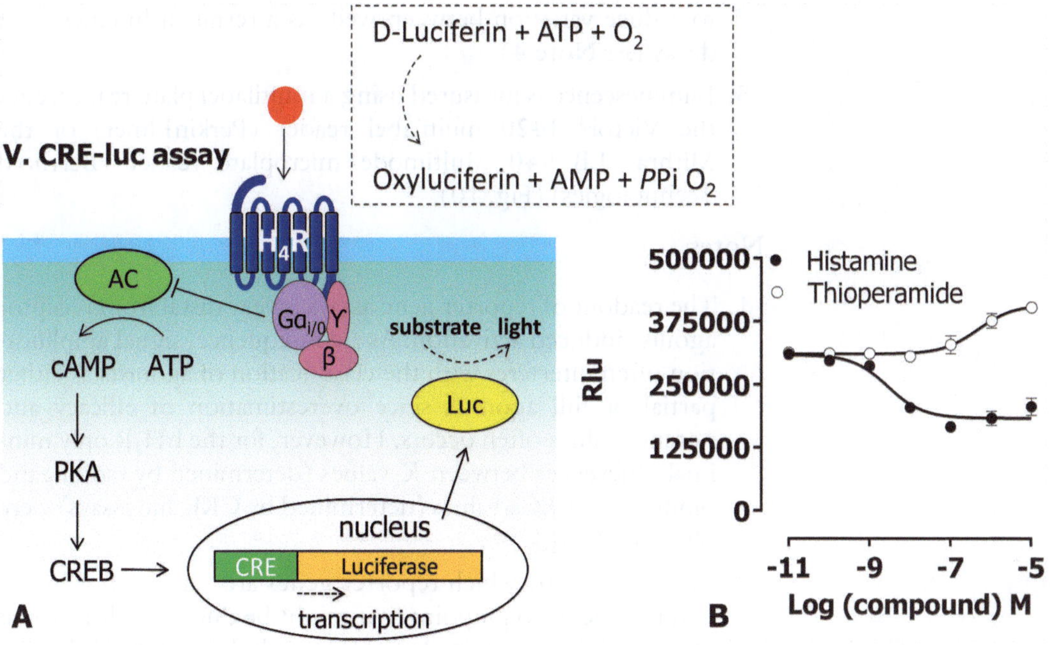

Fig. 10 (**a**) Principle of a CRE-luc reporter gene assay. Activation of the H_4R inhibits the production of adenylyl cyclase (AC) which thereby inhibits the transcription of a luciferase reporter gene. (**b**) HEK293T cells co-transiently transfected with 1 μg of hH_4R and 2.5 μg CRE-luc reporter gene. Cells were stimulated with increasing concentrations of histamine or thioperadmide (10 pM–10 μM) in the presence of 1 μM forskolin. Basal activity is inhibited with thioperamide stimulation

Method

1. HEK293T cells were transiently co-transfected with 1 μg hH_4R and 2.5 μg CRE-luc reporter gene cDNA (Sect. 2.1).
2. 24 h after transfection, cells were seeded as described in Sect. 2.4.1. 96-well plates are coated with PLL if a nonhomogeneous format of the assay is used (*see* **Note 3**).
3. 48 h after transfection, cells are incubated with H_4R ligands diluted in serum-free DMEM supplemented with 1 μM forskolin at 37 °C and 5% CO_2. An incubation of at least 6 h is required for induced firefly luciferase protein expression.
4. Medium is aspirated from the cells (nonhomogeneous format), thereafter 25 μL of luciferase assay reagent (LAR) is added to each well. Alternatively, 25 μL of LAR is added directly on the medium (homogeneous format). As a consequence, the homogeneous format will result in a smaller window of response (measured relative luminescence) compared to the nonhomogeneous format as LAR will be more diluted. In contrast, loss of cells caused by aspiration of medium is prevented. Although luminescence can be measured directly after the addition of LAR, we recommend an incubation period of 30 min at 37 °C

to reduce variation between wells as a result of luminescence decay (*see* **Note 4**).

5. Luminescence is measured using a multilabel plate reader, e.g., the Victor³ 1420 multilabel reader (PerkinElmer) or the Mithras LB 940 Multimode microplate reader (Berthold Technologies) (Fig. 10).

Notes

1. The readout of reporter gene assays is very distal from receptor agonist-induced activation. As a consequence, signal amplification often interferes with the classification of agonists as either partial or full agonists since overestimation of efficacy and potency values often occurs. However, for the hH_4R only minimal differences between K_i values (determined by radioligand binding) and EC_{50} values (determined by CRE-luc assays) were observed [26].
2. The pathway by which reporter genes are activated or inhibited is difficult to pinpoint as it might be due to multifactorial causes, e.g., G protein dependent or independent pathways, cross-talk between pathways, or even receptor independent (off-target) effects [11, 64]. In the case of off-target effects, it is always recommended to include negative control cells devoid of the H_4R to validate if observed effects are receptor mediated.
3. The CRE-luc reporter gene assay is also applicable for high-throughput assay formats. In this case, 24 h post-transfection, cells are seeded in white-bottomed 384-well plates (8000 cells/well) in 20 μL culture medium.
4. Luciferases can be subdivided as either flash-type or glow-type enzymes. Flash-type luciferases induce a rapid burst of light with high signal intensity in the presence of their substrate. This makes the assay highly sensitive. However, rapid decay of the luminescent signal makes this assay more vulnerable for sample variation within the same assay. A more stable luminescent signal is acquired with the use of glow-type luciferases as the decay is slower compared to flash, although sensitivity is reduced. Depending on the experimental procedure/design either glow- or flash-type luciferases can be required.

3 Conclusion

In this chapter, we described some of the main methods applicable and proven to be successful at the H_4R. Elucidation of ligand-binding properties and signaling pathways of the H_4R are important for future drug development, as this receptor has proven to be a designated target for treatment of inflammatory diseases. Main difficulties encountered in practical procedures are often due to slight nuances in protocols, which can be tackled with easy tips or clever tricks if known by the particular scientist. Here, we provide a detailed overview of methods used in our laboratory to determine H_4R expression and study receptor-ligand binding, G protein signaling, and β-arrestin2 signaling. In addition, advantages and pitfalls of methods were discussed.

Acknowledgments

The authors participated in the European COST Action BM0806. ECHO grant (711.013.014) of the Netherlands Organization of Scientific Research supported this work.

References

1. Panula P, Chazot PL, Cowart M et al (2015) International union of basic and clinical pharmacology. XCVIII. Histamine receptors. Pharmacol Rev 67:601–655
2. Arrang J-M, Garbarg M, Schwartz J-C (1983) Auto-inhibition of brain histamine release mediated by a novel class (H_3) of histamine receptor. Nature 302:832–837
3. Black JW, Duncan WAM, Durant CJ et al (1972) Definition and antagonism of histamine H_2-receptors. Nature 236:385–390
4. Wells JA, Morris HC (1945) Observations on the nature of the antagonism of histamine by beta-dimethylaminoethyl benzhydryl ether (benadryl). J Pharmacol Exp Ther 85:122–128
5. Liu C, Ma X, Jiang X et al (2001) Cloning and pharmacological characterization of a fourth histamine receptor (H_4) expressed in bone marrow. Mol Pharmacol 59:420–426
6. Oda T, Morikawa N, Saito Y et al (2000) Molecular cloning and characterization of a novel type of histamine receptor preferentially expressed in leukocytes. J Biol Chem 275:36781–36786
7. Morse KL, Behan J, Laz TM et al (2001) Cloning and characterization of a novel human histamine receptor. J Pharmacol Exp Ther 296:1058–1066
8. Zhu Y, Michalovich D, Wu H et al (2001) Cloning, expression, and pharmacological characterization of a novel human histamine receptor. Mol Pharmacol 59:434–441
9. Nakamura T, Itadani H, Hidaka Y et al (2000) Molecular cloning and characterization of a new human histamine receptor, HH4R. Biochem Biophys Res Commun 279:615–620
10. Nguyen T, Shapiro DA, George SR et al (2001) Discovery of a novel member of the histamine receptor family. Mol Pharmacol 59:427–433
11. Lim HD, Van Rijn RM, Ling P et al (2005) Evaluation of histamine H_1-, H_2-, and H_3-receptor ligands at the human histamine H_4 receptor: identification of 4-methylhistamine as the first potent and selective H_4 receptor agonist. J Pharmacol Exp Ther 314:1310–1321
12. Simons FER, Simons KJ (2011) Histamine and H_1-antihistamines: celebrating a century of progress. J Allergy Clin Immunol 128:1139–1150.e4
13. Scarpignato C (2007) New drugs to suppress acid secretion: current and future developments. Drug Discov Today Ther Strateg 4:155–163
14. Esbenshade TA, Browman KE, Bitner RS et al (2008) The histamine H_3 receptor: an attractive target for the treatment of cognitive disorders. Br J Pharmacol 154:1166–1181
15. Dauvilliers Y, Bassetti C, Lammers GJ et al (2013) Pitolisant versus placebo or modafinil in patients with narcolepsy: a double-blind, randomised trial. Lancet Neurol 12:1068–1075
16. Jemima EA, Prema A, Thangam EB (2014) Functional characterization of histamine H_4 receptor on human mast cells. Mol Immunol 62:19–28
17. Dijkstra D, Leurs R, Chazot P et al (2007) Histamine downregulates monocyte CCL2 production through the histamine H_4 receptor. J Allergy Clin Immunol 120:300–307

18. Dijkstra D, Stark H, Chazot PL et al (2008) Human inflammatory dendritic epidermal cells express a functional histamine H_4 receptor. J Invest Dermatol 128:1696–1703
19. Bäumer W, Wendorff S, Gutzmer R et al (2008) Histamine H_4 receptors modulate dendritic cell migration through skin—immunomodulatory role of histamine. Allergy 63:1387–1394
20. Hofstra CL, Desai PJ, Thurmond RL (2003) Histamine H_4 receptor mediates chemotaxis and calcium mobilization of mast cells. J Pharmacol Exp Ther 305:1212–1221
21. Gantner F, Sakai K, Tusche MW et al (2002) Histamine H_4 and H_2 receptors control histamine-induced interleukin-16 release from human CD8(+) T cells. J Pharmacol Exp Ther 303:300–307
22. Novak N, Mete N, Bussmann C et al (2012) Early suppression of basophil activation during allergen-specific immunotherapy by histamine receptor 2. J Allergy Clin Immunol 130:1153–1158
23. Violin JD, Soergel DG, Boerrigter G et al (2013) GPCR biased ligands as novel heart failure therapeutics. Trends Cardiovasc Med 23:242–249
24. Kingwell K (2015) Pioneering biased ligand offers efficacy with reduced on-target toxicity. Nat Rev Drug Discov 14:809–810
25. Nijmeijer S, Vischer HF, Rosethorne EM et al (2012) Analysis of multiple histamine H_4 receptor compound classes uncovers Gαi protein- and β-arrestin2-biased ligands. Mol Pharmacol 82:1174–1182
26. Nijmeijer S, Vischer HF, Sirci F et al (2013) Detailed analysis of biased histamine H_4 receptor signalling by JNJ 7777120 analogues. Br J Pharmacol 170:78–88
27. Rosethorne EM, Charlton SJ (2011) Agonist-biased signaling at the histamine H_4 receptor: JNJ7777120 recruits β-arrestin without activating G proteins. Mol Pharmacol 79: 749–757
28. Thurmond RL (2015) The histamine H_4 receptor: from orphan to the clinic. Front Pharmacol 6:1–11
29. Kollmeier A, Francke K, Chen B et al (2014) The H_4 receptor antagonist, JNJ 39758979, is effective in reducing histamine-induced pruritus in a randomized clinical study in healthy subjects. J Pharmacol Exp Ther 350:181–187
30. Shin N, Covington M, Bian D et al (2012) INCB38579, a novel and potent histamine H_4 receptor small molecule antagonist with anti-inflammatory pain and anti-pruritic functions. Eur J Pharmacol 675:47–56
31. Dunford PJ, O'Donnell N, Riley JP et al (2006) The histamine H_4 receptor mediates allergic airway inflammation by regulating the activation of CD4(+) T cells. J Immunol 176:7062–7070
32. Cowden JM, Yu F, Banie H et al (2014) The histamine H_4 receptor mediates inflammation and Th17 responses in preclinical models of arthritis. Ann Rheum Dis 73:600–608
33. Varga C, Horvath K, Berko A et al (2005) Inhibitory effects of histamine H_4 receptor antagonists on experimental colitis in the rat. Eur J Pharmacol 522:130–138
34. Adami M, Pozzoli C, Menozzi A et al (2012) Effects of histamine H_4 receptor ligands in a mouse model of mastric ulceration. Pharmacology 89:287–294
35. Murata Y, Song M, Kikuchi H et al (2015) Phase 2a, randomized, double-blind, placebo-controlled, multicenter, parallel-group study of a H_4R-antagonist (JNJ-39758979) in Japanese adults with moderate atopic dermatitis. J Dermatol 42:129–139
36. Connelly WM, Shenton FC, Lethbridge N et al (2009) The histamine H_4 receptor is functionally expressed on neurons in the mammalian CNS. Br J Pharmacol 157:55–63
37. Schneider EH, Seifert R (2015) The histamine H_4-receptor and the central and peripheral nervous system: a critical analysis of the literature. Neuropharmacology:1–13
38. Altinbas B, Yilmaz MS, Savci V et al (2015) Centrally injected histamine increases posterior hypothalamic acetylcholine release in hemorrhage-hypotensive rats. Auton Neurosci 187:63–69
39. Feliszek M, Speckmann V, Schacht D et al (2015) A search for functional histamine H_4 receptors in the human, guinea pig and mouse brain. Naunyn Schmiedebergs Arch Pharmacol 388:11–17
40. Lethbridge NL, Chazot PL (2010) Immunological identification of the mouse H_4 histamine receptor on spinal cord motor neurons using a novel anti-mouse H_4R antibody. Inflamm Res 59:S197–S198
41. Gutzmer R, Diestel C, Mommert S et al (2005) Histamine H_4 receptor stimulation suppresses IL-12p70 production and mediates chemotaxis in human monocyte-derived dendritic cells. J Immunol 174:5224–5232
42. Czerner CP, Klos A, Seifert R et al (2014) Histamine induces chemotaxis and phagocytosis in murine bone marrow-derived macrophages and RAW 264.7 macrophage-like cells via histamine H_4-receptor. Inflamm Res 63:239–247

43. Ling P, Ngo K, Nguyen S et al (2004) Histamine H_4 receptor mediates eosinophil chemotaxis with cell shape change and adhesion molecule upregulation. Br J Pharmacol 142:161–171
44. O'Reilly M, Alpert R, Jenkinson S et al (2002) Identification of a histamine H_4 receptor on human eosinophils—role in eosinophil chemotaxis. J Recept Signal Transduct Res 22:431–448
45. Costa T, Cotecchia S (2005) Historical review: negative efficacy and the constitutive activity of G-protein-coupled receptors. Trends Pharmacol Sci 26:618–624
46. Schneider EH, Schnell D, Papa D et al (2009) High constitutive activity and a G-protein-independent high-affinity state of the human histamine H_4-receptor. Biochemistry 48:1424–1438
47. Bakker RA, Schoonus SBJ, Smit MJ et al (2001) Histamine H_1-receptor activation of nuclear factor-κB: roles for Gβγ- and Gαq/11-subunits in constitutive and agonist- mediated signaling. Mol Pharmacol 60:1133–1142
48. Smit MJ, Leurs R, Alewijnse AE et al (1996) Inverse agonism of histamine H_2 antagonist accounts for upregulation of spontaneously active histamine H_2 receptors. Proc Natl Acad Sci USA 93:6802–6807
49. Moore CAC, Milano SK, Benovic JL (2007) Regulation of receptor trafficking by GRKs and arrestins. Annu Rev Physiol 69: 451–482
50. Marchese A, Paing MM, Temple BRS et al (2008) G protein-coupled receptor sorting to endosomes and lysosomes. Annu Rev Pharmacol Toxicol 48:601–629
51. Nijmeijer S, Engelhardt H, Schultes S et al (2013) Design and pharmacological characterization of VUF14480, a covalent partial agonist that interacts with cysteine 983.36 of the human histamine H_4 receptor. Br J Pharmacol 170:89–100
52. Shenoy SK, Drake MT, Nelson CD et al (2006) beta-arrestin-dependent, G protein-independent ERK1/2 activation by the beta2 adrenergic receptor. J Biol Chem 281:1261–1273
53. Lim HD, Smits RA, Bakker RA et al (2006) Discovery of S-(2-guanidylethyl)-isothiourea (VUF8430) as a potent nonimidazole histamine H_4 receptor agonist. J Med Chem 49:6650–6651
54. De Lean A, Stadel JM, Lefkowitz RJ (1980) A ternary complex model explains the agonist-specific binding properties of the adenylate cyclase-coupled beta-adrenergic receptor. J Biol Chem 255:7108–7117
55. Igel P, Schnell D, Bernhardt G et al (2009) Tritium-labeled N 1 -[3-(1 H -imidazol-4-yl) propyl]- N 2 -propionylguanidine ([3 H] UR-PI294), a high-affinity histamine H_3 and H_4 receptor radioligand. ChemMedChem 4:225–231
56. Nijmeijer S, Leurs R, Smit MJ et al (2010) The Epstein-Barr virus-encoded G protein-coupled receptor BILF1 hetero-oligomerizes with human CXCR4, scavenges Gαi proteins, and constitutively impairs CXCR4 functioning. J Biol Chem 285:29632–29641
57. Hulme EC, Trevethick MA (2010) Ligand binding assays at equilibrium: validation and interpretation. Br J Pharmacol 161:1219–1237
58. Smits RA, Lim HD, van der Meer T et al (2012) Ligand based design of novel histamine H_4 receptor antagonists; fragment optimization and analysis of binding kinetics. Bioorg Med Chem Lett 22:461–467
59. Harrison C, Traynor JR (2003) The [35S] GTPγS binding assay: approaches and applications in pharmacology. Life Sci 74:489–508
60. Bacart J, Corbel C, Jockers R et al (2008) The BRET technology and its application to screening assays. Biotechnol J 3:311–324
61. Salahpour A, Espinoza S, Masri B et al (2012) BRET biosensors to study GPCR biology, pharmacology, and signal transduction. Front Endocrinol 3:1–9
62. Barak LS, Salahpour A, Zhang X et al (2008) Pharmacological characterization of membrane-expressed human trace amine-associated receptor 1 (TAAR1) by a bioluminescence resonance energy transfer cAMP biosensor. Mol Pharmacol 74:585–594
63. Williams C (2004) cAMP detection methods in HTS: selecting the best from the rest. Nat Rev Drug Discov 3:125–135
64. Nordemann U, Wifling D, Schnell D et al (2013) Luciferase reporter gene assay on human, murine and rat histamine H_4 receptor orthologs: correlations and discrepancies between distal and proximal readouts. PLoS One 8:e73961
65. Hill SJ, Williams C, May LT (2010) Insights into GPCR pharmacology from the measurement of changes in intracellular cyclic AMP; advantages and pitfalls of differing methodologies. Br J Pharmacol 161:1266–1275
66. Hill SJ, Baker JG, Rees S (2001) Reporter-gene systems for the study of G-protein-coupled receptors. Curr Opin Pharmacol 1:526–532

Chapter 7

Chemiluminescence: A Sensitive Method for Detecting the Effects of Histamine Receptor Agonists/Antagonists on Neutrophil Oxidative Burst

Ondřej Vašíček, Tomáš Perečko, Viera Jančinová, Silvia Pažoureková, Radomír Nosáľ, and Milan Číž

Abstract

Polymorphonuclear leukocytes (neutrophils) form the first line of defence in humans. After activation, they migrate through vessel walls toward the invading agent. The intruding pathogens are eliminated through the action of released proteases and by production of reactive oxygen species (ROS). Histamine, a biogenic amine with various physiological and pathological effects, is known to modulate the immune response of neutrophils, e.g., it blunts the production of ROS in neutrophils after binding to the histamine-2 receptor. To detect the ROS in neutrophils, various methods are used. Among these, luminophore-enhanced chemiluminescence is a very sensitive and easy tool for studying the effects of various compounds on ROS production in neutrophils. On the other hand, its selectivity is questionable. However, employing cell-free systems producing selective ROS types, the inhibitory effects of tested compounds against distinct ROS may be evaluated. In this chapter, we describe the methods for the evaluation of ROS modulating effects of histamine agonists/antagonists in human neutrophils by using chemiluminescence methods.

Key words Antihistamines, Chemiluminescence, Histamine, Histamine receptor, Neutrophil, Reactive oxygen species

1 Introduction

Histamine is a biogenic amine that plays an essential role in controlling many physiological functions and serves as an important chemical messenger. Most of these physiological effects are mediated through interactions with four histamine receptor subtypes, all of which are members of the larger family of rhodopsin-like class A G-protein coupled receptors (GPCRs) [1]. Histamine can influence most cells of the immune system and selectively recruit them into tissue sites, affecting their maturation, activation, polarization, and effector functions, and leading to chronic inflammation [2].

The H_1R is involved in most of the acute inflammatory responses and antagonists for this receptor have been used as successful drugs

Ekaterini Tiligada and Madeleine Ennis (eds.), *Histamine Receptors as Drug Targets*, Methods in Pharmacology and Toxicology, DOI 10.1007/978-1-4939-6843-5_7,

for treating allergies [3, 4]. The H_2R is mainly involved mainly in gastric acid secretion, in heart contraction, or in regulating various functions such as cell proliferation, differentiation, and immune responses such as the oxidative burst [5–7]. The H_3R is localized primarily in the central nervous system and modulates neurotransmitter levels [4]. H_4R is the latest identified histamine receptor and is preferentially, but not exclusively, identified in hematopoietic cells, especially in basophils, mast cells, eosinophils, T lymphocytes, and dendritic cells. Some authors have also reported H_4R on neutrophils and monocytes [8–10]. Following a challenge by pathogens, histamine secreted from various cells modulates the function (including oxidative burst) of neutrophils and other phagocytes mainly through the activation of H_1R and H_2R [7, 11–14].

H_1-antihistamines belong to the most frequently prescribed medications used by patients suffering from allergic rhinitis, conjunctivitis, or urticaria, as well as in therapy for asthma, atopic dermatitis, and anaphylaxis [15, 16]. Besides blocking histamine effects, their therapeutic effectiveness for allergic diseases has also been suggested as relying on the interfering with one or more components of the inflammatory response, including the activity of immune cells [17, 18]. In neutrophils, H_1-antihistamines decrease the formation of reactive oxygen species (ROS) [19–22], chemotaxis, release of elastase, and liberation of myeloperoxidase [23, 24]. The observed effects were considered beneficial since prolonged or excessive liberation of cytotoxic agents from neutrophils may increase the risk of tissue damage, block resolution, and lead to permanent inflammation [25].

Neutrophils are the predominant immune cell type in the blood stream of humans [26]. In response to injury or infection they migrate to the inflammation loci to neutralize the invading pathogens or to cease tissue injury [27]. Together with monocytes and macrophages, they are called "professional phagocytes" because of their primary function – engulfing and destroying potentially injurious stimuli. Neutrophil recruitment from the bloodstream is triggered by inflammatory stimuli such as inflammatory chemokines, cytokines, or lipid mediators. The inflammatory microenvironment triggers a multi-factorial process leading to the transmigration of neutrophils through the vessel wall, known as extravasation [28]. Recent studies indicate that recruited neutrophils contribute to the overall inflammation [28–30]. After the phagocytosis of invading pathogens, neutrophils die by programmed cell death and are cleared by tissue macrophages [31]. An inflammatory response that lasts for only a few days is called "acute inflammation," while a response of longer duration is referred to as "chronic inflammation." Acute inflammation is usually beneficial. But, in some cases, inflammation may cause injury to the host. Physiologically, acute neutrophilic inflammation is followed by a resolution phase [32]. If these resolving mechanisms

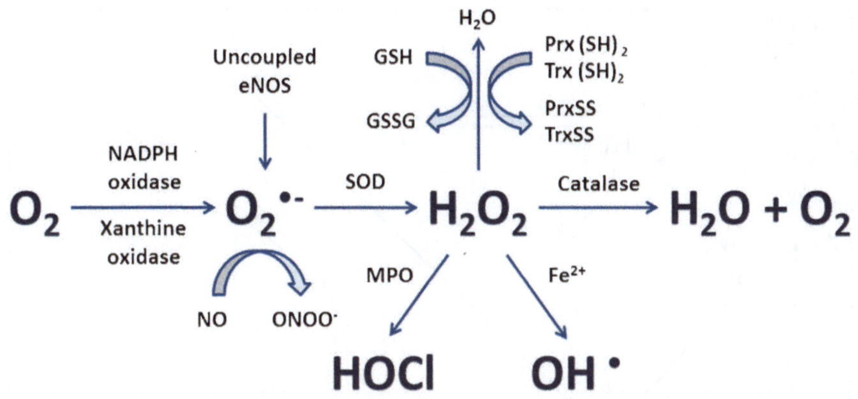

Fig. 1 Cascade of reactive oxygen species generation. *eNOS* endothelial nitric oxide synthase, *GSH* reduced glutathione, *GSSG* oxidized glutathione, *MPO* myeloperoxidase, *Prx* peroxiredoxin, *SOD* superoxide dismutase, *Trx* thioredoxin

are impaired, neutrophils drive chronic inflammation, characterized by the release of oxidants and proteases and leading to tissue injury [26].

ROS (Fig. 1) produced by phagocytes after their activation are critical for protection against invading microorganisms and also seem to have important physiological roles in priming the immune system as second messengers [33–36]. This phenomenon is known as the "respiratory burst" and is due to activation of the enzyme NADPH oxidase [37]. NADPH oxidase is a multicomponent enzyme system composed of heterodimeric membrane-associated flavocytochrome b588 protein, which is composed of gp91phox and p22phox and three cytosolic proteins (p47phox, p67phox, and p40phox) and the small GTPase (Rac1 or Rac2). NADPH oxidase activation is controlled by the recruitment of regulatory proteins to the flavocytochrome b588, including the p40phox, p47phox, and p67phox, of which p47phox and p67phox are essential for activity (Fig. 2).

The development of a methodology for measuring the generation and release of phagocyte-derived ROS is of great importance, and a number of different techniques are currently used for this purpose. One of the basic techniques frequently used is luminol/isoluminol-enhanced chemiluminescence [38, 39]. Allen (1977) [40] described that activated neutrophils are able to produce a chemiluminescence that could be correlated with their oxidative burst. Chemiluminescence is the light energy produced by the neutrophils during their activation and has been demonstrated to correlate well with their antibacterial integrity. Measurement of neutrophil chemiluminescence provides a very sensitive assay of the functional ability of these cells [41]. This technique is a valuable tool to test the effects of drugs on the activity of neutrophils [42]. Chemiluminescence allows the development of simple analytical

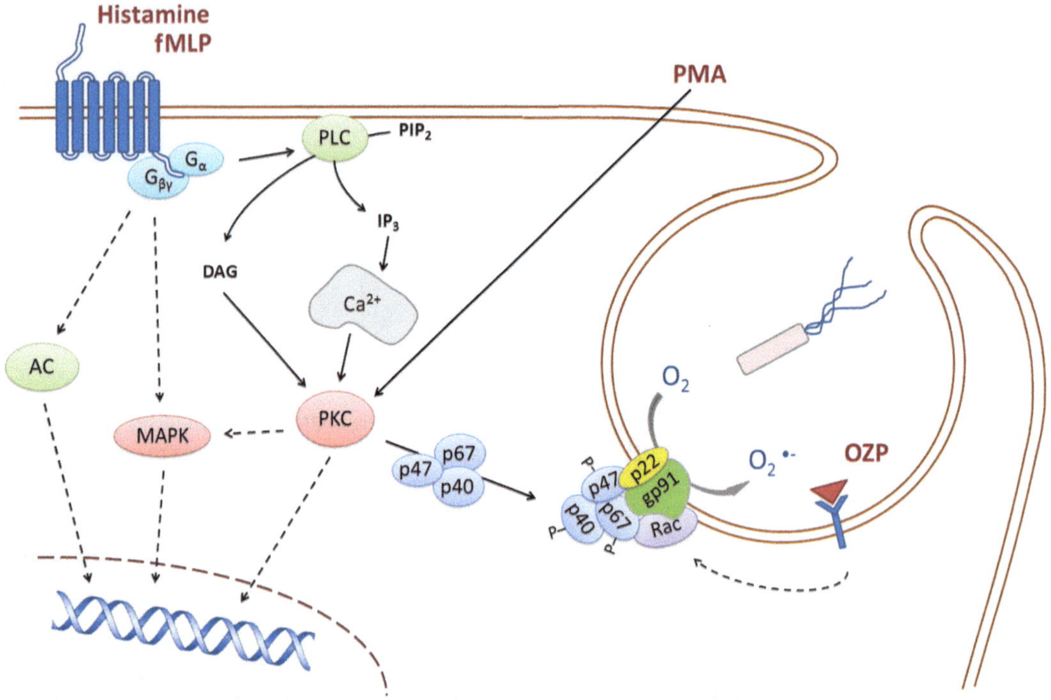

Fig. 2 Signaling pathways leading to the assembly and activation of NADPH oxidase in neutrophils. *AC* adenylate cyclase, *DAG* diacyl-glycerol, *fMLP* N-Formylmethionine-leucyl-phenylalanine, *IP3* inositol trisphosphate, *MAPK* mitogen-activated protein kinases, *OZP* opsonized zymosan particles, *PIP2* phosphatidylinositol 4,5-bisphosphate, *PKC* protein kinase C, *PLC* phospholipase C, *PMA* 4β-phorbol-12β-myristate-13α-acetate

procedures using low cost instrumentation that can be easily controlled by computers. The sensitivity of the method is excellent [43]. On the other hand, it was reported that luminol-dependent chemiluminescence gives very little ability to discriminate between individual ROS. Furthermore, luminol-dependent chemiluminescence used in biological systems is extremely prone to many interferences that are very difficult to control [44].

Luminol- and isoluminol-enhanced chemiluminescence (CL) is a widely used method of measuring ROS. Luminol crosses cellular membranes [45]; thus, it measures overall CL. On the other hand, the amino group in the isoluminol molecule is placed further from the oxygen group, which makes the molecule more polar [20]. As a result, isoluminol is thought not to pass through membranes [46, 47] and therefore detects extracellular CL. Different approaches were developed to differentiate between the intra- and extracellular parts of luminol-enhanced CL (some of them are reviewed in Dahlgren & Karlsson, 1999) [38]. The use of azide to inhibit myeloperoxidase, the addition of azide and horseradish peroxidase (HRP) to recover extracellular CL, and the addition of superoxide dismutase (SOD) and catalase (CAT) to deplete extracellular ROS are processes often applied to isolated phagocytes [46, 48–50].

The luminol/isoluminol-enhanced chemiluminescence method was applied in pharmacological characterization of therapeutically used drugs (H_1 antihistamines) for evaluation of oxidative burst in whole human blood and to differentiate between extra- and intracellular scavenging effect on isolated human neutrophils [20, 22, 51–53]. This method gives a precise differentiation for the ratio between extracellular scavenging and intracellular alteration of ROS important for dual suppression of ROS. An excessive and/or sustained increase in ROS production has been implicated in the pathogenesis of many diseases [54]. Neutrophil functions must be appropriately regulated to achieve host defense and to avoid tissue-damaging inflammation. Development and pharmacological use of neutrophil-targeting agents may therefore be a good therapeutic strategy in regulating neutrophil functions for the control of inflammation and tissue injury [55]. Compounds decreasing the amount of extracellular ROS generation, yet affecting only minimally intracellular ROS generation, are promising for further investigation in vivo [22].

2 Protocols

2.1 Isolation of Human Neutrophils from Venous Blood

2.1.1 Materials

- Heparin: Prepare working solution of heparin (2000 U/mL) in saline. The solution can be stored at 4 °C for several weeks.
- 3% Dextran: Dissolve 30 g/L of dextran 500 (average molecular weight 200,000–500,000) in sterile saline. Heat the solution if necessary to promote dissolution of the dextran, filter the solution with a 0.22 μm syringe filter, and handle the solution using sterile technique.
- Hank's Balanced Salt Solution (HBSS): 5.4 mM KCl, 0.44 mM KH_2PO_4, 0.81 mM, NaCl 136.87 mM, $NaHCO_3$ 4.17 mM, $Na_2HPO_4 \times 12\ H_2O$ 0.335 mM, glucose 5.05 mM, $CaCl_2$ 1.26 mM, pH 7.4.
- Phosphate buffered saline (PBS): 136.9 mM NaCl, 2.7 mM KCl, 8.1 mM Na_2HPO_4, 1.5 mM KH_2PO_4, 1.8 mM $CaCl_2$, and 0.5 mM $MgCl_2.6H_2O$, pH 7.4.

2.1.2 Assay Procedure

1. Draw blood into a syringe containing sufficient preservative-free heparin to have a final concentration of 20 U/mL in the blood sample.
2. Mix the blood with dextran in a 50 mL conical tube—two parts of blood and one part of 3% dextran, i.e., blood:dextran 2:1.
3. Invert the tubes gently five times, and set tubes upright for 30–40 min at room temperature (RT) (*see* **Note 1**).
4. Aspirate the straw-colored, leukocyte-rich, erythrocyte-poor upper layer with a sterile plastic pipette and transfer the aspirate to a sterile 50 mL conical tube (*see* **Note 2**).

5. Pellet leukocytes by centrifugation at 200 × *g* for 7 min at RT; aspirate and discard the supernatant.
6. Resuspend pellets in 10 mL of PBS without Ca^{2+} and Mg^{2+}; shake well but do not vortex.
7. Carefully overlay the leukocyte suspension over 10 mL of Ficoll-Hypaque using a sterile, plastic 10 mL pipette.
8. Centrifuge at 390 × *g* (without acceleration and brake) for 30 min at RT.
9. After centrifugation, two bands should be apparent in the conical tube. The lighter band contains mononuclear cells, whereas the denser band has both granulocytes and erythrocytes. If monocytes are desired, aspirate the less dense band using a sterile plastic pipette and mix with an equal volume of cold sterile saline in a separate conical tube.
10. Aspirate and discard supernatant above the neutrophil-erythrocyte layer, taking care not to lose any of the neutrophil-rich pellet.
11. Resuspend pellet in sterile water and mix well (but do not vortex) for 30 s. Promptly restore tonicity by adding an equal volume of 1.8% saline and mixing (*see* **Note 3**).
12. Centrifuge 200 × *g* for 7 min at RT. Discard supernatant and repeat **step 11** if more lysis is needed, but repeat **step 11** only once.
13. Resuspend cells in 1 mL of PBS or HBSS without Ca^{2+} and Mg^{2+}.
14. Determine the cell concentration by a hemocytometer. The differential cell count for the leukocytes can be assessed by examining a stained slide microscopically.

Notes

1. Adequate mixing of the sample is essential for reproducible sedimentation, presumably to distribute the erythrocytes throughout the suspension and to provide maximal opportunities for rouleaux formation.
2. Once the leukocyte-rich supernatant from the dextran sedimentation has been centrifuged, proceed as quickly as possible with the isolation procedure. Do not leave cell pellets at intermediate steps.
3. The hypotonic lysis of erythrocytes exploits the relative resistance of leukocytes to osmotic stress. This difference is relative, and prolonged or repeated hypotonic lysis will damage neutrophils. More than two cycles of hypotonic lysis must be avoided, as they will not lyse additional erythrocytes but will begin to damage neutrophils.

2.2 Chemiluminescence of Whole Blood or Isolated Neutrophils

2.2.1 Principle of the Method

Detections of ROS produced in whole blood or isolated neutrophils are based on the reaction of luminophore with ROS in the presence of a catalyst. The nonstable intermediate of this reaction is transformed into the end-product by releasing chemiluminescence energy.

2.2.2 Materials

- Luminol-base (3-Aminophthalhydrazide): Dissolve 0.1772 g of luminol-base in 100 mL of borate buffer to obtain 10 mM working solution. Aliquots are stable for 6 months at −20 °C. Keep in the dark (*see* **Note 4**).
- Horseradish peroxidase (HRP): Dissolve HRP in PBS to 40 U/mL. The solution can be stored at 4 °C for several weeks.
- PMA (4β-phorbol-12β-myristate-13α-acetate): Dissolve PMA in 20% dimethyl sulfoxide (DMSO) to 1.6 mM and store in small aliquots at −20 °C. On the day of the experiment, dilute with HBSS to 0.25 μM.
- Opsonized zymosan particles (OZP): Dissolve OZP in HBSS to 250 μg/mL. 500 μg/mL aliquots in PBS are stable for several months at −20 °C.
- N-Formylmethionyl-leucyl-phenylalanine (fMLP): Dissolve 5 mg of fMLP in 1 mL of DMSO and store in small aliquots at −20 °C. On the day of the experiment, dilute with HBSS to a final concentration of 1 μM.
- Tested compounds (e.g., H_1-antihistamines): Dissolve the tested compounds in deionized water to 5 mM and store in small aliquots at −20 °C. On the day of the experiment, dilute with HBSS as required.
- Hank's Balanced Salt Solution (HBSS): 5.4 mM KCl, 0.44 mM KH_2PO_4, 0.81 mM, NaCl 136.87 mM, $NaHCO_3$ 4.17 mM, $Na_2HPO_4 \times 12\ H_2O$ 0.335 mM, glucose 5.05 mM, $CaCl_2$ 1.26 mM, pH 7.4.
- Phosphate buffered saline (PBS): 136.9 mM NaCl, 2.7 mM KCl, 8.1 mM Na_2HPO_4, 1.5 mM KH_2PO_4, 1.8 mM $CaCl_2$ and 0.5 mM $MgCl_2.6\ H_2O$, pH 7.4.
- Borate buffer: 7.628 g of $Na_2B_4O_7 \times 10H_2O$ dissolve in 400 mL of distilled water (40 mM) and mix with 100 mL of 40 mM H_3BO_3 (1.237 g/100 mL), pH 9.
- Human blood or fresh suspension of isolated human neutrophils adjusted to 10^6 cells/mL (*see* **Note 5**).
- Precision pipettes capable of accurately delivering volumes between 10 μL and 1000 μL.
- Multichannel or repetitive pipettes, disposable pipette tips.

- Microtitre plate luminometer equipped with a temperature-controlled sample holder.
- Microtiter flat-bottom strips or 96-well microplates, both made of densely pigmented white polystyrene (*see* **Note 6**).

2.2.3 Assay Procedure

1. Programme luminometer to take an integrated reading of each relevant well and set working temperature to 37 °C (*see* **Note 7**).
2. Pipette the tested compounds; for control samples, use HBSS.
3. Pipette 10× diluted blood in HBSS or isolated neutrophils. The number of neutrophils per well should be 100,000–500,000.
4. Add luminol at a final concentration of 1 mM (*see* **Note 8**).
5. The activator should be added last, immediately before the measurement. For control samples, use HBSS instead of stimulant.
6. Read the chemiluminescence for 30 (fMLP) or 60 (OZP, PMA) min. The integral values of Relative Light Units over time are recorded and evaluated for controls and tested compounds. However, pharmacokinetic parameters such as amplitude or peak time may be also evaluated.

Notes

4. You may use luminol sodium salt. Prepare 1.25 mM solution in HBSS. Aliquots of luminol sodium salt (12.5 mM in PBS) may be prepared. Keep at −20 °C in the dark.
5. Store neutrophils on melting ice until use, maximally for 2 h, as long as control chemiluminescence keeps constant.
6. The use of strips is more practical, as the number of wells (samples) can be adjusted optionally.
7. The time of measurement should be adjusted depending on the stimulus used.
8. In our experiments, the final concentration of luminol sodium salt is 250 μM.
9. Addition of Horse Radish Peroxidase (8 U/mL) is optional for amplification of the signal. Respective controls are needed.

2.2.4 Representative Results

Figure 3 shows representative curves of CL signal of neutrophils stimulated with fMLP (**a**), PMA (**b**), or OZP (**c**). PMA has the highest amplitude in comparison with fMLP or OZP. The fMLP peak is very fast followed by a fast decline of the signal. OZP is comparable with fMLP; however, the CL signal lasts for a longer time.

Figure 4 shows the effects of Dimaprit (H2R agonist), Ranitidine (H2R antagonist), and JNJ10191584 (H4R antagonist) on whole blood ROS production. Dimaprit in a concentration of 10 μM decreased the CL signal to 77% of the control. Ranitidine in the concentration range of 10 nM–10 mM significantly

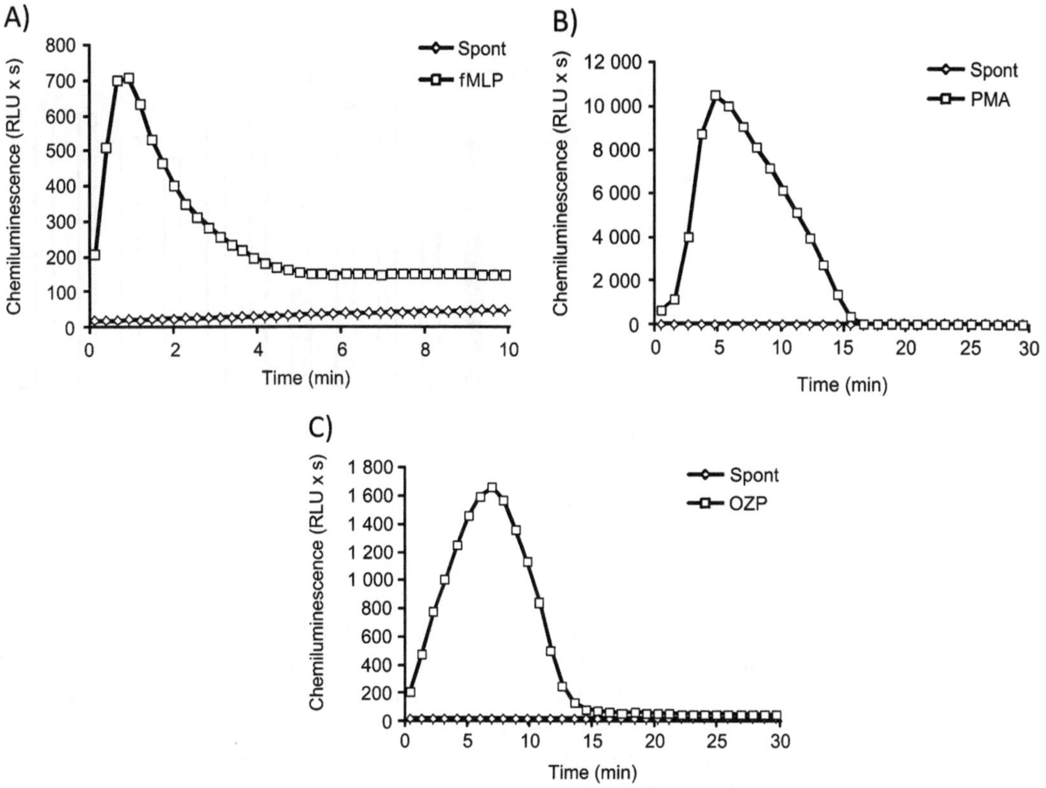

Fig. 3 Representative chemiluminescence curves of neutrophil ROS production activated by (**a**) N-Formylmethionyl-leucyl-phenylalanine (fMLP), (**b**) 4β-phorbol-12β-myristate-13α-acetate (PMA), or (**c**) opsonized zymosan particles (OZP)

reverted the effect of dimaprit in a dose-dependent manner. JNJ10191584 did not reduce the effect of dimaprit in any concentrations.

2.3 Chemiluminescence Measurement of Extra- and Intra-Cellular ROS Production in Isolated Neutrophils

2.3.1 Principle of the Method

The method is based on different abilities of luminol and isoluminol to cross biological membranes [38, 56, 57]. Despite their very similar structure, molecules of these luminophores differ in their physicochemical properties (Fig. 5). The molecule of isoluminol was found to be more polar and more hydrophilic than that of luminol, as indicated by values of lipophilicity parameters, solvation energies, and dipole moments. Moreover, in comparison to luminol, isoluminol possesses a lower capacity to form intramolecular hydrogen bridges (since the aminogroup is further from the oxygen of the phthalazine ring and is less protonated). All these characteristics result in reduced membrane movement and in accumulation of isoluminol outside neutrophils [57]. The extracellular origin of isoluminol chemiluminescence was confirmed by its essential dependence on extracellular peroxidase, as well as by complete blockade in the presence of extracellular scavengers –

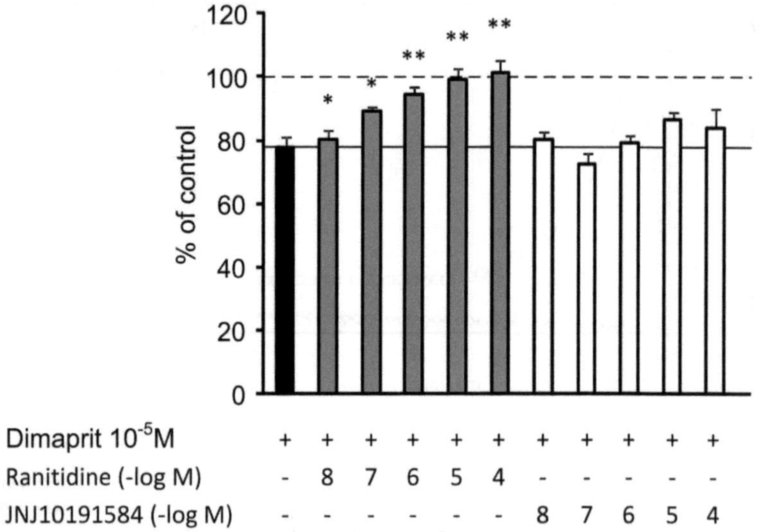

Fig. 4 The effects of H_2R agonist dimaprit alone (*black bar*) and combination of dimaprit with H_2R antagonist ranitidine (*gray bars*) and H_4R antagonist JNJ10191584 (*white bars*). The whole blood with luminol was pre-incubated with ranitidine and/or JNJ10191584 for 10 min. (in the dark, 37 °C). 10 μM dimaprit was added and incubated for 5 min (in the dark, 37 °C). After incubation, opsonized zymosan particles (OZP) were added and the samples were directly measured. The results from five independent experiments were integrated, converted to a percent of the control and expressed as the mean + SEM. Data were statistically analyzed using ANOVA, which was followed by Dunnett's multiple comparison test (**$P < 0.01$, *$P < 0.05$ show the significance against dimaprit effect alone)

superoxide dismutase and catalase (Fig. 6). On the other hand, the physicochemical parameters of luminol and partial resistance of its chemiluminescence to the effect of extracellular inhibitors (Figs. 5 and 6) proved the lipo/hydrophilic character of this luminophore and its ability to produce chemiluminescence also inside neutrophils. This intracellular portion can be selectively recorded in the presence of extracellular scavengers – superoxide dismutase (SOD) and catalase (CAT).

2.3.2 Materials

- Luminol sodium salt (3-Aminophthalhydrazide): Dissolve 1.99 mg of luminol in 1 mL of Tyrode's buffer to obtain 10 mM solution. Dilute with Tyrode's buffer to 25 μM. Prepare fresh on the day of the experiment, keep cooled and protected from light.
- Isoluminol (4-Aminophthalhydrazide): Dissolve 1.77 mg of isoluminol in 10 μL of 1 M NaOH and add 990 μL of Tyrode's buffer. Dilute this 10 mM solution with Tyrode's buffer to 25 μM. Prepare fresh on the day of the experiment, keep cooled and protected from light.

Isoluminol	Luminol
• aminogroup more distant from the oxygen of phthalazine ring	• aminogroup closer to the oxygen of phthalazine ring
• aminogroup less protonated (E = -148.40 kcal/mol)	• aminogroup more protonated (E = -154.30 kcal/mol)
• lower capacity to form intramolecular hydrogen bridges	• higher capacity to form intramolecular hydrogen bridges
• polar (DM = 3.38 D)	• less polar (DM = 2.86 D)
• hydrophilic nature (R_M = -0.67)	• lipo/hydrophilic nature, exists in several forms of dissociation (R_M = 0.09)
• chemiluminescence completely blocked by extracellular scavengers	• chemiluminescence partially resistant to extracellular scavengers
• chemiluminescence essentially dependent on extracellular peroxidase	• chemiluminescence partially dependent on extracellular peroxidase
• accumulation outside cells	• crossing of biological membranes
• **identifies extracellular oxidants**	• **in the presence of extracellular scavengers SOD/CAT, identifies intracellular oxidants**

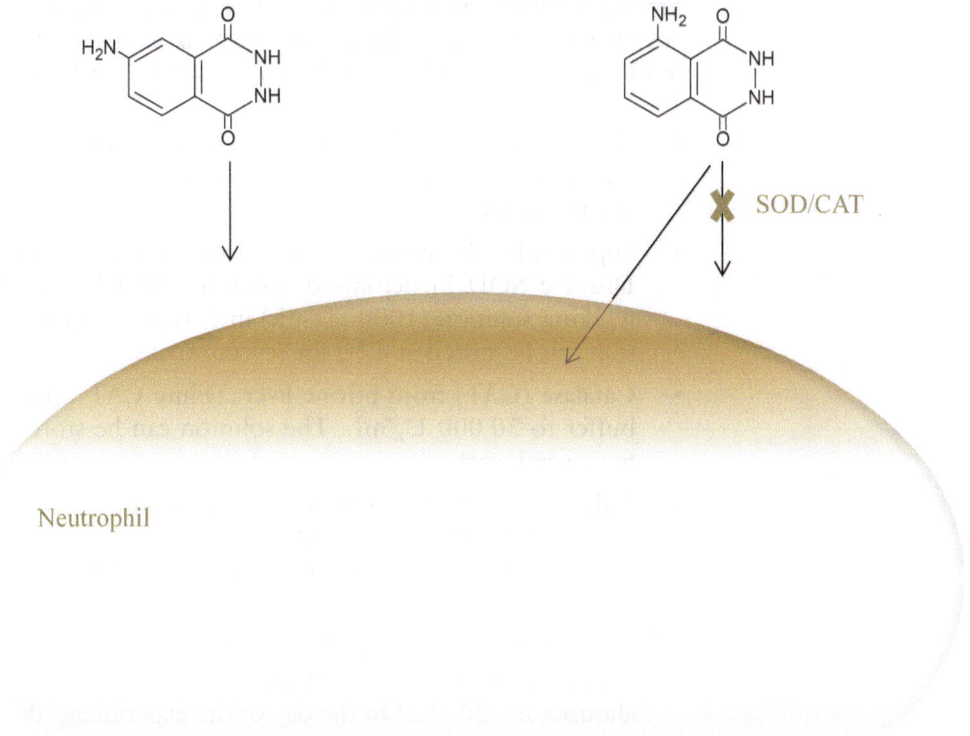

Fig. 5 Physicochemical properties, chemical structures, and membrane permeability of luminol and isoluminol molecules. The principle of identification of extracellular and intracellular oxidants. *E* energy of –NH2 group protonation, *DM* dipole moment, *RM* lipophilicity parameter, *SOD* superoxide dismutase, *CAT* catalase

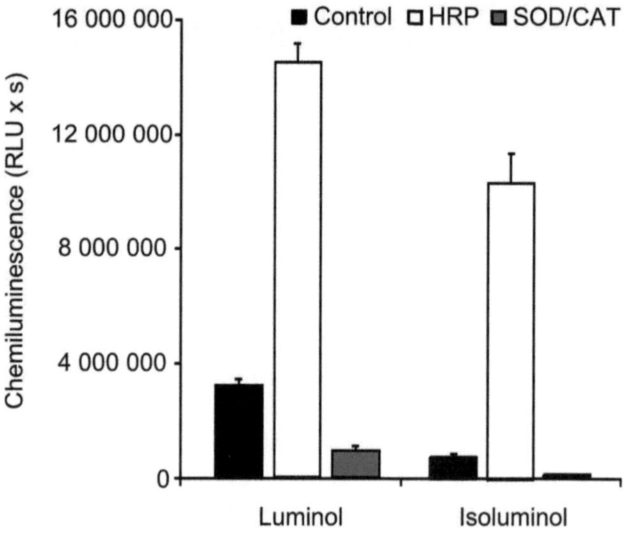

Fig. 6 Effect of extracellular peroxidase (HRP) and extracellular scavengers (SOD/CAT) on luminol- and isoluminol-enhanced chemiluminescence of human neutrophils stimulated with PMA. Data represent mean integral values of chemiluminescence over 1800 s ± SEM obtained from six donors. *HRP* horseradish peroxidase, *SOD* superoxide dismutase, *CAT* catalase, *RLU* relative light units

- Horseradish peroxidase (HRP): Dissolve HRP in Tyrode's buffer to 40 U/mL. The solution can be stored at 4 °C for several weeks.
- Superoxide dismutase (SOD) from bovine erythrocytes: Dissolve SOD in deionized water to 5000 U/mL. Prepare working solution (1000 U/mL) in Tyrode's buffer. The solution can be stored at 4 °C for several weeks.
- Catalase (CAT) from bovine liver: Dilute CAT with Tyrode's buffer to 20,000 U/mL. The solution can be stored at 4 °C for several weeks.
- PMA (4β-phorbol-12β-myristate-13α-acetate): Dissolve PMA in 20% DMSO to 1.6 mM and store in small aliquots at −20 °C. On the day of the experiment, dilute with PBS to 0.25 μM.
- Substances tested (e.g., H_1-antihistamines): Dissolve the substances tested in deionized water to 5 mM and store in small aliquots at −20 °C. On the day of the experiment, dilute with Tyrode's buffer as required.
- Phosphate buffered saline (PBS): 136.9 mM NaCl, 2.7 mM KCl, 8.1 mM Na_2HPO_4, 1.5 mM KH_2PO_4, 1.8 mM $CaCl_2$ and 0.5 mM $MgCl_2.6\ H_2O$, pH 7.4.
- Tyrode's buffer: 136.9 mM NaCl, 2.7 mM KCl, 11.9 mM $NaHCO_3$, 0.4 mM $NaH_2PO_4.2H_2O$, 1 mM $MgCl_2.6\ H_2O$ and 5.6 mM glucose, pH 7.4.

Table 1
Extracellular chemiluminescence assay, volumes, and concentrations of reagents. The schedule involves the measurement of spontaneous and 4β-phorbol-12β-myristate-13α-acetate (PMA) stimulated extracellular chemiluminescence of control neutrophils and neutrophils treated with the compounds tested

		Extracellular chemiluminescence			
		Spontaneous		PMA stimulated	
	Concentration	Control	Compounds	Control	Compounds
Tyrode's buffer		50 μL		50 μL	
Compounds tested	Optionally		50 μL		50 μL
Horseradish peroxidase	40 U/mL	50 μL	50 μL	50 μL	50 μL
Isoluminol	25 μM	50 μL	50 μL	50 μL	50 μL
Neutrophils	10^7/mL	50 μL	50 μL	50 μL	50 μL
PMA	0.25 μM			50 μL	50 μL
PBS		50 μL	50 μL		

PBS phosphate buffered saline

- Fresh suspension of isolated human neutrophils adjusted to 10^7 cells/mL (*see* **Note 5**).
- Precision pipettes capable of accurately delivering volumes between 10 μL and 1000 μL.
- Multichannel or repetitive pipettes, disposable pipette tips.
- Microtitre plate luminometer equipped with a temperature-controlled sample holder.
- Microtiter flat-bottom strips or 96-well microplates, both made of densely pigmented white polystyrene (*see* **Note 6**).

2.3.3 Assay Procedure

1. Programme luminometer to take a 30-min integrated reading of each relevant well and set working temperature to 37 °C (*see* **Note 10**).
2. Pipette reagents and neutrophils into wells of microtiter strips or microplates, according to the schedules specified in Table 1 (extracellular chemiluminescence) or Table 2 (intracellular chemiluminescence). Neutrophils of the same donor should be used in both parts of the measurement (*see* **Note 11**).
3. Insert the samples into the luminometer and initiate the programme (*see* **Note 12**).
4. Evaluate the overall amount of oxidants produced by neutrophils extra- or intracellularly on the basis of integral values of chemiluminescence. Other parameters of chemiluminescence curves –

Table 2
Intracellular chemiluminescence assay, volumes, and concentrations of reagents. The schedule involves the measurement of spontaneous and 4β-phorbol-12β-myristate-13α-acetate (PMA) stimulated intracellular chemiluminescence of control neutrophils and neutrophils treated with the compounds tested

		Intracellular chemiluminescence			
		Spontaneous		PMA stimulated	
	Concentration	Control	Compounds	Control	Compounds
Tyrode's buffer		50 μL		50 μL	
Compounds tested	Optionally		50 μL		50 μL
SOD	1000 U/mL	25 μL	25 μL	25 μL	25 μL
CAT	20,000 U/mL	25 μL	25 μL	25 μL	25 μL
Luminol	25 μM	50 μL	50 μL	50 μL	50 μL
Neutrophils	10^7/ml	50 μl	50 μl	50 μl	50 μL
PMA	0.25 μM			50 μL	50 μL
PBS		50 μL	50 μL		

CAT catalase, *PBS* phosphate buffered saline, *SOD* superoxide dismutase

peak and peak time – should also be analyzed to characterize the time-course of oxidant production in greater detail.

2.3.4 Representative Results

The kinetics of extracellular and intracellular chemiluminescence produced by human neutrophils spontaneously or in response to PMA stimulation are compared in Fig. 7. As indicated by the chemiluminescence curves, intracellular ROS formation is much less pronounced and achieves maximum values later than does external ROS formation. Figures 8 and 9 present significant differences in the activity of H_1-antihistamines, revealed through the combined luminol- and isoluminol-enhanced chemiluminescence method. Brompheniramine reduced preferentially extracellular oxidants with minimal impact on ROS formed inside neutrophils, while loratadine was inhibitory in both compartments. Since extra- and intracellular oxidants are differently involved in neutrophil function and in the regulation of inflammatory reaction, a clearly identified site of action could be useful in assessing the anti-inflammatory activity of H_1-antihistamines.

Notes

10. The time of measurement should be adjusted depending on the stimulus used. For PMA activation, a 30 min period is sufficient to follow the complete kinetics of ROS formation in the great majority of donors.

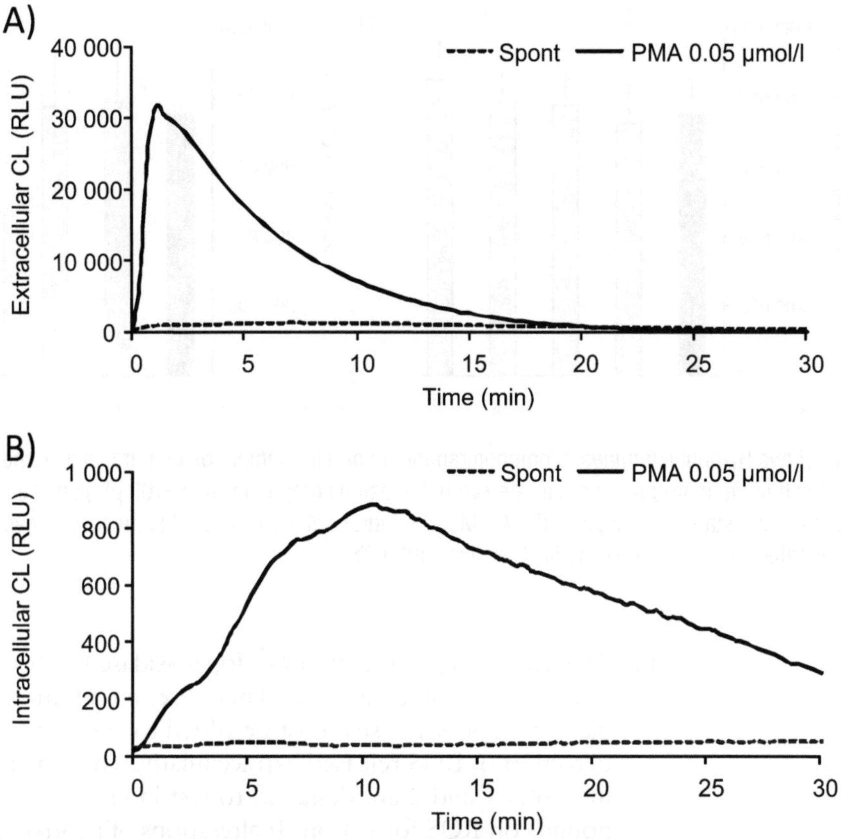

Fig. 7 Representative chemiluminescence curves. The kinetics of extracellular (**a**) and intracellular (**b**) chemiluminescence produced by human neutrophils spontaneously or after 4β-phorbol-12β-myristate-13α-acetate (PMA) stimulation

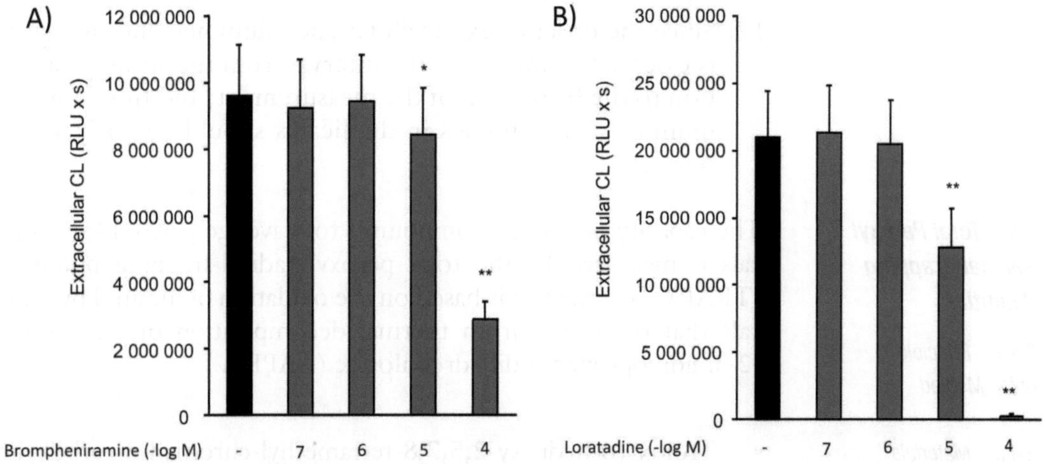

Fig. 8 Effect of two H_1-antihistamines brompheniramine (**a**) and loratadine (**b**) on extracellular chemiluminescence. Isolated human neutrophils were treated with the tested compounds (0.1–100 μM) and stimulated with 4β-phorbol-12β-myristate-13α-acetate (PMA). Mean integral values of chemiluminescence over 1800 s ± SEM are presented; n = 6; *$P < 0.05$; **$P < 0.01$; RLU, relative light units

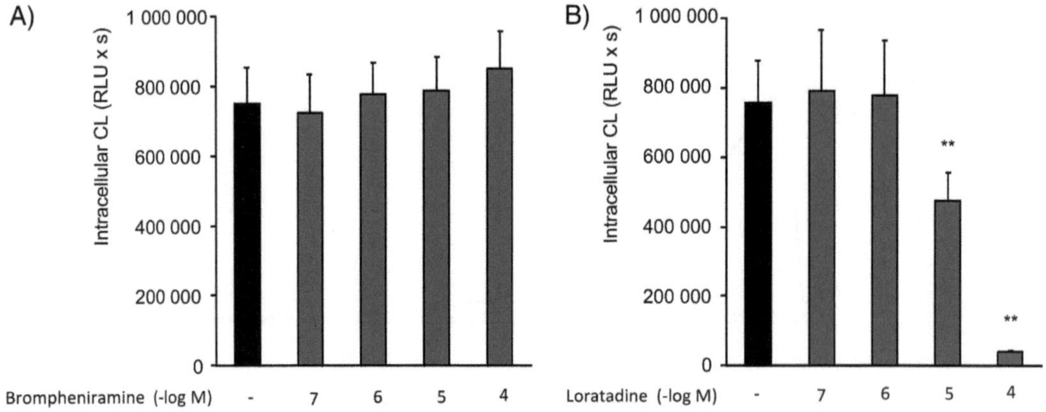

Fig. 9 Effect of two H_1-antihistamines, brompheniramine (**a**) and loratadine (**b**), on intracellular chemiluminescence. Isolated human neutrophils were treated with the tested compounds (0.1–100 μM) and stimulated with 4β-phorbol-12β-myristate-13α-acetate (PMA). Mean integral values of chemiluminescence over 1800 s ± SEM are presented; $n = 6$; $^{**}P < 0.01$; *RLU* relative light units

11. The availability of secreted myeloperoxidase limits the chemiluminescence of isoluminol. Therefore, an additional peroxidase (e.g., horseradish) must be added to ensure the complete detection of ROS released extracellularly. The schedules given in Tables 1 and 2 are designed to test in vitro effects of compounds on ROS formation. If alterations of neutrophil activity are to be studied—for example, under pathological states or during therapy—it is helpful to apply several stimulus concentrations, e.g., 0.005, 0.025, 0.05, 0.25, and 0.5 μM PMA. This dose-response approach can characterize more precisely the capability of neutrophils to form radicals.
12. Since the onset of extracellular chemiluminescence is fast, it is essential to minimize the interval from the stimulus addition to the beginning of the measurement, and thus, a maximum of seven samples in duplicates should be analyzed in one set.

2.4 Total Peroxyl Radical-Trapping Potential

2.4.1 Principle of the Method

The capacity of studied compounds to scavenge peroxyl free radicals is measured by the total peroxyl radical-trapping potential (TRAP). The method is based on the oxidation of luminol by radicals that originated from thermal decomposition of 2,2′-azobis (2-amidinopropane) dihydrochloride (AAPH).

2.4.2 Materials

- Trolox (6-hydroxy-2,5,7,8-tetramethyl-chroman-2-carboxylic acid): Dissolve 5 mg of Trolox in 50 mL of distilled water; mix well. Heat the solution if necessary, to promote dissolution of the trolox. The concentration is 400 μM. Store in small aliquots at −20 °C.

- AAPH (2,2′-azobis(2-amidinopropane) dihydrochloride): Dissolve 108.48 mg of AAPH in 1 mL of PBS (400 mM). Prepare fresh; keep in the fridge.
- Luminol-base (3-aminophthalhydrazide): Dissolve 0.1772 g of luminol-base in 100 mL of borate buffer to obtain 10 mM working solution. Aliquots are stable for 6 months at −20 °C. Keep in the dark.
- Tested compounds (e.g., H_1-antihistamines): Dissolve the tested compounds in deionized water to 5 mM and store in small aliquots at −20 °C. On the day of the experiment, dilute with HBSS as required.
- Phosphate buffered saline (PBS): 136.9 mM NaCl, 2.7 mM KCl, 8.1 mM Na_2HPO_4, 1.5 mM KH_2PO_4, 1.8 mM $CaCl_2$ and 0.5 mM $MgCl_2.6\ H_2O$, pH 7.4.
- Precision pipettes capable of accurately delivering volumes between 10 μL and 1000 μL.
- Multichannel or repetitive pipettes, disposable pipette tips.
- Microtitre plate luminometer equipped with a temperature-controlled sample holder.
- Microtiter flat-bottom strips or 96-well microplates, both made of densely pigmented white polystyrene (*see* **Note 6**).

2.4.3 Assay Procedure

1. Programme luminometer to take a 60-min integrated reading of each relevant well and set working temperature to 37 °C.
2. Pipette 146.6 μL of PBS.
3. Add 16.7 μL of luminol base.
4. Add 20.1 μL of tested compounds. In positive controls, add 20.1 μL of trolox.
5. Incubate for 10 min at 37 °C. Shake the micro-plate before measurement.
6. Add 16.7 μL of AAPH. Read the chemiluminescence signal for 60 min.
7. Data interpretation: The results are interpreted as trolox equivalents (TE). To calculate TE, the following formula is used:

$$\text{TRAP} = \frac{2 \times [\text{trolox}] \times t(\text{sample})}{f \times t(\text{trolox})}$$

2—Stoichiometric factor of trolox; one molecule of trolox is capable of reacting with two molecules of ROS

[trolox]—Concentration of trolox.

t(sample)—Time to reach half-peak of the sample

f—Dilution factor.

t(trolox)—Time to reach half-peak of trolox.

2.5 Luminol-HRP-Hydrogen Peroxide Cell-Free Assay

2.5.1 Principle of the Method

The assay is similar to whole blood or isolated neutrophil assays. However, the neutrophils are replaced by hydrogen peroxide [58].

2.5.2 Materials

- Luminol sodium salt (3-aminophthalhydrazide): Dissolve 1.991 mg of luminol in 800 μL of PBS to obtain 12.5 mM solution. Next, dilute 20 μL of 12.5 mM luminol with 6230 μL of PBS to reach 40 μM luminol working buffer. Prepare fresh on the day of the experiment; keep cooled and protected from light.
- Horseradish peroxidase (HRP): Dissolve 1.32 mg of 181.8 U/mg HRP in 3 mL of PBS, followed by 1/10 dilution to a final concentration of 8 U/mL
- Hydrogen peroxide (H_2O_2): Dissolve 10 μL of 30% stabilized H_2O_2 solution in 990 μL of distilled water to obtain 97.88 mM solution. Next add 10 μL of 97.88 mM H_2O_2 to 969.72 μL of distilled water to obtain 1 mM solution. Finally, prepare 400 μM H_2O_2 working solution in PBS.
- Tested compounds (e.g., H_1-antihistamines): Dissolve the tested compounds in deionized water to 5 mM and store in small aliquots at −20 °C. On the day of the experiment, dilute with PBS as required.
- Phosphate buffered saline (PBS): 136.9 mM NaCl, 2.7 mM KCl, 8.1 mM Na_2HPO_4, 1.5 mM KH_2PO_4, 1.8 mM $CaCl_2$ and 0.5 mM $MgCl_2.6\ H_2O$, pH 7.4.
- Precision pipettes capable of accurately delivering volumes between 10 μL and 1000 μL.
- Multichannel or repetitive pipettes, disposable pipette tips.
- Microtitre plate luminometer equipped with a temperature-controlled sample holder.
- Microtiter flat-bottom strips or 96-well microplates, both made of densely pigmented white polystyrene (*see* **Note 6**).

2.5.3 Assay Procedure

1. Programme luminometer to take a 10-min integrated reading of each relevant well and set working temperature to RT.
2. Pipette 50 μL of tested compounds or PBS as control.
3. Add 50 μL of 8 U/mL HRP (*see* **Note 13**).
4. Add 50 μL of 40 μM luminol sodium salt.
5. The reaction with hydrogen peroxide is very quick; therefore, add hydrogen peroxide just before the reading. In our experiments, we put the micro-plate in the luminometer, prepare the reading, add 50 μL of 400 μM hydrogen peroxide, and read immediately (*see* **Note 14**).

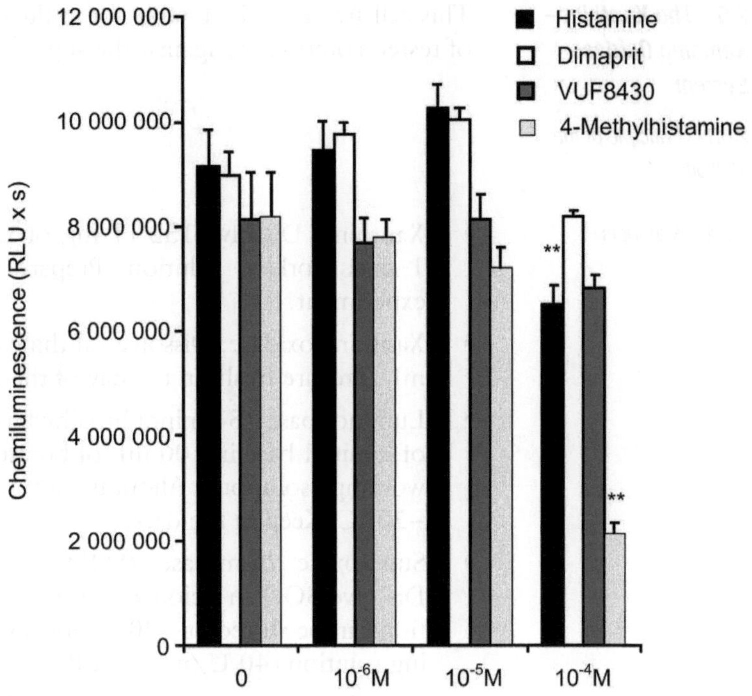

Fig. 10 The antioxidant properties of histamine and its H_2R/H_4R agonists expressed as the mean of CL integral ± SEM. Level of significance was analyzed by ANOVA and followed by Dunnett's multiple comparison test

6. Read the chemiluminescence signal for 10 min at RT.
7. The integral value of positive control (hydrogen peroxide) is compared with tested compounds. The results are then shown as a percentage of positive control or percentage of inhibition.

2.5.4 Representative Results

The luminol–HRP–H_2O_2 cell-free assay showed the significant antioxidant properties of histamine and 4-methylhistamine (potent H_2R and H_4R agonist) in their highest concentration (Fig. 10). 4-methylhistamine was a better antioxidant than histamine. The other compounds, in all concentrations, did not exert any antioxidative effects.

Notes

13. HRP from different manufacturers may have different activity. If the ratio of HRP and hydrogen peroxide described above is not sufficient to provide a significant peak which lasts for 10–15 min, you may titrate your own concentration of hydrogen peroxide or HRP. We use HRP P 8250-25 KU from Sigma-Aldrich.
14. If possible, use a luminometer equipped with an injector.

2.6 The Xanthine–Xanthine Oxidase System

2.6.1 Principle of the Method

This cell-free assay is suitable for evaluation of scavenger activities of tested compounds against the superoxide anion-radical [59].

2.6.2 Materials

- Xanthine: Dissolve 152.11 mg of xanthine in PBS to obtain 1 mM working solution. Prepare fresh on the day of the experiment.
- Xanthine oxidase: Dissolve xanthine oxidase in PBS to 0.5 U/mL. Prepare fresh on the day of the experiment.
- Luminol-base (3-aminophthalhydrazide): Dissolve 0.1772 g of luminol-base in 100 mL of borate buffer to obtain 10 mM working solution. Aliquots are stable for 6 months at −20 °C. Keep in the dark.
- Superoxide dismutase (SOD) from bovine erythrocytes: Dissolve SOD in deionized water to 5000 U/mL. The solution can be stored at −20 °C for several weeks. Prepare working solution (40 U/mL) in PBS before measurement.
- Tested compounds (e.g., H_1-antihistamines): Dissolve the tested compounds in deionized water to 5 mM and store in small aliquots at −20 °C. On the day of the experiment, dilute with PBS as required.
- Phosphate buffered saline (PBS): 136.9 mM NaCl, 2.7 mM KCl, 8.1 mM Na_2HPO_4, 1.5 mM KH_2PO_4, 1.8 mM $CaCl_2$ and 0.5 mM $MgCl_2.6\ H_2O$, pH 7.4.
- Precision pipettes capable of accurately delivering volumes between 10 μL and 1000 μL.
- Multichannel or repetitive pipettes, disposable pipette tips.
- Microtitre plate luminometer equipped with a temperature-controlled sample holder.
- Microtiter flat-bottom strips or 96-well microplates, both made of densely pigmented white polystyrene (*see* **Note 6**).

2.6.3 Assay Procedure

1. Programme luminometer to take a 15-min integrated reading of each relevant well and set working temperature to 37 °C.
2. Pipette 120 μL of tested compounds or PBS.
3. Add 20 μL of xanthine with a final concentration of 0.1 mM.
4. Add 20 μL of luminol with a final concentration of 1 mM.
5. For negative controls, add 20 μL of SOD (final concentration is 4 U/mL).
6. Put the plate in the luminometer, set the temperature for 37 °C, and wait 10 min.

7. Start the reaction by adding 20 μL of xanthine-oxidase (final concentration is 0.05 U/mL), and read the signal for 15 min.
8. Analyze the integral of chemiluminescence signal over 15 min.

2.7 The Hydrogen Peroxide–Ferrous Sulfate System (H_2O_2–$FeSO_4$)

2.7.1 Principle of the Method

To generate the hydroxyl radical, Fenton reaction of Fe^{2+} with hydrogen peroxide is used [59]. Hydrogen peroxide is quickly reduced in the presence of ferrous ions and the hydroxyl radical is generated.

$$H_2O_2 + Fe^{2+} \rightarrow HO^{*} + OH^{-} + Fe^{3+}.$$

2.7.2 Materials

- Fe-EDTA: $FeSO_4$ solution: dissolve 27.8 mg of $FeSO_4$ in 5 mL of distilled water.
- EDTA solution: Dissolve 44.6 mg of EDTA (disodium salt) in 5 mL of distilled water. Mix both solutions 1:1 to obtain 10 mM $FeSO_4$: 12 mM EDTA.
- Luminol-base (3-aminophthalhydrazide): Dissolve 0.1772 g of luminol-base in 100 mL of borate buffer to obtain 10 mM working solution. Aliquots are stable for 6 months at −20 °C. Keep in the dark.
- Hydrogen peroxide (H_2O_2): Dissolve 10 μL of 30% stabilized H_2O_2 solution in 10 mL of distilled water to obtain 10 mM solution.
- Tested compounds (e.g., H_1-antihistamines): Dissolve the tested compounds in deionized water to 5 mM and store in small aliquots at −20 °C. On the day of the experiment, dilute with PBS as required.
- Phosphate buffered saline (PBS): 136.9 mM NaCl, 2.7 mM KCl, 8.1 mM Na_2HPO_4, 1.5 mM KH_2PO_4, 1.8 mM $CaCl_2$ and 0.5 mM $MgCl_2.6\,H_2O$, pH 7.4.
- Precision pipettes capable of accurately delivering volumes between 10 μL and 1000 μL.
- Multichannel or repetitive pipettes, disposable pipette tips.
- Microtitre plate luminometer equipped with a temperature-controlled sample holder.
- Microtiter flat-bottom strips or 96-well microplates, both made of densely pigmented white polystyrene (*see* **Note 6**).

2.7.3 Assay Procedure

1. Programme luminometer to take a 20–60 min integrated reading of each relevant well and set working temperature to RT.
2. Pipette 150 μL of distilled water.
3. Add 60 μL of 10 mM hydrogen peroxide.
4. Add 30 μL of 10 mM luminol base.

5. Pipette 30 μL of tested compounds.
6. Start the reaction with adding 30 μL of Fe-EDTA buffer, measure chemiluminescence for 20–60 min.
7. Analyze the integral of chemiluminescence signal. Compare integral values of the positive controls and tested compounds.

2.8 Western Blot Detection of Phospho- and Total-PKC Isoforms or NADPH-Oxidase Subunits

2.8.1 The Principle of the Method

The whole procedure comprises three steps. The first step is electrophoretic separation of proteins which is dependent on their molecular weight. The second step is transfer of proteins onto a membrane (blotting). Finally, proteins of interest are detected using specific antibodies.

2.8.2 Materials

- PMA (4β-phorbol-12β-myristate-13α-acetate): Dissolve PMA in 20% DMSO to 1.6 mM and store in small aliquots at −20 °C. On the day of the experiment, dilute with HBSS to 0.25 μM.
- Opsonized zymosan particles (OZP): Dissolve OZP in HBSS to 250 μg/mL. 500 μg/mL aliquots in PBS are stable for several months at −20 °C.
- N-Formylmethionyl-leucyl-phenylalanine (fMLP): Dissolve 5 mg of fMLP in 1 mL of DMSO and store in small aliquots at −20 °C. On the day of the experiment, dilute with HBSS to a final concentration of 1 μM.
- Tested compounds (e.g., H_1-antihistamines): Dissolve the tested compounds in deionized water to 5 mM, and store in small aliquots at −20 °C. On the day of the experiment, dilute with HBSS as required.
- 5% Bovine Serum Albumin (BSA) in Tris Buffered Saline with 0.1% Tween (TBST): Dissolve 5 g of BSA in 100 mL of TBST.
- Hank's Balanced Salt Solution (HBSS): 5.4 mM KCl, 0.44 mM KH_2PO_4, 0.81 mM, NaCl 136.87 mM, $NaHCO_3$ 4.17 mM, $Na_2HPO_4 \times 12\ H_2O$ 0.335 mM, glucose 5.05 mM, $CaCl_2$ 1.26 mM, pH 7.4.
- Phosphate buffered saline (PBS): 136.9 mM NaCl, 2.7 mM KCl, 8.1 mM Na_2HPO_4, 1.5 mM KH_2PO_4, 1.8 mM $CaCl_2$ and 0.5 mM $MgCl_2.6\ H_2O$, pH 7.4.
- Lysis buffer: 50 mM TRIS, 1% SDS, 100 mM NaCl, 1 mM EDTA, 10% glycerine, 1 mM PMSF, proteases and phosphatases inhibitor cocktail, pH 7.4.
- Tris Buffered Saline with 0.1% Tween (TBST): 137 mM NaCl, 2.7 mM, 24.8 mM TRIS, pH 7.6) with 0.1% Tween 20.

- 5× Running (Tank) Buffer: 0.124 M Tris, 0.96 M glycine, 0.5% SDS, pH 8.3. Dilute 5× with water.
- Transfer Buffer: 25 mM Tris, pH 8.1–8.5, 192 mM glycine in water, 20% methanol.
- Isolated human neutrophils adjusted to 10^6 cells/mL. Neutrophils are stored on melting ice until use, maximally for 2 h.
- Precision pipettes capable of accurately delivering volumes between 10 μL and 1000 μL.
- Multichannel or repetitive pipettes, disposable pipette tips.
- Microtitre plate luminometer equipped with a temperature-controlled sample holder.
- Microtiter flat-bottom strips or 96-well microplates, both made of densely pigmented white polystyrene (*see* **Note 6**).

2.8.3 Assay Procedure

1. Isolated human neutrophils (2.5 × 10^6 cells) were incubated at 37 °C with tested compounds followed by stimulation with PMA (0.15 μM). Additional controls are needed. Other stimuli may be used.
2. Samples were lysed in lysis buffer and sonicated. Debris from the lysed cells was pelleted by centrifugation and the supernatant was taken for blotting assay. Protein concentration was measured using Bradford Dye Reagent detection kit (Bio-Rad, Hercules, CA, USA). Samples were diluted to equal concentration of proteins by lysis buffer followed by the addition of Laemmli buffer.
3. The molecular weight of phosphorylated or total PKC isoforms are around 70–80 kDa. Selected NADPH-oxidase subunit has a molecular weight of 47 kDa. Therefore, we used 7 or 10% acrylamide gels for protein separation.
4. Load 20 μg of total protein lysates onto the gel. Run electrophoresis with 100 V.
5. Transfer the proteins onto a polyvinyl difluoride membrane with 200 mA for 2 h with cooling.
6. Block the membranes with 5% bovine serum albumin (BSA) in TBST for one hour. If the blocking was not efficient, you may use 1% gelatine in TBST.
7. For the detection of selected phosphorylated or total proteins, the following primary antibodies were used: phospho-PKCα/βII (Cell Signaling Technology–CST 9375) 1:2000, phospho-PKCδ (CST 9374), PKCδ (CST 9616), and phospho-p47phox (CST 4301). All antibodies were prepared in TBST with 5% BSA. As reference protein, we used β-actin (Santa Cruz, sc47778). The membranes were incubated overnight at 4 °C.

8. After washing with TBST, secondary antibodies conjugated with HRP (1:5000, HRP-anti-mouse CST 7076S or HRP-anti-rabbit CST 7074S) according to primary antibodies species were incubated with the membranes for one hour at RT.
9. We wash the membranes in TBST and incubate them with Enhanced Chemiluminescence kit (GE Health Care) for 5 min and then expose them to blue X-ray film (Agfa).
10. For data analysis, films are scanned and the densities of distinct bands evaluated using ImageJ freeware. The densities of the target proteins are normalized to the densities of the reference protein.

Acknowledgments

The study was supported by the MEYS of the Czech Republic (LD14030), Slovak Research and Development Agency (APVV-0052-10), and the Scientific Grant Agency of the Slovak Republic (VEGA 2/0029/16). OV and TP were supported by the project no. LQ1605 from the National Program of Sustainability II (MEYS CR) and by the project FNUSA-ICRC no. CZ.1.05/1.1.00/02.0123 (OP VaVpI).

References

1. Leurs R, Vischer HF, Wijtmans M et al (2011) En route to new blockbuster anti-histamines: surveying the offspring of the expanding histamine receptor family. Trends Pharmacol Sci 32:250–257
2. Alcaniz L, Vega A, Chacon P et al (2013) Histamine production by human neutrophils. FASEB J 27:2902–2910
3. Huang JF, Thurmond RL (2008) The new biology of histamine receptors. Curr Allergy Asthma Rep 8:21–27
4. Shahid M, Walker GB, Zorn SH et al (2009) Asenapine: a novel psychopharmacologic agent with a unique human receptor signature. J Psychopharmacol 23:65–73
5. Bury TB, Corhay JL, Radermecker MF (1992) Histamine-induced inhibition of neutrophil chemotaxis and T-lymphocyte proliferation in man. Allergy 47:624–629
6. O'Reilly M, Alpert R, Jenkinson S et al (2002) Identification of a histamine H4 receptor on human eosinophils—role in eosinophil chemotaxis. J Recept Signal Transduct Res 22:431–448
7. Vasicek O, Lojek A, Jancinova V et al (2014) Role of histamine receptors in the effects of histamine on the production of reactive oxygen species by whole blood phagocytes. Life Sci 100:67–72
8. Oda T, Morikawa N, Saito Y et al (2000) Molecular cloning and characterization of a novel type of histamine receptor preferentially expressed in leukocytes. J Biol Chem 275:36781–36786
9. Morse KL, Behan J, Laz TM et al (2001) Cloning and characterization of a novel human histamine receptor. J Pharmacol Exp Ther 296:1058–1066
10. Zhu Y, Michalovich D, Wu H et al (2001) Cloning, expression, and pharmacological characterization of a novel human histamine receptor. Mol Pharmacol 59:434–441
11. Melmon KL, Khan MM (1987) Histamine and its lymphocyte-selective derivatives as immune modulators. Trends Pharmacol Sci 8:437–441
12. Azuma Y, Shinohara M, Wang PL et al (2001) Histamine inhibits chemotaxis, phagocytosis, superoxide anion production, and the production of TNFalpha and IL-12 by macrophages via H2-receptors. Int Immunopharmacol 1:1867–1875
13. Betten A, Dahlgren C, Hermodsson S et al (2003) Histamine inhibits neutrophil NADPH oxidase activity triggered by the lipoxin A4 receptor-specific peptide agonist Trp-Lys-Tyr-Met-Val-Met. Scand J Immunol 58:321–326
14. Lojek A, Ciz M, Pekarova M et al (2011) Modulation of metabolic activity of phagocytes

by antihistamines. Interdiscip Toxicol 4: 15–19
15. Liu SC, Chu YH, Kao CH et al (2015) Steroids and antihistamines synergize to inhibit rat's airway smooth muscle contractility. Eur Arch Otorhinolaryngol 272(6):1443–1449
16. Scichilone N, Ventura MT, Bonini M et al (2015) Choosing wisely: practical considerations on treatment efficacy and safety of asthma in the elderly. Clin Mol Allergy 13(1):7
17. Leurs R, Church MK, Taglialatela M (2002) H1-antihistamines: inverse agonism, anti-inflammatory actions and cardiac effects. Clin Exp Allergy 32:489–498
18. Church MK, Church DS (2013) Pharmacology of antihistamines. Indian J Dermatol 58:219–224
19. Drabikova K, Nosal R, Jancinova V et al (2002) Reactive oxygen metabolite production is inhibited by histamine and H1-antagonist dithiaden in human PMN leukocytes. Free Radic Res 36:975–980
20. Jancinova V, Drabikova K, Nosal R et al (2006) Extra- and intracellular formation of reactive oxygen species by human neutrophils in the presence of pheniramine, chlorpheniramine and brompheniramine. Neuro Endocrinol Lett 27(Suppl 2):141–143
21. Ciz M, Lojek A (2013) Modulation of neutrophil oxidative burst via histamine receptors. Br J Pharmacol 170:17–22
22. Nosal R, Jancinova V, Drabikova K et al (2015) Molecular pharmacology of antihistamines in inhibition of oxidative burst of professional phagocytes. Gen Physiol Biophys 34:209–216
23. Drabikova K, Jancinova V, Nosal R et al (2006) Extra- and intracellular oxidant production in phorbol myristate acetate stimulated human polymorphonuclear leukocytes: modulation by histamine and H(1)-antagonist loratadine. Inflamm Res 55(Suppl 1):S19–S20
24. Nosal R, Drabikova K, Jancinova V et al (2006) On the pharmacology and toxicology of neutrophils. Neuro Endocrinol Lett 27(Suppl 2):148–151
25. Wright HL, Moots RJ, Bucknall RC et al (2010) Neutrophil function in inflammation and inflammatory diseases. Rheumatology (Oxford) 49:1618–1631
26. Kruger P, Saffarzadeh M, Weber AN et al (2015) Neutrophils: between host defence, immune modulation, and tissue injury. PLoS Pathog 11:e1004651
27. Serhan CN, Brain SD, Buckley CD et al (2007) Resolution of inflammation: state of the art, definitions and terms. FASEB J 21:325–332
28. Mocsai A, Walzog B, Lowell CA (2015) Intracellular signalling during neutrophil recruitment. Cardiovasc Res 107:373–385
29. Scapini P, Lapinet-Vera JA, Gasperini S et al (2000) The neutrophil as a cellular source of chemokines. Immunol Rev 177:195–203
30. Scapini P, Cassatella MA (2014) Social networking of human neutrophils within the immune system. Blood 124:710–719
31. Maderna P, Godson C (2003) Phagocytosis of apoptotic cells and the resolution of inflammation. Biochim Biophys Acta 1639:141–151
32. Serhan CN (2014) Pro-resolving lipid mediators are leads for resolution physiology. Nature 510:92–101
33. Jones DP (2006) Disruption of mitochondrial redox circuitry in oxidative stress. Chem Biol Interact 163:38–53
34. Halliwell B (2007) Biochemistry of oxidative stress. Biochem Soc Trans 35:1147–1150
35. Oktyabrsky ON, Smirnova GV (2007) Redox regulation of cellular functions. Biochemistry (Mosc) 72:132–145
36. Filippin LI, Vercelino R, Marroni NP et al (2008) Redox signalling and the inflammatory response in rheumatoid arthritis. Clin Exp Immunol 152:415–422
37. Babior BM (1999) NADPH oxidase: an update. Blood 93:1464–1476
38. Dahlgren C, Karlsson A (1999) Respiratory burst in human neutrophils. J Immunol Methods 232:3–14
39. Liu L, Dahlgren C, Elwing H et al (1996) A simple chemiluminescence assay for the determination of reactive oxygen species produced by human neutrophils. J Immunol Methods 192:173–178
40. Allen RC (1977) Evaluation of serum opsonic capacity by quantitating the initial chemiluminescent response from phagocytizing polymorphonuclear leukocytes. Infect Immun 15: 828–833
41. Seymour GJ, Whyte GJ, Powell RN (1986) Chemiluminescence in the assessment of polymorphonuclear leukocyte function in chronic inflammatory periodontal disease. J Oral Pathol 15:125–131
42. Fromtling RA, Abruzzo GK (1985) Chemiluminescence as a tool for the evaluation of antimicrobial agents: a review. Methods Find Exp Clin Pharmacol 7:493–500
43. Calokerinos AC, Deftereos NT, Baeyens WR (1995) Chemiluminescence in drug assay. J Pharm Biomed Anal 13:1063–1071
44. Vilim V, Wilhelm J (1989) What do we measure by a luminol-dependent chemiluminescence of phagocytes? Free Radic Biol Med 6:623–629
45. Dahlgren C, Stendahl O (1983) Role of myeloperoxidase in luminol-dependent chemiluminescence of polymorphonuclear leukocytes. Infect Immun 39:736–741

46. Lundqvist H, Kricka LJ, Stott RA et al (1995) Influence of different luminols on the characteristics of the chemiluminescence reaction in human neutrophils. J Biolumin Chemilumin 10:353–359
47. Lundqvist H, Dahlgren C (1996) Isoluminol-enhanced chemiluminescence: a sensitive method to study the release of superoxide anion from human neutrophils. Free Radic Biol Med 20:785–792
48. Dahlgren C (1988) Effects on extra- and intracellularly localized, chemoattractant-induced, oxygen radical production in neutrophils following modulation of conditions for ligand-receptor interaction. Inflammation 12: 335–349
49. Johansson A, Dahlgren C (1989) Characterization of the luminol-amplified light-generating reaction induced in human monocytes. J Leukoc Biol 45:444–451
50. Kopprasch S, Pietzsch J, Graessler J (2003) Validation of different chemilumigenic substrates for detecting extracellular generation of reactive oxygen species by phagocytes and endothelial cells. Luminescence 18:268–273
51. Kralova J, Nosal R, Drabikova K et al (2008) Comparative investigations of the influence of H1-antihistamines on the generation of reactive oxygen species by phagocytes. Inflamm Res 57(Suppl 1):S49–S50
52. Kralova J, Rackova L, Pekarova M et al (2009) The effects of H1-antihistamines on the nitric oxide production by RAW 264.7 cells with respect to their lipophilicity. Int Immunopharmacol 9:990–995
53. Nosal R, Drabikova K, Jancinova V et al (2009) H1-antihistamines and oxidative burst of professional phagocytes. Neuro Endocrinol Lett 30(Suppl 1):133–136
54. Droge W (2002) Free radicals in the physiological control of cell function. Physiol Rev 82:47–95
55. Kori S, Namiki H, Suzuki K (2009) Biphasic regulation of polymorphonuclear leukocyte spreading by polyphenolic compounds with pyrogallol moieties. Int Immunopharmacol 9:1159–1167
56. Dahlgren C, Karlsson A, Bylund J (2007) Measurement of respiratory burst products generated by professional phagocytes. Methods Mol Biol 412:349–363
57. Jancinova V, Drabikova K, Nosal R et al (2006) The combined luminol/isoluminol chemiluminescence method for differentiating between extracellular and intracellular oxidant production by neutrophils. Redox Rep 11:110–116
58. Kucekova Z, Humpolicek P, Kasparkova V et al (2014) Colloidal polyaniline dispersions: antibacterial activity, cytotoxicity and neutrophil oxidative burst. Colloids Surf B Biointerfaces 116:411–417
59. Komrskova D, Lojek A, Hrbac J et al (2006) A comparison of chemical systems for luminometric determination of antioxidant capacity towards individual reactive oxygen species. Luminescence 21:239–244

Chapter 8

Techniques Used in Pharmacological Evaluation of Histamine H_4 Receptor Function on Native Human Eosinophils

Marek Grosicki and Katarzyna Kieć-Kononowicz

Abstract

Most of the research on the histamine receptors in in vitro studies was accomplished using recombinant systems. These biological models proved to be ideal in the determination of the receptors' function, biochemistry, and molecular signaling pathways. Unfortunately, they do not reflect the real biological situation, as the receptors are artificially introduced to host system and usually expressed in high quantity, not regulated as in native cells. Recently in order to overcome the limitations of recombinant systems, several important works were published that focus on the histamine receptors' function in native human cells. For histamine H_4 receptor functional studies immune cells, including human eosinophils, were mainly used. Therefore in this chapter we discuss the tools and provide step-by-step protocols used in the pharmacological evaluation of histamine H_4 receptor function in primary human eosinophils. Methods include: isolation of human eosinophils from peripheral blood, functional determination of the effects of histamine receptors' ligands (including selective histamine receptor agonists and antagonists), and data elaboration. We believe that the described methods may play an important role in future studies because as yet the function of histamine receptors on the other immune cells remains elusive.

Key words Eosinophils, G-protein-coupled receptors, Histamine, Histamine receptors, Histamine H_4 receptor, Histamine receptor ligands

1 Introduction

Human eosinophils are leukocytes known as acidophilic granulocytes. These cells are believed to act as late-phase inflammatory cells, which are involved in host defence against parasitic infections as well as in allergies and asthma. Eosinophils can be activated by different stimuli. When triggered they release a number of cytokines, chemokines, and lipids mediators, followed by degranulation of cytotoxic granules including proteins like: major basic protein (MBP), eosinophil cationic protein (ECP), eosinophil peroxidase (EPO), eosinophil-derived neurotoxin (EDN), and reactive oxygen species (ROS) [1–3]. Furthermore, these cells possess partial

Ekaterini Tiligada and Madeleine Ennis (eds.), *Histamine Receptors as Drug Targets*, Methods in Pharmacology and Toxicology, DOI 10.1007/978-1-4939-6843-5_8, © Springer Science+Business Media LLC 2017

phagocytic activity, act as antigen-presenting cells, and can interact with mast cells, lymphocytes, and endothelial cells [4–6]. These different cellular properties make human eosinophils an interesting pharmacological model in biological assays. Unfortunately due to problematic isolation, very low frequency in the human peripheral blood (1–7% of all leukocytes in healthy donors), low and short time cell viability, and individual-donor-dependent eosinophils diversity, the study of native human eosinophils is very difficult. Despite this human eosinophils together with human neutrophils and mast cells remain the main cellular model used in native histamine receptor research [7].

Histamine is one of stimuli that can lead to eosinophil activation. To date, three histamine receptors subtypes have been described on human eosinophils, these are H_1, H_2, and H_4 histamine receptors [8–10], whose function is summarized in Fig. 1. Activation of the histamine H_1 receptor results in stimulation of eosinophilic superoxide ion generation [10]. Activation of the histamine H_2 receptor induces increase in cellular cAMP concentration, which results in inhibition of eosinophil degranulation [8, 11]. The histamine H_4 receptor plays a general immunomodulatory role in eosinophil activation. This receptor has been extensively studied on human eosinophils and when activated it results in cytoskeleton and cellular shape change, chemotaxis, intracellular calcium change, and adhesion to endothelial cells [9, 12–14]. It must be noted that functional existence of histamine H_1 and H_2 receptors on human eosinophils has been recently questioned. This controversy arose from the fact that only partial characterization of the histamine receptors (on mRNA and protein level) was performed

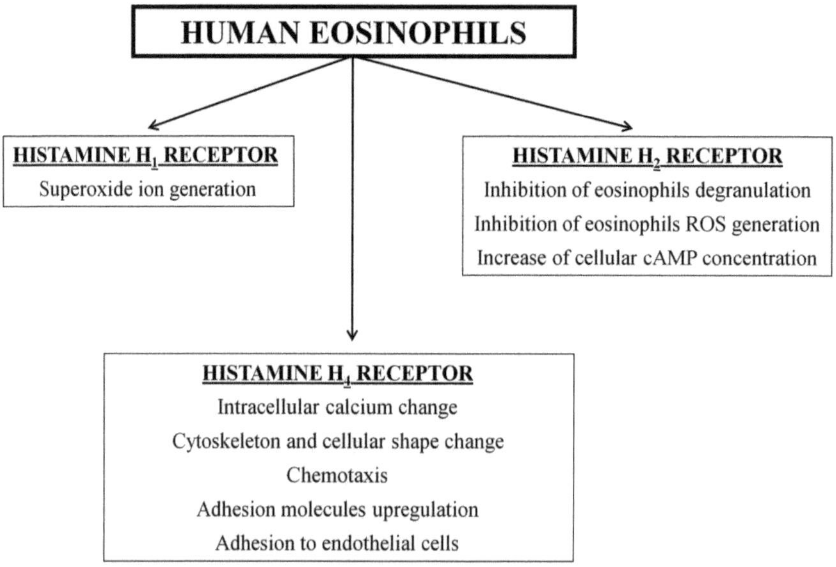

Fig. 1 Histamine receptors functions on the human eosinophils

on human eosinophils. Most of the data were obtained from functional tests. However, some tests were performed before the actual identification of new histamine receptors classes (like H_3 and H_4 receptors), and positive results might come from off target effects [13]. Therefore, the true function of each histamine receptor on human eosinophils must be reevaluated.

In this chapter, we will describe selected techniques used in pharmacological evaluation of histamine H_4 receptor function on human eosinophils. Paragraphs will include: eosinophil isolation from the peripheral blood, reactive oxygen species and eosinophil peroxidase activity measurement, intracellular calcium change, cytoskeleton and cellular shape change assays, chemotaxis and observations of eosinophil adhesion to endothelial cells.

2 Tools Used in Evaluation of Histamine Receptors Functions

The functional studies of histamine receptors are mainly conducted using selective receptor ligands that can alter the receptor or other ligand activity resulting in a biological response. Agonists have the ability to bind to the receptor and stabilize its active conformation, whereas inverse agonists are stabilizing receptor inactive form. Antagonists are ligands that reduce the action of other ligands with agonistic properties. On their own, antagonists have no effect on the receptors active or inactive state [15].

To date, several selective agonists and antagonists have been developed for the histamine receptors study. Examples of these compounds are listed in Table 1.

Most of the histamine receptor antagonists and agonists exhibit some degree of affinity for the other histamine receptor classes.

Table 1
Indicative selective histamine receptor ligands

Histamine receptor			
H_1	H_2	H_3	H_4
Agonists	*Agonists*	*Agonists*	*Agonists*
Histamine [29]	Histamine [29]	Histamine [29]	Histamine [29]
Methylhistaprodifen [30] Histaprodifen [34]	Amthamine [31]	Methimepip [32] Immethridine [36]	VUF 8430 [33] 4-methylhistamine [35]
Antagonists	*Antagonists*	*Antagonists*	*Antagonists*
Diphenhydramine [29]	Ranitidine [29]	Thioperamide [37]	Thioperamide [37]
Loratadine [38]	Famotidine [39]	Pitolisant [39]	JNJ7777120 [40]
Pyrilamine [39]	Cimetidine [41]	Clobenpropit [35]	JNJ39758979 [42]

This lack of absolute specificity sometimes makes receptor function evaluation very difficult. Therefore, it is very important when examining the function of each of the histamine receptors to use a set of structurally different histamine receptor ligands specific to one receptor class. Histamine receptors differ not only in function but also in the affinity toward the natural agonist histamine. Histamine H_1 and H_2 receptors are considered low affinity receptors with pK_i values of 4.2 and 4.3 respectively, whereas histamine H_3 and H_4 receptors are high affinity receptors with pK_i values of 8.0 and 8.2 respectively [14]. Therefore, it is important when testing the effects of histamine receptor agonists or antagonists to use both low and high concentrations of compounds to include/exclude each histamine receptors subclass activation.

A number of the investigated compounds demonstrate paradoxical and unexpected effects when studied using different biological assays. This for example refers to JNJ7777120 activity. This compound described as selective histamine H_4 receptor antagonist exhibits unusual stimulatory effects in some experimental systems acting as partial agonist, full antagonist, or inverse agonist [16–18]. Additionally, JNJ7777120 possesses biased ligand features, which apart from the antagonistic effect on the histamine H_4 receptor, exert partial agonistic effect on the β-arrestin pathway [16]. This might be the proof that histamine receptors exhibit ligand functional selectivity, in which any histamine receptor ligand can activate its specific receptor conformation [7]. This concept however still needs to be confirmed using native human cells.

3 Isolation of Eosinophils from Human Peripheral Blood

In healthy human individuals eosinophils constitute 1–7% of all blood circulating leukocytes. Due to their low number and very short lifespan, immunomagnetic separation methods are the best choice for the isolation of eosinophils. These methods are relatively fast and result in highly purified cellular populations. In this protocol, the negative immunomagnetic selection of eosinophils from whole blood will be described using the column-based Miltenyi Biotec system. Before magnetic separation, an enriched granulocyte population is obtained through red blood cells depletion and Ficoll-Paque Plus density gradient separation. The granulocytes are incubated with a mixture of biotin-conjugated monoclonal antibodies: anti-CD2, CD14, CD16, CD19, CD56, CD123, CD235a that are targeted against multiple surface antigens of non-eosinophils blood cells and anti-biotin antibodies conjugated to MicroBeads. An overview of the entire isolation procedure is presented in Fig. 2.

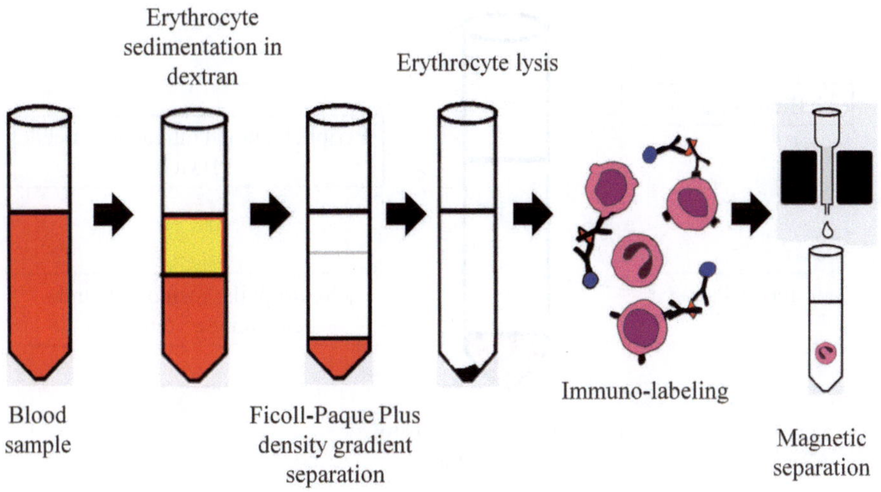

Fig. 2 Overview of the eosinophils isolation methodology from human peripheral blood

3.1 Materials

Eosinophils are obtained from human whole blood through venipuncture. Blood (10 mL) is collected in heparin-coated tubes. The reagents and materials are:

- 6% dextran from Leuconostoc spp. 500 000 dissolved in Dulbecco's phosphate buffered saline (DPBS).
- Ficoll-Paque Plus d = 1.077 g/mL.
- Eosinophil isolation kit #130-092-010 (Miltenyi Biotec).
- Separation buffer containing DPBS, 2 mM EDTA and 10% (v/v) fetal bovine serum (FBS).
- Distilled water.
- Incubation medium containing RPMI 1640 with L-glutamine and 10% FBS for isolated cells.
- Conical polypropylene centrifuge tubes (15 mL).
- Disposable transfer pipettes.
- Tubes (1.5 mL).
- Cell separation magnetic columns (for this protocol size MS).
- Magnet for cell separation with stand.
- Hemocytometer for cell counting.
- Centrifuge.

3.2 Methods

3.2.1 Blood Pretreatment in Order to Eliminate Red Blood Cells and Granulocyte Enrichment

1. The solution of 6% dextran and Ficoll-Paque Plus should be brought to room temperature (RT), the remaining reagents (separation buffer, distilled water and antibodies) must be kept on ice (*see* **Note 1**).
2. Transfer 10 mL venous blood to 15 mL conical tube filled with 2 mL of 6% dextran solution, blood should be mixed with dextran.

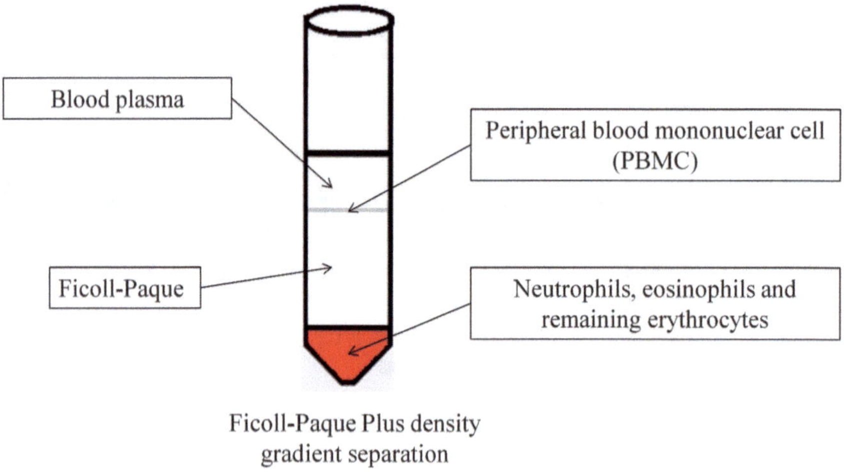

Fig. 3 Blood sample after Ficoll-Paque Plus density gradient separation

3. Centrifuge mixture at 50 × *g*, for 7 min at RT, without centrifuge brake. This will speed up the erythrocytes' sedimentation process. After centrifugation, the blood mixture will divide into two phases: lower red phase containing erythrocytes and upper, yellow with leukocytes.
4. The upper layer should be transferred to a new 15 mL conical tube, over 5 mL Ficoll-Paque Plus (ρ = 1.077 g/mL). When collecting the upper layer care should be maintained not to take any part of the red cell layer to minimize red cell contamination, which would greatly affect the outcome of the purification procedure. The upper layer must be transferred slowly not to destroy Ficoll-Paque gradient.
5. The mixture is centrifuged at 400 × *g* for 12 min at RT in a swinging bucket rotor without brake. The sample will divide into four layers (Fig. 3). The bottom one will contain granulocytes and remaining erythrocytes. After centrifugation, plasma, peripheral blood mononuclear cell (PBMC), and Ficoll interface should be discarded, leaving only the last bottom layer.
6. The remaining erythrocytes from the granulocyte sample can be removed by hypotonic shock lysis for 30 s in 1 mL distilled water. Lysis should be stopped by adding 5 mL of RPMI 1640/10% (v/v) FBS cell culture medium, followed by centrifugation at 300 × *g* for 5 min (*see* **Note 2**). At this step number of isolated cells should be estimated using a hemocytometer.

3.2.2 Immunomagnetic Separation of Eosinophils

1. For magnetic labeling 1 × 10^7 cells (cell count obtained in Sect. 3.2.1, **step 6**) should be resuspended in 40 μL separation buffer (*see* **Note 3**).

2. To the cellular mixture add 10 μL of Miltenyi biotin-antibody cocktail, then incubate the cell solution for 10 min at 4 °C. After incubation, 30 μL of separation buffer should be added to cell sample.
3. Add 20 μL of Miltenyi anti-biotin microbeads, incubate sample for additional 15 min at 4 °C.
4. After the final incubation cells should be washed in cold DPBS and resuspended in 500 μL separation buffer.
5. During the washing step, prime the MS magnetic column with 500 μL separation buffer. The empty column should be placed into the magnet, attached to appropriate stand (provided by manufacturer). Add the separation buffer into the upper part of the column. Liquid should be allowed to pass passively through the column. Discard flow-through.
6. Place new 1.5 mL probe at the bottom of the column (this will be the probe in which the eosinophils will be collected). The enriched population of granulocytes labeled with microbeads antibodies, resuspended in 500 μL separation buffer, should be placed into the upper part of primed column. Place column in the magnetic field (on magnet). Collect effluent (*see* **Note 4**).
7. Wash the column two times with separation buffer (500 μL), collect effluents.
8. Isolated eosinophils will be present in the collected effluents, as the unlabeled cells. The rest of the non-eosinophilic cells will be retained on the column (*see* **Notes 5** and **6**).

4 Eosinophils Reactive Oxygen Species Generation Assay

Human eosinophils possess the ability to synthesize reactive oxygen species including superoxide ($O_2^{\bullet -}$) and hydrogen peroxide (H_2O_2) [1]. This ability can be used to determine the functional properties of eosinophils as well as in the evaluation of specific ligand effects on eosinophil activation. The experimental data indicate that histamine can inhibit fMLP-induced production of reactive oxygen species by eosinophils [11]. One of the methods used in superoxide quantification is the measurement of ferricytochrome c reduction to ferrocytochrome c. During that process the spectroscopic spectrum of ferrocytochrome c is changed, the absorbance at 550 nm is increased, whereas absorbance at 540 nm and 560 nm remains unaltered. Researchers should keep in mind that the reduction of ferricytochrome c is not specific for $O_2^{\bullet -}$ but might result from direct reduction by electrons donated from enzymes or other substances. Therefore in order to confirm the effect of superoxide in ferricytochrome c reduction, the experiments must be performed in the presence and absence of superoxide dismutase (SOD).

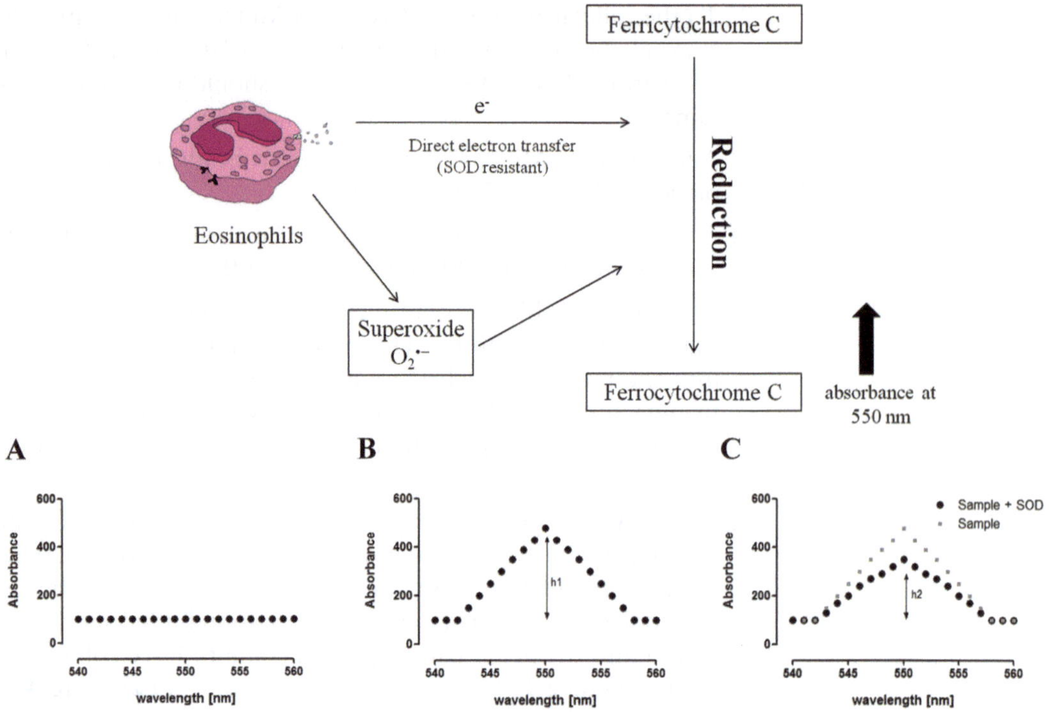

Fig. 4 Ferricytochrome c reduction to ferrocytochrome c. The reduction of ferricytochrome c can occur through direct electron transfer or by reaction with superoxide. Amount of superoxide radicals is proportional to ferrocytochrome c absorption. Sample background absorption (nonactivated eosinophils). (**a**) Eosinophils activation (sample absorption). (**b**) Absorption of superoxide-mediated reduction of ferricytochrome c. (**c**) Superoxide dismutase (SOD) is used to differentiate between a direct reduction of ferricytochrome c or mediated by superoxide

This enzyme catalyzes the transformation of the superoxide radical into either oxygen or hydrogen peroxide. Only the SOD-inhibitable signal can be used to calculate the amount of superoxide radicals in the sample (Fig. 4) [19].

4.1 Materials

- The reaction buffer consists of: 1 mM $CaCl_2$, 0.3 μg/mL cytochalasin B, and 100 μM ferricytochrome c.
- The eosinophil buffer contains: DPBS, 1 mM $CaCl_2$, 1 mM $MgCl_2$, and 0.5% (w/v) bovine serum albumin (BSA).
- For activation and control, fMLP and superoxide dismutase are used.

4.2 Methods

1. Prepare 96-well microplate containing 10 μL of 20-fold concentrated reagent (e.g., histamine or histamine receptor ligands) and 80 μL reaction buffer per well (*see* **Note** 7).
2. Resuspend eosinophils in eosinophil buffer; prepare the cell suspension at density appropriate for experimental setup.
3. Cell suspension should be added into the experimental plate in volume of 100 μL/well with cell density of 1×10^5 cells/mL.

4. Pre-incubate the cell mixture with the reagents for 5 min at 37 °C.
5. The reaction is started by adding 10 μL fMLP (final concentration of fMLP is 1 μM) (*see* **Note 8**).
6. Superoxide radical production should be measured with continuous kinetics analysis over 30 min. The microplate reader should be set up for absorbance measurement at 540 nm and 560 nm, as well as of superoxide dismutase-inhibitable reduction of ferricytochrome c at 550 nm.
7. The difference of the absorbance at 550 nm between the beginning and the end of the experiment is used to determine the amount of superoxide radicals produced (*see* **Note 9**).

5 Eosinophil Peroxidase Activity Measurement

Eosinophil peroxidase (EPO) is released from human eosinophil secondary granules upon cellular activation [20]. Histamine inhibits the degranulation of human eosinophil peroxidase via histamine H_2 receptor activation [8, 13]. There are a number of methods to quantify the concentration of peroxidase in biological samples. Here, the fluorometric Amplex Red method will be described. Amplex Red reagent (10-acetyl-3,7-dihydroxyphenoxazine) in the presence of peroxidase enzymes reacts with H_2O_2 in a 1:1 stoichiometry to produce red fluorescent compound—resorufin (Fig. 5). Resorufin is a fluorescent compound with high fluorescence emission at 590 nm, and therefore can be easily quantified [21].

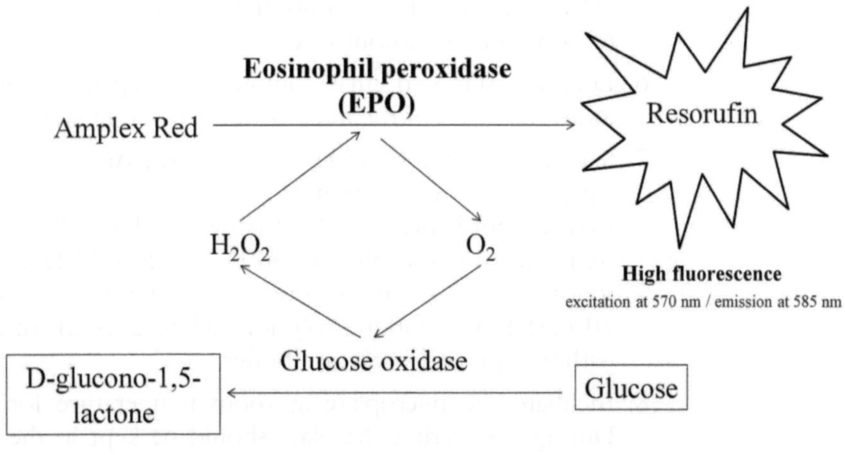

Fig. 5 Principle of eosinophil peroxidase (EPO) detection using Amplex Red reagent

5.1 Materials

- Eosinophil buffer (*see* Sect. 4.1) supplemented with 5 μg/mL cytochalasin B.
- For eosinophil activation, calcium ionophore A23187, phorbol 12-myristate 13-acetate (PMA), fMLP, and eotaxin can be used.
- Reagents for peroxidase quantification originate from Amplex Red Hydrogen Peroxide/Peroxidase Assay (Thermofisher). The kit consists of 5× reaction buffer, 10 mM Amplex Red reagent stock solution, DMSO, 10 U/mL Horseradish Peroxidase (HRP) stock solution, and ~3% H_2O_2 reagent (*see* **Notes 10** and **11**).

5.2 Methods

1. Prepare 96-well microplate. Each microplate well should be filled with different histamine ligands, and eosinophil activators in total volume of 100 μL per well. It must be noted that substrates in microplate will be diluted 2-fold in the final reaction volume.
2. Before eosinophil activation add cytochalasin B to the cells at a final concentration of 5 μg/mL.
3. Primed eosinophils with cytochalasin B should be transferred into the 96-well microplate at a concentration of 1×10^5 cells per well, in a volume of 100 μL (*see* **Note 12**).
4. The microplate should be incubated for 30 min at 37 °C. Thereafter, centrifuge the microplate at 430 × *g* for 5 min, 20 °C. A 50 μL aliquot of each well should be transferred into a new 96-well plate.
5. Before the actual assay, peroxidase standard curve and negative controls should be prepared. For the standard curve dilute 10 U/mL horseradish peroxidase (HRP) stock solution in 1× reaction buffer into concentrations ranging from 0 to 2 mU/mL HRP (each in volume of 50 μL). For negative control use 1× reaction buffer without HRP.
6. Load the standard curve samples and negative controls into individual wells of the microplate prepared in **step 4** above.
7. Start the reaction by adding 50 μL of the Amplex Red reagent with excess concentration of H_2O_2 to each well. The Amplex Red reagent is prepared by mixing 50 μL of 10 mM Amplex Red reagent stock solution, 500 μL of 20 mM H_2O_2 working solution and 4.45 mL of 1× reaction buffer. In order to prepare 20 mM H_2O_2 working solution, dilute 22.7 μL of 3% H_2O_2 with 977 μL of 1× reaction buffer.
8. Incubate the microplate at room temperature for 30 min. During this period the plate should be kept in the dark (*see* **Note 13**).
9. Measure the fluorescence of each well using a microplate reader. Measurements should be performed at an excitation of 530 nm and fluorescence emission at 590 nm.

10. For each measurement point, the obtained value should be subtracted from mean non-HRP control. The amount of eosinophil peroxidase in the sample should be calculated from the HRP standard curve (*see* **Note 14**).

6 Intracellular Calcium Change Assay

G protein-coupled receptors including histamine receptors can trigger an increase in cytosolic calcium concentration (calcium flux). Agonist binding to GPCR receptors results in the activation of phospholipase C (PLC) via Gαq or Gβγ subunits. This leads to the generation of inositol 1,4,5-trisphosphate (InsP 3), which reaches the endoplasmic reticulum, provoking the opening of InsP 3-sensitive calcium channels and release of stored calcium into the cellular cytosol [22]. The cellular calcium responses are rapid with the maximal peak response reached after few seconds. The response is transient, it quickly declines to reach a plateau (Fig. 6). Cytosolic calcium concentration change has been recognized as one of the fundamental mechanisms of cell signaling. Therefore, several assays as well as calcium dyes have been developed, including fura-2-AM. Fura-2-AM calcium-sensitive fluorescent dyes (excitation at 340–380 nm, emission at 510 nm) possess the ability to migrate through cellular membranes as an ester. In the cell this dye is hydrolyzed to the acidic form and it becomes trapped inside the cellular cytosol. Fluorescence measurement of calcium bound fura-2 dye is possible using a fluorometric scanning imaging plate reader with integrated fluids transfer workstation [22]. When studying the effect of the agonist on cellular calcium signaling, it is

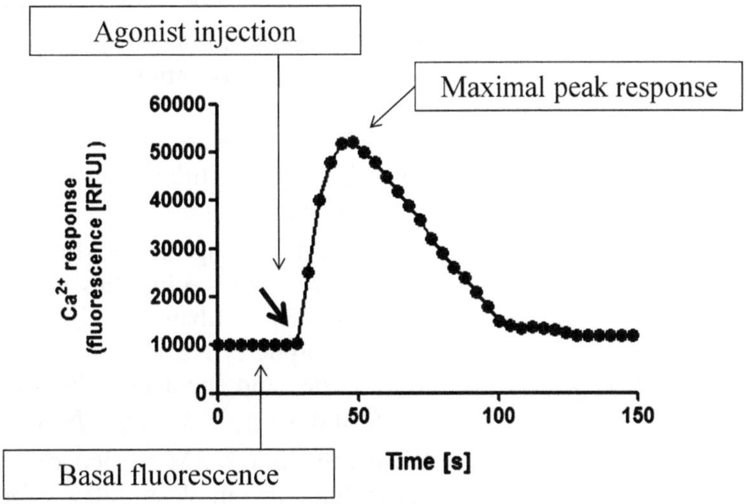

Fig. 6 Kinetics of intracellular calcium change (*bold arrow* indicates agonist addition)

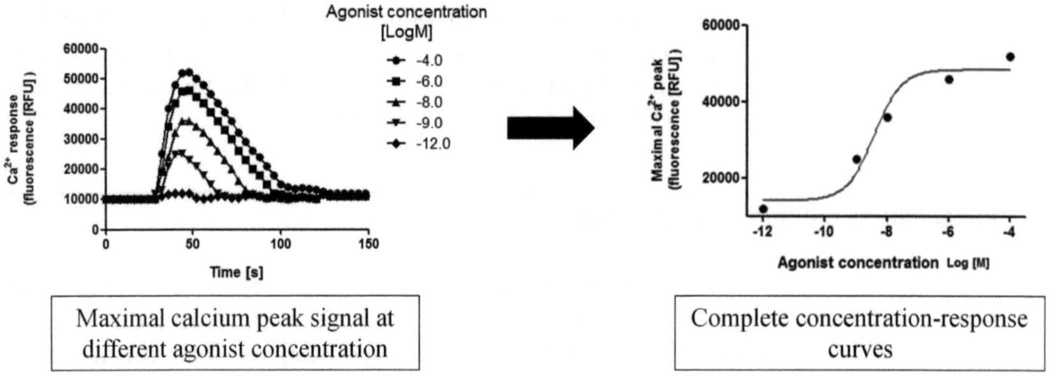

Fig. 7 Calculation of complete concentration-response curves based on maximal calcium peak in each investigated agonist concentration

possible to create complete concentration-response curves when investigating different concentrations of agonists. Curves can be generated from the data obtained from agonist responses using either peak calcium or area under the curve (Fig. 7).

The effect of histamine on calcium signaling in human eosinophils has been investigated by several authors [9, 13]. Histamine rapidly triggers (10–20 s) calcium flux by activation of phospholipase C, in concentrations from 10 nM to 100 μM. Activation of histamine-mediated intracellular calcium change can be blocked by selective histamine H_4 receptor antagonists indicating its direct involvement in eosinophils activation [13].

6.1 Materials

- For assay buffer see eosinophil buffer (*see* Sect. 4.1).
- Fura-2-AM loading dye.
- 96-well clear-bottom black-welled plates.
- Fluorometric scanning imaging plate reader with integrated fluids transfer workstation (dispenser).

6.2 Methods

1. Prepare eosinophils at a dilution of 5×10^5 cells/probe (in 15 mL conical centrifuge tube). Cells should be suspended in assay buffer in volume of 500 μL.
2. Fura-2-AM loading should be performed as follows: Add Fura-2-AM to the eosinophils at a final concentration of 4 μM (*see* **Note 15**), incubate cells for 10 min at 37 °C and 5% (v/v) CO_2 atmosphere. Next dilute cell mixture up to 1 mL with assay buffer and incubate cells for an additional 30 min at 37 °C and 5% (v/v) CO_2 (*see* **Note 16**).
3. Wash the Fura-2-AM loaded cells with 2 mL assay buffer (centrifuge the sample at 250 × *g* for 5 min, 20 °C).
4. Resuspend the washed cells in 10 mL of assay buffer, cells should be protected from light and stored at RT for a maximum of 2 h.

5. The fluorescence of the loaded cells should be measured with an excitation wavelength of 340–380 nm and emission of 510 nm.
6. In order to evaluate the effects of selective histamine receptors ligands, selective compounds should be incubated with cells for 3 min. The basal fluorescence of the cells should be measured for 1 min.
7. After the preincubation step, the stimulatory compound should be added. The change of fluorescence should be measured immediately after compound addition for another 5 min.
8. In order to calibrate the Fura-2 fluorescence, Triton X-100 should be added to the Fura-2 loaded cells samples (to a final concentration of 5 mM). The saturated signal of Fura-2-AM (Fmax) should be recorded for 1 min.
9. After estimation of Fmax, EGTA solution should be added to Fmax sample (**step 8** above) to a final concentration of 6 mM, in order to determine the quenched calcium-induced fluorescence signal (Fmin).
10. The concentration of intracellular calcium should be calculated using the equation:

$$[Ca^{2+}]_i = Kd \times [(F \times Fmin)/(Fmax \times F)]$$

Kd is the dissociation constant of Fura-2 (224 nM)

7 Eosinophils Cytoskeleton and Cellular Shape Change Assay

Eosinophil locomotion and chemotaxis into the site of inflammation requires cytoskeleton rearrangement and cellular shape change. This phenomenon can be investigated using microscopic imaging or flow cytometry analyses. In this paragraph, flow cytometry assays for cytoskeleton and cellular shape change will be discussed, based on studies with histamine and histamine receptors ligands [9, 12]. Changes in the cytoskeleton require the polymerization of cytoplasmic monomeric actin (G-actin) to microfilamentous actin (F- actin) [23, 24]. The rapid induction of actin polymerization can be measured with FITC labeled phalloidin, which has a high affinity toward F-actin. Eosinophil shape change can be measured by flow cytometry analysis in the gated autofluorescence forward scatter (GAFS) assay. The quantitative measurement of cellular shape change induced by histamine receptors ligands can be expressed as percentage of increase in forward scatter (FSC) events counts, compared to unstimulated cells [12].

7.1 Materials

- Reaction buffer: DPBS without Ca^{2+} and Mg^{2+}, supplemented with 0.1% (w/v) BSA, 10 mM glucose and 10 mM HEPES.

- Fixing buffer: DPBS without Ca^{2+} and Mg^{2+}, 4% (w/v) formaldehyde, 125 ng/mL L-α-lysophatidylcholine palmitoyl and 100 nM FITC phalloidin.
- For actin polymerization measurement flow cytometer will be used in FITC channel [FL1] Ex. 488 nm, Em. 525 nm.

7.2 Methods

7.2.1 Actin Polymerization in Human Eosinophils

1. Suspend isolated eosinophils in a concentration of 1 × 10^6 cells/mL in reaction buffer. Eosinophils should be divided into samples containing 1 × 10^5 eosinophils.
2. Selective antagonists of histamine receptors should be added into the samples in appropriate concentration, with a total sample volume of 90 μL. Cells should be incubated with compounds for 15 min at 37 °C and 5% (v/v) CO_2.
3. For eosinophil stimulation, the histamine receptor agonist (e.g., histamine) should be added to the samples in volume of 10 μL (resuspended in reaction buffer) (*see* **Note 17**). Cells should be mixed gently. Incubation with agonist should last for 5–10 s (for maximal cellular response) (*see* **Note 18**).
4. Reaction should be stopped with the addition of 200 μL fixing buffer.
5. Eosinophils that have been fixed, permeabilized and with FITC labeled F-actin should be analyzed in flow cytometry. Eosinophils can be gated according to side scatter (SSC) and forward scatter (FSC) characteristics. Effect of histamine ligands on actin polymerization can be expressed as percentage increase in fluorescence of FITC labeled phalloidin compared to unstimulated cells.

7.2.2 Eosinophils Shape Change Assay [Gated Autofluorescence Forward Scatter (GAFS) Assay]

This protocol was introduced by Ling et al., 2004 [12]. In the original version, the GAFS assay was performed using human polymorphonuclear leukocytes (PMNL), prepared from Ficoll-Paque separation methods. The quantitative flow cytometry measurement of cellular shape change induced by chemoattractants was expressed as the percentage increase in forward scatter (FSC) events counts, compared to unstimulated cells. Eosinophils were selected from other polymorphonuclear cells based on their high autofluorescence in PE (FL2) channel (*see* **Note 19**) (Fig. 8).

1. Prepare polymorphonuclear leukocytes (PMNL) cells in assay buffer. Cells should be divided into 80 μL aliquots containing 5 × 10^5 PMNC cells.
2. Appropriate histamine receptor antagonists in different concentrations should be added to cellular mixture in volume of 10 μL. Samples should be pretreated with histamine receptor ligands for 10 min at RT (*see* **Note 20**).
3. Eosinophil stimulation is performed via 10 μL addition of histamine agonists, e.g., histamine to a final sample volume of

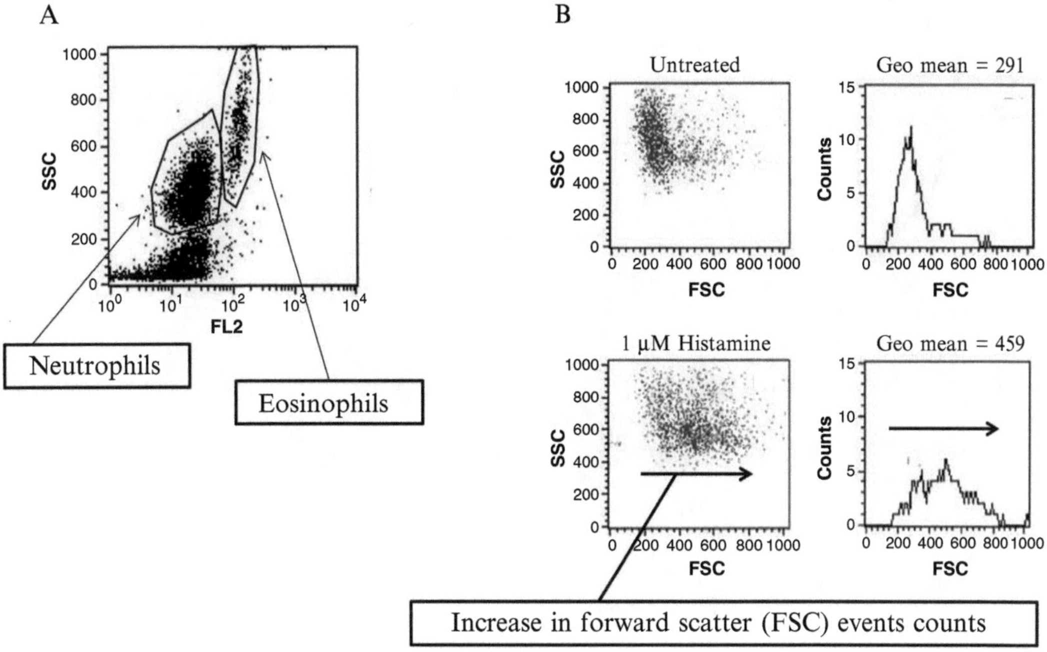

Fig. 8 Gated autofluorescence forward scatter (GAFS) assay. Eosinophils were selected from other polymorphonuclear leukocytes (PMNL) based on high autofluorescence in PE (FL2) channel and side scatter (SSC) signal (**a**). Shape change was measured by increase in forward scatter (FSC) events counts (**b**)

100 µL. Samples should be incubated for 10 min at 37 °C (*see* **Note 21**).

4. After the incubation time, the samples should be immediately transferred to an ice-water bath. Ice-cold fixative reagent (250 µL) should be added to terminate the reaction and to maintain the cell shape change (*see* **Note 22**).
5. The cell shape change is analyzed with the flow cytometer. Eosinophils in PMNL are gated based on their high autofluorescence relative to that of neutrophils in FL2 channel (575 nm emission or PE channel). Cell shape change is monitored using the increase in forward scatter signals (*see* **Note 23**) (Fig. 8).
6. The quantitative measurements of cellular shape change induced by chemoattractants are expressed as a percentage increase in forward scatter (FSC) events counts, compared to unstimulated cells.

8 Eosinophil Chemotaxis Assay

Cellular chemotaxis studies are usually based on a two-chamber system, known as Boyden or transwell system. In these assays cells are placed in one chamber and the chemical signal known as the chemoattractant in the other, usually separated with appropriate

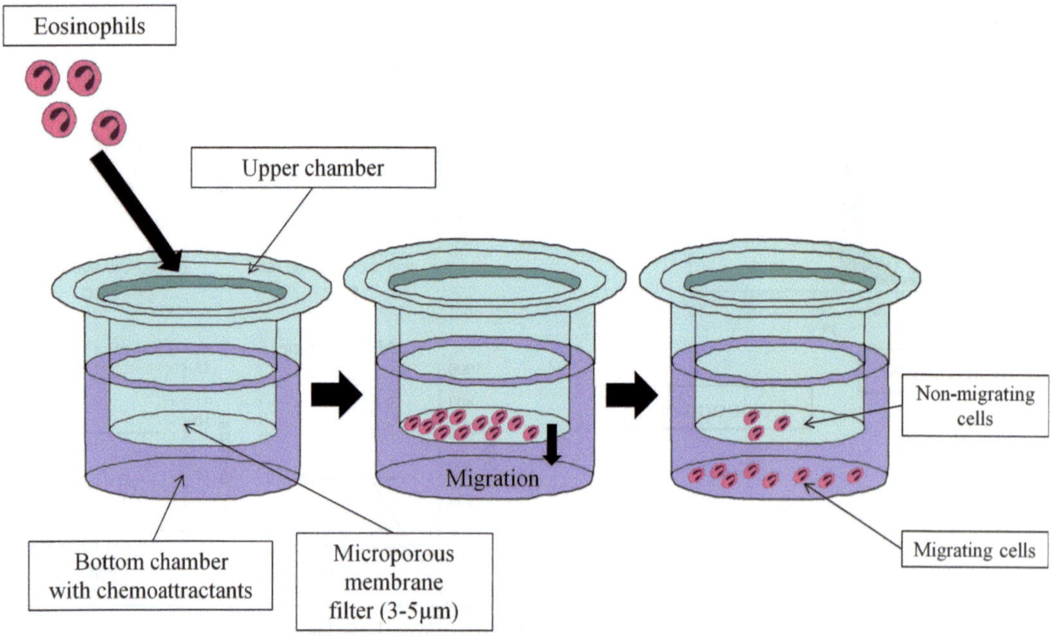

Fig. 9 Overview of transwell migration system (chemotaxis assay)

pore size filter. This creates a chemoattractant gradient in which cells migrate. The movement of the cells from control side to the side containing chemical signal results from either chemokinesis (cellular random movement) or chemotaxis (cellular directional movement up a chemoattractant gradient, which requires cellular polarity and shape change) [25]. In this protocol the transwell system is described. This system consists of two upper and bottom compartments positioned between tissue-culture-treated microporous membrane through which cells migrate sensing the source of the chemoattractants. If the investigated compound is not chemotactic, or chemotactic response of the cells has been blocked the majority of the cells will remain on the membrane. If the ligands are chemotactic, then the cells will migrate through the membrane into the bottom chamber (Fig. 9).

Histamine in 1 μM concentration was reported to induce eosinophil chemotaxis by Clark and coworkers in 1975 [26]. Interestingly, this effect could not be blocked by selective H_1 and H_2 histamine receptors antagonists known at that time. Histamine-mediated eosinophil chemotaxis can by blocked only by selective histamine H_4 receptor antagonists [13]. In comparison with other known eosinophils chemoattractants like fMLP or eotaxin, histamine is a very weak chemotactic factor.

8.1 Materials

- Transwell system consisting of top and bottom chambers separated by filter with 3–5 μm filter pore, in a 24-well plate format.
- Transwells are coated with human fibronectin.
- Chemotaxis assay buffer: RPMI 1640 with 0.5% (w/v) BSA.

8.2 Methods

1. Before experimentation, 24-well plate transwells with 3–5 μm filter pore size should be coated with 100 μL of 100 ng/mL human fibronectin for 2 h at RT. Excess fibronectin should be removed from transwells after the incubation time (*see* **Note 24**).
2. Prepare different concentrations of histamine receptor agonists (e.g., histamine) or other chemotactic compounds in chemotaxis assay buffer. Solutions should be added to the transwells bottom chambers in a volume of 450 μL.
3. Isolated eosinophils (100 μL of 1×10^6 cells/mL) should be added to the upper transwell chamber.
4. When testing the effects of selective histamine receptors antagonists, eosinophils should be pre-incubated with appropriate histamine receptor ligands for 10 min at 37 °C and 5% (v/v) CO_2, before cell addition to the upper transwell compartment.
5. Incubate the transwell plate for 2 h at 37 °C and 5% (v/v) CO_2. This will allow cells to migrate toward the underside of the insert and the bottom compartment. After incubation time upper chamber should be removed (*see* **Note 25**). Centrifuge bottom chamber cells at 430 × *g* for 5 min, 20 °C.
6. The cells in the bottom transwell chamber can be quantified using microscopic imaging, automated cell-counting devices, or by flow cytometric analyses (*see* **Notes 26** and **27**).

9 Eosinophil Adhesion to Endothelium

Leukocytes including eosinophils possess the ability to transmigrate from the peripheral blood into the site of inflammation. This feature requires close interaction with endothelial cells in a process known as leukocyte adhesion [27]. Previously, it has been shown that histamine through activation of histamine H_4 receptor upregulates certain adhesion proteins on human eosinophils [12]. In our experiments histamine could increase the number of adherent human eosinophils in a dose-dependent manner. The histamine-induced adhesion process could be blocked by the selective histamine H_4 receptor antagonist JNJ7777120, suggesting the involvement of H_4 receptor in cellular adhesion (Fig. 10). In the presented protocol, we describe eosinophil adhesion to EA.hy926 endothelial cell line assay. Adherent cells are counted using automated fluorescent microscope-based imaging platform. Eosinophils can be distinguished from endothelial cells based on their small size nuclei (Fig. 11).

9.1 Materials

- Endothelial cell culture medium: Dulbecco's modified Eagle medium (DMEM) with L-glutamine, 10% (v/v) FBS and 1x HAT supplement.
- Assay medium: RPMI 1640 medium supplemented with 10% (v/v) FBS.

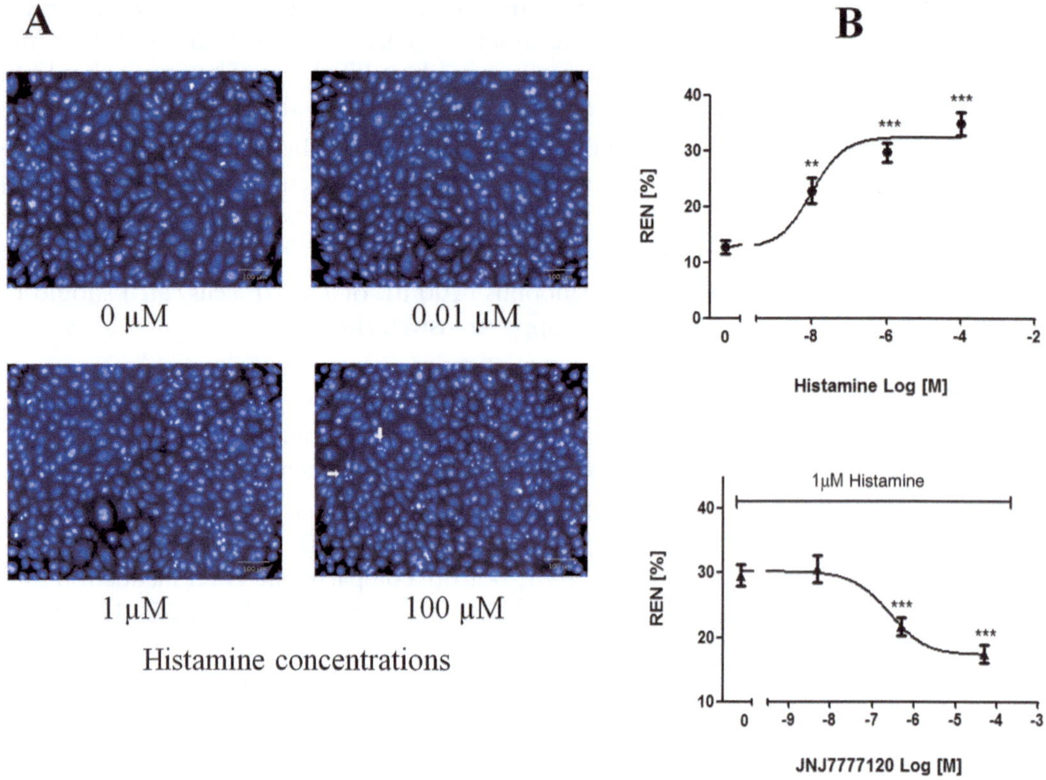

Fig. 10 Histamine effect on eosinophil adhesion to endothelium (**a**), effect of histamine H_4 receptor ligands on eosinophils adhesion (histamine–H_4 receptor agonist, JNJ7777120–H_4 receptor antagonist) (**b**)

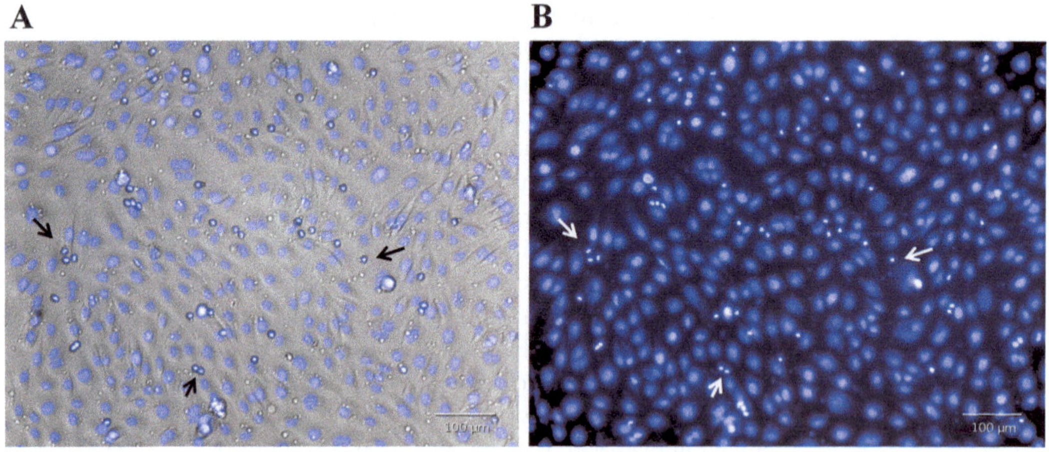

Fig. 11 Microscopic images of adherent eosinophils to EA.hy926 endothelial cell line. Image of adherent cells made in transient light (**a**); fluorescence image of adherent cells nuclei (**b**). *Arrows* indicate eosinophils

- For washing use DPBS.
- Hoechst 33342 dye is prepared through dissolving 4 μL of Hoechst 33342 trihydrochloride staining reagent in 8 mL of RPMI 1640 medium with 10% (v/v) FBS.

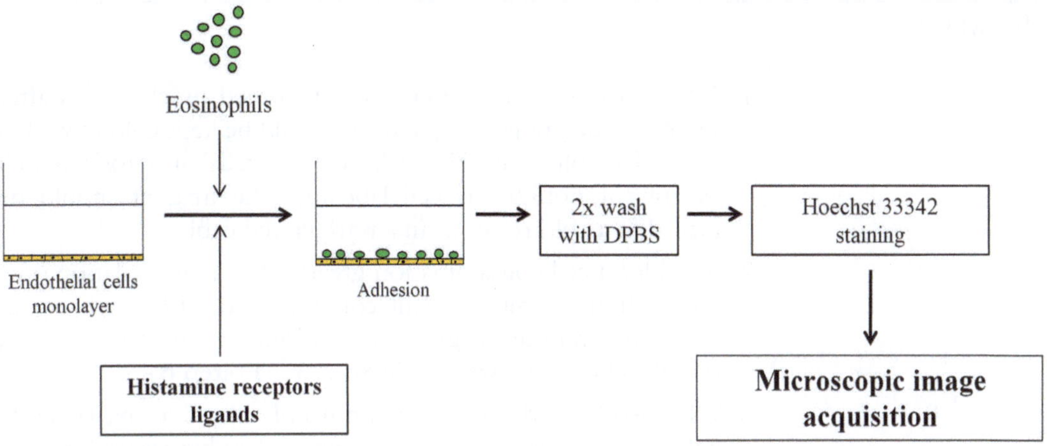

Fig. 12 The experimental setup of eosinophils adhesion to endothelium (DPBS, Dulbecco's phosphate buffered saline)

9.2 Methods

1. An overview of adhesion experiments with eosinophils is shown in Fig. 12.
2. 48 h before the adhesion assay, EA.hy926 endothelial cells should be seeded on a 24-well tissue culture plate at 5×10^5 cells per well in endothelial cell culture medium. Cells should be incubated at 37 °C and 5% (v/v) CO_2 until they reach full confluence.
3. Immediately after eosinophil isolation, wash the endothelial cells with DPBS.
4. Histamine receptor ligands should be added to each well in volume of 100 μL. Compounds should be resuspended in assay medium (*see* **Note 28**).
5. Adjust the eosinophil number to 1.5×10^6 cells in 3.75 mL assay medium. Cells should be added to each well in volume of 150 μL (each well contains 6×10^4 eosinophils) (*see* **Note 29**).
6. Mix cells and incubate for 5 min at 37 °C and 5% (v/v) CO_2.
7. Add 50 μL of selective histamine receptor agonists (e.g., histamine).
8. Allow eosinophils to adhere to the endothelial cells for 30 min at 37 °C and 5% (v/v) CO_2 (*see* **Note 30**).
9. After incubation remove nonadherent eosinophils by gentle plate wash. For that wash each plate well two times with 200 μL DPBS.
10. Stain the remaining cells' nuclei with Hoechst 33342 dye for 10 min (keep cells at 37 °C and 5% (v/v) CO_2).
11. Adherent cells can be counted using an automated fluorescent microscope-based imaging platform. Eosinophils can be detected as cells with small (nuclei area of 40–90 μm^2) nuclei in contrast to endothelial cells with single-shape, round, and big nuclei (nuclei area of 200–260 μm^2) (*see* **Notes 31** and **32**) (Fig. 11).

10 Notes

1. Isolation procedures should be performed quickly, cells after Ficoll-Paque gradient separation should be kept cold as well as precooled solutions. This will slow the cells' apoptosis as well as prevent nonspecific cell labeling. The magnet should be placed in a cold room or in a refrigerated cabinet.
2. Red blood cell contamination greatly affects the isolation outcome. If the sample is still contaminated with erythrocytes before the immunomagnetic separation, perform an additional red blood cell lysis step (as in Sect. 3.2.1, **step 6**).
3. When working with a greater number of cells, scale up all reagent volumes and total volumes accordingly. Use bigger probes.
4. Cells should be kept in single-cell suspension, as the cellular aggregates can block the separation column.
5. Eosinophil purity can be estimated with flow cytometric analysis, using CD16 Mouse Anti-Human mAb FITC antibody. Suspend 1×10^5 isolated cells in 500 μL DPBS/10% FBS (v/v). Add 10 μL CD16 Mouse Anti-Human mAb FITC conjugated antibody to the cells and mix. After a 10 min incubation at 4 °C wash the cell suspension with DPBS. Cells should be then resuspended in 250 μL DPBS/10% FBS (v/v). Analyze the cell population in flow cytometer. Eosinophils are detected as the CD16-negative cells, whereas neutrophils are CD16-positive cells (Fig. 13) [28].

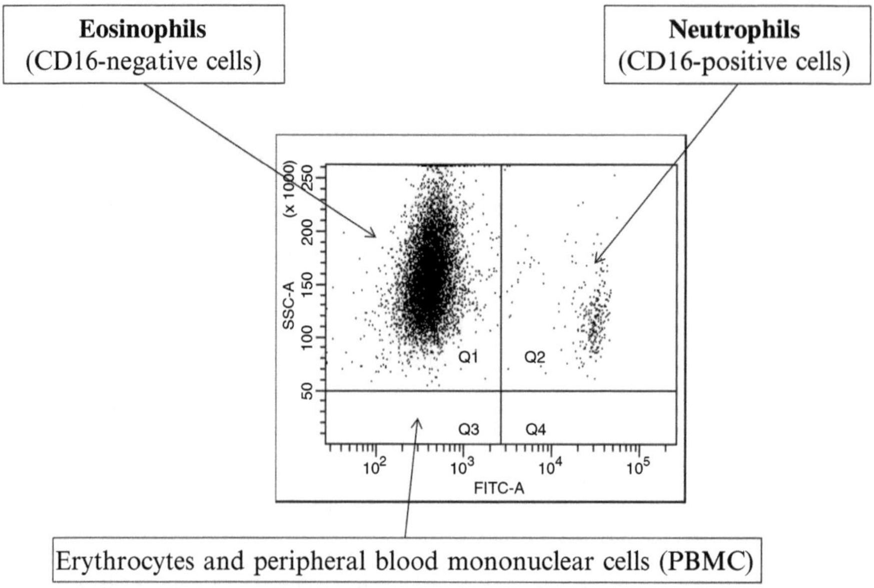

Fig. 13 Flow cytometric analysis of isolated eosinophils from the peripheral blood (erythrocytes and PBMC cells have been depleted completely during isolation steps)

6. After isolation, the viability of isolated cells should be examined. This can be performed using trypan-blue staining or flow cytometric apoptosis analyses.
7. Experimental setup should contain the wells with and without 10 U/mL SOD as the control.
8. Control samples without fMLP should be included.
9. To calculate the amount of superoxide radicals, subtract the average absorbance at 540 and 560 nm from absorbance at 550 nm (calculated in Sect. 4.2, **step** 7).

   The amount of $O_2^{\bullet -}$ is calculated from the formula:

   $O_2^{\bullet -}$ [mmol / l^{-1}] = (ΔOD without SOD – ΔOD with SOD) / 21.1 mmol/L^{-1} cm^{-1}

   where ΔOD with and without SOD represent the difference in absorbance at 550 nm and the average of absorbance at 540 and 560 nm.
10. Amplex Red reagent is unstable in the presence of thiols.
11. Resorufin fluorescence is pH-dependent. The reaction should be performed at pH 7–8.
12. The detection limit for peroxidase detection using Amplex Red assay is estimated as 1×10^{-5} U/mL of HRP. If the detection limit is reached during the assay use higher numbers of cells.
13. The Amplex Red reagent is air and light sensitive. Once the Amplex Red reagent is prepared it should be used on the same day. Light can itself promote the conversion of Amplex Red reagent to resorufin, contributing to incorrect results, consequently samples should be always kept in the dark.
14. Extremely high levels of peroxidase in the samples (e.g., 100 mU/mL) can produce lower fluorescence signal than samples with a lower peroxidase content. This can happen through the oxidation of resorufin to resazurin, which does not fluoresce. Therefore in the preliminary studies it is important to determine the optimal dilution of the samples added to reaction. Sample dilution should be done in 1× reaction buffer.
15. The final working concentrations of AM ester dyes are between 1 and 10 μM. Dye concentration should be kept low to reduce overloading effects.
16. AM esters exhibit low-toxicity, the dye manufacturer advises to use a dispersing agent such as Pluronic F127 to facilitate cell loading.
17. Histamine has been reported to activate actin polymerization in a dose-dependent manner from 0.01 to 10 μM [9].
18. The reaction is very fast, the best results can be obtained 5 s after eosinophil stimulation. Fluorescence signal will decrease with longer incubation times.

19. To further identify eosinophils from PMNL, cells can be stained with FITC-conjugated anti-CCR3 or anti-CD16 antibodies (*see* **Note 5**: eosinophils purity estimation).
20. Antagonists of H_1, H_2, and H_3 histamine receptors have no effect on cellular shape change, whereas histamine H_4 antagonist JNJ7777120 abolishes histamine-dependent cellular shape change.
21. Maximal eosinophil shape change is observed when cells are treated with 0.3 μM histamine. High histamine concentrations, e.g., 100 μM do not increase shape change measurements. The minimal histamine concentration that causes a change in eosinophils shape has been estimated as 0.01 μM [9, 12].
22. Cellular shape change induced by histamine is rapid and transient. It is detected by flow cytometry 1 min after stimulation. Maximal response is observed 5 min after treatment.
23. After histamine stimulation eosinophils gradually return to their original shape. No cellular shape change is detected 40 min from histamine addition. After longer periods of time eosinophils become insensitive to histamine.
24. When merging the transwell upper compartment with the bottom one it is essential that no air bubbles are trapped between the insert membrane and the medium.
25. The filter membrane should be removed in one steady motion. This will prevent cellular debris from passing through filter pores.
26. Cell can also be counted from the downside of transwell filter using microscopic imaging. For this the upper side of the filter membrane needs to be gently cleared from nonmigrated cells. The removal of cellular debris should be performed gently, using cotton towels. Swiping should be in one direction only. Cells on the lower side of the insert can be fixed with 5% glutaraldehyde for 10 min.
27. Data can be expressed as migration index (the number of cells that migrated in response to agonist relative to the number of cells that migrated randomly), as percentage of migrated cells (the number of cells that migrated to total number of cells) or total migrated cells.
28. It is very important not to destroy the endothelial cells monolayer, or to detach the adherent cells. Therefore, extreme care should be ensured when adding compounds, cells or performing washing steps.
29. After the addition of eosinophils, the plate should be mixed to achieve good cellular dispersion in the well.
30. Adhesion assays should not be carried out for longer than 1 h as the adherent cells will detach.

31. Number of adherent eosinophils can be analyzed with specialized computer software, such as Columbus 2.4.2 image data storage and analysis system software (PerkinElmer).
32. Data can be presented as the direct adherent cells count or as percentage of adherent cells (the number of cells that adhere in one sample experiment to the total number of cells observed in the experiment).

Acknowledgments

This work was supported by the Polish National Science Center grant: "Research on human eosinophils as a potential therapeutic target" DEC/2014/13/N/NZ7/00897 and "Histamine H_3/H_4 receptors as an attractive target for the search of biologically active compounds" DEC/2011/02/A/NZ4/00031.

References

1. Rothenberg ME, Hogan SP (2006) The eosinophil. Annu Rev Immunol 24:147–174
2. Rosenberg HF, Dyer KD, Foster PS (2013) Eosinophils: changing perspectives in health and disease. Nat Rev Immunol 13:9–22
3. Kita H (2011) Eosinophils: multifaceted biological properties and roles in health and disease. Immunol Rev 242:161–177
4. Piliponsky AM, Gleich GJ, Bar I et al (2002) Effects of eosinophils on mast cells: a new pathway for the perpetuation of allergic inflammation. Mol Immunol 38:1369–1372
5. Ben-Zimra M, Bachelet I, Seaf M et al (2013) Eosinophil major basic protein activates human cord blood mast cells primed with fibroblast membranes by integrin-β1. Allergy 68:1259–1268
6. Weller PF (1994) Eosinophils: structure and functions. Curr Opin Immunol 6:85–90
7. Seifert R (2013) Functional selectivity of G-protein-coupled receptors: From recombinant systems to native human cells. Biochem Pharmacol 86:853–861
8. Ezeamuzie CI, Philips E (2000) Histamine H(2) receptors mediate the inhibitory effect of histamine on human eosinophil degranulation. Br J Pharmacol 131:482–488
9. Buckland KF, Williams TJ, Conroy DM (2003) Histamine induces cytoskeletal changes in human eosinophils via the H(4) receptor. Br J Pharmacol 140:1117–1127
10. Pincus SH, DiNapoli AM, Schooley WR (1982) Superoxide production by eosinophils: activation by histamine. J Invest Dermatol 79:53–57
11. Reher TM, Brunskole I, Neumann D et al (2012) Evidence for ligand-specific conformations of the histamine H 2-receptor in human eosinophils and neutrophils. Biochem Pharmacol 84:1174–1185
12. Ling P, Ngo K, Nguyen S et al (2004) Histamine H4 receptor mediates eosinophil chemotaxis with cell shape change and adhesion molecule upregulation. Br J Pharmacol 142:161–171
13. Reher TM, Neumann D, Buschauer A et al (2012) Incomplete activation of human eosinophils via the histamine H_4-receptor: evidence for ligand-specific receptor conformations. Biochem Pharmacol 84:192–203
14. Grosicki M, Kieć-Kononowicz K (2015) Human eosinophils-potential pharmacological model applied in human histamine H_4 receptor research. Curr Med Chem 22:1–13
15. Neubig RR, Spedding M, Kenakin T et al (2003) International union of pharmacology committee on receptor nomenclature and drug classification. XXXVIII. Update on terms and symbols in quantitative pharmacology. Pharmacol Rev 55:597–606
16. Seifert R, Schneider EH, Dove S et al (2011) Paradoxical stimulatory effects of the "standard" histamine H_4-receptor antagonist JNJ7777120: the H4 receptor joins the club of 7 transmembrane domain receptors exhibiting functional selectivity. Mol Pharmacol 79:631–638
17. Nijmeijer S, Vischer HF, Sirci F et al (2013) Detailed analysis of biased histamine H_4 receptor signalling by JNJ 7777120 analogues. Br J Pharmacol 170:78–88

18. Rosethorne EM, Charlton SJ (2011) Agonist-biased signaling at the histamine H_4 receptor: JNJ7777120 recruits β-arrestin without activating G proteins. Mol Pharmacol 79:749–757
19. Dikalov S, Griendling KK, Harrison DG (2007) Measurement of reactive oxygen species in cardiovascular studies. Hypertension 49:717–727
20. Adamko DJ, Wu Y, Gleich GJ et al (2004) The induction of eosinophil peroxidase release: improved methods of measurement and stimulation. J Immunol Methods 291:101–108
21. Zhou M, Diwu Z, Panchuk-Voloshina N et al (1997) A stable nonfluorescent derivative of resorufin for the fluorometric determination of trace hydrogen peroxide: applications in detecting the activity of phagocyte NADPH oxidase and other oxidases. Anal Biochem 253:162–168
22. Charlton SJ, Vauquelin G (2010) Elusive equilibrium: the challenge of interpreting receptor pharmacology using calcium assays. Br J Pharmacol 161:1250–1265
23. Cooper JA (1987) Effects of cytochalasin and phalloidin on actin. J Cell Biol 105:1473–1478
24. Kernen P, Wymann MP, von Tscharner V et al (1991) Shape changes, exocytosis, and cytosolic free calcium changes in stimulated human eosinophils. J Clin Invest 87:2012–2017
25. Blow N (2007) Cell migration: our protruding knowledge. Nat Methods 4:589–594
26. Clark RA, Gallin JI, Kaplan AP (1975) The selective eosinophil chemotactic activity of histamine. J Exp Med 142:1462–1476
27. Ley K, Laudanna C, Cybulsky MI et al (2007) Getting to the site of inflammation: the leukocyte adhesion cascade updated. Nat Rev Immunol 7:678–689
28. Thurau AM, Schylz U, Wolf V et al (1996) Identification of eosinophils by flow cytometry. Cytometry 23:150–158
29. Parsons ME, Ganellin CR (2009) Histamine and its receptors. Br J Pharmacol 147: 127–135
30. Seifert R, Wenzel-Seifert K, Burckstummer T et al (2003) Multiple differences in agonist and antagonist pharmacology between human and guinea pig histamine H_1-receptor. J Pharmacol Exp Ther 305:1104–1115
31. Kraus A, Ghorai P, Birnkammer T et al (2009) N(G)-acylated aminothiazolylpropylguanidines as potent and selective histamine H(2) receptor agonists. ChemMedChem 4:232–240
32. Kitbunnadaj R, Hashimoto T, Poli E et al (2005) N-substituted piperidinyl alkyl imidazoles: discovery of methimepip as a potent and selective histamine H_3 receptor agonist. J Med Chem 48:2100–2107
33. Lim HD, Smits RA, Bakker RA et al (2006) Discovery of S-(2-guanidylethyl)-isothiourea (VUF 8430) as a potent nonimidazole histamine H_4 receptor agonist. J Med Chem 49: 6650–6651
34. Pertz HH, Elz S, Schunack W (2004) Structure-activity relationships of histamine H_1-receptor agonists. Mini Rev Med Chem. 4:935–940
35. Lim HD, van Rijn RM, Ling P et al (2005) Evaluation of histamine H_1-, H_2-, and H_3-receptor ligands at the human histamine H_4 receptor: identification of 4-methylhistamine as the first potent and selective H_4 receptor agonist. J Pharmacol Exp Ther 314:1310–1321
36. Kitbunnadaj R, Zuiderveld OP, Christophe B et al (2004) Identification of 4-(1H-imidazol-4(5)-ylmethyl)pyridine (immethridine) as a novel, potent, and highly selective histamine H(3) receptor agonist. J Med Chem 47:2414–2417
37. Liu C, Ma X, Jiang X et al (2001) Cloning and pharmacological characterization of a fourth histamine receptor (H(4)) expressed in bone marrow. Mol Pharmacol 59:420–426
38. Janssens F, Leenaerts J, Diels G et al (2005) Norpiperidine imidazoazepines as a new class of potent, selective, and nonsedative H_1 antihistamines. J Med Chem 48:2154–2166
39. Mahdy AM, Webster NR (2011) Histamine and antihistamines. Anaesth Intensive Care Med 12:324–329
40. Jablonowski JA, Grice CA, Chai W et al (2003) The first potent and selective non-imidazole human histamine H_4 receptor antagonists. J Med Chem 46:3957–3960
41. Beukers MW, Klaassen CH, De Grip WJ et al (1997) Heterologous expression of rat epitope-tagged histamine H2 receptors in insect Sf9 cells. Br J Pharmacol 122:867–874
42. Ohsawa Y, Hirasawa N (2014) The role of histamine H_1 and H_4 receptors in atopic dermatitis: from basic research to clinical study. Allergol Int 63:533–542

Chapter 9

Assessment of the Efficacy of Histamine Receptor Antagonists in Murine Models of Atopic Dermatitis

Kristine Roßbach, Hanna Köchling, Tomoki Fukuyama, Jenny Wilzopolski, Manfred Kietzmann, and Wolfgang Bäumer

Abstract

Atopic dermatitis is a common allergic skin disease characterized by eczematous lesions and pruritus. Experimental animal models are essential tools to study the underlying pathogenic mechanisms of atopic dermatitis. This chapter describes a mouse model with spontaneous manifestation of atopic dermatitis-like skin lesions (NC/Nga mice) and a protein-induced mouse model of atopic dermatitis (ovalbumin model) and discusses the role of the histamine receptor (HR) H_1R and H_4R antagonists in these models.

Key words Atopic dermatitis, Histamine 1 receptor, Histamine 4 receptor, Mouse model, NC/Nga mice, Ovalbumin-induced dermatitis

1 Introduction

Atopic dermatitis is a chronic allergic skin disease characterized by eczematous lesions and pruritus. It is one of the most prevalent allergic skin diseases in humans and dogs [1, 2]. Experimental animal models are essential tools to study the underlying pathogenic mechanisms and to predict the efficacy of pharmacological interventions with potential new drug targets. Four basic types of animal models are used in atopic dermatitis research: spontaneous models, induced models, genetically engineered models, and humanized mouse models [3]. This chapter describes a mouse model with spontaneous manifestation of atopic dermatitis-like skin lesions (NC/Nga mice) and a protein-induced mouse model of atopic dermatitis [ovalbumin (OVA) model].

NC/Nga mice are frequently used to test new possible treatment options for atopic dermatitis. It is still not entirely clear how the mice develop atopic-like lesions. Some mutations on chromosome 9 have been described, which are linked to increased immunoglobulin E (IgE) production [4]. In the very first reports it has

Ekaterini Tiligada and Madeleine Ennis (eds.), *Histamine Receptors as Drug Targets*, Methods in Pharmacology and Toxicology, DOI 10.1007/978-1-4939-6843-5_9,

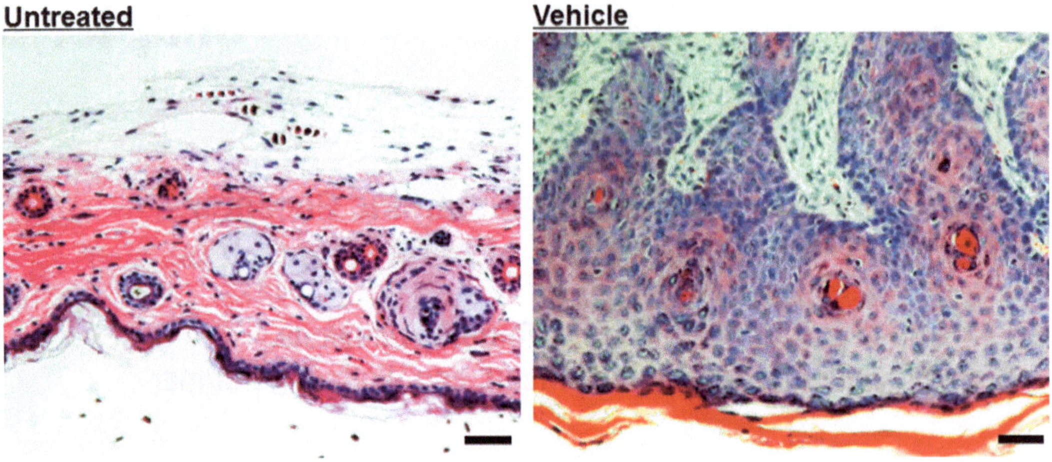

Fig. 1 Histological evaluation of back skin of NC/Nga mice. *Left* is untreated back skin of age-matched NC/Nga mice *right* is back skin of mice 12 weeks after starting challenge with HDM antigen. "Vehicle" means topical treatment with a hydrogel

been stated that it is just enough to bring these mice from a SPF facility into "conventional" environment to induce atopic-like skin lesions. However, this could not be reproduced by other laboratories and we also see no development of lesions in mice that are not challenged with an antigen although the mice are kept under non-SPF conditions. This allowed us to sacrifice some untreated mice, which were age matched with house dust mite antigen challenged mice. These did not show lesions in skin (see histology Fig. 1) or increased levels of total IgE (see Fig. 2). There are different protocols for sensitization of NC/Nga mice, some with haptens like dinitrochlorobenzene or picryl chloride [5, 6] and some with house dust mite antigen [7]. We tend to use the latter, as house dust mite antigen is a relevant allergen in atopic dermatitis patients.

The epicutaneous sensitization with chicken OVA was first described by Spergel and coworkers [8] and Wang and coworkers [9]. This model shows many aspects of human atopic dermatitis, including elevated antigen-specific IgE and atopic dermatitis-like skin lesions [3, 8]. Epicutaneous sensitization is more prone to elicit a Th2 response compared with intraperitoneal sensitized mice [8, 10]. Interestingly, epicutaneously sensitized mice developed asthma-like symptoms after a single exposure to OVA aerosol [8]. However, genetic predisposition or skin barrier dysfunction is not reported for this model [3].

Classical histamine 1 receptor (H_1R) antagonists show insufficient efficacy in the treatment of atopic dermatitis [11] and also in mouse models of allergic dermatitis H_1R antagonists have only limited effects [for detailed review, see [12]]. H_4R antagonists have been tested in several mouse models of allergic dermatitis [6, 13–17]; however, results of these studies are conflicting and partially

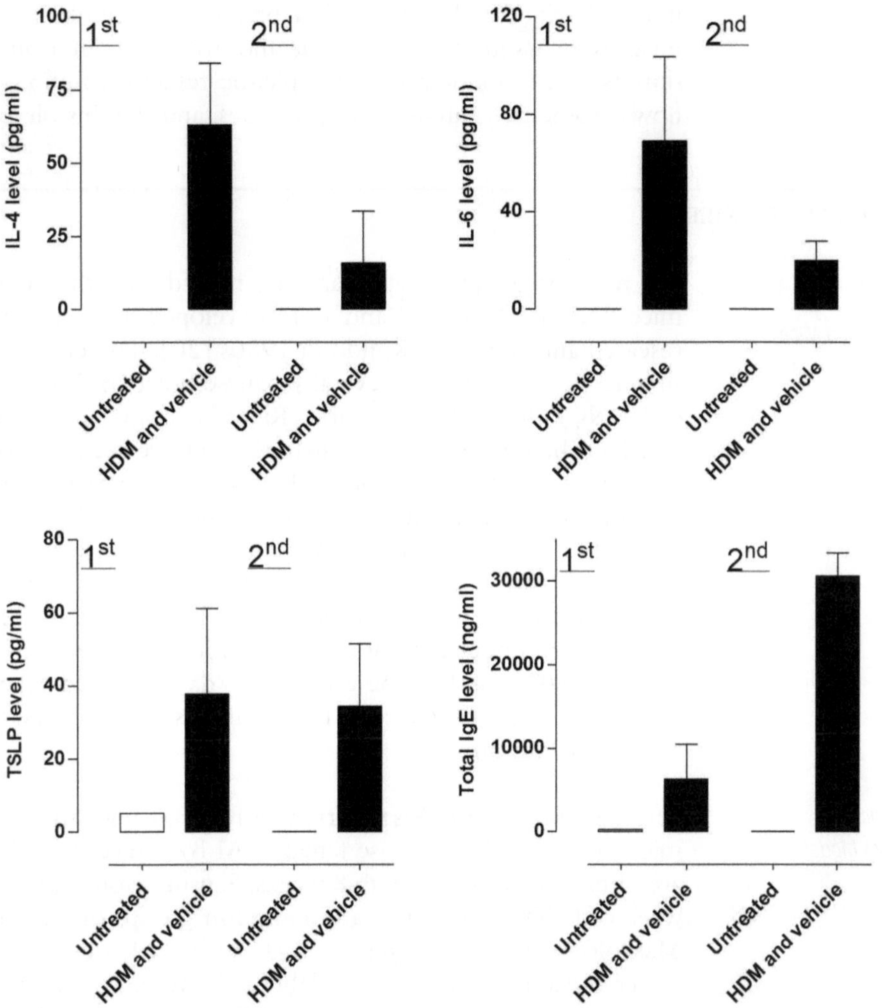

Fig. 2 Cytokines (IL-4, IL-6, and TSLP) and total IgE in serum of NC/Nga mice challenged with house dust mite (HDM) antigen twice weekly. Mice were sacrificed for the first determination after 7 weeks and for the second determination after 11 weeks. Note the steady increase in total IgE over time. $n = 5$ for vehicle, $n = 1$ for untreated control for each time point. Vehicle means topical treatment with a hydrogel

heterogeneous [18]. The most prominent effects were found in chronic allergic contact dermatitis and acute allergic contact dermatitis with predominant Th2 milieu, but in lesions of acute allergic contact dermatitis with predominant Th1 milieu, the H_4R seems to play only a marginal role [6, 13, 14, 16, 19]. Moreover, results of our latest study indicate that it is necessary to block the H_4R during ontogeny and development of the allergic inflammation [19].

In this chapter, we describe the sensitization of NC/Nga mice with house dust mite allergen and the epicutaneous sensitization of BALB/c mice with OVA. Moreover, we describe the observation (scoring of skin lesions, measuring of ear thickness, monitoring of itch behavior) and examination parameters (cytokine and IgE measurements in serum, cytokine and histamine determination in skin tissues, cytokine release by splenocytes and lymph node cells, flow cytometric analysis of lymph nodes, and skin histology).

2 Materials and Animals

2.1 Mice

2.1.1 NC/Nga Mice

NC mice originate in Japan and are named after the favorite pet mice "Nishiki Nezumi" and were developed as an experimental research animal by Dr. Kondo in 1950s [20]. Therefore, it is possible to get NC mice via several Japanese breeders. We are able to order NC/Nga mice via Charles River Japan or Japan SLC, Inc., and NC/Jic mice via CLEA Japan, Inc. However, NC/Nga mice in Charles River, Laboratories (Kanagawa, Japan) would be the only option to be able to order from outside Japan. It is prohibited to use the mice for breeding. We only worked with female mice. The animals are housed in groups of two to four animals in plastic cages that are fixed into stainless-steel racks. Animals are kept in an animal room under the following conditions: temperature :22 °C, humidity:50%, and lighting cycle :12 h/day. Certified pellet diet is supplied to the animals freely from stainless-steel feeders. Water is available ad libitum.

2.1.2 Mice for the OVA Model

Sensitization with OVA is reported for BALB/c mice and C57BL/6 mice [10, 21]. We only use female BALB/c mice. BALB/c mice are obtained at the age of 6–8 weeks. Sensitization starts after one week of habituation. Mice are housed in groups of six animals in Makrolon® Type III cages at 22 °C with a 12 h light/dark cycle. Water and a standard diet is available ad libitum. To our knowledge the OVA protocol is only reported for female mice. We do not know if the sex or age of the mice influences the outcome of the OVA-induced dermatitis model.

2.2 Materials

- Sensitization of NC/Nga mice with house dust mite allergen: House dust mite allergen (*Dermatophagoides farinae*, RMB83M/86142; Greer laboratories), mineral oil light (O 121-1) and phosphate buffered saline (PBS), depilation cream.
- OVA model: OVA (synonym: albumin from chicken egg white) Grade V and Grade VI (Sigma Aldrich), PBS, elastic fixation bandage (Peha-haft® Color Latex Free Cohesive Conforming Bandage, Hartmann), surgical tape (Blenderm™ (3M™; 5.0 cm × 4.6 m), gauze bandage, electric clippers, depilation cream, and scissors.
- Measuring of ear thickness: Cutimeter (Mitutoyo, Neuss, Germany), forceps.
- Monitoring of itch behavior: Clear cages and a video camera.

- Dissection instruments for the preparation of skin specimen, spleens, lymph nodes, and blood collection: Dissection board, scissors, scalpel, forceps, and fine forceps.
- Cytokine and histamine determination in skin tissues: Liquid nitrogen, mortar and pestle, RPMI 1640 medium, Pefabloc, 1.5 reaction tubes, DC protein assay kit (BIO-RAD), ELISAs [like interleukin (IL)-1β, -4, -6, TSLP, and histamine ELISAs].
- Cytokine and IgE measurements in serum: Isoflurane and equipment for inhalational anesthesia, 25-gauge needle, 1 ml syringe, serum sample tube, centrifuge, 1 mL reaction tube, OVA-specific IgE ELISA (BioLegend), BD OptEIA Mouse IgE ELISA (Becton).
- Single-cell suspension of lymph nodes: 70-μm nylon cell strainer or glass potter, RPMI 1640 medium, fetal calf serum (FCS), streptomycin, penicillin, centrifuge, sterile vials, Cellometer, or Neubauer chamber.
- CD4+ isolation from lymph node cells: EasySep™ Mouse CD4+ T Cell Isolation Kit and the EasyEights™ EasySep™ Magnet or CD4+ T Cell Isolation Kit II and the autoMACS Separator.
- Flow cytometric analysis: Polystyrene round-bottom 12 × 75 mm tubes, PBS, FCS, mouse BD Fc Block, centrifuge, monoclonal antibodies like anti-mouse CD3 (rat IgG2bk, FITC-conjugated, clone 17A2), CD11c (hamster IgG, APC-conjugated, N418), CD19 (rat IgG2ak, PE-conjugated, clone 6D5) and CD40 (rat IgG2ak, PE-conjugated, clone NLDC-145), flow cytometer.
- Single-cell suspensions of spleens: 70-μm nylon cell strainer, hemolysis buffer: 8.3 g NH_4CL, 0.04 g Na_2EDTA, 0.84 g $NaHCO_3$ and 1000 mL aqua bidestillata (pH 7.3), plunger end of a 5 mL syringe or small pestle, RPMI 1640 medium, FCS, streptomycin, penicillin, centrifuge, sterile vials, cellometer or Neubauer chamber.
- Cytokine determination in cell culture supernatants: 48-well plates (for lymph node cells), 12-well plates (for splenocytes) concanavalin A (Con A), OVA Grade VI, cytokine ELISA kits.
- Skin histology: Bouin's fluid fixation: 75 mL saturated aqueous solution of picric acid, 25 mL formalin (40% aqueous solution of formaldehyde), 5 mL glacial acetic acid (add shortly before use); glass vials, ethanol (100%, 96%, 90%, 80%, 70%), xylol, paraffin wax, wax blocks, foam pads, histology cassettes, microtome, floating bath, drying oven, acid alcohol: 100 mL ethanol 70% + 1 mL HCL, hemalum, eosin, Giemsa stain, glass slides, mounting medium.

3 Methods

3.1 Sensitization of NC/Nga Mice with House Dust Mite Allergen

We ordered the mice at an age of 4 weeks; they arrived aged 5 weeks and had to be in quarantine for another 2 weeks. Mice were 7 weeks of age, when sensitization began. House dust mite allergen is applied topically twice a week for up to 11 weeks. During the experimental period, body weight, scratching behavior, ear thickness, and clinical scores are monitored every week on Tuesdays and/or Fridays. Mice are sacrificed 7 and 11 weeks after the initiation of the procedure. The rostral neck skin, ear auricle, auricular lymph nodes, and serum are removed from each mouse and stored until used for histology, cytokine determination, IgE determination, and FACS analysis.

Protocol

1. Depilate rostral neck of the NC/Nga mice with electric clippers.
2. Dilute house dust mite allergen in mineral oil (500 μg/20 μL).
3. Strip skin at the rostral neck with adhesive tape (ten times with five different tapes).
4. Apply house dust mite suspension topically onto the stripped skin (20 μL onto 1 × 2 cm area) and on ear auricle (10 μL) twice a week (for example Tuesdays and Thursdays every week).

3.2 Sensitization and Challenge of BALB/c Mice with OVA

Mice have a total of three 1-week exposures to OVA V separated from each other by 2-week intervals. Two weeks after the last treatment with OVA V (sensitization), mice receive identical patches with OVA VI (*see* **Note 1**) for 1 week (1. challenge week; Fig. 3). We have performed up to three challenges (separated from each other by 2-week intervals). During the experimental period, scratching behavior and clinical scores are monitored on day 7 of each challenge week. After the last challenge mice are sacrificed and abdominal skin, draining lymph nodes of the skin, the spleen, and serum are removed from each mouse and stored until used for histology, cytokine determination, OVA-specific IgE determination, and FACS analysis.

Protocol (*see* **Note 1**)

1. Treat abdominal skin of the mice with depilatory cream.
2. Prepare OVA solution at a concentration of 1 mg/mL PBS.
3. Prepare patches of gauze consisting of three layers of gauze placed on surgical tape and then cut gauze/tape combination into 1.5 × 1.5 cm pieces (one for each mouse).
4. Cut elastic fixation bandage to a length of 10–12 cm and a width of 2 cm (one for each individual).

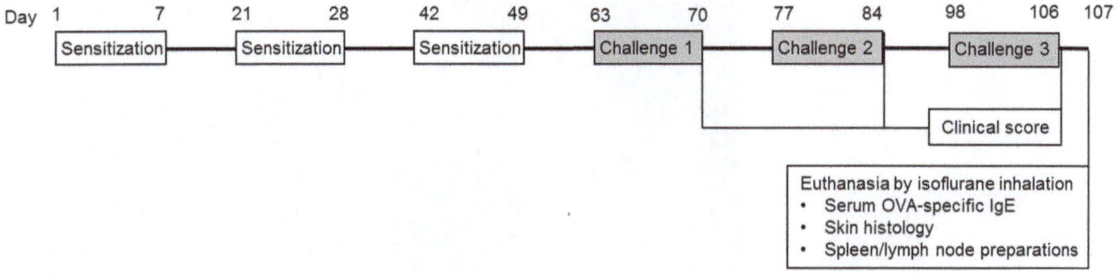

Fig. 3 Sensitization and challenge with OVA. Mice have a total of three 1-week exposures to OVA V separated from each other by 2-week intervals (sensitization). Two weeks after the last treatment with OVA V, mice receive identical patches with OVA VI for 1 week (challenge week)

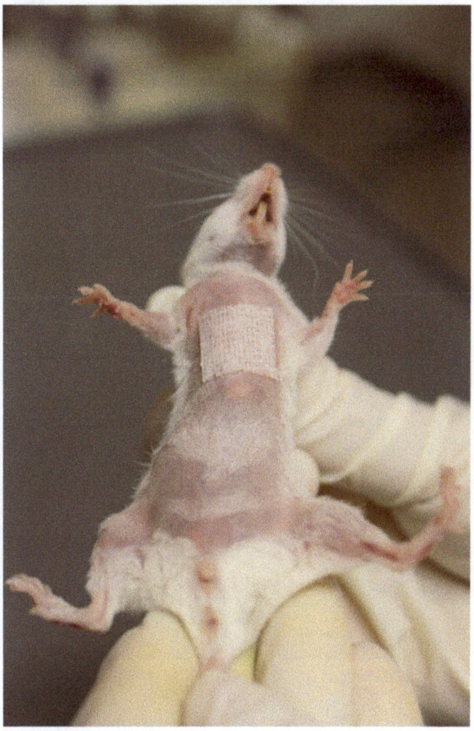

Fig. 4 A patch of gauze soaked with OVA solution (100 μg OVA/100 μL PBS) is placed onto the abdominal skin

5. Four hours after depilation, place a patch of gauze soaked with 100 μL OVA solution (100 μg OVA/100 μL PBS) onto the abdominal skin (between the forelegs, Fig. 4).
6. Tie mice with elastic fixation bandage to fix the gauze patch onto the skin (Fig. 5).
7. Fix the end of the elastic fixation bandage with a piece of surgical tape (Fig. 6a).

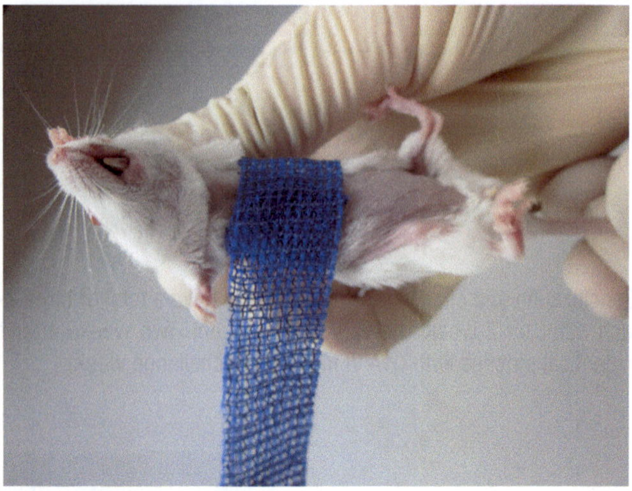

Fig. 5 Peha-haft® bandage is tied around the abdomen of the mouse to fix the gauze patch onto the skin

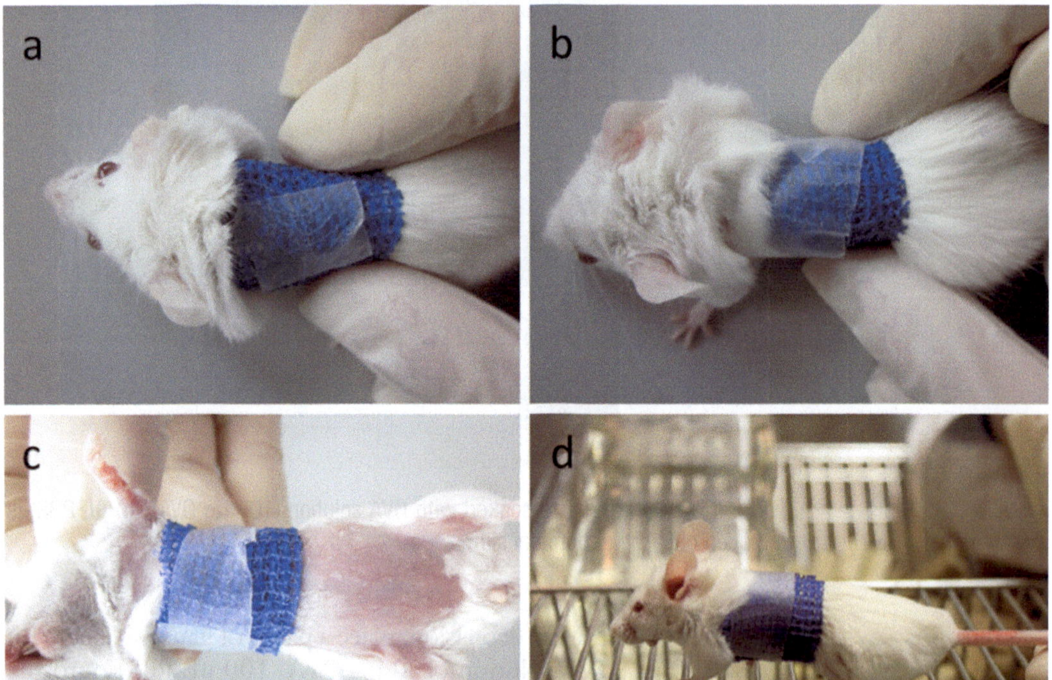

Fig. 6 The fur in the neck (**a**) has to be covered with a piece of Blenderm™ (**b**, **d**). The ends of the Blenderm™ have to be fixed at the site of the abdomen with another piece of Blenderm™ (**c**)

8. Cover the fur in the neck with surgical tape (1.5 × 5 cm; Fig. 6b). Fix the ends of the surgical tape on the abdominal site with another piece of surgical tape (Fig. 6c).
9. Renew patches and bandages after 4 days.
10. Remove OVA patch at day 7 of each sensitization or challenge week respectively.

3.3 Administration of Histamine Receptor Antagonists

In the OVA model, H_4R knockout mice developed less severe skin lesions, a reduced epidermal hyperproliferation and a diminished inflammatory cell influx at lesional skin sites, a significant lower OVA-specific IgE level cell influx, and a reduced number of splenocytes and lymph node cells (with less CD4+ T cells) compared to wild-type mice [19]. The H_4R antagonist JNJ-28307474 (20 mg/kg) given twice daily during the challenge phase did not show an anti-inflammatory effect in the OVA model. However, the anti-inflammatory effect could partially be mimicked when JNJ-28307474 (20 mg/kg) was given twice daily during sensitization and challenge phase. Mice treated during sensitization and challenge with JNJ-28307474 had a significantly reduced number of splenocytes, about 30% less lymph node cells and reduced the inflammatory cell influx at lesional skin sites compared to vehicle-treated mice [19]. In NC/Nga mice, the H_4R antagonists JNJ-7777120 (10 mg and 30 mg/kg) and JNJ-28307474 (10 mg and 30 mg/kg) did not show significant amelioration of dermatitis, nor inhibited scratching behavior induced by house dust mite allergen ointment [17]. However, the H_4R antagonists were only given three times per week. The half-life in mice of JNJ-28307474 (20 mg/kg) is 4.3 h and for JNJ-7777120 (after oral treatment) about 1 h; thus, a dosing only three times per week is most likely insufficient [22, 23]. The pharmacokinetic and pharmacodynamic properties of a substance have to be considered before testing it in an animal model. Moreover, in case of animal models of allergic dermatitis, the concentration of a drug in the skin is most likely important for the clinical efficacy and additional topical treatment might be beneficial [24]. In addition, according to Neumann and coworkers [25], the use of histamine receptor subtype selective ligands has to be interpreted with caution with regard to specificity, efficacy, and potency.

3.4 Scoring of Skin Lesions

NC/Nga mice are scored once a week. Figures 7 and 8a show typical results in vehicle-treated and house dust mite challenged NC/Nga mouse skin lesions. Visible lesions are expected to occur after 4–6 weeks.

OVA mice are scored 6–8 h after the removal of the OVA patches at day 7 of each challenge week. Mice develop first signs of dermatitis after the first challenge. Skin lesions are more severe after two or three challenges than after just one challenge (Fig. 9).

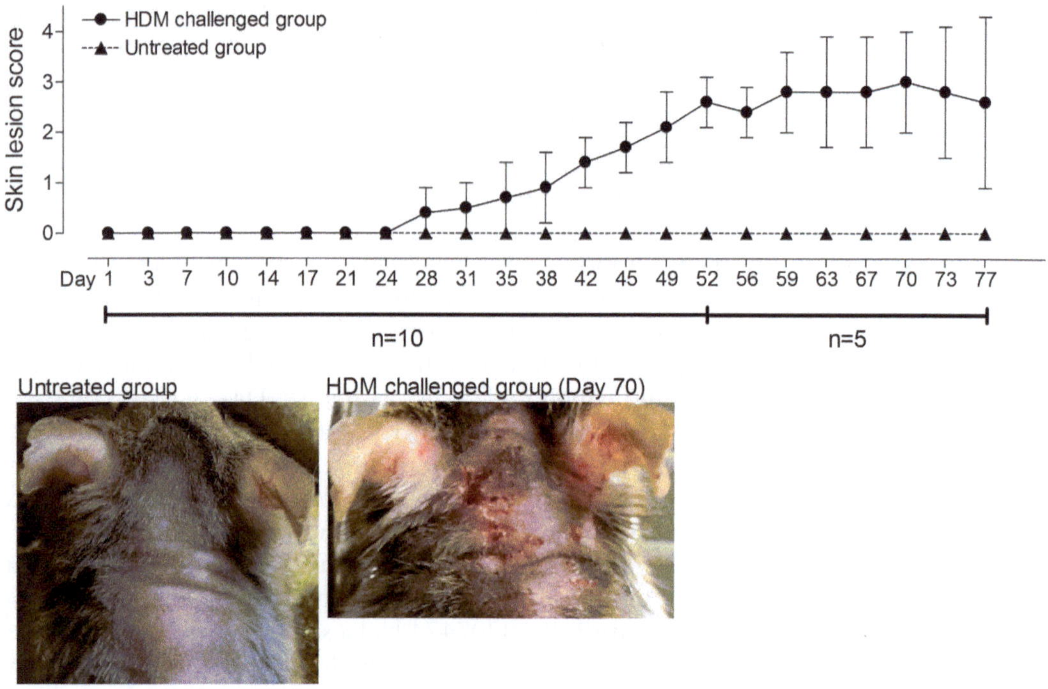

Fig. 7 Typical time course and pictures of development of lesions over time after twice weekly administration of house dust mite (HDM) antigen. This study was started with n = 10 and 5 mice/group were sacrificed after 52 days. A pharmacological intervention can start, when lesions already progress (e.g., day 45) as a "therapeutic" setting or it can be started directly at the beginning of a sensitization in a "preventive" manner

Typical lesions seen in the OVA model and examples of the scoring system are shown in Fig. 8b.

Protocol

1. Skin score should be assessed by one or two blinded investigators.
2. A standardized skin score is used in both mouse models of atopic dermatitis.
   (a) No symptoms.
   (b) Mild symptoms.
   (c) Moderate symptoms.
   (d) Severe symptoms.
   (e) Extreme symptoms.
3. OVA model: Clinical measures analyzed are
   (a) scaling (0–4).
   (b) erythema (0–4).
   (c) erosion/excoriation (0–4).

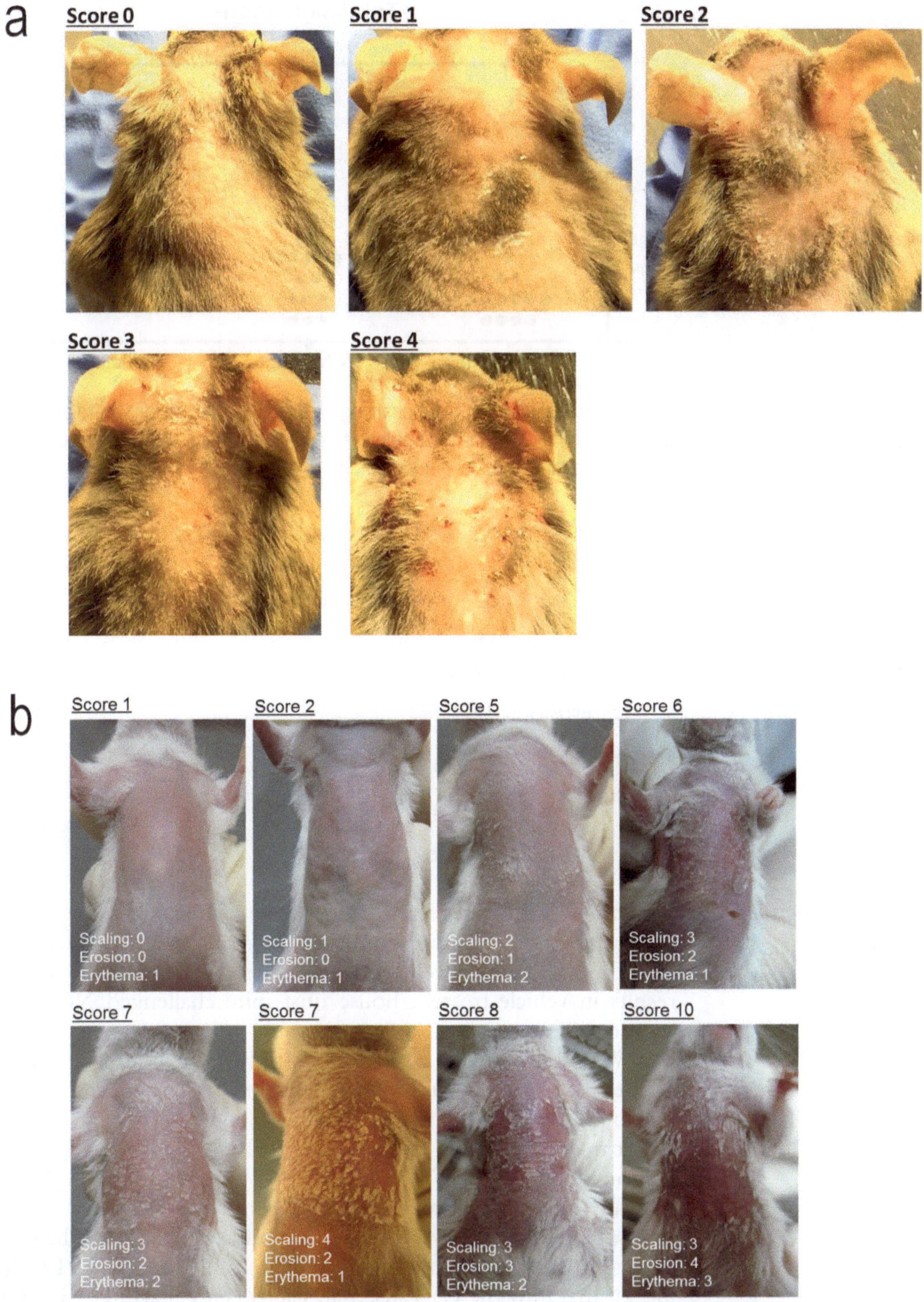

Fig. 8 (**a**) House dust mite challenged Nc/Nga mice. (**b**) OVA-challenged BALB/c mice. Pictures give examples of our scoring system. Please note that erythema cannot be assessed from a picture. Mice with a total skin score (score) from 1, 2, and 5 were challenged once with OVA Grade VI, the other mice had a total of three challenges with OVA Grade VI

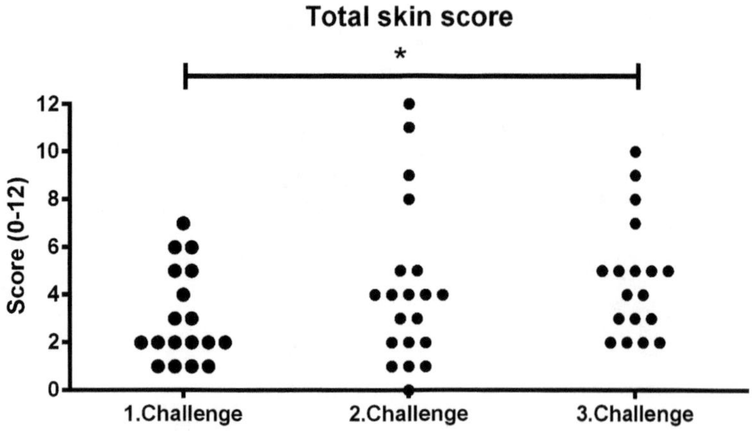

Fig. 9 Total skin score in mice challenged with OVA. Skin lesions were scored 6 h after the removal of the OVA patch at day 7 end of each challenge week. Data pooled from three independent settings

Total skin score (0–12) is calculated as sum of scores of scaling, erythema, and excoriation.

4. NC/Nga mice: Clinical measures analyzed are
   (a) skin dryness (0–4).
   (b) erythema (0–4).
   (c) erosion (0–4).
   (d) edema (0–4).

Skin lesion score is calculated as average of skin dryness, erosions, edema, and erythema. This means a score of 4 is the most severe outcome possible.

3.5 Measuring of Ear Thickness

Ear thickness is measured with a cutimeter. This measurement can be an easy and reliable readout for inflammation and edema, but only if performed by well-trained persons. See Fig. 10 for typical results in vehicle-treated, house dust mite challenged NC/Nga mouse ears.

We investigated in a small pilot study, if application of OVA Grade VI onto the ear to OVA-sensitized mice induces an ear swelling. Application of OVA Grade VI onto the ear and subsequent treatment with a microneedle roller did not induce inflammation of the ear. OVA solution (100 μg/20 μL) was applied topically onto the ear and afterward a microneedle roller with a needle length of 200 μm was rolled in four axes radial over the skin surface. In contrast, intradermal injection of OVA Grade VI (100 μg/20 μL) into the ear caused an ear swelling starting 3 h after injection with a maximum after 48 h. About 72 h after injection, ear swelling started to decrease.

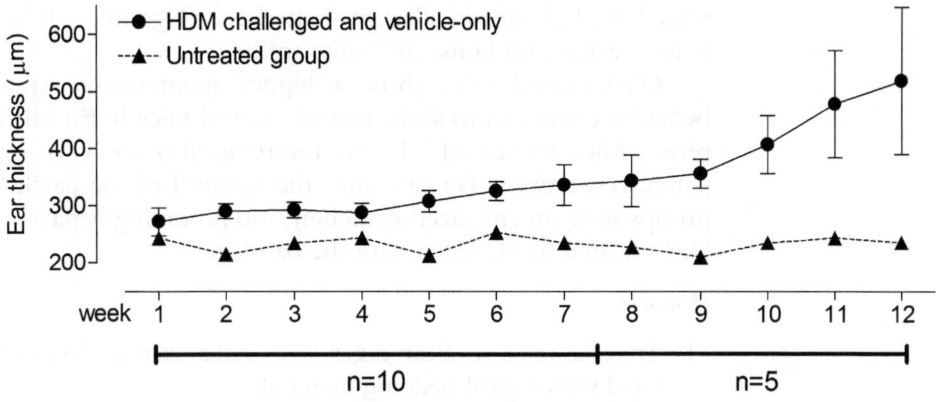

Fig. 10 Time course of ear thickness in mice treated topically with house dust mite (HDM) antigen twice weekly. Please note the increase of ear swelling occurs later than the development of lesions. The increase is variable among the mice, thus to see an inhibitory effect in ear thickness, the inhibitory potential of the drug must be pronounced. We only used ear thickness as a secondary parameter and had a major focus on development of lesions in the rostral neck

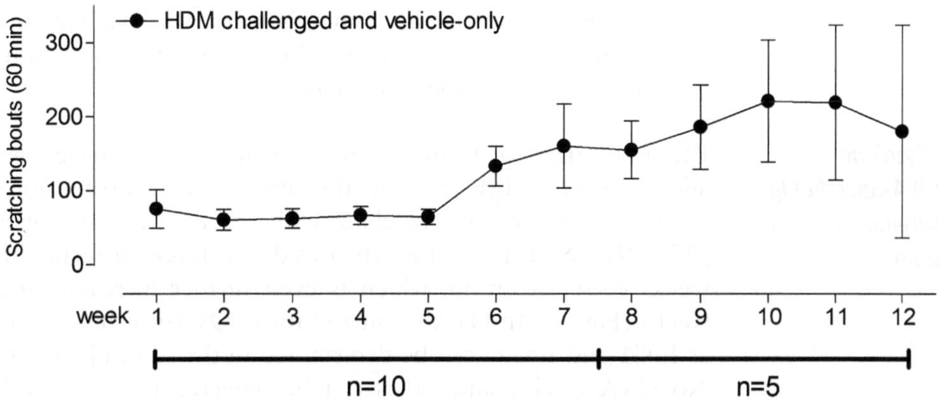

Fig. 11 Time course of scratching behavior in NC/Nga mice challenged with house dust mite (HDM) antigen twice weekly. Please note the quite high frequent scratching behavior from the very beginning. For comparison, e.g. BALB/c mice, which are not challenged, show spontaneous scratching behavior between 10 and 20 bouts/h. This study was started with $n = 10$ and 5 mice/group that were sacrificed after 7 weeks

Protocol (*see* **Note 2**)

1. An assistant has to place the mouse onto the grid cage top and grab a skin fold at the rear of the neck (close to the ears) with thumb and forefinger (grip the skin properly to prevent the animal from turning its head).
2. Hold the ear with anatomic forceps.
3. Measure ear thickness with a cutimeter.

3.6 Monitoring of Itch Behavior

As an indicator of pruritus, the scratching behavior of mice can be determined. Scratching behavior of NC/Nga mice is monitored once a week for 1 h. Figure 11 displays a typical time course of scratching behavior in allergen-treated NC/Nga mice challenged twice weekly with house dust mite antigen.

OVA-treated mice show a higher spontaneous scratching behavior compared to sham-treated control mice in the challenge phase. Mice are scored 7 h after the removal of the OVA or PBS patch, respectively. Directly after the removal of the patch, both groups show an enhanced scratching and grooming behavior most likely related to the removal of the bandage.

Protocol

1. Transfer mice to clear cages (two mice/cage). Cages can be filled with typical bedding material.
2. Record mice on video for 1 h.
3. Leave the observation room to avoid distraction.
4. Video analysis: Count scratching bouts with the hind paws directed against the house dust mite antigen-treated ear and neck region (Nc/Nga mice) or against the abdomen and lateral body site (OVA model). A bout is over, when the hind paw reaches the floor again. Analysis is performed in a blinded manner, the person, who analyzes the itch behavior, should not be aware of the treatment the mice received.

3.7 Cytokine and (OVA-Specific) IgE Measurements in Serum

Patients suffering from atopic dermatitis often have elevated allergen-specific IgE levels in the serum [26]. Furthermore, the severity of the disease correlates with the IgE level in the serum [27]. NC/Nga mice show enhanced IgE levels in serum after 7 weeks of sensitization, which is even further increased after 11 weeks (Fig. 2). In OVA-sensitized mice, OVA-specific IgE as well as IgG1 and IgG2a can be determined in the serum [10, 19, 28]. No OVA-specific antibodies can be detected in sham-sensitized control mice.

Protocol

1. Anesthetize mouse by isoflurane inhalation.
2. Test for reaction by toe pinch.
3. Place animal on back (dorsal recumbency) and open the thorax.
4. Collect blood (0.5–0.75 mL) by cardiac puncture with a 25-gauge needle with 1 mL syringe from the ventricle slowly to avoid collapsing of heart.
5. Transfer blood samples from the syringe quickly into a serum sample tube.
6. Remove the heart to ensure that animal is deceased.
7. Centrifuge blood samples within 2 h of collection at 10,000 × *g* for 5 min at room temperature.

8. After centrifugation, remove the serum and place it into reaction tubes.
9. Store serum at −20 or −40 °C until analysis.
10. Perform ELISAs (IgE, OVA-specific IgE) according to manufacturer's instructions.

Blood can also be collected from the inferior vena cava directly after euthanasia of the mice.

1. Euthanize mice.
2. Open the abdomen with a "Y"- or "V"-shaped cut.
3. Remove intestines.
4. Push the liver forward.
5. The posterior vena cava can be identified between the kidneys.
6. Insert a 25-gauge needle into the vein to collect the blood.

This procedure has to be repeated up to four times to collect more blood volume.

3.8 Histological Analysis of the Skin

Acute skin lesions of atopic dermatitis patients are characterized by marked epidermal intercellular edema (spongiosis), hyper- and focal parakeratosis, and a marked accumulation of CD4+ T cells in the dermis. Chronic lesions show a strong epidermal hyperplasia with hyperkeratosis, parakeratosis, and acanthosis. The chronic lesions contain lymphocytes predominantly CD4+ T cells, mast cells, macrophages, and eosinophils in the dermis and IgE-bearing Langerhans cells and inflammatory dendritic epidermal cells in the epidermis [3, 29].

Skin lesions of Nc/Nga mice show hyperparakeratosis, hyperplasia, and spongiosis and an infiltration of dermal mast cells, eosinophils and lymphocytes (CD4+ T cells) and macrophages [30]. In the OVA-induced mouse model of atopic dermatitis, a significant dermal and epidermal thickening and an infiltrate of inflammatory cells (consisting of T cells, eosinophils, and mast cells) can be found [10, 28].

3.8.1 Sample Preparation (Paraffin Processing of Tissue)

Protocol

1. Separate lesional skin sites (NC/Nga mice: rostral neck; OVA model: abdomen).
2. Slice skin into a piece of about 1 × 1.5 cm.
3. Place skin in glass vials filled with Bouin's fluid fixation for 48 h (minimum 6 h) (*see* **Note 3**).
4. Transfer tissue between two foam pads and place the specimen into a histology cassette.

5. For dehydration, pass specimen through a series of graded ethanol baths.
   (a) 70% ethanol 24 h (or longer).
   (b) 80% ethanol 24 h (or longer).
   (c) 96% ethanol 2 h.
6. Incubate specimen for 2 h in xylol.
7. Incubate specimen for 2 h in fresh xylol.
8. Infiltrate specimen overnight with paraffin wax.
9. Embed the infiltrated tissues into wax blocks.
10. Cut paraffin sections with a microtome at a thickness of 7 μm.
11. Float sections on the surface of warm water (50 °C) in a flotation bath to flatten them and then pick up the slices onto microscope slides.
12. Dry slides overnight at 60 °C in a drying oven.
13. Proceed to staining.

3.8.2 Hematoxylin and Eosin Stain (HE Stain)

The HE stain is used for staining of inflammatory cells and determination of epidermal thickness. Cell nuclei are stained blue while cytoplasm, smooth muscle, collagen, and other components are stained in shades of pink.

Protocol

Place slide in a staining dish and submerge them with:

1. Xylol 2 min.
2. Xylol 2 min.
3. Ethanol 100% 2 min.
4. Ethanol 96% 2 min.
5. Ethanol 90% 2 min.
6. Ethanol 80% 2 min.
7. Ethanol 70% 2 min.
8. *Aqua destillata* 5 min.
9. Hemalum 8 min.
10. Acid alcohol 2 sec.
11. Rinse in running tap water for 5 min.
12. Eosin (0.5%, prepare fresh) 2 min.
13. Tap water 30 s.
14. Ethanol 70% 20 s.
15. Ethanol 80% 20 s.
16. Ethanol 90% 20 s.

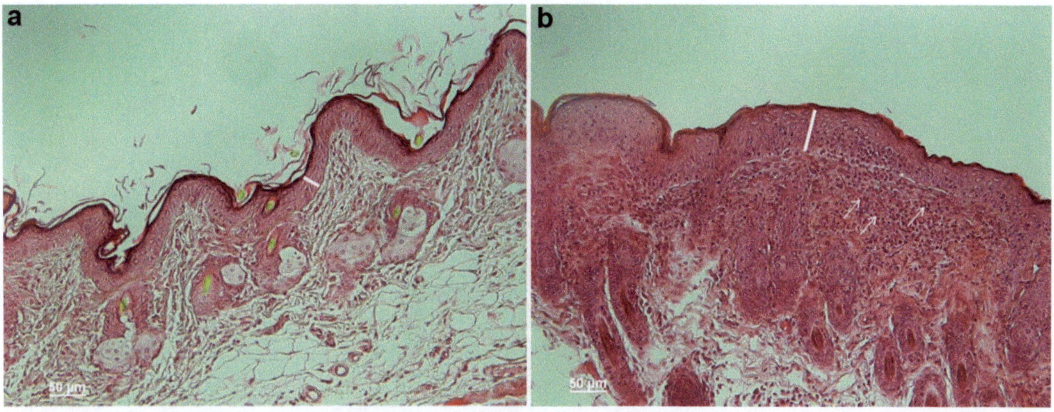

Fig. 12 Histological evaluation (HE stain) of abdominal skin of BALB/c mice treated with PBS (**a**) or OVA (**b**) after the two challenges. The *white line* marks the epidermis. *Arrows* indicate inflammatory cells in the dermis exemplary

17. Ethanol 100% 20 s.
18. Xylol 20 s.
19. Xylol 20 s.
20. Blot excess xylol from the slide without letting tissue dry.
21. Mount slides with mounting medium for microscopy.

Determination of Inflammatory Cell Influx and Edema

Sections are analyzed under light microscopy by a blinded observer. Total inflammatory cell influx is determined by a semi-quantitative examination (0, no influx, no edema; 1, mild; 2, moderate; and 3, severe influx, severe edema). Figure 12 shows abdominal skin of a mouse treated with PBS or OVA respectively. Compared to the OVA-treated mouse no inflammatory cell influx or epidermal hyperproliferation is visible in the PBS-treated mouse, whereas the OVA-treated mouse shows a high cell influx and the epidermal thickness is increased (Fig. 12).

Determination of Epidermal Thickness

Epidermal thickness is analyzed under light microscopy by a blinded observer. Epidermal thickness is determined in ten randomly selected areas using a digital image processing software (for example Axiovision 4.8 software). The distance from the basal membrane to the stratum corneum is measured (Fig. 12). The *stratum corneum* itself cannot be measured, since it often partially or completely detaches during sectioning. Figure 1 shows a histological section of back skin of NC/Nga mice. Note the strong epidermal hyperproliferation that is manifested as lichenification, a typical symptom seen in chronic AD lesions.

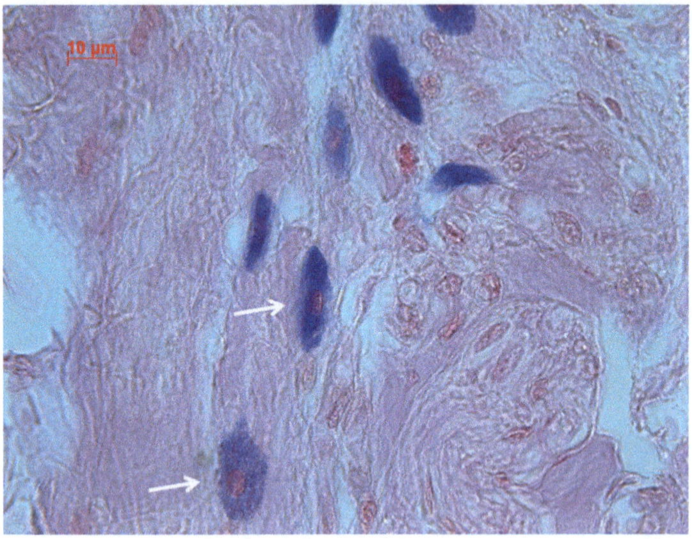

Fig. 13 Giemsa stain of the abdominal skin of a mouse treated with OVA (second challenge). *Arrows* indicate mast cells

3.8.3 Giemsa Stain

The Giemsa stain is used for staining of mast cells. Mast cell granules (Fig. 13) and basophils are stained purple, eosinophils are stained bright pink and lymphocytes blue.

Protocol

Place slide in a staining dish and submerge them with:

1. Xylol 2 min.
2. Xylol 2 min.
3. Ethanol 100% 2 min.
4. Ethanol 96% 2 min.
5. Ethanol 90% 2 min.
6. Ethanol 80% 2 min.
7. Ethanol 70% 2 min.
8. *Aqua destillata* 5 min.
9. Giemsa stain (prepare fresh, filtrated) 5 min.
10. Acetic acid 0.1% 20 s.
11. Acetic acid 0.1% (slew staining dish until no stain will come of the slides anymore).
12. *Aqua destillata* 10 s.
13. Isopropanol 20 s.
14. Isopropanol 20 s.

15. Isopropanol (slew staining dish until no stain will come of the slides anymore).
16. Xylol 5 min.
17. Xylol 5 min.
18. Blot excess xylol from the slide without letting tissue dry.
19. Mount slides with mounting medium for microscopy.

Determination of Mast Cell Number

Sections are analyzed under light microscopy by a blinded observer. Mast cells are counted in ten parts of high-power fields (HPF) at 400 × magnification. Figure 13 shows mast cells in the skin of an OVA-treated mouse.

3.9 Cytokine and Histamine Determination in Skin Tissue

The skin has to be homogenized at first and the total protein concentration of each skin specimen has to be determined to normalize the protein content between multiple samples. Cytokines and histamine concentrations are measured by ELISA. Cytokine determination for ear tissue is performed according to [31]. Cytokine profiles (IL-1β, IL-4, IL-6, and TSLP) in skin tissues (rostal neck and ear) of NC/Nga mice are shown in Fig. 14. Level of histamine in skin tissues of NC/Nga mice 7 weeks after initiation of house dust mite antigen challenge is shown in Fig. 15. In OVA-sensitized mice, elevated levels of IL-4, IL-5, and IFN-γ mRNA can be found [28].

Protocol

1. Take one part of the ear tissue and the rostral neck skin (NC/Nga mice) or abdominal skin (OVA mice) tissue and shock-freeze it in liquid nitrogen.
2. Store at −80 °C until use.
3. Cool down mortar and pestle to −80 °C.
4. Homogenize ear tissue under liquid nitrogen using mortar and pestle.
5. Place skin tissue on the bottom of the cooled mortal and add ~2 mL of liquid nitrogen to the mortar.
6. Crush samples by the pestle.
7. Scratch the crushed samples together by means of a pipette tip.
8. Repeat the procedure.
9. Scratch the homogenates again together to the bottom of the mortar.
10. Transfer homogenates to a 1.5 mL reaction tube filled with 200 μL RPMI 1640 medium containing 1 mmol/l Pefabloc (protease inhibitor).
11. Vortex the samples thoroughly.
12. Store samples for 30 min on ice.

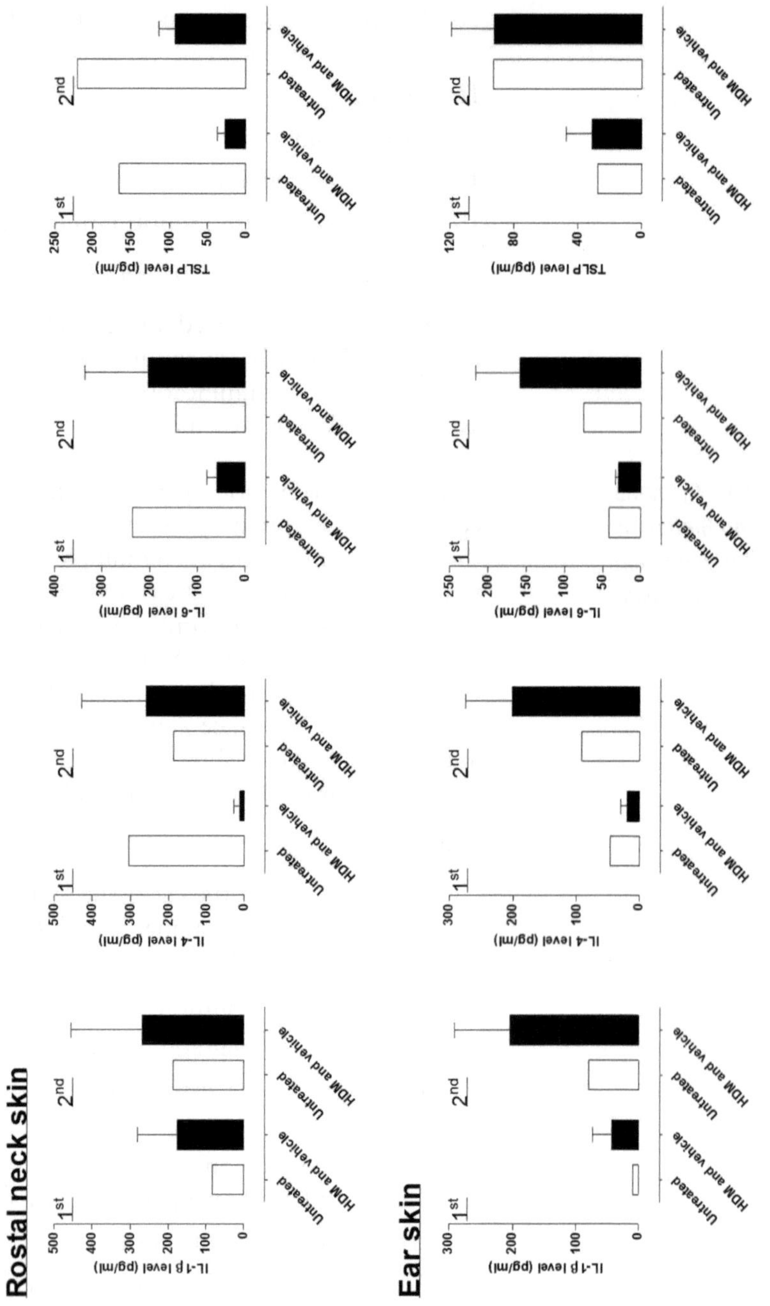

Fig. 14 Cytokine profile (IL-1β, IL-4, IL-6, and TSLP) in skin tissues (rostal neck and ear) of NC/Nga mice challenged with house dust mite (HDM) antigen twice weekly. Mice were sacrificed for the first determination after 7 weeks and for the second determination after 11 weeks. The levels of IL-1β in both skin tissues were increased by HDM treatment; however, the levels of IL-4, IL-6, and TSLP in skin tissue 8 weeks after initiation of study were decreased by HDM treatment. Interestingly, although the level of TSLP 12 weeks after initiation of study was increased by house dust mite, the levels of IL-4 and IL-6 were decreased by HDM treatment. n = 5 for vehicle (treatment with a hydrogel), n = 1 for untreated control for each time point

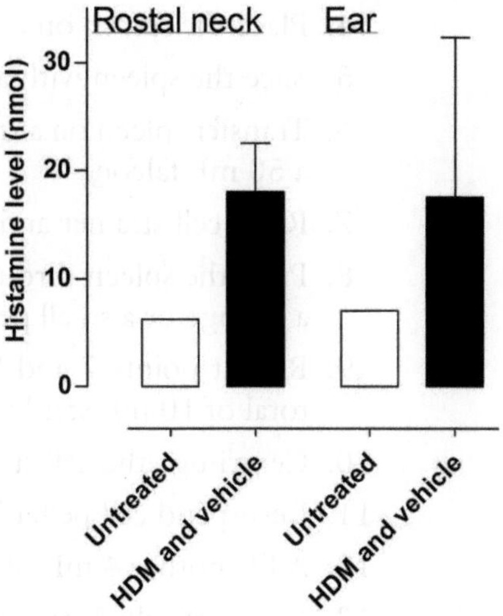

Fig. 15 Level of histamine in skin tissues (rostal neck and ear) of NC/Nga mice 7 weeks after initiation of house dust mite (HDM) antigen challenge. $n = 5$ for vehicle, $n = 1$ for untreated control

13. Centrifuge homogenate at 3000 × *g* for 10 min at 4 °C.
14. Collect the supernatants.
15. Determine protein content with a protein assay kit according to manufacturer's instructions.
16. Dilute samples with RPMI 1640 medium to the desired concentration (normalize samples).
17. Store samples at −20 °C until analysis.
18. Measure cytokines and histamine by ELISA.

3.10 Single-Cell Preparation of Spleens

The spleen is a rich source of lymphocytes, antigen-presenting cells (macrophages, dendritic cells), and erythrocytes. Because erythrocytes may interfere with in vitro assays, they are eliminated with hemolysis buffer during the single-cell preparation. In case of an ongoing immune response, the cell number in the spleen increases. OVA-sensitized H_4R-knockout mice have a significant lower number of splenocytes compared to wild-type mice after one and three challenges with OVA [19]. In addition, mice treated with the H_4R antagonist JNJ-28307474 twice daily during sensitization and challenge with OVA also have a significant lower number of splenocytes compared to vehicle-treated mice [19].

Protocol

1. Place the animal on a clean dissection board.
2. Incise the abdominal cavity.
3. Remove the spleen (located to the left side of the abdomen, inferior to the stomach).

4. Place the spleen on a sterile petri dish.
5. Slice the spleen with a scalpel in four pieces.
6. Transfer spleen on a sterile 70-μm nylon cell strainer placed on a 50 mL falcon.
7. Rinse cell strainer and spleen with 1 mL sterile PBS.
8. Press the spleen through the strainer using the plunger end of a syringe or a small pestle.
9. Repeat points 7 and 8 until spleen has been perfused with a total of 10 mL sterile PBS.
10. Centrifuge the cell suspension at 1000 × *g* for 10 min.
11. Resuspend cell pellet in 1 mL hemolysis buffer.
12. Add another 4 mL of the hemolysis buffer.
13. Incubate cells 5 min at room temperature.
14. Add 45 mL of sterile PBS.
15. Centrifuge the cell suspension at 1000 × g for 10 min.
16. Resuspend pellet in 1 mL RPMI 1640 + 10% FCS + 100 μg/mL streptomycin and 100 U/mL penicillin.
17. Add another 4 mL RPMI 1640 + 10% FCS + 100 μg/mL streptomycin and 100 U/mL penicillin.
18. Determine cell count by means of a cellometer or Neubauer chamber.

3.10.1 Determination of Cytokine Release by Splenocytes

Splenocytes of OVA-challenged mice, which have been in vitro restimulated with OVA Grade VI, produce significantly more IL-4, IL-10, and interferon (INF)-γ than splenocytes restimulated with PBS (Fig. 16). Also levels of IL-5 and IL-13 are increased in splenocytes from OVA-sensitized mice in response to OVA restimulation [8].

Protocol

1. Seed splenocytes (3 million/mL RPMI 1640 + 10% FCS + 100 μg/mL streptomycin and 100 U/mL penicillin) in 12-well plates.
2. Stimulate splenocytes for 96 h with OVA VI (100 μg/mL).
3. Collect cell culture medium and store at −20 °C until analysis.
4. Determine levels of cytokines (like IL-4, IL-10, and INF-γ) in the supernatants by ELISA.

3.11 Preparation of Lymph Nodes

Of interest are the draining lymph nodes of the ear auricle ("auricular") node in NC/Nga mice and the draining lymph nodes of the skin (*Ln. axillaris proprius*). In healthy mice, lymph nodes are hardly distinguishable from the surrounding fat and connective tissue [32]. However, when ear tissue or the skin is inflamed, the

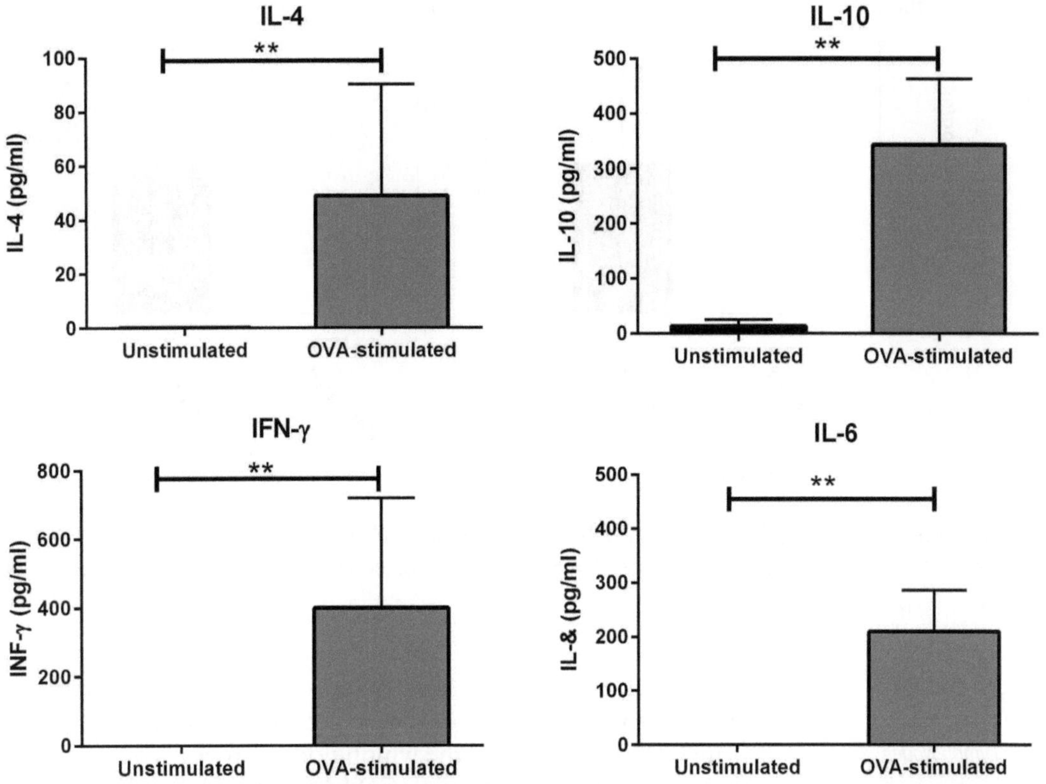

Fig. 16 Levels of IL-10, IL-4, and INF-γ in supernatants of splenocytes isolated from OVA-challenged mice (two challenges). Cells have been restimulated with OVA (100 μg/mL) for 96h. $^{**}p < 0.01$ Mann-Whitney test

draining lymph nodes are enhanced and easily visible. For the preparation of the draining lymph nodes of the ear auricle, place the mouse on a clean dissection board and separate the skin below the ear into the direction of the neck by fine scissors and prepare cautiously from the superficial tissue. The lymph node is visible caudo-ventral to the masseter. For the preparation of the *Ln. axillaris proprius* cut the skin into the direction of the forepaws by fine scissors and prepare cautiously from the superficial tissue. Fix the skin flap below the leg. The *Ln. axillaris proprius* is now visible medial to the shoulder, at the junction between the lateral thoracic vein and the axillary vein. For a schematic drawing of the localization of the lymph nodes in the mouse, see [32].

3.11.1 Single-Cell Preparation of Lymph Node Cells

Protocol

1. Pick up the lymph nodes with fine forceps.
2. Carefully remove connective tissue if necessary.
3. Passage lymph nodes through a sterile 70-μm nylon cell strainer in 1 mL RPMI 1640 supplemented with 5% FCS (*see* **Note 4**).
4. Determine cell count by means of a cellometer or Neubauer chamber.

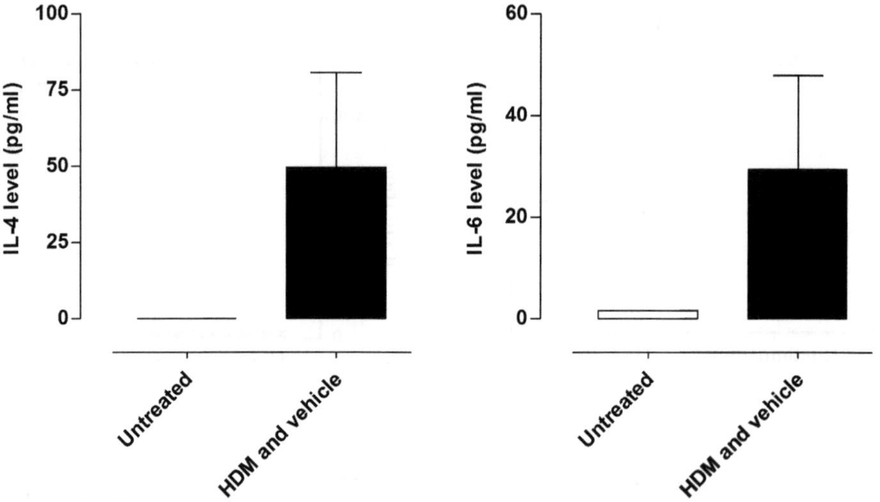

Fig. 17 Concentrations of IL-4 and IL-6 in lymph node supernatants of NC/Nga mice 11 weeks after initiation of house dust mite (HDM) antigen challenge. $n = 5$ for vehicle (treated with a hydrogel), $n = 1$ for untreated control

3.11.2 Isolation from CD4+ T Cells from Lymph Nodes

OVA-sensitized H_4R knockout mice have a significantly reduced number of CD4+ T cells compared to wild-type mice [19]. To isolate CD4+ T cells from the lymph nodes, process single-cell suspension from lymph nodes with CD4+ T Cell Isolation Kits according to manufacturer's instructions. The manufacturers provide detailed step-by-step protocols. These kits can also be used to isolate CD4+ T cells from single-cell suspensions of splenocytes or other tissues by negative selection. We had a purity of the sorted cells greater than 98% with the EasySep™ Mouse CD4+ T Cell Isolation Kit.

3.11.3 Cytokine Determination of Lymph Nodes

Lymph node cells isolated from house dust mite challenged NC/Nga mice secrete IL-4 and IL-6 whereas IL-4 and IL-6 could not be detected in supernatants of Con A-stimulated lymph nodes cells of an untreated Nc/Nga mouse (Fig. 17). In OVA-stimulated lymph node cells isolated from OVA-challenged mice, no IL-6, IL-10, or INF-γ could be detected and only very small amounts of IL-4 (Fig. 18). CD4+ T cells isolated from lymph nodes of OVA-challenged mice and then restimulated with OVA Grade VI produced significantly more IL-4 and IL-10 than CD4+ T cells that have been restimulated with PBS (Fig. 19). INF-γ could not be detected in supernatants of CD4+ T cells.

Protocol

1. Centrifuge lymph nodes cells at 300 × *g*, 5 min, 4 °C.
2. Take up cells in RPMI 1640 + 10% FCS + 100 μg/mL streptomycin and 100 U/mL penicillin.

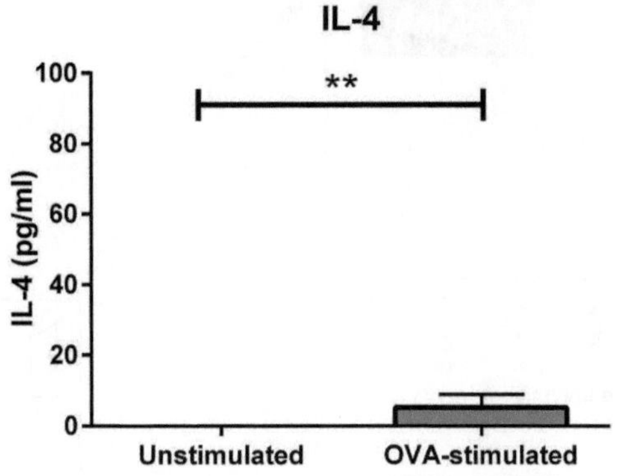

Fig. 18 Concentration of IL-4 in lymph node supernatants of OVA-challenged mice (two challenges). Cells have been restimulated with OVA (100 μg/mL) for 96h. $n = 6$ mice per group. $^{**}p < 0.01$ Mann-Whitney test

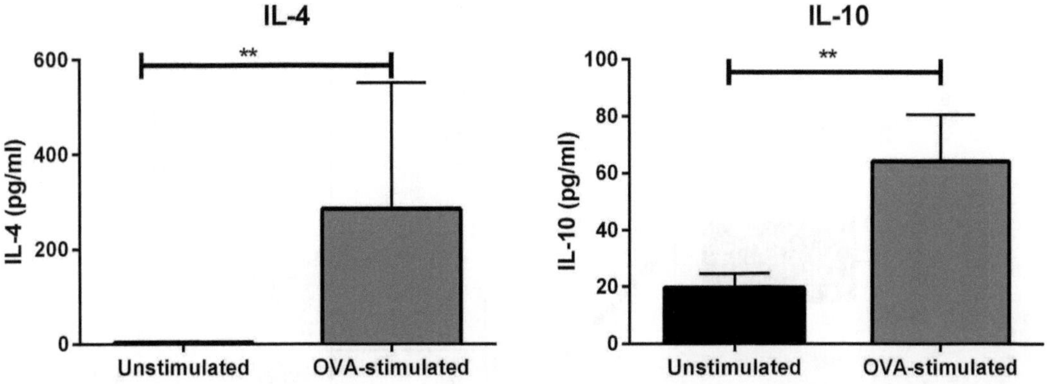

Fig. 19 Concentration of IL-4 in CD4+ T cell supernatants of OVA-challenged mice (one challenge). Cells have been restimulated with OVA (grade VI 100 μg/mL) for 96h. $n = 6$ mice per group. $^{**}p < 0.01$ Mann-Whitney test

3. Transfer 5×10^5 cells/well into a 48-well plate.
4. NC/Nga mice: Stimulate cells for 24 or 96 h with Con A (5 μg/mL) at 37 °C in a 5% CO^2 atmosphere

   OVA model: Stimulate cells for 96 h with OVA VI (100 μg/mL) at 37 °C in a 5% CO^2 atmosphere.
5. The levels of cytokines (like IL-4 and IL-6) in cell culture medium can be measured by using an ELISA.

3.11.4 Flow Cytometric Analysis of Lymph Node Cells

Total cell numbers of CD3+ T cell, CD11c+ CD40+ dendritic cell, CD19+ B cell, and CD19+ IgG1+ B cell counts in auricular lymph nodes of NC/Nga mice are shown in Fig. 20.

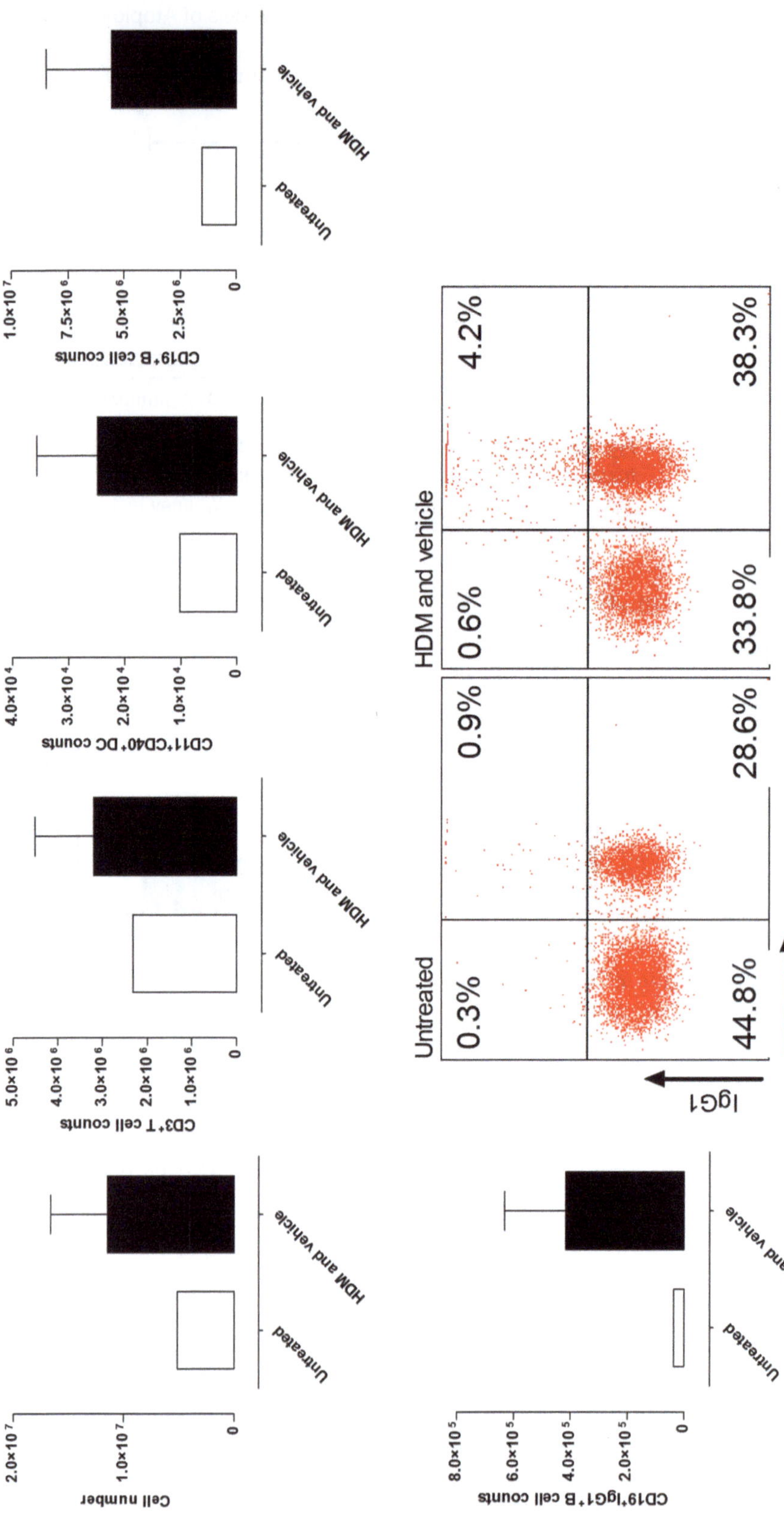

Fig. 20 Total cell number, CD3+ T cell, CD11c+ CD40+ dendritic cell, CD19+ B cell, and CD19+ IgG1+ B cell counts in auricular lymph node of NC/Nga mice 11 weeks after initiation of house dust mite (HDM) antigen challenge. $n = 5$ for vehicle (hydrogel treated), $n = 1$ for untreated control

Protocol

1. Transfer 5 × 10^5 cells/200 μL PBS in polystyrene round-bottom 12 × 75 mm tubes (*see* **Note 5**).
   (a) One sample per mouse.
   (b) One control sample without antibodies ("unstained control") to determine autofluorescence.
   (c) Isotype controls are essential to exclude nonspecific binding.
   (d) One sample for each fluorochrome used in the antibody cocktail as compensation controls to determine the extent of fluorochrome spectral overlap.
2. To avoid nonspecific binding, incubate cells with 1 μg mouse BD Fc Block for 5 min at 4°C.
3. Wash cells.
   (a) Centrifuge cells (300 × *g*, 5 min, 4 °C).
   (b) Aspirate supernatant and resuspend cells in 200 μL 5% FCS in PBS.
   (c) Centrifuge cells (300 × *g*, 5 min, 4 °C).
   (d) Aspirate supernatant and resuspend cells in 200 μL 5% FCS in PBS.
4. Prepare a master mix of all antibodies needed (2 μL/antibody and probe).
5. Incubate cells with the monoclonal antibodies cocktail for 30 min at 4 °C in the dark.
6. Wash cells.
   (a) Centrifuge cells (300 × *g*, 5 min, 4 °C).
   (b) Aspirate supernatant and resuspend cells in 200 μL 5% FCS in PBS.
   (c) Centrifuge cells (300 × *g*, 5 min, 4 °C).
   (d) Aspirate supernatant and resuspend cells in 500 μL PBS.
7. Analyze cells on a flow cytometer (we analyze 10,000 events for expression of antigens) as soon as possible (on the same day).

4 Notes

1. The fixation of the OVA patch and the bandage needs training. Special care has to be taken not to restrict the breathing of the mice by wrapping the bandage too tight around the abdomen. However, if you wrap it too loosely it most likely will come off again. That is why it is important to fix the fur in the neck with

a piece of surgical tape; otherwise, the mouse will easily slough off the bandage. During the challenge phases you have to use OVA Grade VI. Visible skin lesions only occur with challenge with OVA Grade VI and not with OVA Grade V. It is very important to depilate the mice on the same day the OVA patch is applied to the skin (during sensitization and challenge). The depilation will disrupt the skin barrier and enhance the antigen (OVA) uptake. Mice that had been depilated 24 h before the application of the OVA patch (during sensitization and challenge) did not develop skin lesions. Mice even did not develop skin lesions when they were depilated during the sensitization phase 24 h before OVA patch application, but in the challenge phases on the same day.

2. Measurement of ear thickness needs some training as the ear must not be placed within the cutimeter for too long. The pressure would then artificially reduce the ear thickness. Best training outcome is by repeating the ear measurement two to three times. If the variation from determination to determination is bigger than 10 μm, the person needs more training to determine the ear thickness.
3. For fixation of skin specimen for histology, the skin can also be placed in 10% neutral buffered formalin or 4% paraformaldehyde solution.
4. An alternative method for the preparation of single-cell suspensions from lymph nodes is to transfer lymph nodes to a sterile glass potter filled with 500 μL RPMI 1640 supplemented with 5% FCS. By cautious screwing the pestle up and down for roughly five times the lymph nodes get disintegrated into a single-cell suspension. Add 500 μL RPMI 1640 supplemented with 5% FCS and count the cells in a Cellometer or Neubauer chamber.
5. Staining for flow cytometric analysis can also be performed in a 96-well round-bottom plate. When you have more than 20 samples this is time saving. Therefore, place 5×10^5 cells/100 μL PBS/well. Leave several empty wells between your samples to avoid contaminations between the probes. Discharge the supernatants after the washing steps by inverting the plate over the sink and shake the plate for about three times. After the last wash step, resuspend cells in 100 μL PBS and transfer cells to FACS tubes containing 400 μL PBS.

References

1. Spergel JM, Paller AS (2003) Atopic dermatitis and the atopic march. J Allergy Clin Immunol 112(6 Suppl):S118–S127
2. Hillier A, Griffin CE (2001) The ACVD task force on canine atopic dermatitis (I): incidence and prevalence. Vet Immunol Immunopathol 81:147–151
3. Gutermuth J, Ollert M, Ring J et al (2004) Mouse models of atopic eczema critically evaluated. Int Arch Allergy Immunol 135:262–276

4. Matsumoto M, Ra C, Kawamoto K et al (1999) IgE hyperproduction through enhanced tyrosine phosphorylation of Janus kinase 3 in NC/Nga mice, a model for human atopic dermatitis. J Immunol 162:1056–1063
5. Segawa S, Hayashi A, Nakakita Y et al (2008) Oral administration of heat-killed Lactobacillus brevis SBC8803 ameliorates the development of dermatitis and inhibits immunoglobulin E production in atopic dermatitis model NC/Nga mice. Biol Pharm Bull 31:884–889
6. Ohsawa Y, Hirasawa N (2012) The antagonism of histamine H_1 and H_4 receptors ameliorates chronic allergic dermatitis via anti-pruritic and anti-inflammatory effects in NC/Nga mice. Allergy 67:1014–1022
7. Murota H, El-latif MA, Tamura T et al (2010) Olopatadine hydrochloride improves dermatitis score and inhibits scratch behavior in NC/Nga mice. Int Arch Allergy Immunol 153:121–132
8. Spergel JM, Mizoguchi E, Brewer JP et al (1998) Epicutaneous sensitization with protein antigen induces localized allergic dermatitis and hyperresponsiveness to methacholine after single exposure to aerosolized antigen in mice. J Clin Invest 101:1614–1622
9. Wang LF, Lin JY, Hsieh KH et al (1996) Epicutaneous exposure of protein antigen induces a predominant Th2-like response with high IgE production in mice. J Immunol 156:4077–4082
10. Spergel JM, Mizoguchi E, Oettgen H et al (1999) Roles of TH1 and TH2 cytokines in a murine model of allergic dermatitis. J Clin Invest 103:1103–1111
11. Akdis CA, Akdis M, Bieber T et al (2006) Diagnosis and treatment of atopic dermatitis in children and adults: European Academy of Allergology and Clinical Immunology/American Academy of Allergy, Asthma and Immunology/PRACTALL consensus report. J Allergy Clin Immunol 118:152–169
12. Ohsawa Y, Hirasawa N (2014) The role of histamine H_1 and H_4 receptors in atopic dermatitis: from basic research to clinical study. Allergol Int 63:533–542
13. Rossbach K, Wendorff S, Sander K et al (2009) Histamine H_4 receptor antagonism reduces hapten-induced scratching behaviour but not inflammation. Exp Dermatol 18:57–63
14. Seike M, Furuya K, Omura M et al (2010) Histamine H(4) receptor antagonist ameliorates chronic allergic contact dermatitis induced by repeated challenge. Allergy 65:319–326
15. Hirasawa N, Ohsawa Y, Katoh G et al (2009) Modification of the picryl chloride-induced allergic dermatitis model in mouse ear lobes by 12-O-tetradecanoylphorbol 13-acetate, and analysis of the role of histamine in the modified model. Int Arch Allergy Immunol 148:279–288
16. Cowden JM, Zhang M, Dunford PJ et al (2010) The histamine H4 receptor mediates inflammation and pruritus in Th2-dependent dermal inflammation. J Invest Dermatol 130:1023–1033
17. Kamo A, Negi O, Tengara S et al (2014) Histamine H(4) receptor antagonists ineffective against itch and skin inflammation in atopic dermatitis mouse model. J Invest Dermatol 134:546–548
18. Gutzmer R, Gschwandtner M, Rossbach K et al (2011) Pathogenetic and therapeutic implications of the histamine H_4 receptor in inflammatory skin diseases and pruritus. Front Biosci (Schol Ed) 3:985–994
19. Rossbach K, Schaper K, Kloth C et al (2016) Histamine H_4 receptor knockout mice display reduced inflammation in a chronic model of atopic dermatitis. Allergy 71:189–197
20. Wakasugi N, Tomita T and Kondo K (1967) Differences of fertility in reciprocal crosses between inbred strains of: DDK, KK and NC. J. Reprod. Fert. 13: 41–50
21. Yanaba K, Kamata M, Asano Y et al (2013) CD19 expression in B cells regulates atopic dermatitis in a mouse model. Am J Pathol 182:2214–2222
22. Cowden JM, Yu F, Challapalli M et al (2013) Antagonism of the histamine H4 receptor reduces LPS-induced TNF production in vivo. Inflamm Res 62:599–607
23. Thurmond RL, Desai PJ, Dunford PJ et al (2004) A potent and selective histamine H_4 receptor antagonist with anti-inflammatory properties. J Pharmacol Exp Ther 309: 404–413
24. McClain RW, Yentzer BA, Feldman SR (2009) Comparison of skin concentrations following topical versus oral corticosteroid treatment: reconsidering the treatment of common inflammatory dermatoses. J Drugs Dermatol 8:1076–1079
25. Neumann D, Schneider EH, Seifert R (2014) Analysis of histamine receptor knockout mice in models of inflammation. J Pharmacol Exp Ther 348:2–11
26. Novak N, Bieber T (2003) Allergic and nonallergic forms of atopic diseases. J Allergy Clin Immunol 112:252–262
27. Laske N, Niggemann B (2004) Does the severity of atopic dermatitis correlate with serum IgE levels? Pediatr Allergy Immunol 15:86–88

28. Dahten A, Koch C, Ernst D et al (2008) Systemic PPARgamma ligation inhibits allergic immune response in the skin. J Invest Dermatol 128:2211–2218
29. Leung DY, Bieber T (2003) Atopic dermatitis. Lancet 361:151–160
30. Matsuda H, Watanabe N, Geba GP et al (1997) Development of atopic dermatitis-like skin lesion with IgE hyperproduction in NC/Nga mice. Int Immunol 9:461–466
31. Bäumer W, Seegers U, Braun M et al (2004) TARC and RANTES, but not CTACK, are induced in two models of allergic contact dermatitis. Effects of cilomilast and diflorasone diacetate on T-cell-attracting chemokines. Br J Dermatol 151:823–830
32. Van den Broeck W, Derore A, Simoens P (2006) Anatomy and nomenclature of murine lymph nodes: descriptive study and nomenclatory standardization in BALB/cAnNCrl mice. J Immunol Methods 312:12–19

Chapter 10

Methodological Approaches to Study Histamine Pharmacology in the Kidney: From Cell Culture and Cell Imaging to Functional Assays and Electron Microscopy

Alessandro Pini, Eleonora Veglia, Cristina Grange, and Arianna Carolina Rosa

Abstract

The best approach to study the complexity of renal pathophysiology is to use living organisms. However, to limit the number of animal experiments undertaken and obtain first in humans results, in vitro models can be extremely helpful options. Moreover, in vitro assays allow us to characterize a new pharmacological target, defining also the selectivity, efficacy, and potency of ligands in a specific cell type. This chapter aims to describe the steps taken to obtain a suitable model to study histamine pharmacology in renal cells, starting from the cell isolation to the morpho-functional assays. The in vitro system herein reported mostly reflects the in vivo situation as demonstrated by our previously published data.

Key words Cell imaging, Electron microscopy, Mesangial cells, Permselectivity, Podocytes, Renal cells, Time-resolved fluorescence resonance energy transfer (TR-FRET), Tubular epithelial cells

1 Introduction

To date, few pharmacological interventions have been developed specifically for treating the kidney with most of the pharmacological therapy for renal patients therefore relying on the treatment of comorbidities. One of the most relevant challenges in renal-targeted drug development is to find a suitable preclinical model. Renal physiology and pathology are complex systems that are best studied in whole living organisms. However, to limit the number of animal experiments undertaken and obtain first on humans results, in vitro models can be used as surrogates [1]. In vitro assays allow us to characterize a new pharmacological target as well as define the selectivity, efficacy, and potency of ligands in a specific cell type. The first step in deciding which in vitro assays to use is to define the system. A physiologic or pharmacologic observation spurs questions to further investigate the broader role of a receptor

Ekaterini Tiligada and Madeleine Ennis (eds.), *Histamine Receptors as Drug Targets*, Methods in Pharmacology and Toxicology, DOI 10.1007/978-1-4939-6843-5_10,

Table 1
Histamine receptor (H_xR) expression in the human renal cortex [3–7]

	H_1R	H_2R	H_3R	H_4R
Glomeruli Podocytes Mesangial cells	✓✓	✓		?✓
Tubules Tubular epithelial cells HK-2 cells	✓✓	✓✓	✓	✓✓

in a specific organ system [2]. Under this task, the expression, the binding of specific ligand or substrates, and functional activity of a receptor should be demonstrated. Within this chapter we describe the major techniques to characterize histamine receptor expression and function in suitable renal cells in in vitro models. The in vitro system herein reported mostly reflects the in vivo histamine receptor (H_xR) presence and distribution along the nephron, as demonstrated by our previously published data (Table 1) [3–7]. Thereby, renal cells represent a unique system to study histamine pharmacology in native cells.

1.1 Renal Cellular Models

The adult kidney is composed of 26 different cell types deriving from the ureteric bud and the metanephrogenic mesenchyme [8]. The differentiated cells are organized into functional structures called nephrons. Each nephron, composed of regions of different morphology, can be further divided into two main functional structures: the renal corpuscle and the tubules. Within these structures the cells are characterized by an elaborated shape and lateral interdigitating processes. However, each cell can be considered highly specialized for function and morphology, thus an in vitro study on renal pharmacology has to involve different cell types.

The renal corpuscle has some resemblance to a balloon (the capsule), with a fist (the capillaries) punched into it. The outer wall of the capsule is called the parietal layer while the inner is the visceral (glomerular) layer, which closely embraces the entire network of glomerular capillaries and consists of complex-shaped cells called podocytes. Between podocytes and the capillaries there is an extracellular layer, the glomerular basement membrane (GBM). The anastomizing capillary network forms a lobule supported by a region called the mesangial. All this structure forms the functional filtration unit: the glomerulus.

The nephron structure immediately adjacent to the glomerulus of the kidney is a tubule formed by a single layer of epithelial cells into which the glomerular filtrate passes after it has reached the Bowman's capsule. The tubule is traditionally divided into three functional regions: proximal tubule, loop of Henle (composed of a descending and an ascending tract), and distal tubule. The distal tubules converge onto collecting ducts, which forms the papillary region. Notably, although the collecting duct embryonic derivation is from the ureteric bud, for many years physiologists and anatomists have viewed the collecting duct as an integral portion of the nephron regardless of its embryonic origin [9].

Renal epithelial cells are the single layer of cells lining the nephron, including the glomerulus, the proximal and distal convoluted tubules, and the collecting ducts. Recognition among the different subtypes is difficult and morphological characteristics vary depending on the place of origin within the nephron. It is now clear that morphology alone is not sufficiently discriminating to assess cell purity or ensure that a homogenous population of cells has been isolated. Antibodies to specific cell-surface and cytoskeletal markers need to be used to confirm cell identity and purity. Table 2 shows the main markers used to differentiate between the glomerular and tubular cell types present in culture [10–18].

Human renal cells are usually isolated from specimens obtained from the normal pole of kidneys surgically removed from patients with renal carcinoma. Traditional culture performed with primary cells offers characteristics more close to their organs of origin [19]. But the shortcomings of this approach include the problem of obtaining enough cells for large-scale screens and the rapid loss of important protein and gene expression profiles usually within 48 h. Therefore, having to resort to immortalized cell lines is often necessary, although these cells are prone to genotypic and phenotypic drifting and cell lines can lose tissue-specific functions and acquire molecular phenotypes quite different from cells in vivo. Thereby, whatever it is possible, data generated by primary and immortalized or transformed cell lines should be combined.

1.1.1 Glomerular Cells

It emerges that the complex anatomical structure of the glomerulus contains many different cell types, including visceral and parietal epithelial cells, mesangial cells, and fenestrate endothelial cells, which form the simple squamous layer of the renal capillary endothelium and have complex processes extending into the capillary lumen. These cells have long been recognized as distinct entities, because they occupy defined anatomical locations and have distinguishable morphological and cytochemical features. Mesangial cells and their matrix form the central stalk of the glomerulus and are part of the functional unit interacting closely with endothelial cells and podocyte epithelial cells. Several studies have been based on mixed populations of glomerular cell cultures [20–24]. However, the specific glomerular compartmentalization and several anatomical characteristics such as endothelial fenestrations and epithelial pedicels are lost in culture [25, 26], where cells may undergo de-differentiation.

Table 2
Examples of key markers for glomerular and tubular cell types

	Podocytes	Mesangial cells	Tubular cells			
			Proximal tubule	*Loop of Henle*	*Distal tubule*	*Collecting duct*
α-SMA		✓				
myosin		✓				
vimentin	✓	✓				
podocyin	✓					
nephrin	✓					
synaptopodin	✓					
P-cadherin	✓					
E-cadherin					✓	
cytokeratin 19			✓			
cytokeratin 18			✓		✓	
CD10			✓			
CD13			✓			
desmin			✓			
gamma-glutamyl transferase			✓			
aminopeptidase M			✓			
megalin			✓			
AQP-1			✓			
AQP-2						✓
AQP-3						✓
AQP-4						✓
Na-K-ATPase			✓		✓	
promin 1			✓			
promin 2				✓	✓	✓
NKCC1					✓	
NKCC2				✓		
THP				✓	✓	
SGLT-2			✓			

SMA smooth muscle actin; PDGFR; CD10, neutral endopeptidase; CD13, aminopeptidase N; AQP, acquaporin; NKCC, $Na^+/K^+/Cl^-$ Symporters; THP, Tamm–Horsfall glicoprotein; *SGLT* sodium-glucose linked transporter

Despite these limitations, studies on mixed populations of glomerular cells contributed to clarify many important aspects of renal (patho)-physiology at the cellular level [27]. Notably, the use of human glomerular suspension was the basis of one of the first observations supporting the role of histamine in influencing glomerular function. Indeed, Sedor and Abbound [28] demonstrated that human glomeruli have histamine H_2 receptors, which mediate enhanced cyclic adenosine monophosphate (cAMP) accumulation, and that glomeruli are major sites of histamine production in the human kidney [28]. With the advances in cellular isolation and culturing techniques, the different glomerular cells have been isolated, propagated, and cell lines generated by viral or nonviral oncogenic transformation [22, 29–31]. Indeed, for most of the glomerular cell types, glomerular cell lines have now been established [31–34]. These lines provide advantages of a longer life span, the possibility of cell proliferation also for non-proliferating cells such as podocytes, but they usually result in cellular transformation to a less differentiated phenotype.

The "Mosaic Theory" [35], according to which separate populations of cells can be obtained from a mixed population of cells based on their different growth rates or culture requirements, is the principle of isolation of glomerular cells. Whatever glomeruli are sieved to be free of tubule contamination, directly seeded into culture flasks or enzymatically dissociated, the first cells to emerge are epithelial cells, which have a distinctive "cobblestone" appearance [36] and, for the first 7–10 days of outgrowth, are the most common cell type in a mixed population of glomerular cells. Endothelial cells and mesangial cells may then present at this stage. Mesangial cells become more evident later in culture, have a stellate appearance, grow vigorously, in multilayers and are subject to contact inhibition [17]. Therefore after 30 days of growth, the cultures are nearly pure mesangial cells [35]. Homogeneity of cells can be improved by using cloning rings and repeated cloning but the yield of cells is less and they do de-differentiate with passage number. Podocytes are largely obtained by culturing glomerular cells after sieving [37] or microbead embolization [38] under optimized conditions to enrich them [39], but also by magnetic sorting [40]. However, such approaches require 1 or 2 weeks for podocyte outgrowths from individual glomeruli plated on dishes. As podocytes are terminally differentiated cells [41], they have a very low proliferative potential, and they have been reported to irreversibly arrest their proliferation as early as day 5 of primary culture [42]. Immortalized podocyte cell lines could circumvent these important limitations of primary culture [31, 43–45]. However, these cell lines should be carefully managed to maintain desirable differentiation, and the expression levels of podocyte-specific molecules [39]. Indeed, changes induced by immortalization processes and the alteration in cellular physiology due to continuous proliferation are implicit limits in their use. Thereby, data obtained from these cells should be interpreted with caution and the parallel and comparative use of both primary and immortalized cells should be pursued.

1.1.2 Tubular Cells

The epithelial tubular cells are the single layer of cells lining the entire tubules from the proximal to the collecting tubules. Their recognition is mostly based on the morphological and functional characteristics varying on the place of origin. The proximal tubule consists of two parts—tortuous (*pars convoluta*) and straight (*pars recta*). It is lined by simple cuboidal epithelium, whose cells are relatively largely engaged in absorption and ion transport. Their brush border in the apical domain contains alkaline phosphatase. The infoldings on the basal surface contain different ion pumps and mitochondria. Basically, the proximal tubular cells are relatively large, ovoid, or elongated granular cells, which may be mistaken for small or fragmented granular casts. The loop of Henle, structurally resembling the distal tubule, consists of two limbs: the descending, thin, penetrates the medulla and is lined by simple squamous epithelium; and the ascending, thick, hands back to the cortex and is lined by simple cuboidal epithelium. The distal tubule lined by simple cuboidal cells that are responsible for active ion transport under hormonal control (e.g., aldosterone) and exhibit prominent infoldings. The absence of a brush border and the relatively clear cytoplasm in the cells of the distal convolution, together with the scattered microvilli, permit an easy identification of this segment of the nephron. Finally, the collecting tubule is lined by a simple cuboidal epithelium within which two different types, the darker intercalated cells with numerous mitochondria and the pale-staining principal cells, which are affected by antidiuretic hormone, are present.

Although a dissection and cell isolation from the cortex, the medulla and the papilla is possible, the most characterized and commonly used are the tubular cells from the cortex. Generally, the protocols are based on preparing a suspension of non-glomerular cortical cells and isolating them by size or density. In addition, different techniques used to obtain tubular renal cell populations for culture include selective culture media [46], membrane substrates [47], free flow electrophoresis [48], flow cytometry [49], immune-isolation [50], and microdissection [51]. All these techniques have the common limitation that they do not distinguish among the different cell tubular subtypes, for which magnetic sorting is required. However, the mixed population could be considered an interesting model recapitulating not only the features of a single tract of the nephron, but its entirety. Obviously, if this heterogeneity confers to this model the features of a co-culture system, the limits of the co-cultures are implied. Actually, especially in terms of human cells, the most represented tubular pure culture is the proximal one, for which human-transformed cell lines exist. For example, the commercially available SV40-transformed HKC cell line was developed by Loraine Racusen in 1997 [52] and the HPV E6/7-transformed HK-2 cell line was developed by Ryan and coworkers in 1994 [53]. Although extremely useful, both these cells lines have limitations in their phenotypic resemblance to primary counterparts; for example, HKC clone 8 does not express tight junctions while HK-2 cells do not tolerate being grown to confluence [1]. For these reasons, primary cells, also from a mixed tubular suspension, offer a reliable model for the tubular epithelial cells that can be used independently or to confirm results previously obtained from immortalized cell lines.

1.2 Receptor Cellular Topography

The first step for an in vitro pharmacological approach is to define the system by the desired target. To investigate the role of a receptor in a specific organ system, the first demonstrations have to be its expression, binding of specific ligand or substrates, and functional activity [2]. Obviously, the system chosen should reflect the in vivo situation. Histamine receptors belong to the G-protein coupled receptors (GPCRs) family. Considering the influence of the GPCRs density on small molecule activity as a partial or full agonist, antagonist, or inverse agonist [54], great care has to be taken to define the receptor cellular topography. Actually, the idea that greater mRNA expression level, as well as total protein expression level evaluated by immunoblotting, does not imply greater physiological importance is nowadays well recognized [2]. Often the choices for both binding and functional studies are limited to having to transfect the receptor into HEK-293 or CHO-Kl cells, but the cellular context (e.g., distinct functional tract of the nephron) is not explored in that way and critical information may be missed by assaying the receptor activation/inhibition in an inappropriate cell type [2]. Therefore, whenever it is possible, immortalized cell lines for comparison, and eventually primary cultures of the tissue of choice, should be used.

Against that background, the importance of a contemporary qualitative and quantitative analysis is implicit. Although western blotting is one of the semiquantitative techniques most used to investigate the expression of a protein of interest derived from a cell culture or tissue culture sample, it fails to provide real subcellular compartmentalization. All the protocols developed to obtain subcellular fractioning for protein expression analysis [55–57] do not reach the potential of immunofluorescence detection. The use of antibodies to localize structures in cell cultures and tissue sections is an extremely powerful method and is responsible for many important discoveries [58]. Immunofluorescence is a powerful technique that utilizes fluorescent-labeled antibodies to detect specific target antigens. Immunocytochemistry began when Albert Coons and coworkers reported the use of a fluorescent-labeled antibody to localize pneumococcal antigen in liver sections [59]. Indirect immunofluorescence utilizes a two-step technique: a primary, unlabeled antibody binds to the target, and a fluorophore-labeled secondary antibody, directed against the Fc portion of the primary, is used to detect the first one. Requiring two incubation periods, this technique is more complicated and time consuming than direct immunofluorescence; however, it is more sensitive because more than one secondary antibody can bind to each primary antibody, which amplifies the fluorescence signal [60].

Actually, immunofluorescence is more often used to detect the subcellular localization of a receptor and to gauge information as to whether two or more proteins are likely to interact physically in the same cell (co-immunolocalization). A double immunofluorescence procedure can be carried out to examine the co-distribution of different antigens: for two antigens present in the same cellular compartment co-localization is marked by a mixed color; on the contrary when two antigens are located in different cellular compartments (e.g., nucleus-cytoplasm, nucleus-cell membrane, cytoplasm-cell membrane), co-localization should be observed as two separate colors. Primary antibodies raised in different species can be used either in parallel (in a mixture) or in a sequential way.

Appropriate choice of fluorophores-labeled secondary antibodies is critical for unambiguously identifying each component in a co-localization experiment. Basically, organic fluorophores offer an increased photostability and photon output. The choice of fluorophore is coupled to the optical design of the co-localization microscope since a different laser may be necessary to excite each fluorophore and fluorophore emission may need to be monitored individually [61]. The most widely used fluorophores are: green-fluorescent dye with excitation ideally suited to the 488 nm laser (Alexa488™), orange-fluorescent dye excited using the 532 nm laser line (Cy3), red-fluorescent dye excited using 594 nm laser line (Alexa594™), and far-red-fluorescent dye with excitation suited for the 633 nm line (Cy5).

1.3 Functional and Pharmacological Receptor Identification

It is well accepted that protein identification only by immunolabeling is not sufficient to provide solid evidence of its expression and function in cells, thus compromising the translation to in vivo studies. Indeed, major questions around antibody selectivity [62] compel scientists to complement cytoimmunofluorescence studies with functional and pharmacological evidence. This issue of general relevance to GPCRs is true also for histamine receptors. Thereby, the presence of active histamine receptors on renal cells has to be confirmed by functional and pharmacological studies. In order to meet this task, the measurement of second messengers is a suitable and reliable strategy. Notably, this approach allows us also to characterize the affinity and potency of different ligands to the renal histamine receptors. The activation of a single GPCRs protein can affect the production of different second messenger molecules; one of the common targets is adenylyl cyclase that catalyzes the synthesis of cAMP; another common target is the phospholipase C (PLC) that catalyzes the synthesis of diacylglycerol (DAG) and inositol 1,4,5-trisphosphate (IP3) from phosphatidylinositol (PI). Therefore cAMP and IP3 are the canonical second messengers to be evaluated, although it is now recognized that histamine receptors could activate alternative pathways such as the β-arrestin recruitment from H_4R [63]. For decades, the traditional technique for studying GPCRs was radioligand binding; this technique involves the incubation of cells or membranes with a radioactively labeled specific ligand, followed by separation of bound and free radioligand and subsequent quantification of the bound radioactivity. But, these assays have, at least, two major disadvantages: first, radioactivity implies safety and disposal concerns and precautions, and, moreover, these assays have only limited spatial and temporal resolution [64]. To overcome these issues, nonradioactive assays using fluorescent methods have been developed [65, 66]. Among these, fluorescence resonance energy transfer (FRET) requires two fluorophores, where the emission spectrum of the donor overlaps with the excitation spectrum of the acceptor. If the two are in close proximity (usually <10 nm), excitation of the donor can result in emission by the acceptor [67, 68]. This emission of the acceptor, as well as the reduced emission of the donor, can be measured to give an FRET ratio (Fig. 1). The FRET method is based on the competitive binding process executed by original antigen (sample antigen) and add-in antigen, so that the energy transferred is inversely proportional to the sample-antigen quantity. An evolution of FRET was the time-resolved FRET (TR-FRET), in which lanthanides have been used as donors in FRET applications [66]. The two lanthanides most frequently used are europium (Eu^{3+}) or terbium (Tb^{3+}), on which the cAMP TR-FRET kits and the inositol 1-monophosphate (IP1) TR-FRET are usually based, respectively. Because the lanthanides exhibit a very weak absorption, which is 104-fold lower compared with conventional organic fluorophores, they need an organic chromophore as an antenna, which transfers the energy to the lanthanide [68]. The cryptates are the most frequently used chelates for lanthanides: they prevent quenching and broadening of the emission peaks as well as leading to a kinetically stable acid-resistant complex [69]. The emission occurs with a significant time delay, and thus a delay window is used for recording during which the autofluorescence of the sample has decayed [68]. The lanthanides are excited at 340 to 360 nm wavelength in the UV and emit characteristic, almost atom-like spectra at very discrete wavelengths [69].

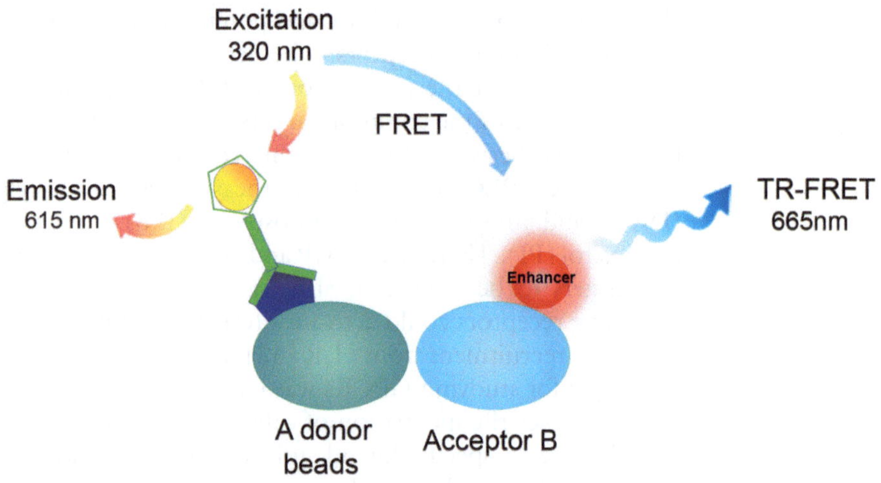

Fig. 1 TR-FRET assay principles. TR-FRET is based on the transfer of energy between two molecules. When the two fluorophore labels are brought together, energy can be transferred from donor to acceptor. As a consequence, excitation of the donor fluorophore will result in emission from the acceptor fluorophore (or enhancer). The level of light emitted from the acceptor fluorophore is proportional to the degree of donor-acceptor complex formation

1.4 Renal Epithelial Junctional Functionality

In the kidney, junction structures have been demonstrated to be variable along the entire nephron. The establishment and maintenance of epithelial cell polarity and the barrier function of the epithelia can be attributed to intercellular junctions and particularly to the tight junctions [70]. Their complexity could be roughly equated with the paracellular permeability of the different segments. Within the glomerulus, mature podocytes develop specialized junctions between the cell body and the GBM (focal adhesion complex) and junctions between interdigitating foot processes (slit diaphragm, SD). The maintenance of this cell in its specialized state and its ability to sustain the filtration barrier is based on the functional and morphological integrity of the junctions. Along the tubules, the unique junctional array in the different tracts is responsible for the paracellular permeability decreases from the proximal tubule to the collecting duct [71].

Numerous renal disease processes involve the functional integrity of the intracellular junctions. In particular, the critical role of the SD for the size-selective filtration barrier of the kidney has been clearly demonstrated. Junctional dysfunction has been extensively correlated to proteinuria, in both inherited and acquired diseases [72]. The importance of these findings led to the recognition of specialized contacts between adjacent podocytes as major candidate targets for albuminuria. Thereby, evaluation of the functional integrity of the renal junctions is a major issue when approaching to the identification of new targets in the kidney. Notably, histamine has been already reported to affect junctional integrity in some epithelial cells [73]. Measurement of the functional status of a junction required the need to set up an ad hoc model recapitulating the paracellular transport through the intercellular space. The three most closely analyzed parameters quantifying barrier function, first developed for endothelial studies, are: (1) the permeability to (macro-)molecular probes; (2) the permeability to water, and (3) the permeability to small inorganic ions described by the transendothelial electrical resistance (TER) [74]. The translation of these models from endothelial cells to podocytes, but also to tubular cells, provides the opportunity to perform a system to study the effect of molecules, such as histamine, on renal barriers. Among the different approaches described above, the permeability to (macro-)molecular probes is the best characterized in cultured podocytes [75–78]. Actually, the use of florescent-labeled macromolecules such as albumin allows to recapitulate one of the most important in vivo renal dysfunctions: namely albumin filtration. Using permeable supports with microporous membranes, the Transwell, first developed for migration assays, has become a standard method for such studies. These permeable supports have allowed significant improvements in culturing polarized cells since these permeable supports permit cells to uptake and secrete molecules on both their basal and apical surfaces and thereby carry out metabolic activities in a more natural fashion. In particular, podocytes grown on the Transwell supports and the trans-membrane flux of fluorescent-labeled albumin are easily recorded measuring the fluorescence in the two compartments with a fluorescence plate reader [78]. The techniques can be considered high-throughput being a multiplexing assay that can provide fast and reliable readouts; however, the high costs of the disposable plates limit the use of this system as a routine screening strategy.

1.5 Renal Epithelial Junctional Morphology

The analysis of the functional integrity of renal cell junctions strictly correlates with the morphological aspect and it has to be complemented by the evaluation of their morphological integrity. From a morphological perspective, along its route through the filtration barrier, the filtrate has to pass the open pores of the glomerular endothelium, the highly hydrated collagenous network of the GBM, and the SD [79–81]. The glomerular SD is the junctional structure linking the interdigitating foot processes from neighboring podocytes and consists of transmembrane-bridging proteins networking with a juxtaposed cytoplasmic platform of protein complexes, which in turn is linked to the actin cytoskeleton [82].

This architecture is associated with high permeability for water, small solutes, and ions but impermeability to plasma proteins and other large molecules, resulting in a virtually protein-free glomerular filtrate. Since adjacent foot processes are derived from different podocytes, the SD bridging foot processes can be considered a highly developed variant of the cell junctions. This concept belongs to the observation by Schnabel and coworkers [83] that the slit diaphragm is a variant of the tight junction, because the tight junction protein zonula occludens (ZO)-1 is localized on the cell surface at the insertion point of the slit diaphragm [84]. This traditional vision of the SD has been progressively changed over time leading to the idea that the intercellular gap of the SD is wider than that of the tight junction. Indeed, some morphological features of the SD, such as the presence of the central dense line observed in grazing sections, are common with those of the adherens junction [84]. Moreover, ZO-1, originally thought to be specific for the tight junction, is also present in adherence junctions [85]. On this basis a more prominent role for P-cadherin and adherents junction has been recognized [86].

Independently of the contribution of single molecules to the SD composition and function, the most reliable experimental approach to clarify the effects of different stimuli, such as histamine, is the morphological one. Indeed, evaluation only of gene and/or protein expression, without a clear cellular localization, does not completely reflect the in vivo SD composition and structure. Taking into account the immunofluorescence technique, its limitation lies in the a priori selection of a validated specific target, which does not provide a general view of the junctional structures. Actually, an in vitro model with a high transferability potential needs to reflect the whole in vivo SD structure and to take advantages of suitable methods to evaluate it. This kind of analysis can be pursued with both transmission and scanning electron microscope (TEM or SEM, respectively), which, differently from the light microscope, enables the examination of fine detail within the whole structure. Indeed, the electron microscope can offer a broad and unique range of characterization techniques with high spatial and analytical resolution, coupled with a completely quantitative understanding of the observed ultrastructures. The TEM allow magnification of a specimen to 120,000×, enabling researchers to attain structure nearly down to the molecular level, making it possible to analyze structure and texture and providing topographical, morphological, and compositional information [87]. The SEM integrates the feature of a TEM with the three-dimensional image capture. Electron microscopy examination is a useful tool to study the ultrastructural morphology of renal cells, in particular podocytes and tubular epithelial cells, and it can be employed to evaluate ultrastructural alterations caused by histamine exposure. Indeed, as histamine has been shown to induce alterations of ZO-1 expression, modifying tight-junction structure [88], the electron microscopic examination can be used to perform qualitative and semiquantitative evaluation of the resultant junctions.

2 Materials

2.1 Cell Isolation and Cell Culture

- Cell dishes and flasks, sterile sharp scissors, centrifuge sterile tubes.
- Stainless-steel filters of 50, 100, and 200 μm mesh size.
- 125, 106, 70, 63, and 45 μm sieves.
- RPMI (Rosewell Park Memorial Institute) 1640 wash medium: supplement 500 mL of RPMI 1640 with 1% of penicillin/streptomycin (10,000/10,000 UI/mL) and 1% of l-glutamine 200 mM. Store at 4 °C for up to 1 month.
- Trypsin EDTA 1X.
- De-complemented fetal bovine serum (FBS): gently and gradually thaw purchased fetal bovine serum (kept frozen at −20 °C until needed). Once serum is completely thawed, incubate serum in 37 °C bath to equilibrate (generally 15 min are enough) before raising the temperature setting of the bath to 56 °C. Incubate serum for 30 min at 56 °C, thereafter cool at room temperature (RT). Aliquot 50 mL of treated serum into conical tubes to avoid repeated thawing and refreezing as it may cause serum denaturation.
- RPMI 1640 culture medium: supplement 500 mL of RPMI 1640 with 15% of filtered (0.22 μm pore size filter, to remove small gram-negative bacteria) de-complemented FBS, 1% of penicillin/streptomycin (10,000/10,000 UI/mL), 1% of l-glutamine 200 mM, and 0.5% of Mycozap™ (to prevent mycoplasma contamination). Store at 4 °C for up to 1 month.
- Fibronectin: reconstitute to 1 mg/mL in sterile double distilled water (dd H_2O), and dilute to 10 μg/mL in RPMI 1640 wash medium. Store at −20 °C in aliquots. Coat flasks at 5 μg/cm^2 leaving solution to bind for at least 30 min before discharging the excess. Coated dishes/flasks are also commercially available.
- Phosphate-buffered saline (PBS): to prepare 1 l of 10X solution, dissolve 87.66 g of NaCl and 17.799 g of Na_2HPO_4 in 800 mL dd H_2O. Adjust pH to 7.4 with HCl. Adjust volume to 1 l with additional dd H_2O. Use diluted at 1:10 (PBS 1X) after sterilization by autoclaving.
- Dulbecco's modified eagle's medium (DMEM)-D-valine culture medium: supplement 500 mL of DMEM 1 mg/l glucose medium with 20% of filtered de-complemented FBS, 1% of penicillin/streptomycin (10,000/10,000 UI/mL), 1% of l-glutamine 200 mM, and 92 mg/l in which 56.06 mg of D-valine, to prevent fibroblast proliferation [19], were dissolved. Store at 4 °C for up to 1 month.

- Complete low glucose cell culture medium: supplement 500 mL of DMEM 1 mg/l glucose medium with 10% filtered de-complemented FBS, 1% of penicillin/streptomycin (10,000/10,000 UI/mL), and 1% of l-glutamine 200 mM. Store at 4 °C for up to 1 month.
- Complete high glucose cell culture medium: supplement 500 mL of DMEM 4.5 mg/l glucose medium with 10% filtered de-complemented FBS, 1% of penicillin/streptomycin (10,000/10,000 UI/mL), and 1% of l-glutamine 200 mM. Store at 4 °C for up to 1 month.
- Collagen type I from calf skin 0.1% (w/v) solution. Alternatively, collagen type I coated tissue culture flasks are commercially available.
- 10% dimethyl sulfoxide (DMSO) in FBS: add 5 mL of DMSO to 45 mL of de-complemented FBS. Store at 4 °C for up to 1 month.
- Hematoxylin solution.
- Tris phosphate buffer (TBS) 1X: dissolve 6.05 g of Tris–HCl and 8.76 g NaCl in 800 mL of dd H_2O. Adjust pH to 7.5 with HCl and make volume up to 1 l with dd H_2O. TBS is stable at 4 °C for 3 months.
- Dako Envision horseradish peroxidase (HRP): Envision HRP (rabbit/mouse) polymer reagent; 3,3'diaminobenzidine tetrahyrochloride (DAB) chromogen solution in the Envision staining Kit: add 20 μL of DAB chromogen to 1 mL of substrate solution.
- Aqueous mounting medium.
- Blocking solution Triton X–100: dissolve 0.5 mL of goat serum in PBS 1× and then add 20 μL of Triton X–100.
- Parathyroid hormone (PTH): dissolve 942.4 μg of the powder in 1 mL dd H_2O to produce100 μM. Aliquot and store at –20 °C. Use at the final concentration of 100 nM.
- Vasopressin: dissolve 108.4 μg of the powder in 1 mL dd H_2O to produce 100 μM. Aliquot and store at –20 °C. Use at the final concentration of 1 μM.
- Calcitonin: dissolve 343.1 μg of the powder in 1 mL dd H_2O to produce 1 μM. Aliquot and store at –20 °C. Use at the final concentration of 100 nM.
- Forskolin: dissolve 41.05 mg of the powder in 10 mL DMSO to obtain 10 mM. Aliquot and store at –20 °C. Use at the final concentration of 10 μM.

2.2 Cell Imaging

- Coverslips and microscope slides.
- Absolute ethanol.

- 4% paraformaldehyde (PAF) solution: paraformaldehyde 4 g is dissolved in 100 mL of PBS 1X in chemical fume hoods (*see* **Note 1**).
- CellMask™ Orange plasma membrane stain (Invitrogen) solution: dilute the stain in complete medium at 5 μg/mL.
- Blocking solution: dissolve 0.15 g of bovine serum albumin (BSA) in 10 mL of PBS 1X.
- Antibody dilution buffer: dissolve 10 mg of BSA in 10 mL of PBS 1X.
- Commercially available antibodies against the histamine receptor anti-H_1R (e.g., Santa Cruz H300, sc-20633) anti-H_2R (e.g., Santa Cruz A20, sc-33973).
- Anti-hH_3R (349–358) and anti-hH_4R (374–390) antibodies produced and validated for detecting both human and rodent H_4R in the School of Biological and Biomedical Sciences, Durham University [89–97].
- Commercially available antibodies for endoplasmic reticulum (ER; anti-calnexin) or nuclear envelop staining (anti-lamin A/C).
- Alexa-Conjugated secondary antibodies.
- Aqueous mounting medium.

2.3 Functional Assays

- 96-well flat-bottom white plate.

2.3.1 IP1 Evaluation

- IP-One HTRF® assay kit (Cisbio).
- Ready-to-use lysis buffer.
- Stimulation buffer: once diluted 1/5 in dd H_2O, it contains Hepes 10 mM, $CaCl_2$ 1 mM, $MgCl_2$ 0.5 mM, KCl 4.2 mM, NaCl 146 mM, glucose 5.5 mM, LiCl 50 mM, pH 7.4.
- IP1-d2 working solution: add 5 volumes of lysis buffer to 1 volume of IP1-d2 stock solution prepared by dissolving the lyophilized in 0.5 mL of dd H_2O (aliquot and store at −20 °C for long storage). Prepare fresh before each test.
- Ab-cryptate working solution: add 5 volumes of Lysis buffer to 1 volume of IP1-d2 stock solution prepared by dissolving the lyophilized material in 0.5 mL of dd H_2O (aliquot and store at −20 °C for long storage). Prepare fresh before each test.

2.3.2 cAMP Evaluation

- LANCE® Ultra cAMP Kit (PerkinElmer).
- 3-Isobutyl-1-methylxanthine (IBMX): dissolve 5.556 g of IBMX in 50 mL of DMSO; the stock solution can be stored at −20 °C.
- Stimulation buffer: add 10 μL of IBMX (final concentration 0.5 mM) to 10 mL complete DMEM medium.

- 4X Eu-cAMP tracer: just before the use, dilute at 1:50 the Eu-cAMP tracer stock solution in cAMP detection buffer in the kit. The working solutions can be stored up to 24 h at 4 °C.
- 4X Ulight-anti-cAMP working solution: just before the use, dilute at 1:150 the Ulight-anti-cAMP stock solution in cAMP detection buffer in the kit. The working solutions can be stored up to 24 h at 4 °C.

2.4 Permeability Assay

- HTS transwell inserts 3 μm pore size, 24-well plate.
- 24-well flat-bottom black plate.
- Wash buffer: PBS 1X supplemented with 1 mM $MgCl_2$ and 1 mM $CaCl_2$ (*see* **Note 2**), dissolve 4.75 mg of $MgCl_2$ and 5.5 mg of $CaCl_2$ in 50 mL of PBS 1X. Filter the solution with 0.22 μm pore size filter.
- Fluorescein isothiocyanate (FITC)-labeled BSA solution: dissolve 10 mg of albumin-FITC conjugate in 1 mL complete high glucose medium.

2.5 TEM

- Millicell culture plate inserts.
- Sodium cacodylate buffers 0.2M: dissolve 4.28 g of sodium cacodylate in 100 mL of dd H_2O. Prepare a solution of HCl by adding 1.6 mL of HCl 36% to 98.4 mL with dd H_2O. Mix 20 mL of the obtained sodium cacodylate solution with 1.4 mL of the stock HCl solution, pH 7.3.
- Paraformaldehyde 8%: mix 2 g paraformaldehyde with 25 mL of dd H_2O in a 125 mL Erlenmyer flask. Heat to 60 °C on a stir plate. When moisture forms on the sides of flask, add 3–5 drops of sodium hydroxide 1 M and stir until the solution clears. Cool solution under the faucet. Filter.
- Karnovsky's glutaraldehyde fixative: mix 10 mL of sodium cacodylate buffers 0.2 M with 2 mL of glutaraldehyde 25%, 5 mL of paraformaldehyde 8% (2 g paraformaldehyde with 25 mL of dd H_2O), 2 mL of dd H_2O, pH 7.3.
- Washing buffer: add 25 mL of sodium cacodylate buffers 0.2 M to 25 mL of sucrose 0.44 M (dissolve 15 g of sucrose in 100 mL of dd H_2O).
- Solution A: dissolve 0.27 g of sodium phosphate monobasic in 200 mL of dd H_2O.
- Solution B: dissolve 0.71 g of sodium phosphate dibasic dodecahydrate in 200 mL of dd H_2O.
- Osmium tetroxide: mix 7.5 mL of Solution A with 42.5 of Solution B and add 0.4 g of NaCl. Add 1 osmium tetroxide vial, pH 7.4.
- NaCl 0.5% solution: dissolve 0.05 g of NaCl in 6 mL dd H_2O. Then adjust volume to 10 mL with additional dd H_2O.

- Acetone.
- Ethanol 100%.
- Propylene oxide.
- Epon 812.
- Glass Petri dish.
- Toluidine blue solution: dissolve 0.1 g of toluidine blue in 100 mL of dd H_2O.
- Gadolinium triacetate: dissolve 2.5 g of gadolinium triacetate in 100 mL of dd H_2O.
- Alkaline lead citrate: place 1.33 g lead nitrate and 1.76 g sodium citrate into a 50 mL volumetric flask and add 30 mL dd H_2O. Shake vigorously for 1 min. Allow to stand at RT for 30 min with intermittent shaking. The solution will be a milky white color. Add 8.0 mL of 1 N NaOH and the solution will turn clear. Make up to 50 mL with boiled, cooled, and filtered double-deionized water. Do not use until day 3.

3 Methods

3.1 Cell Isolation

We describe the method to consistently obtain different subtypes of primary cells from human renal cortex. This procedure minimizes the number of donors, with an explicit ethical advantage. The tissue is derived from specimens obtained from the normal pole of kidneys surgically removed from patients with renal carcinoma (*see* **Note 3**). The tissue should be taken from the pole distant to the tumor and identified as macroscopically tumor-free by a consultant histopathologist. The culture process should then be started straightaway for maximum cell yield. The samples can be stored at 4 °C overnight, but this will reduce the number of viable cells obtained. The cells obtained with this protocol can be used as a substrate to generate the counterpart immortalized cell line. All procedures should be carried out using aseptic technique in a laminar flow hood. Handling human tissue, appropriate precautions such as disposable gloves should be used and immunization against hepatitis B is recommended. Although not described here, there is now a potential to culture podocytes and tubular cells from urine as a new and promising method for monitoring the activity of some glomerular-associated diseases such as diabetic nephropathy [98]. Once isolated, cells have to be characterized to ensure that the correct phenotype has been obtained in a reasonably pure culture.

1. Place the tissue in a sterile Petri dish containing RPMI 1640 wash medium to remove as much blood as possible. No FBS should be used during the isolation procedure, since it may initiate clotting due to blood products present in the tissue.

2. Remove any adherent renal capsule and fat using autoclaved surgical tools.
3. Select the lesion-free pole of the kidney and cut the outer (paler) cortex.
4. Move the selected tissue to a new Petri dish containing 2 mL of RPMI 1640 wash medium.
5. With sharp scissors mince the tissue into small cortical fragments (>2 mm^3) and suspend each in RPMI 1640 wash medium.
6. Mesh the small cortical fragments through a graded series of stainless-steel filters (50, 100, and 200 μm mesh) using an inverted plunger from a sterile syringe; connective tissue is retained in this sieve. The resulting cell suspension is then washed with a generous amount (50–100 mL) of RPMI 1640 wash medium through a 125 μm sieve. This results in the separation of glomeruli from renal tubules, interstitium, and vasculature. In particular, the red particulate matter retained in this sieve can be identified as glomeruli by optical microscopy. Within the latter sieve the Bowman's capsule is also striped from most of the glomeruli (*see* **Note 3**).
7. Recover decapsulated glomeruli with 50 mL of RPMI 1640 wash medium and collect the 200-mesh-filtered kidney cell suspension and continue to Sect. 3.1.3 for tubular cell isolation.
8. Pass the filtrate through a 106 μm sieve, and rinse the retained glomeruli with approximately 50 mL RPMI 1640 wash medium to eliminate any tubular fragments eventually still present.
9. Collect in a 50 mL sterile tube and centrifuge at 984 × *g* for 5 min at RT, the glomeruli retained on the sieve by inverting it over a Petri dish and washing with RPMI 1640 wash medium. Glomeruli remaining on the sieve should be collected washing with a 1 mL pipette tip using FCS 100% to avoid the attachment of glomeruli on the pipette wall.
10. Centrifuge at 984 × *g* for 5 min at RT, resuspend the pellet in RPMI 1640 culture medium, and transfer the glomeruli to a fibronectin-coated culture flask at a concentration of approximately 300 glomeruli/cm^2 (*see* **Note 4**).
11. Culture glomeruli at 37 °C in 95% air/5% CO_2 humidified incubator for at least 24 h to allow good attachment of glomeruli. Continue to Sect. 3.1.2 if podocytes are desired.

3.1.1 Mesangial Cell Isolation

Mesangial cells, which are now commercially available as primary cells (ScienCell Research Laboratories), are the easiest glomerular cells to be grown due to their minimal growth requirements and high proliferative capacity. They show a stellate phenotype, preserved when cultured.

1. Once the glomeruli have adhered to the flask, change the medium every 4–5 days. The first cells to grow out of the glomeruli core are epithelial cells, which can be used for podocyte isolation as described in Sect. 3.1.2, while after a further 2 weeks, a mixed stromal/parenchymal population is observed. After 2–3 weeks more of culture, a mesangial cell overgrow is observed (*see* **Note 5**).
2. Remove the medium washing twice with PBS 1X and resuspend the cells in DMEM-D-valine culture medium to inhibit any fibroblast growth (*see* **Note 6**).
3. Once the cells have grown to confluence, split them 1:1 using Trypsin EDTA 1X and culture them in uncoated tissue culture grade dishes/flasks in complete low glucose cell culture medium according to Sect. 3.2. Cells should be used between passages 3 and 8 (*see* **Notes 5** and 7) after being fully characterized.
4. At passage 3 characterize mesangial cells by morphology, immunolabeling, and functional criteria (*see* **Note 8**). These cells can be slowly expanded and frozen in aliquots. In particular, for immunolabeling, after having prepared the cellular sample as described in Sect. 3.3.1 until step 12, fix the coverslip in 0.3 mL of acetone at 4 °C, incubating it on ice for 10 min.
5. Remove the acetone and let the coverslip dry at RT.
6. Prepare the antibodies, diluting them to the optimal concentration (*see* Table 2) in PBS 1× added with 1.5% of BSA.
7. Rehydrate the coverslip pipetting 0.8 mL of TBS 1X per well (two washes of 5 min).
8. Remove the TBS 1× from the well and lay on the coverslips on microscope slides facing upward in a wet chamber to prevent samples from drying.
9. Add 200 μL of the primary monoclonal antibody and incubate the coverslip for 1 h at RT.
10. Wash the coverslips three times for 2 min in TBS 1X .
11. Add 200 μL of Envision HRP (rabbit/mouse) polymer reagent and incubate for 30 min at RT.
12. Wash with TBS 1X for three times for 2 min each and rinse in dd H_2O.
13. Prepare the DAB chromogen solution and immediately incubate the coverslips at RT for 5–7 min (if the cells are positive for that marker, they become brown).

14. Rinse the coverslips in dd H_2O.
15. Counterstain nuclei pipetting 500 μL of hematoxylin solution. Incubate for 30 s at RT.
16. Wash the coverslips in running tap water for 10 min.
17. Wash the coverslips in dd H_2O for 5 min.
18. Mount the coverslips in aqueous mounting medium with a glass cover slip.
19. Assess for positivity (brown) or negativity (−) of the immunoreactions by microscopical observation, in order to evaluate the cell positive percentage for each marker, establishing the purity of cell cultures.
20. Then these cells can be slowly expanded and frozen in aliquots.

3.1.2 Podocyte Isolation

Podocytes are terminally differentiated cells retaining this feature when cultured. Thereby, an extensive use of [41] podocyte cell lines was initiated to circumvent this important limitation. However, changes induced by immortalization processes and the alteration in cellular physiology due to continuous proliferation could affect the transferability of data generated with these models.

1. Once the glomeruli, prepared as described in Sect. 3.1.1, have adhered to the culture plate or flask, change the medium every 4–5 days. Epithelial cells can be seen growing out of the glomeruli around 7–10 days. This time may vary and generally it takes longer to see cellular outgrowth in glomeruli prepared from kidneys from older patients.
2. After 10–15 days, once sufficient epithelial cells are identified (these have a polygonal, cobblestone appearance), pour off the unbound glomeruli, and gently rinse the bound glomeruli/cells in PBS 1X.
3. Collect the epithelial cells in the filtrate in a 50 mL sterile tube; glomeruli are retained on the sieve. Rinse the sieve several times with a volume of around 10 mL culture medium to stop the trypsin EDTA action ensuring maximum epithelial cell recovery.
4. Pellet the cells passing through the sieve by centrifugation at 984 × *g* for 5 min at RT and then resuspend in complete high glucose cell culture medium.
5. Plate the cells into the tissue culture flasks previously coated with type I collagen at a concentration of 10 μg/cm^2 (*see* **Note 4**).
6. After approximately 1 week, when the epithelial cells have reached confluence (*see* **Note 5**), split them using trypsin EDTA 1×. Plate the trypsinized cells onto culture grade

dishes/flasks without type I collagen. At confluence, the cells will be homogeneous and display a cobblestone appearance. Within 2–3 weeks, the subcultured cobblestone cells transform into individual arborized cells and show positivity for Wilms' tumor-1 (WT-1) antigen.

7. Characterize the culture by morphology, immunolabeling, and functional criteria (*see* **Note 9**). In particular, for immunolabeling, after having prepared the cellular sample as described in Sect. 3.3.1, step 12, fix the coverslip in 0.3 mL of acetone at 4 °C, incubating it on ice for 10 min.
8. Remove the acetone and let the coverslip dry at RT.
9. Prepare the antibodies, diluting them to the optimal concentration (*see* Table 2) in PBS 1X added with 1.5% of BSA.
10. Rehydrate the coverslip pipetting 0.8 mL of TBS 1X per well (two washes of 5 min).
11. Remove the TBS 1X from the well and lay on the coverslips on microscope slides facing upward in a wet chamber to prevent let samples drying.
12. Add 200 μL of primary monoclonal antibody and incubate the coverslip for 1 h at RT.
13. Wash the coverslips three times for 2 min in TBS 1X.
14. Add 200 μL of Envision HRP (rabbit/mouse) polymer reagent and incubate for 30 min at RT.
15. Wash with TBS 1X for three times for 2 min each and rinse in dd H_2O.
16. Prepare the DAB chromogen solution and immediately incubate the coverslips at RT for 5–7 min (In this time, if the cells are positive for that marker the cells appear brown).
17. Rinse the coverslips in dd H_2O.
18. Counterstain nuclei pipetting 500 μL of hematoxylin solution. Incubate for 30 s at RT.
19. Wash the coverslips in running tap water for 10 min.
20. Wash the coverslips in dd H_2O for 5 min.

3.1.3 Tubular Cell Isolation

The epithelial tubular cells are the single layer of cells lining the entire tubules from the proximal to the collecting tubules. Actually, especially in terms of human cells, the most represented pure tubular culture is the proximal, for which a number of human-transformed cell lines are commercially available. In comparison, primary renal cells from mixed tubular suspensions offer a reliable model of tubular epithelial cells. Indeed, although not described here, they could be the substrate for subsequent purification by magnetic sorting.

1. Sequentially wash the 200-mesh-filtered kidney cell suspension from step 7 in Sect. 3.1 through sieves of 106, 70, and 45 μm pores with RPMI 1640 wash medium. The material retained in the 45 μm sieve should be predominantly tubular fragments.
2. Transfer the tubular sediment to a sterile 15 mL centrifuge tube containing RPMI 1640 wash medium and centrifuge at 984 × *g* for 5 min at RT.
3. Discharge the supernatants and resuspend cells in complete low glucose cell culture medium.
4. Centrifuge for at 984 × *g* for 5 min at RT.
5. Discharge the supernatants, resuspend cells in complete low glucose cell culture medium containing Mycozap™ (1:500; 20 μL in 10 mL) to prevent mycoplasm contamination, and seed them.
6. At the first medium change replace the medium with complete low glucose cell culture medium without Mycozap™.
7. Characterize the culture by morphology, immunolabeling, and functional criteria (*see* **Note 10**). In particular, for immunolabeling, after having prepared the cellular sample as described in Sect. 3.3.1, tow the coverslips and remove them from the wells using tweezers, you may need to pipet 1 mL/well of PBS 1X to facilitate this process.
8. Place the coverslips on microscope slides facing upward in a wet chamber to prevent samples from drying and delimit the sample edges with a pap-pen.
9. Saturate any nonspecific binding sites by incubating the coverslips with the Blocking solution Triton X–100 for 20 min at RT.
10. Dilute the primary antibodies in PBS 1X at the desired concentration (anti-vimentin 1:40, anti-pan-cytokeratin 1:400).
11. Incubate cellular slices with the primary antibodies at 4 °C overnight or at RT for 1 h.
12. Wash the slices three times with PBS 1X for 5 min each to remove the excess free antibody.
13. Dilute the conjugate sary fluorescent antibodies 1:200 in PBS 1X ensuring protection from light exposure. For the label control, expose the slice to PBS 1X only.
14. Incubate all the cellular slices with the conjugate secondary fluorescent antibody for 30 min at RT in the dark.
15. Wash the slices three times with PBS 1X for 5 min each to remove the excess free antibody.
16. Mount the coverslips on microscope slides with an aqueous mounting.
17. Let the slides dry and store them at 4 °C protected from light.

18. Evaluate for positivity (fluorescence signal) or negativity (no signal) of the immunofluorescence, in order to evaluate the cell positive percentage for each marker, to establish the purity of cell cultures.
19. For functional analysis, follow the protocol described in Sect. 3.4.2. Exposing the cells to vehicle; PTH, vasopressin, calcitonin, or forskolin for 30 min at 37 °C. Forskolin is used as positive control as it directly activates adenylyl cyclase.
20. Once confluent, the obtained cells can be cultured, trypsinized, and split as described in Sect. 3.2. As a primary pure culture, these cells continue to retain phenotype for three to four passages. These cells can be slowly expanded and frozen in aliquots.

3.2 Cell Culture

The protocol herein included can be used for both the primary and the immortalized renal cells. As a general principle cell cultures should be 75–100% confluent when selected for subculture. The subsequent passages permit obtaining cellular subcultures and long-term storage. Growth in monolayer cultures will be adversely affected if cells are allowed to become overgrown. In particular, mesangial cells are highly subject to contact inhibition, thus they have to be constantly monitored to avoid a confluence higher than 80%. Tubular cell cultures usually do not reach monolayer confluent as they usually arrange around open spaces in the attempt to recapitulate their polarity around the tubular lumen. Therefore, they eventually grow in a multilayer, with the risk of overgrowth until contact inhibition occurs. Passaging cells too early will result in a longer lag time before subcultures are established. Moreover, cells may require to proliferate in a medium conditioned by their self-generated growth factor. Thereby, too few cells may cause an inhibition of growth and proliferation. Aseptic technique and working in a laminar flow hood or biosafety cabinet is required for cell culture. No cell dishes or flask treatment is required. The following protocol describes how to obtain a subculture from a previously established culture.

1. Wash the cells with PBS 1X twice to remove cell debris and to completely remove any FBS residue that can inactivate trypsin digestive enzyme.
2. Incubate cells with trypsin EDTA 1X in a volume sufficient to cover the monolayer (for a T-75 flask usually 1–1.5 mL is enough) for 2–5 min at 37 °C in a 95% air/5% CO_2 humidified incubator (*see* **Note 11**).
3. Add at least the same amount of serum or complete cell culture medium to stop the trypsin enzymatic reaction.
4. Collect the cell suspension in a 15 mL centrifuge tube.
5. Count cells with the Burker chamber.

6. Centrifuge at 984 ×*g* for 5 min at RT to obtain cell pellet.
7. Discard supernatant and collect the pellet.
8. Resuspend in a volume of complete culture medium suitable to obtain a cell confluency of 20% (usually split the original culture into three subcultures). Take care to use the appropriate medium for each cell culture: complete high glucose cell culture medium for podocyte, and complete low glucose cell culture medium for both mesangial and tubular cells.
9. Plate the cells in new cell culture dishes or flasks ensuring that the medium covers the cellular layer (usually 10–12 mL is enough for a T-75 flask) and culture them at 37 °C in a 95% air/5% CO_2 humidified incubator or store them by freezing as described in step 12.
10. Take note of the cell passage number to reduce de-differentiation with increasing passage number (generically, for immortalized cells it is suggested to not use cells over the 15th passage).
11. If long-term storage is desired, freeze cells resuspending the pellet adding 1 mL of 10% DMSO in FBS; alternative complete medium plus 10% DMSO could be used, thus to prevent crystallization of water that will cause cells to lyse during cryo-preservation and during the thawing process and cells are not going to be starved of nutrients.
12. Transfer the suspension in cryogenic vials and freeze them overnight at −80°, insulated with paper towels and placed into a freezing container (e.g., Nalgene® Mr. Frosty, Sigma Aldrich).
13. Transfer vials to liquid N_2 tank for indefinite storage.
14. Whenever cells have to be thawed, remove vial from the liquid N_2 tank and hold in 37 °C water bath to ensure a quick thawing.
15. Transfer the cell suspension in a 15 mL centrifuge tube containing at least 1 mL of serum or complete medium.
16. Centrifuge at 984 × *g* for 5 min at RT to obtain the cell pellet.
17. Once the pellet is collected, add fresh complete medium and seed cells in a new cell dish or flask.
18. Change media the day after washing cells twice with PBS 1X to remove cell debris (*see* **Note 12**).

3.3 Cell Imaging

Cell imaging techniques aim to detect a specific target and define its topographical distribution within a cell. Therefore, this permits not only determining the presence of the histamine receptors in human renal cells, but, more importantly, determining their eventual localization on the cell membrane surface or in the cytoplasm. The topographical distribution allows the researcher to generate a solid hypothesis on functional activity of the histamine receptor. Indeed, being GPCRs, their membrane localization is predictive of their functional status. Moreover, an intracellular localization, even more so in the ER, can suggest possible receptor trafficking. Although some GPCRs, such as those of angiotensin II [99], have been demonstrated to be expressed on the nuclear membrane, no clear data have yet been generated on a similar distribution for histamine receptor subtypes. Whether cell marker staining or specific antibodies are used, different protocols should be applied. Both the protocol to identify the cytoplasmic membrane localization by a cell membrane staining, the CellMask™ Orange plasma membrane stain (Invitrogen; *see* Sect. 3.3.2), and the immune-colocalization protocol (*see* Sect. 3.3.3) of histamine receptors specific marker of cellular compartments are reported herein.

3.3.1 Sample Preparation

1. Design the experiment taking into account the necessary negative controls for each primary antibody used (*see* **Note 13**).
2. Sterilize the coverslips submerging them in ethanol 100% for 1–2 h or by autoclavating them.
3. Let the ethanol evaporate and the coverslip dry in a hood.
4. Insert the coverslip onto cells in 6-multi-well plate (one coverslip/well) using sterile tweezers.
5. Cover the coverslip with Collagen 0.1% solution (for 6-well plate 500 μL/well is sufficient) and incubate for 5 min at RT (*see* **Note 14**).
6. Discharge the excess Collagen solution and let the coverslips dry.
7. Collect cells in a 15 mL centrifuge tube by trypsinization (*see* Sect. 3.2).
8. Count cells with the Burker chamber.
9. Centrifuge at 984 × *g* for 5 min at RT to obtain a cell pellet.
10. Discard supernatant and resuspend cells in fresh Medium to obtain a final concentration of 45,000 cells/mL and seed 1 mL of cell suspension on each coverslip.
11. Let cells adhere onto coverslip and maintain the culture for 24 h at 37 °C in a 95% air/5% CO_2 humidified incubator. If a pharmacological treatment is desired, incubate cells seeded on the coverslips with the test compound(s) at the required concentration.
12. Wash cells once with PBS 1X. If the plasma membrane is desired continue to Sect. 3.3.2, otherwise follow the subsequent protocol (*see* **Note 15**).
13. Cover the coverslips with 500 μL of PAF 4% and incubate the plate at 37 °C in a 95% air/5% CO_2 humidified incubator.

14. Wash cells twice with PBS 1× 5 min to remove the excess of fixative used.
15. Let the coverslip dry.
16. Store the plate with the coverslips at −20 °C for at least 24 h.

3.3.2 Plasma Membrane Staining

1. After having washed the cells with PBS 1X as described in Sect. 3.3.1, step 12, incubate cells with CellMask™ Orange plasma membrane solution for 5 min at 37 °C in a 95% air/5% CO_2 humidified incubator (*see* **Note 15**).
2. Wash cells twice with PBS 1× for 5 min to remove the unbound excess staining.
3. Fix cells with PAF 4% as described in Sect. 3.3.1, washing cells once with PBS 1X and letting the coverslip dry before freezing the plate with the coverslips at −20 °C for at least 24 h.
4. Thaw the coverslips and remove them from the wells using tweezers; pipette 1 mL/well of PBS 1× to facilitate this process.
5. Lay the coverslips on microscope slides facing upward in a wet chamber to prevent samples from drying out and delimit the sample edges with a pap-pen.
6. Block any nonspecific binding site by incubating the coverslips with the blocking solution described in Sect. 2.3, for 20 min at RT.
7. Dilute the primary antibody(ies) in antibody dilution buffer at the desired concentration (*see* **Note 16**).
8. Incubate cellular slices with the primary antibody overnight at 4 °C. For both the secondary antibody and label controls, expose the slice to antibody dilution buffer only (*see* **Note 13**).
9. Wash the slices three times with PBS 1X for 5 min each to remove the excess free antibody.
10. Dilute the conjugate secondary fluorescent antibody(ies) in antibody(ies) dilution buffer at the desired concentration (*see* **Note 17**) ensuring protection from the light exposure. For the label control, expose the slice to antibody dilution buffer only (*see* **Note 13**).
11. Incubate all the cellular slices with the conjugate secondary fluorescent antibody for 2 h at RT in the dark.
12. Wash the slices three times with PBS 1X for 5 min each to remove the excess free antibody.
13. Mount the coverslips on microscope slides with an aqueous mountant, taking care of avoiding bubbles and mounting solution excess (*see* **Note 18**).
14. Let the slides dry and store them at 4 °C protected from the light.

15. Evaluate the protein expression and its co-localization with a confocal microscope.

3.3.3 Immune-Co-Localization

1. Thaw samples previously prepared according to Sect. 3.3.1 and remove the coverslips from the wells using a tweezer, laying them on microscope slides facing upward in a wet chamber to not let samples dry and mark the borders with a pap-pen.
2. Saturate any nonspecific binding sites by incubating the coverslips with the blocking solution containing Triton X−100 at 0.5% (dissolve 50 μL Triton X−100 in 10 mL PBS 1X; *see* **Note 19**), for 20 min at RT.
3. Dilute the primary antibody(ies) against the tested receptor in antibody dilution buffer at the desired concentration (*see* **Note 16**).
4. Incubate cellular slices with the primary antibody overnight at 4 °C. For both the secondary antibody and label controls, expose the slice to antibody dilution buffer only (*see* **Note 13**).
5. Wash the slices three times with PBS 1X for 5 min each to remove the excess free antibody.
6. Dilute the conjugate secondary fluorescent antibody in antibody(ies) dilution buffer at the desired concentration (*see* **Note 17**) protection from light exposure. For the label control, expose the slice to antibody dilution buffer only (*see* **Note 13**).
7. Incubate all the cellular slices with the conjugate secondary fluorescent antibody for 2 h at RT in the dark.
8. Wash the slices three times with PBS 1X for 5 min each to remove the excess free antibody.
9. Block again to avoid nonspecific binding sites by incubating the coverslips with the Blocking solution containing Triton X−100 at 0.5% for 20 min at RT.
10. Dilute the primary antibody(ies) directed against the cellular compartment in antibody dilution buffer at the desired concentration (*see* **Note 20**) and incubate cellular slices overnight at 4 °C. For both the secondary antibody and label controls, expose the slice to antibody dilution buffer only (*see* **Note 13**).
11. Wash the slices three times with PBS 1X for 5 min each to remove the excess free antibody.
12. Dilute the conjugate secondary fluorescent antibody in antibody(ies) dilution buffer at the desired concentration (*see* **Note 17**) ensuring to protect it from light exposure, and incubate cellular slices for 2 h at RT. For the label controls, expose the slice to Antibody dilution buffer only (*see* **Note 13**).
13. Wash the slices three times with PBS 1X for 5 min each to remove the excess free antibody.

14. Mount the coverslips on microscope slides with an aqueous mounting medium, taking care to avoid bubbles and excess of the mounting solution (*see* **Note 18**).
15. Let the slides dry and store them at 4 °C protected from light.
16. Evaluate the protein expression and its co-localization with a confocal microscope.

3.4 Functional Assays

To functionally and pharmacologically evaluate the presence of active histamine receptors on renal cells the measurement of messenger production has to be evaluated. Moreover, this evaluation can be used to characterize the pharmacological activity of classical and new antihistamines in human renal cells. As the four subtypes of histamine receptors couple with different G proteins the production of at least two different messengers has to be assessed. However, biased signals, such as β-arrestin recruitment by H_4R [63], are also important to evaluate. The TR-FRET method to evaluate both IP-1 and cAMP is subsequently described. As the assay is based on the competitive binding process displayed by original antigen (sample antigen) and add-in antigen, the TR-FRET signal is inversely proportional to the second messenger produced by cells.

3.4.1 IP1 Evaluation

Agonist stimulation of GPCR coupled to Gαq leads to the activation of PLC-β followed by production of D-myo-IP3. IP3 leads to the release of intracellular stored Ca^{2+}, but it is rapidly degraded to IP2, and then to IP1. So to overcome these disadvantages, IP1, final step of the inositol phosphate cascade, can be easily measured by a TR-FRET assay, such as the one developed by Cisbio (IP-One HTRF®). Basically, this assay allows the accumulation of intracellular IP1 avoiding its degradation through the presence of LiCl.

1. Design the experimental scheme for a 96-multi-well white plate (*see* **Note 21**) taking into account using a Negative control as well as an Assay positive control (*see* **step 9**) and the standard curve of at least seven points (blank included; *see* **step 6**).
2. Determine the number of cells taking into account that 50,000 cells/well are needed.
3. Collect the cells in a 15 mL centrifuge tube gently scraping them in their culture medium without washing (*see* **Note 22**).
4. Count cells with the Burker chamber, and transfer the amount of cells required in the experiment in one or more new 15 mL centrifuge tubes (one vial for each different compound treatment is suggested).
5. Centrifuge for 5 min at 984 × *g* to obtain a cell pellet.

6. Discard supernatant and collect the cell pellet.
7. In the meantime prepare the desired stimuli in a volume of stimulation buffer to obtain a double concentration of the final expected one (for a 96-well plate 15 μL/well is the minimum volume required). If an antagonist is used, pretreat cells for 10 min before adding the stimulus (*see* **Note 23**).
8. Prepare serial dilutions of the IP1 standard through serial titration from 11,000 nM to 0 using stimulation buffer.
9. Resuspend cell pellet with the stimulation buffer (*see* Sect. 2.3.1) alone or with the final expected concentration of antagonist prepared according to step 4, to pretreat cells for 10 min at RT.
10. Pipette into the assay plate the serial dilutions of the IP1 prepared as standard curve (*see* **step 5**; for a 96-well plate 30 μL/well is the minimum volume required).
11. Pipette into the assay plate stimulation buffer alone as both negative control and assay control (for a 96-well plate 30 μL/well is the minimum volume required).
12. After the pretreatment incubation, pipette into the assay plate the cell suspension (for a 96-well plate 15 μL/well is the minimum volume required).
13. Add to cell suspension the Stimulation buffer with compound previously prepared as described in step 5 (for a 96-well plate 15 μL/well is the minimum volume required).
14. Gently mix and shake the plate on a rocker shaker and check for the absence of air bubbles.
15. Incubate for 1 h at RT covering the plate with a TopSeal.
16. Prepare the IP1d2 working solution and the antibody-cryptate working solution as described in Sect. 2.3.1 (for a 96-well plate 15 μL/well of each reagent is the minimum volume required).
17. Pipette the IP1d2 working solution in each well except the negative control.
18. Pipette lysis buffer alone in the negative control.
19. Pipette the antibody-cryptate working solution in each well of the assay plate.
20. Incubate for 1 h at RT. Cover the microplate with a TopSeal.
21. Measure the energy transfer by exciting at 320 nm and check the emission at both 620 and 665 nm using aTR-FRET compatible reader (*see* **Note 24**).
22. Results are calculated from the 665/620 nm ratio and usually expressed in ratio. The ratio so determined is inversely proportional to the concentration of IP1 in the sample (*see* **Note 25**).

3.4.2 cAMP Evaluation

Agonist stimulation of GPCRs coupled led to the dissociation of the trimer formed by the α subunit plus the β-γ dimer, into Gα and Gβγ, Gαi and Gβγ, respectively. Therefore, Gαs activation is involved in adenylyl cyclase stimulation, while Gαi and Gβγ in adenylyl cyclase inhibition, so that in both cases cAMP basal levels are affected. In this regard, cAMP is the canonical second messenger coupled with H_2R, H_3R, and H_4R. For Gαs-coupled receptors, such as H_2R, agonist stimulation of cells results in an increase in cAMP levels, while for Gαi-coupled receptors, such as H_3R and H_4R, agonist stimulation of cells results in decreased cAMP. In the presence of a selective antagonist, a reverse response is achieved.

1. Design the experimental scheme for a 96-multi-well white plate taking into account having a standard curve of at least 12 points (*see* **Note 21**).
2. Collect the cells in a 15 mL centrifuge tube gently scraping them in their culture medium without washing (*see* **Note 22**).
3. Centrifuge for 5 min at 984 × *g* to obtain a cell pellet.
4. Discard supernatant and collect the cell pellet.
5. In the meantime prepare the desired stimuli in a volume of stimulation buffer to obtain a double concentrate of the final test concentration (for a 96-well plate 15 μL/well is the minimum volume required). If an antagonist is used, pretreat cells for 10 min before adding the stimulus (*see* **Notes 23** and **26**).
6. Prepare serial dilutions of the cAMP standard through serial titration from 1 mM to 0 using stimulation buffer.
7. Resuspend the cell pellet with the stimulation buffer (*see* Sect. 3.3.2) alone or with the final test concentration of antagonist prepared according to step 4, and pretreat cells for 10 min at RT.
8. Pipette into the assay plate the serial dilutions of the cAMP prepared as standard curve (*see* **step 5**; for a 96-well plate 30 μL/well is the minimum volume required).
9. Pipette into the assay plate the cell culture medium alone as a negative control (for a 96-well plate 30 μL/well is the minimum volume required).
10. After the pretreatment incubation, pipette into the assay plate the cell suspension (for a 96-well plate 15 μL/well is the minimum volume required).
11. Add to cell suspension the cell culture medium with compound previously prepared as described in point 5 (for a 96-well plate 15 μL/well is the minimum volume required).
12. Gently mix and shake the plate on a rocker shaker and check for the absence of air bubbles.
13. Incubate for 30 min at RT covering the plate with a TopSeal.

14. Pipette the 4X Eu-cAMP working solution (*see* Sect. 3.3.2) in each well of the assay plate (for a 96-well plate 15 μL/well of each reagent is the minimum volume required).
15. Pipette the 4X Ulight-anti-cAMP working solution (*see* Sect. 3.3.2) in each well of the assay plate (for a 96-well plate 15 μL/well of each reagent is the minimum volume required).
16. Incubate for 1 h at RT. Cover microplate with a TopSeal.
17. Measure the energy transfer by exciting the Eu^{3+} at 320 nm and record the allophycocyanin emission at both 620 and 665 nm using a TR-FRET compatible reader (*see* **Note 24**).
18. Results are calculated from the 665/620 nm ratio and usually expressed as a ratio. The ratio so determined is inversely proportional to the concentration of cAMP in the sample (*see* **Note 25**).

3.5 Permeability Assay

Tight junctions form a morphological and functional border between the lateral cell surface domains. In renal epithelial cells they directly contribute to maintaining the cell surface polarity, forming a barrier that prevents the diffusion of macromolecules, such as albumin, in the outer leaflet of the plasma membrane [100]. Paracellular permeability can be monitored with compounds that are fluorescently labeled. Thus, podocytes and tubular cells permselectivity to albumin can be analyzed by the use of FITC-labeled albumin. In particular, a model of the glomerular filtration function by cultured podocytes is described below.

1. Design the experimental scheme for a 24 black multi-well plate (*see* **Note 27**).
2. Prepare the receiver plate by adding 1 mL of high glucose cell culture medium.
3. Add the transwell insert to the well by merging the bottom of the insert into the medium in the lower compartment. Make sure of sterility preservation by using sterile tweezers and ensure that no air bubbles are trapped between the insert membrane and the medium.
4. Allow transwell inserts, equilibrate for 15 min at 37 °C in a 95% air/5% CO_2 humidified incubator.
5. Collect podocytes in a 15 mL centrifuge tube as described in Sect. 3.2.
6. Count cells with the Burker chamber.
7. Centrifuge at 984 × *g* for 5 min at RT to obtain a cell pellet.
8. Discard supernatant and resuspend cells in complete high glucose cell culture medium to obtain a final concentration of 50,000 cells/300 μL.

9. Gently add 300 μL/well of cells to the upper compartment and let the cells adhere to the membrane support by culturing for 26–24 h at 37 °C in a 95% air/5% CO_2 humidified incubator.
10. After testing for monolayer confluence, wash cells once with wash buffer (*see* **Note 2**) aspirating from the bottom side first and then from the top side (while, to replace the media or wash buffer, proceed in the opposite order; upper then lower), taking care of avoiding the cell culture surface damage (*see* **Note 28**).
11. Add 300 μL/well of fresh complete high glucose medium with the tested compound at the final required concentration in the upper compartment.
12. Replace the medium from the bottom compartment with 500 μL/well FITC-labeled BSA solution.
13. Conduct the assay at 37 °C in a 95% air/5% CO_2 humidified incubator.
14. At the selected time-point(s) quantify the trans-membrane flux of FITC-BSA measuring with a fluorescence plate reader (excitation: 495 nm, emission: 520 nm) the fluorescence activity of the medium in the top chamber corresponding to the podocyte monolayer permeability (Fig. 2).
15. Express the data as fold-change with respect to the control mean. Alternatively, determine the trans-membrane flux of FITC-BSA in micrograms/h, calculating the BSA concentration in the upper chamber using fluorescent arbitrary units of the albumin solution added to the bottom compartment, taking into account the volume of the upper one [101].

3.6 TEM

Among the different organs in body, the kidney is one of the most extensively investigated by electron microscopy, which is even considered to be an essential component of human diagnostic

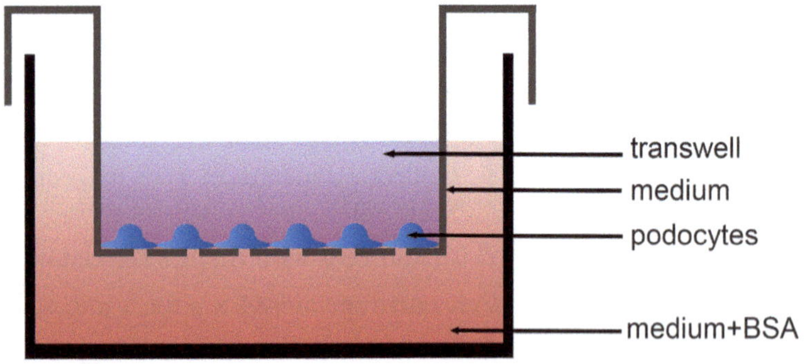

Fig. 2 Podocyte permeability assay. Podocyte permeability is evaluated with FITC-BSA assay using Transwell permeable supports. FITC-BSA is added into the bottom chamber medium. The monolayer permeability is assessed by measuring the fluorescence signal in the top chamber medium

renal pathology. Electron microscopic examination is a useful tool to study the ultrastructural morphology of renal cells, in particular podocytes and tubular epithelial cells, and it could be employed to evaluate ultrastructural alterations caused by histamine exposure. The techniques of fixing, dehydrating, and embedding specimens in the preparation for ultra-thin sectioning and electron microscopy are similar, in principle, to those used in preparing sections for light microscopy, with some modifications at each stage of the procedures because of the different requirements of the light and electron microscopes and the need to reduce even minor artifactual alterations of the sample to be observed. The fixation process profoundly affects the cell structural visualization; therefore, it must be carefully chosen. Formerly, osmium tetroxide, a good fixative and excellent stain for membrane lipids, was used in electron microscopy both as a fixative and a heavy metal stain to enhance the image contrast. However, some intracellular structures are lost in samples fixed with osmium tetroxide and, in the current methods, aldehyde fixation, using glutaraldehyde or a combination of glutaraldehyde and paraformaldehyde (i.e., Karnovsky's fixative), is performed. As some components of aldehyde-fixed cells, such as membranes, are extracted during dehydratation, a primary aldehyde fixation is usually followed by treatment with an osmium tetroxide solution (post-fixation). On the other hand, when the sample has to be prepared for immune-electron microscopy, it must be considered that osmium tetroxide negates immunogenicity of most tissue macromolecules and post-fixation should be omitted. For the same reason, divalent aldehydes such as glutaraldehyde induce more distortion of the tertiary structure of proteins than does formaldehyde, which should be preferred for immune-electron microscopy fixation protocols. Herein, it is described a simple method to embed podocytes grown as a thin layer without scraping them, thus allowing not only the study of the intracellular structure, but also the evaluation of the intercellular network.

3.6.1 Fixation of Cell Monolayers

1. Place the Millicell® culture plate inserts in a 24-multi-well plate and coat them with 300 μL of collagen 0.1% sterile solution. Collect podocytes in a 15 mL centrifuge tube as described in Sect. 3.2.
2. Count cells with the Burker chamber.
3. Centrifuge at 984 × g for 5 min at RT to obtain a cell pellet.
4. Discard supernatant and resuspend cells in complete high glucose cell culture medium.
5. Gently pipette 400 μL of culture medium into each insert and 600 μL into each well.

6. Seed 40,000 cells onto the inside of each insert above the membrane and place the multiwell into the cellular incubator.
7. After cell adhesion (generally 24 h of incubation at 37 °C in a 95% air/5% CO_2 humidified incubator), wash cells once and replace the medium with fresh complete high glucose medium containing the tested compound at the final expected concentration in the upper compartment.
8. Gently remove the culture medium and wash with 1% PBS to remove the excess protein derived from the culture.
9. Gently pipette 400 μL of Karnovsky's glutaraldehyde fixative in each insert. Incubate for at least 2 h at RT or overnight at 4 °C.
10. Rinse the membrane inserts with 1 mL of washing buffer; repeat three times. The sample can be stored in washing buffer at 4 °C for 4 days.
11. Cut the membranes along the insert border with plastic set of scissors. Do not use metal tool because metal ions react with aldehydes.
12. Post-fixate the membranes with phosphate-buffered 1% osmium tetroxide solution (*see* **Note 29**) for 1 h at RT.
13. Gently rinse the membranes in a 0.5% NaCl solution.

3.6.2 Dehydration

1. Dehydrate the samples (*see* **Notes 30** and **31**), as described in Table 3.

3.6.3 Infiltration and Embedding in Epoxy Resin

1. Embed in epoxy resin (e.g., Epon 812; *see* **Note 32**) as described in Table 4.
2. Prepare the embedding molds by placing small paper labels (with numbered codes in pencil) at the top of capsules.

Table 3
Dehydration procedure

30% acetone	**10 min**
40% acetone	10 min
50% acetone	10 min
60% acetone	10 min
70% acetone	10 min
80% acetone	10 min
90% acetone	20 min
100% acetone	2 changes of 20 min each

Table 4
Embedding procedure

1:1 mix of acetone:propylene oxide	2 changes of 10 min each
100% propylene oxide	2 changes of 20 min each
1:1 mix of propylene oxide:epon resin	2 changes of 20 min each
Epon resin	4 °C O/N
Fresh epon resin	45 °C for 1 h

3. Transfer each block into a capsule, orientate it, and then pipette resin to fill the capsule.
4. The blocks are polymerized at 60 °C for 48 h in a vacuum chamber.

3.6.4 Ultramicotome Sectioning

1. Trim the block to a trapezoid-shaped pyramid with the section area being as small as possible to include the part of the specimen (*see* **Note 33**).
2. Place the block into the specimen holder of the ultramicrotome and make sure that the block is firmly fastened.
3. Cut a semithin section of 0.5–1 μm thick with a glass knife.
4. Use a paint brush to transfer the semithin section to a drop of water on a microscope slide.
5. Place the slide on a hot plate to flatten the section, making it adherent to the slide.
6. Stain the section on a 70 °C hot plate with toluidine blue solution for 10 s until a gold rim is visible around the drop of stain. Wash off the section with dd H_2O and dry on the hotplate. This procedure allows observing the cellular structure into the section at the optical microscope to choose the area of interest.
7. Select the area of interest and trim the face of the block to a trapezium shape of approximately 0.4 mm^2, the longer side downward for ultra-thin sectioning.
8. Place a diamond knife in the knife holder of the ultramicrotome and check that it is tightly fastened and at a clearance of 6 degree angle.
9. Align the block face to the knife.
10. Fill the knife tray with either filtered dd H_2O or 10% ethanol so as to obtain a silvered reflection off the surface of the liquid (*see* **Note 34**).
11. Adjust the section thickness settings to 70 nm.

12. Either cut individual sections by hand or activate the motor (if the ultramicrotome has this function) and begin cutting continuous sections. Carefully lower the uncoated grid, dull side downward, onto the sections. The grid must be lowered parallel with the surface of the liquid in the tray and slowly push-over the kept sections to the center of the grid (*see* **Note 35**).
13. Place grids in a filter paper-lined Petri dish with the sections facing upward. Using uncoated grids the liquid will be absorbed through the grid mesh.
14. Allow the grids to properly dry for 24 h on the filter paper before staining.

3.6.5 Staining Ultra-Thin Sections

1. Place one drop of gadolinium triacetate per section onto wax in a 100 mm Petri dish.
2. Place the grid with the sections downward onto the drop, cover the Petri dish, and incubate for 20 min at RT.
3. Wash the grid with dd H_2O.
4. Pipet 2 mL of alkaline lead citrate into a 30 mm Petri dish.
5. Submerge the grids with the sections facing upward into alkaline lead citrate.
6. Cover the Petri dish and incubate for 10 min at RT. Do not breathe over the lead citrate stain to avoid CO_2 contamination.
7. Pick the grid out and carefully wash it with dd H_2O by either drop wash or immersing.
8. Allow the grids to properly dry for 24 h at 45 °C.

3.6.6 Micrographic Acquisition of Cell-Cell Junctions

1. Under the electron microscope, set the magnification at 10,000X.
2. Identify a cell-cell contact area of the cells cultured and take a photo, tacking care to overlay the scale bar.
3. Set the tight junction structure to the center of video-area and select the magnification at 70,000X. Focus the image and take a photo, tacking care to overlay the scale bar.
4. Collect at least ten images per section at both the magnifications, taking care not to pass by the same structure twice.
5. Repeat this procedure for each experimental group.

3.6.7 Qualitative and Semiquantitative Evaluation of Tight-Junction

1. Qualitative analysis of tight-junctions can be performed on the low-power TEM micrograph (10,000X), evaluating the length of the tight-junction and the content of electron-dense material located at the cytoplasmic insertion as well as the maintenance of the regular cell-cell contact area between adjacent cells.

2. Quantitative analysis of tight-junction should be carried out on high-power TEM micrograph (at least 70,000X), measuring the intercellular gap.
3. Launch ImageJ software (available at http://imagej.nih.gov/ij/download.html).
4. Open all the images collected.
5. Choose *analyze*; set measurements and select perimeter. Then click OK.
6. To set the scale, use the straight line selection tool to drag out a line across the scale bar over-laid on the photo. Select *analyze* and then *set scale*. The distance measured in pixels will be displayed. Enter the known distance (corresponding to that shown in the scale bar) and the unit of length. Then select *global*, to maintain the scale across all the images.
7. For each cell-cell contact area, using the straight line selection tool, drag out a line across the intercellular space bridged by the tight-junction, exactly perpendicular to the cellular edge. Then choose *analyze*; *measure*.
8. Repeat the procedure for each image collected.
9. Analyze the outputs with a suitable statistical software.

4 Notes

1. Paraformaldehyde crystals or powder dissolved in solution give off toxic formaldehyde vapors; ready-to-use solutions are strongly recommended. Use gloves and protective clothing. Handling and waste disposal should be done according to the guidelines of the local authorities.
2. 1 mM $MgCl_2$ and 1 mM $CaCl_2$ are added to the normal PBS 1X to preserve the cadherin-based junctions [75]. Such preservation has to be considered for every experiment involving adherent junctions.
3. When using nephrectomy samples, care should be taken to avoid using renal tissue adjacent to tumor and all local ethical permissions should be in place before tissue is obtained. The characteristics of the medical history of the individuals subjected to kidney removal that may interfere with the properties of the obtained cultures have to be taken into account. More specifically, for studies on histamine the possible induction of the amine by other relevant pathology in the medical history of each patient enrolled or by drugs has to be verified. Whether it is possible, measure circulating and tissue histamine levels.
4. Alternatively, collagenase digestion can be used for glomeruli dissociation [36]. In this case, incubate the specimens with

collagenase from *Clostridium histolyticum* type D at 0.5 mg/mL for 30 min at 37 °C before meshing the glomeruli remnants to meshes for glomerular fragmentation. On the basis of the sieve used, single cells can be separated and plate for mesangial cells and podocytes culture. This technique improves the efficiency of cell recovery, but the risk of over-digestion could affect podocytes' viability.

5. The phenotypic properties of cells are strictly dependent on the extracellular matrix composition. Both fibronectin and collagen greatly improve the initial adherence of mesangial and epithelial cells; however, these cells can be cultured in the absence of such matrices.
6. Epithelial cells are subject to contact inhibition. Therefore, they have to be split at sub-confluence. After the passage 3 their proliferative activity decreases and cells may adopt a spindle-like structure due to dedifferentiation which compromise their experimental use.
7. Substitute D-valine for L-valine prevents and arrests fibroblast growth, as this latter cell type does not contain the D-amino-acid-oxidase enzyme necessary to convert the D- to the L-isoform [102].
8. Mesangial cells phenotypic changes usually occur after about ten passages, when angiotensin II receptors are lost and no contraction to vasoactive hormones is achieved [103]. At this point the morphology changes with the development of stress fibers.
9. According to published criteria [32, 104–106], mesangial cells cultures grow as stellate cells in interwoven bundles. For immunohistochemical analysis: this cell type is positive for vimentin, alfa-SMA, myosin, PDGF-Rbeta and negative for GLEPP1, WT-1, cytokeratin 18, cytokeratin 19, FVIIIr:Ag, PECAM-1 (for a more complete list of key markers, *see* Table 2). Mesangial cells contract after stimulation with 100 ng/mL angiotensin II [32, 107, 108] and show phagocytosis of IgG-coated latex beads [32].
10. According to published criteria [36, 44, 106, 109] podocytes are polyhedral cells with a cobblestone-like appearance when confluent. For immunohistochemical analysis: this cell type is positive for cytokeratins 8, 18, and 19, vimentin, and laminin, while lack of reactivity with antibodies to smooth muscle-type myosin, CD45, and FVIIIr:Ag (for a more complete list of key markers, *see* Table 2). Lastly, podocytes show cytotoxicity and cytoskeletal alterations [110] in response to puromycin aminonucleoside (10, 20, and 50 mg/mL) or adriamycin (1, 2, and 5 mg/mL).

11. Tubular cells show marked positive staining for cytokeratin 19, minimal for desmin, and negative for FVIIIr:Ag and vimentin [1, 109, 111] (for a more complete list of key markers, *see* Table 2). Tubular cells are positive for alkaline phosphatase (determined by the naphtol AS-MX method) and show enhanced cAMP production after stimulation with 100 nM parathyroid hormone, but not with 1 mM antidiuretic hormone [109, 112].
12. The time required by trypsin EDTA 1X to remove adherent cells from a culture surface can depend on differences in trypsin activity or potency and on different cell line adhesion properties. Thus, a dose-titration when a new trypsin or cell type is cultured is strictly recommended. Incubating cells with too high a trypsin concentration for too long a time period will damage cell membranes and lead to cell death. Trypsin EDTA is inactivated by Ca^{2+} or Mg^{2+}.
13. Medium changes keep the cells healthy by providing fresh nutrients. The medium appearance has to be monitored. The medium color is due to the phenol red as pH indicator: when it turns to yellow the pH is reduced (acidic environment), when it turns to purple the pH is increased (alkaline environment, cell growth is inhibited). In both situations, the medium should be changed and/or cells need to be split. Cells require self-produced growth factor for optimal culturing. Thereby, if a rapid medium change is required (e.g., the day after thawing), collect the medium from the cell culture in a centrifuge tube and centrifuge for 3 min at 984 × *g*. After washing cells twice with PBS 1X refill the culture with two-thirds of fresh medium and one-third of old one, taking care not to pipette any cell pelleted-debris into the dishes/flasks.
14. Control samples are required to show whether label localization is correct. In particular, three types of controls are required. The primary antibody control shows the specificity of primary antibody binding to the antigen (positive control). The secondary antibody control shows the label is specific to the primary antibody label. This control is achieved by either eliminating the primary antibody or replacing it with the same amount of normal serum from the same species. With no primary antibody to bind the secondary antibody, no labeling should be seen. The secondary antibody control needs to be run in parallel with each experiment and for each antibody used. The label control shows the labeling is the result of label added during the procedure and not endogenous labeling or reaction products. Include a sample of cultured cells that is incubated in all of the buffers and detergents used in the experiment but no antibodies. These controls should be performed with each new sample or fixation or change in incubation condition [58].

15. Collagen coating allows an enhanced growth of cells on glass, alternatively other coating, such as polylysine, polyornithine, fibronectin, or laminin, can be used. Moreover, polylysine-coated coverslips are commercially available.
16. The CellMask™ plasma membrane stains provide staining in live cells due to the amphipathic molecules providing a lipophilic moiety for excellent membrane loading and a negatively charged hydrophilic dye for "anchoring" of the probe in the plasma membrane. The staining pattern is maintained after fixation with formaldehyde. Fixation has to be performed after the staining to avoid CellMask™ plasma membrane stain from entering the cytoplasm. The working solution should be freshly prepared.
17. A dilution titration could be necessary to set the specific condition for the antibody(ies) used. For anti-H_1R (H300, sc-20633) use 1.3 μg/mL; for anti H_2R (A20, sc-33973) use 1.3 μg/mL; for anti-hH_3R antibody use 1 μg/mL; anti-hH_4R (374–390) antibody use 2 μg/mL.
18. When Alexa-Conjugated secondary antibodies are employed, use a 1:350 dilution.
19. Different mounting media exist; however, an 80% glycerol in dd H_2O solution could be alternatively used, but extra time for drying is required and nailpolish can be used to seal the coverslip on the microscope slide. Any bubbles on the sample can drastically affect the fluorescence signal.
20. Triton X–100 can be added to the Blocking buffer to obtain a more efficient plasma membrane permeabilization necessary for the detection of intra-cellular targets.
21. A dilution titration can be necessary to set the specific condition of the antibody(ies) used. For anti-calnexin (AF18, sc-23954) and anti-lamin A/C (636, sc-7292) use a 2 μg/mL and 0.28 μg/mL concentration, respectively.
22. Crosstalk can be an issue in reading absorbance and fluorescence measurements. White plates reflect light and will maximize light output signals. For these reasons, white plates are commonly used for luminescent assays such as TR-FRET. In a multiplexing assay use a multichannel pipette or, even better a repetitive pipette for time-saving and minimizing systematic errors.
23. Collect the cells with a scraper instead of using Trypsin EDTA 1X enables assays to be performed with in-suspension cells preserving the transmembrane receptor integrity. Alternatively, the test can be performed on adherent cells, but white plates do not allow cell confluence to be checked.
24. If a reversible agonist is used, it has to be maintained in the medium also during the agonist stimulation. In this case,

prepare Stimulation buffer with either the antagonist at the final expected concentration or both the agonist and the antagonist at a double concentration or the final expected, respectively. In contrast, if an irreversible antagonist is used, after the pretreatment it has to be removed from the medium.

25. The generated signal is stable over a 24 h period at RT. If a delayed recording is performed take care not to expose the plate to direct light.
26. Alternatively, use the standard curve for a quantitative analysis of the IP-1 ng/mL or cAMP μg/mL produced. The use of software is recommended to minimize errors and for time-saving.
27. Generally, when the effect of an antagonist on cAMP levels has to be measured forskolin is used to induce the adenylyl cyclase activity. However, to study histamine in our renal cells, where more than one histamine receptor subtype is present, the use of forskolin is unnecessary; moreover, it can generate false-negative or positive data.
28. Crosstalk can be an issue in reading absorbance and fluorescence measurements, black plates absorb light and reduce background. When multiplexing a fluorescent assay, the use of a black plate would reduce fluorescent signal crosstalk and background with a reduction in luminescence. As the black plate does not allow the microscope visualization of cells, it is recommended to use a standard transparent plate till the assay is performed. When a reversible antagonist is used, it has to be maintained in the medium also during the agonist stimulation. In this case, prepare Stimulation buffer either with the antagonist at the final expected concentration or both the agonist and the antagonist at a double of the final expected concentration, respectively. In contrast, if an irreversible antagonist is used, after the pretreatment it has to be removed from the medium.
29. Take care not to allow pipette tips to come in contact with the fragile membrane when removing or adding cells, medium or wash buffer to the insert.
30. Since Osmium Tetroxide is toxic and volatile, all work should be performed in a fume hood using gloves and protective clothing. Handling and waste disposal should be done according to the guidelines of the local authorities.
31. Since propylene oxide is much more volatile than acetone, be careful not to allow the sample to be exposed to the air as damage will occur due to the rapid evaporation of the solvent.
32. The dehydrating times should be adjusted to size of sample. The purpose of the embedding medium is to provide a stable, hard matrix throughout a sample in order that very thin sections may be cut.

33. Epoxy-resin embedding offers the best results in terms of plasticity during ultra-sectioning, transparency, and thermal resistance under the electron beam. On the other hand, polymerized epoxy-resin are hydrophobic and therefore unsuited for immuno-electron microscopic studies because they heavily interfere with antigen-antibody interactions. Whenever a sample is prepared for immuno-electron microscopic purposes, hydrophilic acrylic resins should be substituted for epoxy resins.
34. At the ultramicrotome binoculars, using a clean razor blade, trim away the excess resin from each of the four sides of the block to obtain a trapezoid-shaped pyramid. Initially, leave a margin of resin around the specimen. Once a trapezoid shape has been achieved, use a dry glass knife to trim the front surface of the block until reaching the specimen. At this stage, semithin sections can be cut to view the whole specimen front section and select a particular of interest.
35. To manage shrinkage during sectioning, the sections can be easily expanded by floating in 10% ethanol put in the knife tray. If the sections still appear shrunken, they can be expanded with chloroform or acetone vapor. Use a cotton swab soaked in solvent and gently wave it over the sections. Be careful not to over-expand the sections as this can lead to damage to the embedding resin.
36. There are different techniques for collecting the sections, the easiest way to collect the sections onto a grid is to use uncoated grids and carefully lower the grid, dull side downward, onto the sections. If the grid is not lowered parallel with the sections floating over the surface of the liquid in the tray, the sections will be bunched up onto the side of the grid by surface tension effects. Placing a few good sections on a single grid and collecting multiple grids is preferable than trying to gather numerous sections onto the same grid. An alternative method is possible by putting the grid under the liquid in the knife tray, the glossy side upward, and gently surfacing the grid under the sections. Use uncoated grids to allow the liquid to drain through the grid holes; with coated grids, the liquid flows over the surface and may carry the sections away as it is raised under the sections.

References

1. Sharpe CC, Dockrell ME (2012) Primary culture of human renal proximal tubule epithelial cells and interstitial fibroblasts. Methods Mol Biol 806:175–185
2. Moreland RB (2006) In vitro models: research in physiology and pharmacology of the lower urinary tract. Br J Pharmacol 147(Suppl 2):S56–S61
3. Rosa AC, Grange C, Pini A et al (2013) Overexpression of histamine H(4) receptors in the kidney of diabetic rat. Inflamm Res 62:357–365

4. Veglia E, Moggio A, Pini A et al (2014) Histamine reduces ZO-1 tight-junction protein expression in human immortalized podocytes. In: Society BP (ed) Pharmacology 2014, London.
5. Pini A, Chazot PL, Veglia E et al (2015) H3 receptor renal expression in normal and diabetic rats. Inflamm Res 64:271–273
6. Veglia E, Grange C, Pini A et al (2015) Histamine receptor expression in human renal tubules: a comparative pharmacological evaluation. Inflamm Res 64:261–270
7. Veglia E, Pini A, Moggio A et al (2015) Histamine affects the glomerular slit diaphragm integrity through H_1R. Inflamm Res 64(Suppl1):S41
8. Al-Awqati Q, Oliver JA (2002) Stem cells in the kidney. Kidney Int 61:387–395
9. Tisher CC, Madsen MK, Verlander JW (1991) Functional morphology of the nephron. In: Hatano M (ed) Nephrology, vol I. Springer Japan, pp 19–38
10. Stewart KN, Hillis G, Roy-Chaudhury P et al (1995) Integrin distribution in normal kidney and cultured human glomerular cells. Exp Nephrol 3:140–141
11. Coleman RA, Wu DC, Liu J et al (2000) Expression of aquaporins in the renal connecting tubule. Am J Physiol Renal Physiol 279:F874–F883
12. Rahmoune H, Thompson PW, Ward JM et al (2005) Glucose transporters in human renal proximal tubular cells isolated from the urine of patients with non-insulin-dependent diabetes. Diabetes 54:3427–3434
13. Baer PC, Bereiter-Hahn J, Schubert R et al (2006) Differentiation status of human renal proximal and distal tubular epithelial cells in vitro: Differential expression of characteristic markers. Cells Tissues Organs 184:16–22
14. Muller T, Myrtek D, Bayer H et al (2006) Functional characterization of histamine receptor subtypes in a human bronchial epithelial cell line. Int J Mol Med 18:925–931
15. Zhai XY, Fenton RA, Andreasen A et al (2007) Aquaporin-1 is not expressed in descending thin limbs of short-loop nephrons. J Am Soc Nephrol 18:2937–2944
16. Jaszai J, Farkas LM, Fargeas CA et al (2010) Prominin-2 is a novel marker of distal tubules and collecting ducts of the human and murine kidney. Histochem Cell Biol 133:527–539
17. Wilson HM, Stewart KN (2012) Glomerular epithelial and mesangial cell culture and characterization. Methods Mol Biol 806: 187–201
18. Mount DB (2014) Thick ascending limb of the loop of Henle. Clin J Am Soc Nephrol 9:1974–1986
19. Pan C, Kumar C, Bohl S et al (2009) Comparative proteomic phenotyping of cell lines and primary cells to assess preservation of cell type-specific functions. Mol Cell Proteomics 8:443–450
20. Fish AJ, Michael AF, Vernier RL et al (1975) Human glomerular cells in tissue culture. Lab Invest 33:330–341
21. Holdsworth SR, Glasgow EF, Atkins RC et al (1978) Cell characteristics of cultured glomeruli from different animal species. Nephron 22:454–459
22. Holdsworth SR, Glasgow EF, Thomson NM et al (1978) Normal human glomerular cells in culture. J Pathol 126:231–237
23. Foidart JM, Foidart JB, Mahieu PR (1980) Synthesis of collagen and fibronectin by glomerular cells in culture. Ren Physiol 3:183–192
24. Kreisberg JI, Karnovsky MJ (1983) Glomerular cells in culture. Kidney Int 23:439–447
25. Krtil J, Platenik J, Kazderova M et al (2007) Culture methods of glomerular podocytes. Kidney Blood Press Res 30:162–174
26. Mene P, Stoppacciaro A (2009) Isolation and propagation of glomerular mesangial cells. Methods Mol Biol 466:3–17
27. Striker LJ, Doi T, Elliot S et al (1989) The contribution of glomerular mesangial cells to progressive glomerulosclerosis. Semin Nephrol 9:318–328
28. Sedor JR, Abboud HE (1984) Actions and metabolism of histamine in glomeruli and tubules of the human kidney. Kidney Int 26:144–152
29. Scheinman JI, Fish AJ, Brown DM et al (1976) Human glomerular smooth muscle (mesangial) cells in culture. Lab Invest 34:150–158
30. Ardaillou R (1996) Biology of glomerular cells in culture. Cell Biol Toxicol 12:257–261
31. Saleem MA, O'Hare MJ, Reiser J et al (2002) A conditionally immortalized human podocyte cell line demonstrating nephrin and podocin expression. J Am Soc Nephrol 13:630–638
32. Camussi G, Turello E, Tetta C et al (1990) Tumor necrosis factor induces contraction of mesangial cells and alters their cytoskeletons. Kidney Int 38:795–802
33. Doublier S, Ruotsalainen V, Salvidio G et al (2001) Nephrin redistribution on podocytes

is a potential mechanism for proteinuria in patients with primary acquired nephrotic syndrome. Am J Pathol 158:1723–1731
34. Coppo R, Fonsato V, Balegno S et al (2010) Aberrantly glycosylated IgA1 induces mesangial cells to produce platelet-activating factor that mediates nephrin loss in cultured podocytes. Kidney Int 77:417–427
35. Soukupova M, Holeckova E (1964) The latent period of explanted organs of newborn, adult and senile rats. Exp Cell Res 33:361–367
36. Striker GE, Striker LJ (1985) Glomerular cell culture. Lab Invest 53:122–131
37. Akis N, Madaio MP (2004) Isolation, culture, and characterization of endothelial cells from mouse glomeruli. Kidney Int 65:2223–2227
38. Takemoto M, Asker N, Gerhardt H et al (2002) A new method for large scale isolation of kidney glomeruli from mice. Am J Pathol 161:799–805
39. Shankland SJ, Pippin JW, Reiser J et al (2007) Podocytes in culture: past, present, and future. Kidney Int 72:26–36
40. Murakami A, Oshiro H, Kanzaki S et al (2010) A novel method for isolating podocytes using magnetic activated cell sorting. Nephrol Dial Transplant 25:3884–3890
41. Pavenstadt H, Kriz W, Kretzler M (2003) Cell biology of the glomerular podocyte. Physiol Rev 83:253–307
42. Mundel P, Reiser J, Kriz W (1997) Induction of differentiation in cultured rat and human podocytes. J Am Soc Nephrol 8:697–705
43. Delarue F, Virone A, Hagege J et al (1991) Stable cell line of T-SV40 immortalized human glomerular visceral epithelial cells. Kidney Int 40:906–912
44. Ardaillou N, Lelongt B, Turner N et al (1992) Characterization of a simian virus 40-transformed human podocyte cell line producing type IV collagen and exhibiting polarized response to atrial natriuretic peptide. J Cell Physiol 152:599–616
45. Rosa AC, Rattazzi L, Miglio G et al (2012) Angiotensin II induces tumor necrosis factor-alpha expression and release from cultured human podocytes. Inflamm Res 61:311–317
46. Taub ML, Yang IS, Wang Y (1989) Primary rabbit kidney proximal tubule cell cultures maintain differentiated functions when cultured in a hormonally defined serum-free medium. In Vitro Cell Dev Biol 25:770–775
47. Yang AH, Gould-Kostka J, Oberley TD (1987) In vitro growth and differentiation of human kidney tubular cells on a basement membrane substrate. In Vitro Cell Dev Biol 23:34–46
48. Heidrich HG, Dew ME (1977) Homogeneous cell populations from rabbit kidney cortex. Proximal, distal tubule, and renin-active cell isolated by free-flow electrophoresis. J Cell Biol 74:780–788
49. Hammond TG (1992) Analysis and isolation of renal tubular cells by flow cytometry. Kidney Int 42:997–1005
50. Stanton RC, Mendrick DL, Rennke HG et al (1986) Use of monoclonal antibodies to culture rat proximal tubule cells. Am J Physiol 251:C780–C786
51. Wilson PD, Dillingham MA, Breckon R et al (1985) Defined human renal tubular epithelia in culture: growth, characterization, and hormonal response. Am J Physiol 248(3 Pt 2):F436–F443
52. Racusen LC, Monteil C, Sgrignoli A et al (1997) Cell lines with extended in vitro growth potential from human renal proximal tubule: characterization, response to inducers, and comparison with established cell lines. J Lab Clin Med 129:318–329
53. Ryan MJ, Johnson G, Kirk J et al (1994) HK-2: an immortalized proximal tubule epithelial cell line from normal adult human kidney. Kidney Int 45:48–57
54. Kenakin T (2003) Predicting therapeutic value in the lead optimization phase of drug discovery. Nat Rev Drug Discov 2:429–438
55. Abdolzade-Bavil A, Hayes S, Goretzki L et al (2004) Convenient and versatile subcellular extraction procedure, that facilitates classical protein expression profiling and functional protein analysis. Proteomics 4:1397–1405
56. Cox B, Emili A (2006) Tissue subcellular fractionation and protein extraction for use in mass-spectrometry-based proteomics. Nat Protoc 1:1872–1878
57. Murray CI, Barrett M, Van Eyk JE (2009) Assessment of ProteoExtract subcellular fractionation kit reveals limited and incomplete enrichment of nuclear subproteome from frozen liver and heart tissue. Proteomics 9:3934–3938
58. Burry RW (2011) Controls for immunocytochemistry: an update. J Histochem Cytochem 59:6–12
59. Coons AH, Chreech HJ, Jones RN et al (1942) The demonstration of pneumococcal antigen in tissues by the use of fluorescent antibody. J Immunol 45:159–170
60. Odell ID, Cook D (2013) Immunofluorescence techniques. J Invest Dermatol 133:e4

61. Larson JD, Rodgers ML, Hoskins AA (2014) Visualizing cellular machines with colocalization single molecule microscopy. Chem Soc Rev 43:1189–1200
62. Seifert R, Strasser A, Schneider EH et al (2013) Molecular and cellular analysis of human histamine receptor subtypes. Trends Pharmacol Sci 34:33–58
63. Seifert R, Schneider EH, Dove S et al (2011) Paradoxical stimulatory effects of the "standard" histamine H4-receptor antagonist JNJ7777120: the H4 receptor joins the club of 7 transmembrane domain receptors exhibiting functional selectivity. Mol Pharmacol 79:631–638
64. Emami-Nemini A, Roux T, Leblay M et al (2013) Time-resolved fluorescence ligand binding for G protein-coupled receptors. Nat Protoc 8:1307–1320
65. Cottet M, Faklaris O, Maurel D et al (2012) BRET and time-resolved FRET strategy to study GPCR oligomerization: from cell lines toward native tissues. Front Endocrinol 3:92
66. Lohse MJ, Nuber S, Hoffmann C (2012) Fluorescence/bioluminescence resonance energy transfer techniques to study G-protein-coupled receptor activation and signaling. Pharmacol Rev 64:299–336
67. Mathis G (1999) HTRF(R) technology. J Biomol Screen 4:309–314
68. Bazin H, Trinquet E, Mathis G (2002) Time resolved amplification of cryptate emission: a versatile technology to trace biomolecular interactions. J Biotechnol 82:233–250
69. Degorce F, Card A, Soh S et al (2009) HTRF: A technology tailored for drug discovery—a review of theoretical aspects and recent applications. Curr Chem Geneomics 3:22–32
70. Brown D (2000) Tight junctions: guardians of the paracellular pathway. Kidney Int 57:2652–2653
71. Denker BM, Sabath E (2011) The biology of epithelial cell tight junctions in the kidney. J Am Soc Nephrol 22:622–625
72. Benzing T (2004) Signaling at the slit diaphragm. J Am Soc Nephrol 15:1382–1391
73. Takeuchi K, Kishioka C, Ishinaga H et al (2001) Histamine alters gene expression in cultured human nasal epithelial cells. J Allergy Clin Immunol 107:310–314
74. Wegener J, Seebach J (2014) Experimental tools to monitor the dynamics of endothelial barrier function: a survey of in vitro approaches. Cell Tissue Res 355:485–514
75. Awad AS, Rouse M, Liu L et al (2008) Activation of adenosine 2A receptors preserves structure and function of podocytes. J Am Soc Nephrol 19:59–68
76. Bondeva T, Ruster C, Franke S et al (2009) Advanced glycation end-products suppress neuropilin-1 expression in podocytes. Kidney Int 75:605–616
77. Jin X, Wang W, Mao J et al (2014) Overexpression of Myo1e in mouse podocytes enhances cellular endocytosis, migration, and adhesion. J Cell Biochem 115:410–419
78. Li SY, Huang PH, Yang AH et al (2014) Matrix metalloproteinase-9 deficiency attenuates diabetic nephropathy by modulation of podocyte functions and dedifferentiation. Kidney Int 86:358–369
79. Mundel P, Kriz W (1995) Structure and function of podocytes: an update. Anat Embryol 192:385–397
80. Shapiro L, Fannon AM, Kwong PD et al (1995) Structural basis of cell-cell adhesion by cadherins. Nature 374:327–337
81. Yonemura S, Itoh M, Nagafuchi A et al (1995) Cell-to-cell adherens junction formation and actin filament organization: similarities and differences between non-polarized fibroblasts and polarized epithelial cells. J Cell Sci 108:127–142
82. Lee DB, Huang E, Ward HJ (2006) Tight junction biology and kidney dysfunction. Am J Physiol Renal Physiol 290:F20–F34
83. Schnabel E, Anderson JM, Farquhar MG (1990) The tight junction protein ZO-1 is concentrated along slit diaphragms of the glomerular epithelium. J Cell Biol 111: 1255–1263
84. Drumond MC, Deen WM (1995) Hindered transport of macromolecules through a single row of cylinders: application to glomerular filtration. J Biomech Eng 117:414–422
85. Kestila M, Lenkkeri U, Mannikko M et al (1998) Positionally cloned gene for a novel glomerular protein—nephrin—is mutated in congenital nephrotic syndrome. Mol Cell 1:575–582
86. Reiser J, Kriz W, Kretzler M et al (2000) The glomerular slit diaphragm is a modified adherens junction. J Am Soc Nephrol 11:1–8
87. Gordon RE (2014) Electron microscopy: a brief history and review of current clinical application. Methods Mol Biol 1180: 119–135
88. Gardner TW, Lesher T, Khin S et al (1996) Histamine reduces ZO-1 tight-junction protein expression in cultured retinal microvascular endothelial cells. Biochem J 320:717–721

89. Chazot PL, Hann V, Wilson C et al (2001) Immunological identification of the mammalian H3 histamine receptor in the mouse brain. Neuroreport 12:259–262
90. van Rijn RM, Chazot PL, Shenton FC et al (2006) Oligomerization of recombinant and endogenously expressed human histamine H_4receptors. Mol Pharmacol 70:604–615
91. Cannon KE, Chazot PL, Hann V et al (2007) Immunohistochemical localization of histamine H3 receptors in rodent skin, dorsal root ganglia, superior cervical ganglia, and spinal cord: potential antinociceptive targets. Pain 129:76–92
92. Dijkstra D, Leurs R, Chazot P et al (2007) Histamine downregulates monocyte CCL2 production through the histamine H_4receptor. J Allergy Clin Immunol 120:300–307
93. Baumer W, Wendorff S, Gutzmer R et al (2008) Histamine H_4receptors modulate dendritic cell migration through skin--immunomodulatory role of histamine. Allergy 63:1387–1394
94. Dijkstra D, Stark H, Chazot PL et al (2008) Human inflammatory dendritic epidermal cells express a functional histamine H_4receptor. J Invest Dermatol 128:1696–1703
95. Grandi D, Shenton FC, Chazot PL et al (2008) Immunolocalization of histamine H_3receptors on endocrine cells in the rat gastrointestinal tract. Histol Histopathol 23:789–798
96. Morini G, Becchi G, Shenton FC et al (2008) Histamine $H_3$and H_4 receptors are expressed on distinct endocrine cell types in the rat fundic mucosa. Inflamm Res 57:S57–S58
97. van Rijn RM, van Marle A, Chazot PL et al (2008) Cloning and characterization of dominant negative splice variants of the human histamine H_4 receptor. Biochem J 414: 121–131
98. Oliveira Arcolino F, Tort Piella A, Papadimitriou E et al (2015) Human urine as a noninvasive source of kidney cells. Stem Cells Int 2015:362562
99. Erdmann B, Fuxe K, Ganten D (1996) Subcellular localization of angiotensin II immunoreactivity in the rat cerebellar cortex. Hypertension 28:818–824
100. Matter K, Balda MS (2003) Functional analysis of tight junctions. Methods 30:228–234
101. Macconi D, Abbate M, Morigi M et al (2006) Permselective dysfunction of podocyte-podocyte contact upon angiotensin II unravels the molecular target for renoprotective intervention. Am J Pathol 168:1073–1085
102. Gilbert SF, Migeon BR (1975) D-valine as a selective agent for normal human and rodent epithelial cells in culture. Cell 5:11–17
103. Kreisberg JI, Venkatachalam M, Troyer D (1985) Contractile properties of cultured glomerular mesangial cells. Am J Physiol 249: F457–F463
104. Biancone L, Tetta C, Turello E et al (1992) Platelet-activating factor biosynthesis by cultured mesangial cells is modulated by proteinase inhibitors. J Am Soc Nephrol 2:1251–1261
105. Davies M (1994) The mesangial cell: a tissue culture view. Kidney Int 45:320–327
106. Moutabarrik A, Nakanishi I, Zaid D et al (1994) Interleukin-1-beta activation of cultured glomerular epithelial cells. Exp Nephrol 2:196–204
107. Ausiello DA, Kreisberg JI, Roy C et al (1980) Contraction of cultured rat glomerular cells of apparent mesangial origin after stimulation with angiotensin II and arginine vasopressin. J Clin Invest 65:754–760
108. Singhal PC, Scharschmidt LA, Gibbons N et al (1986) Contraction and relaxation of cultured mesangial cells on a silicone rubber surface. Kidney Int 30:862–873
109. Biancone L, David S, Della Pietra V et al (1994) Alternative pathway activation of complement by cultured human proximal tubular epithelial cells. Kidney Int 45: 451–460
110. Coers W, Huitema S, van der Horst ML et al (1994) Puromycin aminonucleoside and adriamycin disturb cytoskeletal and extracellular matrix protein organization, but not protein synthesis of cultured glomerular epithelial cells. Exp Nephrol 2:40–50
111. Conaldi PG, Biancone L, Bottelli A et al (1997) Distinct pathogenic effects of group B coxsackieviruses on human glomerular and tubular kidney cells. J Virol 71:9180–9187
112. Detrisac CJ, Sens MA, Garvin AJ et al (1984) Tissue culture of human kidney epithelial cells of proximal tubule origin. Kidney Int 25:383–390

Chapter 11

Histamine and the Kidney: In Vivo Animal Models

Alessandro Pini, Eleonora Veglia, and Arianna Carolina Rosa

Abstract

Animal models have been, and for the foreseeable future, will remain pivotal to bridge the gap between the test tube and the human condition. In particular, the use of an animal model provides the unique chance to study the onset and the progression of renal disease, approaching it simultaneously at the functional, morphological, and biochemical levels. Thereby, in vivo models offer the ideal opportunity to develop effective therapy for the optimal management of renal diseases. More specifically, the evaluation of renal functional and morphological parameters can be used to investigate the role of histamine and its receptors in renal (patho)-physiology and to validate histamine receptors as new pharmacological targets in renal diseases. Within this chapter a suitable in vivo model to study diabetic nephropathy and some of the most important parameters to monitor the functional and morphological integrity of the kidney are described.

Key words Animal models, In vivo, Kidney, Renal function, Renal morphology

1 Introduction

Research involving animals is a critical step in understanding physiology, pathophysiology, and the development of therapies in both humans and animals. For decades animal models have provided valuable insights into kidney biology and the pathogenesis of acute and chronic kidney disease, ranging from hypertension and diabetes, to renal manifestations of systemic disease such as lupus and diseases primarily affecting the kidney such as glomerulonephritis and tubular necrosis [1]. Indeed, although different in vitro, ex vivo organ culture [2] and on-chip [3] systems have been developed, the whole living organism remains the most suitable and reliable model to study the complex systems underling renal physiology and pathology. Relevant anatomical and functional differences do exist between animals and humans. For instance, important structural issues include the unilobular-unipapillary structure of rodent, rabbit, and dog kidneys compared with the multipapillary kidney of humans, pigs, and sheep [4] and the gender-related renal anatomical dimorphism found in mice [1]. Thereby, animal renal phenotypes are greatly influenced by species

Ekaterini Tiligada and Madeleine Ennis (eds.), *Histamine Receptors as Drug Targets*, Methods in Pharmacology and Toxicology, DOI 10.1007/978-1-4939-6843-5_11, © Springer Science+Business Media LLC 2017

and strain. Consequently, the choice of the most appropriate animal models is a critical point. The most popular species for modeling human disease are rodents. In particular, mice are one of the most used because of their small size and their ability to be genetically manipulated. The possibility of generating genetically defined strains permits the generation of metabolic or immunological variants leading to spontaneous disease models. However, different limitations implied with the use of mice must be taken in account. Surgical manipulations are widely used to model human disease. These may reproduce the injury that causes renal disease (e.g., ureteric obstruction), reproduce the consequences of renal injury (e.g., renal ischemia, reduction in renal mass), or involve collection of specimens from microenvironments [1]. The small size of mice may lead to more difficult procedures, such as blood pressure measurement [5]. Despite these limitations in transferability, the ongoing technical advances, with new and efficient gene transfer techniques [6] and the use of human mouse transgenic animals [7], may help close the gap. Moreover, animal models of renal disease faithfully reproduce all aspects of the human pathophysiology and clinical syndromes, whereas many models of reproducing particular aspects of kidney disease also exist [8].

1.1 The Kidney

The kidneys are paired retroperitoneal bean-shaped organs belonging to the urinary system. Their complex anatomical different structures reflect their functional role in filtration and reabsorption. Their primary function is the excretion of waste products resulting from protein metabolism and muscle contraction.

Each kidney is surrounded by a thin layer of fibrous connective tissue, the renal capsule, which provides a stiff outer shell to maintain the shape of the soft inner tissues. Macroscopically, the kidney is distinguished into cortex, with a granular appearance, and medulla with a striated appearance. The cortical area is clearly defined from the inverted conical or pyramid-shaped medulla, whose apex protrudes into the renal calyces. These protrusions are called renal papillae. Within these structures, several hundred thousand functionally independent units called nephrons can be distinguished. Each nephron is composed of a glomerulus, the Bowman's capsule, the proximal tubule, the loop of Henlé, the distal tubule, and the collecting tubule. Along each tract of the nephron several different and compelling processes to regulate water and soluble substances in the blood by filtering and reabsorbing take place.

The glomerulus is composed of a capillary tuft surrounded by Bowman's capsule, which together constitute the renal corpuscle. Within the spaces between glomerular, capillaries mesangium can be observed. The Bowman's capsule consists of a visceral layer, formed by podocytes, surrounding the glomerulus and a parietal layer bordering the renal corpuscle. Between these two layers is the urinary space where primary urine is produced. Pedicles of adjacent podocytes interact with the glomerular basement membrane (GBM) and communicate through signaling at the slit diaphragm (SD). This unique architecture is essential for blood plasma ultrafiltration. All molecules below the molecular size of albumin (that is, 68 kDa) pass the filter and enter the tubule, whereas a high osmotic gradient concentrates the filtrate [9].

The proximal tubule consists of a pars convoluta and a pars recta. Its simple cuboidal epithelium is responsible for absorption of amino acids, proteins, glucose, ions, water thanks to their brush border. The proximal tubule is contiguous to the loop of Henlé, a U-shaped loop consisting of a descending portion, highly permeable to water, and an ascending portion, which actively transports ions. The distal tubule follows the loop of Henlé. The cells of its lining epithelium are responsible for active transport of ions under hormonal control (e.g., aldosterone). Finally, the collecting tubule is responsible for water reabsorption under vasopressin and the antidiuretic hormone (ADH), acting on intercalated cells and principal cells, respectively.

1.2 Renal Diseases

Kidney diseases have different manifestations and aetiologies. A first diversification distinguishes between Acute Kidney Injury (AKI), which generally reverts with no long-term consequences, and Chronic Kidney Disease (CKD), which normally progresses toward the end-stage renal disease (ESRD). However, their evaluation is similar. Urine analysis is not considered very appropriate for differentiating AKI from CKD. The most definitive method to distinguish acute from chronic disease is histological findings. AKI is characterized by a rapid decline in the glomerular filtration rate (GFR) and retention of nitrogenous waste products such as blood urea nitrogen (BUN) and creatinine [10, 11]. For diagnosis and management, AKI can be divided into: (1) disease characterized by renal hypoperfusion, in which the integrity of renal parenchymal tissue is preserved; (2) diseases involving renal parenchymal tissue; (3) diseases associated with the acute obstruction of the urinary tract. Most AKI is caused by ischemia or nephrotoxins and is associated with acute tubular necrosis.

CKD is defined as kidney damage with or without decreased GFR. However, its staging is based on GFR estimation [12]. Notably, CKD has been recognized as a risk factor for both progression to end-stage renal disease (ESRD) and cardiovascular morbidity and mortality [13–15]. The two main causes of chronic kidney disease are diabetes and high blood pressure, which are responsible for up to two-thirds of the cases. In particular, diabetic nephropathy is a major cause of illness and death in diabetes, being the single most common cause of ESRD worldwide. The hallmark of diabetic nephropathy is persistent albuminuria (>300 mg/24 h). Moreover, it has been recognized that microalbuminuria (>30 mg/24 h) strongly predicts the development of diabetic nephropathy in both type 1 and type 2 diabetes [16, 17]. Histologically, thickening of the GBM can be observed as well as afferent and efferent glomerular arteriolar hyalinosis. Another key feature is mesangial expansion, primarily due to absolute and relative increases in mesangial matrix [18]. In contrast, interstitial expansion is primarily due to an increase in the cellular component of this renal compartment [19].

1.3 In Vivo Models of Acute Kidney Injury (AKI)

AKI is a syndrome that arises through many triggering events in clinical situations, including nephrotoxic therapeutic drugs, environmental contaminants and poisons, urinary tract obstructions, bacterial toxins, ischemic episodes and, frequently in clinical practice, a sequential or concomitant presence of several of these factors. Since the different aetiologies of AKI are multifold, a large number of animal models have been developed to mimic the clinical conditions of renal failure [20]. Among the different models, glycerol-induced renal failure closely mimics the rhabdomyolysis; ischemia/reperfusion-induced AKI simulates the hemodynamic changes; drug-induced-AKI (e.g., gentamicin, cisplatin, NSAID, ifosfamide, and radio contrast agents) mimics the renal failure secondary to drug administration; sepsis-induced AKI simulates infection-induced renal failure. Conventional AKI models are the result of kidney ischemia/reperfusion (pre-renal cause progressing to parenchymal AKI), exposure to endogenous or exogenous toxins (including those released in sepsis), and urinary tract obstruction (post-renal cause progressing to parenchymal AKI) [21]. Clinically, the leading cause of AKI is ischemia, which may result from a variety of conditions, such as decreased cardiac output, renal vascular occlusion or obstruction, and kidney transplantation.

One of the main causes of AKI, namely ischemia/reperfusion, triggers functional and structural alterations affecting mainly proximal tubular cells and the endothelium [22, 23], finally leading to inflammatory cells recruitment. The most widely used model is warm renal ischemia/reperfusion, either bilateral (the most frequent clinical situation) or unilateral, the latter with or without contralateral nephrectomy [20, 21, 24]. Many species (pigs, dogs, rabbits, rats, and mice) have been used to study ischemia/reperfusion, with rats among the most widely chosen animals. For comparison, the unilateral ureteral obstruction (UUO) model does not induce any increase in serum creatinine, being unilateral. This model is generally used to investigate mechanisms involved in the AKI-to-CKD transition [25]. This model is reproducible across laboratories and mice strains, there is an internal control in each mouse (the contralateral, non-obstructed kidney), and time to reach the main features of CKD is short (2 weeks), allowing easy testing of therapeutic approaches [26], although it is more useful to study the molecular mechanisms for CKD.

Drug- or toxin-induced AKI studies belong to the field of toxicology. A variety of exogenous (mainly drugs such as cisplatin, folic acid) or endogenous (e.g., heme-containing proteins) toxins cause AKI in humans and in experimental animals [20, 24]. Among the different models developed, the glycerol-induced AKI is one of the most used and better characterized. This model closely mimics the clinical conditions of rhabdomyolysis in humans, as the intramuscular injection of glycerol into both hind legs of rats or mice promotes abrupt rhabdomyolysis and AKI [27] due to ischemic injury and tubular nephrotoxicity, inflammation, and oxidative stress caused by myoglobin and tubular obstruction by casts [28]. The renal injury induced by glycerol is maximal after 3 days and is reversible within 8 days.

Animal models of sepsis-associated AKI use either injection of bacterial lipopolysaccharide (LPS) or cecal puncture and ligation [29]. The first is an acute model lasting 72–96 h characterized by a high reproducibility. However, the induced damage does not reproduce bacterial proliferation. To circumvent this limit, the less reproducible model of cecal-puncture and ligation, where bacteria are released into the peritoneum, can be performed.

1.4 In Vivo *Models of Chronic Kidney Disease (CKD)*

Chronic kidney diseases result from recurrent or progressive injuries in glomeruli, tubules, interstitium, and/or vasculature. In order to study pathogenesis, mechanisms, and effects of therapeutic approaches, many animal models have been developed, including spontaneous, genetic, and induced models. However, these models do not exactly simulate human diseases, and most of them are strain-, gender-, or age-dependent [30]. Thereby, choosing the correct model to address specific hypotheses is critical. The huge number of existing models does not allow a fully comprehensive review, and only some selected examples will be discussed herein. Subtotal (5/6) nephrectomy has been extensively used to study glomerulosclerosis. This non-immunological model is the equivalent to humans having lost part of the kidney functional mass and progressing despite removal of the original cause of kidney injury. The advantages of this model include robust functional parameters (e.g., proteinuria, GFR, and secondary hypertension), reliable induction in rodents, which display progressive glomerular and tubulo-interstitial injury, loss of remnant nephrons, and development of systemic and glomerular hypertension. However, limitations of the model include surgical intervention, with a high mortality rate, especially in mice.

The different forms of glomerulonephritis can be divided into acquired (e.g., focal segmental glomerulosclerosis, membranous nephropathy, IgA nephropathy, lupus nephritis, amyloidosis) and hereditary [e.g., Alport syndrome model [31]].

Chronic tubulointerstitial nephritis is characterized by tubular atrophy, interstitial fibrosis, and interstitial inflammation in the absence of significant glomerular disease [32]. Although models to induce chronic tubulointerstitial nephritis are usually secondary to ischemia, proteinuria, AKI, or other models appropriately titrated, a specific model can be generated by feeding mice with adenine for 16 weeks [33, 34] or watering with lead acetate over 90 days [35].

Renal endothelial cell injury includes hemolytic uremic syndrome and preeclampsia. The first can be modeled by shiga toxin intraperitoneal injection, although the full spectrum of hemolytic uremic syndrome with this model is achieved only in baboons [36]. Therefore, H-deficient mice transgenically generated are preferred. Preeclampsia can be surgically induced by aortic and bilateral ovarian artery constriction, which results in reduced uterine perfusion pressure in pregnant rats by gestational day 14. This model is characterized by hypertension, proteinuria, small pup size, and functional and histological renal damage [37, 38].

Particular and specific consideration has to be given to diabetic nephropathy. Diabetic nephropathy is a major microvascular complication of both Type 1 and Type 2 diabetes mellitus, being one of the most important causes of end-stage renal disease (ESRD) in Western nations. About one-third of diabetic patients start to show persistently high urinary albumin excretion, thus being at high risk to develop in primis diabetic ESRD, but also cardiovascular diseases and premature mortality, even without progression to ESRD [39]. Notably, although the natural history of diabetic renal disease differs between Type 1 and Type 2 diabetes, microalbuminuria and the progression to overt proteinuria are the most common clinical features [40]. Indeed, the renal risk is currently equivalent and the time to proteinuria from the onset of diabetes and the time to ESRD from the onset of proteinuria are similar in the two types of diabetes [41, 42]. Diabetic nephropathy is defined by persistent albuminuria (>300 mg/d or >200 μg/min), progressive decline in the glomerular filtration rate (GFR), or both. Different in vivo models of diabetes can be performed to induce diabetic nephropathy. These include Type 1 and Type 2 diabetes models that can be chemically or genetically induced. Although a large number of murine models of DN including artificially induced, spontaneous, and genetically engineered (knockout and transgenic) animal models have been developed, it should be taken into account that none of them develops renal changes sufficiently reflecting those seen in humans. Thereby, the Animal Models of Diabetic Complications Consortium (AMDCC) recommends the constant search for new validated models to replicate a more than 50% decline in GFR over the lifetime of the animal; a greater than 10-fold increase in albuminuria compared with controls for that strain at the same age and gender; mesangial sclerosis (a 50% increase in mesangial volume), any degree of arteriolar hyalinosis, a GBM thickening >25% increase compared with baseline, and tubulointerstitial fibrosis. In the absence of more accurate models, the choice between chemically inbred and genetically modified mice has to be performed. In this regard, one of the best characterized and most extensively studied is the streptozotocin (STZ)-induced model. Within this model, which is associated with reliable and consistent structural and functional deficits, hyperglycemia occurs because of the toxin-induced destruction of pancreatic Beta-islet cells [43]. This is a Type I diabetes chemically induced model, but the development and progression of diabetic nephropathy has been widely demonstrated to be closely associated with hyperglycemia. From this perspective, diabetic nephropathy development does not significantly differ between the two main types of diabetes and the use of a unique reproducible and well-validated animal model of diabetic nephropathy to obtain significant results in a very new field represents the best ethical choice. The STZ model can be performed by two different protocols: single high-dose intraperitoneal injection and multiple low-dose injection. This latter approach induces only a partial damage of pancreatic islets, triggering an inflammatory process that causes the further loss of β-cell activity, which ultimately results in insulin deficiency and hyperglycemia. This response more closely resembles the pathogenesis and morphological changes associated with Type 1 diabetes and is more appropriate to study diabetic nephropathy than the single high-dose approach. Most notably, the low-dose approach minimizes the acute nephrotoxicity induced by STZ and which can be considered an important basis to evaluate potential pharmacological strategies [44]. On the other hand, relevant hierarchical differences (DBA/2 < C57BL/6 < BALB/c) in STZ sensitivity among strains have been documented [45]. Therefore, although the DBA/2 strain is preferred, when another strain is used a tritiation of STZ doses or a second re-administration of STZ after 7 weeks of diabetes should be performed. The detailed protocol for the multiple low-dose STZ-diabetes induction is described in Sect. 3.1. In comparison to chemically induced diabetes, genetically engineered murine models provide valuable insights into the role of pathogenetic genes and molecular mechanisms responsible for diabetic nephropathy. Among the different genetically induced models of diabetic nephropathy, the more robust models currently available are the OVE26 and the eNOS$^{-/-}$/db/db mice, which develop kidney injury most closely resembling that seen in humans.

1.5 Renal Integrity Assessment

Among the current tools used to evaluate renal function, biochemical measurements are the most commonly used and include evaluation of creatinine clearance, by analyzing the serum, plasma, and albumin to creatinine ratio (ACR). Urine analysis of laboratory animals has been possible since the introduction of metabolic cages. The metabolic cage was developed to be able to control total intake of food and water and the excretion of urine and feces. In addition, it is possible to efficiently collect non-contaminated samples of urine and feces. The fundamental aspects of urine collection are: (1) ease of collection, (2) quality of sample, (3) prevention of contamination, (4) severity of procedures used, (5) minimal levels of pain caused to the animal, and (6) refinement of methods to reduce stress or distress [46]. In this regard, metabolic cages offer unquestionable advantages, although animal distress cannot be ruled out. Evidence exists to suggest altered neurohumoral control in rodents housed in metabolic cages [47–50] and sustained changes in cardiovascular function have also been demonstrated, which could potentially affect renal function [51]. Metabolic cages allow a 24-h urine collection, the best choice for a quantitative urine analysis [46]. A spot urine collection could be suitable for a qualitative analysis, but it is largely influenced by body hydration. Quantitative urine analysis includes the estimation of protein excretion, urinary-albumin concentration, albumin (protein) to creatinine ratio (ACR and APR respectively), and creatinine clearance. In particular, albumin should be considered the best parameter to evaluate podocyte detachment and podocyte loss (podocytopenia). So far, since albuminuria rather than proteinuria is the hallmark of glomerular disease, the measurement of total proteinuria only is not sufficient but has to be complemented with albumin urinary content. In particular, albuminuria and microalbuminuria have been recognized as specific biomarkers of diabetic nephropathy. Virtually no albumin is present in the urine when the kidneys are functioning properly. However, albumin may be detected in the urine even in the early stages of kidney disease. As protein and consequently albumin concentration varies with the volume of urine eliminated, the APR or even better the ACR (expressed as μg/mg) is preferentially measured to correct for urine dilution [52]. Creatinine is a by-product of muscle metabolism eliminated almost exclusively in urine and the conversion to creatinine proceeds at a constant rate. Moreover, the creatinine clearance determination can be used as a reliable method to measure the estimated glomerular filtration rate (eGFR). GFR is generally accepted to reflect the number of normally functioning glomeruli in the kidney [53]. eGFR measurement, by creatine clearance, is the less expensive method even if it is approximate because of the problems of accurate urine collection and a risk of overestimation. The use of creatinine measurement as a tool to evaluate renal function in mice has been called into question since Meyer et al. (1985) reported that creatinine levels in the blood (plasma) of mice measured by the Jaffe´ alkaline picrate method yielded significantly higher levels (three to five times) than those measured by high performance liquid chromatography (HPLC) [54]. These studies concluded that the Jaffé method is affected by noncreatinine chromogens [55]. Indeed, HPLC is considered the standard for creatinine measurement instead of the colorimetric, employing alkaline picrate and enzymatic assays [56]. Actually, the gold standard for GFR measurement is inulin GFR, but it is a complex and expensive procedure.

The clinical manifestations of diabetic nephropathy are strongly related to morphological changes. The relationship between structural abnormalities and kidney function is best defined using light and electron microscopic morphometric analysis [57]. In particular, GBM thickening represents the first detectable morphological change in diabetic nephropathy and, in parallel, a thickening of tubular basement membrane (TBM) could appear. These changes are appreciable and measurable using electron microscopy. The same technique allows experimenters to evaluate the degree of mesangial expansion by extracellular matrix deposition and increased mesangial cellularity [57]. Diffuse mesangial expansion, commonly termed diffuse diabetic glomerulosclerosis, can be associated with nodular lesions, named Kimmelstiel-Wilson nodules. The sclerotic nodules are usually peripherally located and are generally positive for the periodic acid Schiff (PAS) stain. Moreover, PAS staining can be used to identify the brush border loss of the proximal convoluted tubules and the eventual cast formation. In contrast to the mesangium, initial interstitial expansion is primarily due to an increase in the cellular component of this renal compartment [19]; increase in fibrillar collagen is measurable with the picro-siuris red staining method. This histological technique can be used to identify also the tubulointerstitial fibrosis consequent to the ability of injured proximal tubular cells to release fibrogenic signals to cortical fibroblasts [58]. Afferent and efferent arteriolar hyalinosis are exudative lesions in which plasma proteins, especially immunoglobulins, complement, fibrinogen and albumin may ultimately replace the smooth muscle cells and the severity of arteriolar hyalinosis. Their onset is significantly correlated with percent sclerosed glomeruli [59] and can be detected by light microscopy, or even better by electron microscopy based on their electron dense appearance. Abnormalities of the glomerular-tubular junction (GTJA) as late manifestations of the disease [60] come from the glomerulus detachment of the tubule from the glomerulus (atubular glomerulus). Podocyte detachment from GBM and the consequent podocyte loss could in part explain or result from increased albuminuria. This phenomenon is associated with foot processes effacement and can easily be detected by electron microscopy.

To study the role of histamine in renal (patho-)physiology, the presence and contribution of mast cells must not be excluded. The first evidence of renal mast cells was already generated in the 1960s and 1970s, but as mast cells were not easily detected by routine histochemical staining, they were ignored or forgotten by nephrologists for a long time. Nowadays, the astra blue staining method can demonstrate the presence of mast cells due to its affinity for glycosaminoglycans (GAG) in mast cell granules [57].

1.6 Histamine in Renal Diseases

The presence of histamine in the kidney has been reported for decades, in keeping with the demonstrated ability of this organ to produce histamine. In humans the renal histamine content markedly exceeds plasma levels ($<10^{-8}$ M in plasma *vs* about 10^{-6} M in glomeruli) [61]. It can derive from resident mast cells [62, 63], glomerular cells, which have been reported as a major site of intrarenal histamine synthesis and accumulation [62, 64], and from proximal tubular epithelial cells, where the expression of HDC has also been demonstrated [64, 65]. Indirect evidence sustains the hypothesis that histamine could be involved in renal physiology in humans. In healthy subjects, the administration of loading doses of L-histidine led to an increase of histamine concentration in urine, but not in blood [65, 66]. In renal transplant patients, the urinary and blood levels of histamine are also elevated [66].

On the basis of the well-described ability of histamine to affect microcirculation, independent studies have examined the effects of histamine on renal function. Interestingly, histamine has been previously reported to decrease the ultrafiltration coefficient (K_f) [67].

Using a model of puromycin aminonucleoside nephrosis on increase of histamine in the renal cortex, predominantly in glomeruli, an increase in urinary histamine excretion has been demonstrated [62]. The effect of histamine was also evaluated in anti-GBM glomerulonephritis models. In rats histamine has been reported to decrease glomerular permeability, and concurrent infusion of H_1R antagonists has been reported to abolish the detrimental effect of histamine, showing aggravation of renal function by histamine H_1R action [68]. Moreover, in mice, the H_2R antagonist cimetidine has been reported to decrease the glomerular permeability coefficient 45 min after anti-GBM antibody administration [69]. More recently, Tanda et al. (2007) demonstrated that histamine ameliorates anti-GBM glomerulonephritis, suggesting the possible involvement of the H_4R [70], through its regulatory action on immune responses in inflammatory cell recruitment [71]. Finally, intravenous injection of thioperamide has been demonstrated to suppress the protective effect of l-carnosine in a model of renal ischemia/reperfusion [72].

More intriguingly, some evidence is suggestive of a possible role of histamine in the development of diabetic nephropathy. The very first evidence on this topic arose from studies performed in STZ-diabetic rats showing, consistent with a generalized effect of diabetes on inducing an increase in histamine, a greater content of histamine in the kidney of diabetic animals compared to that of controls [73, 74]. This increase has been related to a significantly greater tissue HDC activity of diabetic rats than controls without a concomitant decrease in histaminase activity [74]. Notably, a reduced prevalence of hyperglycemia in $HDC^{-/-}$ NOD mice in comparison with the wild-type counterpart [75] has recently been demonstrated. In addition, independent studies indicate that histamine regulates the renal microcirculation, by increasing salt and water excretion [67, 76, 77], decreasing the ultrafiltration coefficient by reducing the total filtration surface area [67], and increasing renin release [78]. In the last few years, we have provided the field with convergent lines of evidence strongly supporting the conclusions that all four histamine receptors are present and functional in the human nephron, although with a differential anatomical topology [79], thus furnishing new evidence for a possible direct detrimental effect of histamine on renal integrity and function. In particular, using the model of STZ-induced diabetes in rats, we have demonstrated that both H_3R and H_4R are profoundly upregulated at the tubular level in STZ-treated rats, which also displayed parallel renal damage (again mostly at the tubular level) [80, 81]. Overall, these data suggest a role of histamine in renal (patho)-physiology, but the actual contribution of the amine and respective receptors requires clarification. In this chapter, we describe a suitable in vivo model to study diabetic nephropathy and some of the most important parameters to monitor the functional and morphological integrity of the kidney.

2 Materials

2.1 In Vivo Model of Diabetes

- Mice (*see* **Note 1**) 7–8 weeks old.
- Citrate Buffer pH 4.5: for a 50 mM citrate buffer solution dissolve 1.47 g of sodium citrate in 50 mL of double-distilled water (dd H_2O). Test pH with pH meter, adjusting to 4.5 pH with monohydrate sodium citrate solution if necessary. Sterilize by autoclaving or by filtering with a 0.22 μm filter to avoid bacterial contamination. The buffer should be freshly prepared for every group of injections.
- STZ solution: dissolve the appropriate amount of STZ to obtain a final concentration in the citrate buffer equal to 7.5 mg/mL and place this into an aluminum covered tube (STZ is light sensitive). The STZ-citrate buffer solution should be prepared immediately before injection as the drug degrades after 15–20 min in the citrate buffer.
- Sterile 23–25 gauge needle.
- Sterile 1–3 mL syringe.
- Sucrose water 10%: dissolve 50 g of sucrose in 500 mL of water.
- Blood glucose meter.
- Blood glucose test strips.

2.2 Renal Function Assessment

2.2.1 Urine Collection

- Centrifuge tubes and microtubes for urine collection.
- Cover: large, vented, keeps animal securely in cage. It can be removed for easy access to animal.
- Upper chamber: made of transparent polycarbonate (PC). Surface is smooth, gnaw-proof, noiseless. It can be cleaned easily with warm soapy water or detergent solution.
- Feeder Chamber: stainless-steel (SS) chamber located outside cage. Size discourages rodent from nesting or sleeping inside.
- Feeder drawer: PC drawer slides out for easy filling without disturbing animal. It is ideal for slurries, liquids, or powders. It is not designed for food in pellet form (*see* **Note 2**). Rear portion helps to catch spilled food to prevent contamination of feces.
- Feces Collection Tube: made of non-wetting polymethylpentene (PMP). Pellets roll down sides of funnel to be collected in tube. It unlocks with single twist from outside the cage without disturbing the animal.
- Urine collection tube: made of water-resistant PMP and graduated in cubic centimeters. It unlocks from outside the cage without disturbing the animal. It can be cooled with an ice bath.
- Lower chamber: made of PC, can be removed without disturbing the animal. It can be cleaned with warm soapy water or detergent solution.
- Collection funnel and separating cone: water-resistant PMP ensures immediate, complete separation of feces and urine.
- Support grid: SS grid lets excreta pass through the widely spaced bars. Grids have handles for easy transport of cage without stand.
- Water bottle support: SS support.
- Water bottle: calibrated PC bottle with SS cap and sipper tube.
- Water spillage tube: collects any water that animals spill, facilitates accurate collection of fluid intake data.
- Stand: SS stand or rack.
- pH test strips.

2.2.2 Blood Collection

- Suitable anesthesia.
- Heparin or any other suitable anticoagulant (*see* **Note 3**).
- Sterile 23–25-gauge needle.
- Sterile 1–3 mL syringe.
- 1.5 mL microtubes.

2.2.3 Urinary Protein Determination

- 96 multi-well plates.
- Bradford reagent (Sigma Aldrich) (*see* **Note 4**).
- Albumin (BSA) standard solution.

2.2.4 Urinary Albumin Determination

- 96 multi-well plates.
- Mouse albumin ELISA quantitation set (Bethyl Laboratories, Inc): the kit contains affinity purified goat anti-mouse albumin coating antibody, mouse reference serum (standard), and horseradish peroxidase (HRP) conjugated goat anti-mouse albumin detection antibody.
- Elisa coating buffer: dissolve 0.32 g of sodium carbonate and 0.58 g of sodium bicarbonate in 100 mL of dd H_2O to obtain a final 0.05 M carbonate-bicarbonate solution. Check the pH that should be 9.6. The solution can be stored at 4 °C but must be equilibrated to room temperature (RT) before use.
- ELISA wash solution: dissolve 6.057 g of Tris–HCl and 8.18 g NaCl in 1 L of dd H_2O. Once completely dissolved, add 0.5 mL of Tween 20. The pH should be 8.0. The solution can be stored at 4 °C but must be equilibrated to RT before use.
- Elisa blocking buffer: to prepare 20 mL of blocking buffer dissolve 0.121 g of Tris–HCl and 0.164 g of NaCl in 20 mL of dd H_2O. Once completely dissolved, add 0.2 g of BSA. The solution can be stored at 4 °C but must be equilibrated to RT before use.
- Sample diluent: to prepare 100 mL of blocking buffer dissolve 0.121 g of Tris–HCl and 0.164 g of NaCl in 20 mL of dd H_2O. Once completely dissolved, add 0.1 g of BSA and 50 μL of Tween 20. The solution can be stored at 4 °C but must be equilibrated to RT before use.
- 3,3′,5,5′-Tetramethylbenzidine (TMB) substrate systems.
- Stop solution: prepare a solution of HCl 1 N diluting 8.3 mL fuming HCl to 91.7 mL dd H_2O. Alternatively, a 0.18 M sulfuric acid could be used.

2.2.5 Creatinine Determination

- 1.5 microtubes.
- Acidified acetonitrile (ACN): add 50 μL of HPLC grade glacial acetic acid to 10 mL of HPLC grade ACN.
- Hamilton syringe or an autosampler.
- Column: Zorbax SCX, strong cation exchange (Aglient, Wilmington, DE), 50 × 2.1 mm, 5 μm particle size. Five micron in-line filter and SCX guard column placed in front of analytical column.

- Mobile phase: prepare 2 L of a 5 mM sodium acetate solution by dissolving 820 mg of the powder in dd H_2O and adjusting to pH 4.2 with HPLC grade glacial acetic acid (1.4 mL). Filter the solution through a 0.22 μm nylon filter and add 80 mL of methanol and 20 mL of ACN to make a total volume of exactly 2.10 mL. Degas the solution before use.

2.3 Renal Morphology Assessment

2.3.1 Tissue Collection

- Surgical scissors.
- Dissecting scissors.
- Scalpel.
- Surgical tweezers.
- Micro needle/needle holder.
- Suture kit.
- Blades.
- Dental wax.
- dd H_2O.
- Phosphate-buffered saline (PBS): to prepare 1 L of 10× solution, dissolve 87.66 g of NaCl and 17.799 g of Na_2HPO_4 in 800 mL dd H_2O. Adjust to pH 7.4 with HCl. Adjust volume to 1 L with additional dd H_2O. Use diluted at 1:10 (PBS 1×) after sterilization by autoclaving.
- Plastic cassettes.

2.3.2 Tissue Fixation

- Fixation solution: dissolve 40 g of formaldehyde in 1 L of PBS 1×.

2.3.3 Tissue Processing

- Absolute ethanol, 95% ethanol (add 190 mL to 10 mL of dd H_2O), 75% ethanol (add 150 mL to 50 mL of dd H_2O), 50% ethanol (add 100 mL to 100 mL of dd H_2O).
- Xylene.
- Paraffin wax.
- Oven.
- Forceps.
- Molds.
- Paraffin dispenser.
- Cold plate.

2.3.4 Hematoxylin/Eosin (H/E) Staining

- Mayer alum hematoxylin: <u>Solution A</u>: dissolve 200 g of aluminum ammonium sulfate in 2.8 L of the dd H_2O and mix with a stirrer until the salt dissolves. <u>Solution B</u>: dissolve 20 g of hematoxylin powder in 40 mL of absolute ethanol by shaking for a few minutes. Mix the solution B with the solution A and stir overnight. Dissolve 4 g of sodium iodate in the obtained solution, add 80 mL of acetic acid, and then 1.2 L of glycerol. Mix well, bring solution to boil and cool, and filter. Plug loosely the solution and store at least 15 days before using it.

- 0.3% Acid alcohol: add 12 mL of hydrochloric acid to 1.2 L of dd H_2O in a sufficiently large container and mix carefully. Add 2.8 L of absolute ethanol and mix thoroughly. The generation of fine bubbles is an indication that mixing is thorough.
- Prepare the stock solutions first, and then create the working solution as needed. 1% of Eosin Stock Solution: dissolve 1 g of eosin Y in 100 mL of dd H_2O. 1% of phloxine stock solution: dissolve 1 g of phloxine B in 100 mL of dd H_2O. Add eosin-phloxine B working solution; mix 100 mL of 1% eosin stock solution with 10 mL of 1% phloxine stock solution, 780 mL of ethanol 95% and 4 mL of glacial acetic acid. Mix well.

2.3.5 PAS Reaction

- Periodic acid solution 0.5%: dissolve 50 mg of periodic acid in 10 mL of dd H_2O.
- Schiff reagent.
- Sulfurous water: add 5 mL of potassium metabisulfite 10% in 90 mL of dd H_2O and mix well. Add 5 mL of hydrochloric acid.

2.3.6 Astra Blue Staining

- Mota fluid: dissolve 0.5 g of basic lead acetate in 24.75 mL of dd H_2O, then add 0.25 mL of acetic acid and 25 mL of absolute ethanol.
- Astra blue solution: Mix the solution A (dissolve 2 g of magnesium chloride and 0.1 g of Pararosaniline hydrochloride in 80 mL of 95% ethanol) with the solution B (dissolve 0.5 g of blue astra in 10 mL of dd H_2O) and let the solution become blue by adding HCl.
- Washing solution: add 5 mL of hydrogen chloride to 95 mL of 70% ethanol (add 30 mL of dd H_2O to 70 mL of absolute ethanol).

2.3.7 Picro-Sirius Red Staining

- Picro-sirius red solution.
- Acetic acid solution (add 0.5 mL of acetic acid to 99.5 mL of dd H_2O).

2.3.8 Electron Microscopy

For details, refer to the Chap. 10, Sect. 2.5.

3 Methods

The use of the mouse as an experimental tool has provided investigators with a portal to define and follow the progression of renal disease by functional analysis, histologic parameters, and molecular profiling [82]. These parameters can help clarify the role of histamine and its receptors in renal (patho)-physiology and to validate histamine receptors as new pharmacological targets in renal diseases. A suitable in vivo model to study diabetic nephropathy and some of the most important parameters to monitor the functional and morphological integrity of the kidney are reported. Animal experiments require reliable breeding and holding facilities. All experimental protocols using live animals must first be reviewed and approved by an Institutional Animal Care and Use Committee (IACUC) and must comply with the guidelines as established by the IACUC regarding the care and use of laboratory animals in scientific experiments.

3.1 In Vivo *Model of Diabetes*

Among the different causes of ESRD, diabetic nephropathy is one of the most important in Western nations. A large number of murine models of diabetes, and consequently diabetic nephropathy exist. Nowadays, the different models vary from the artificially induced to the spontaneous and genetically engineered (knockout and transgenic) animal models. Although none of them develops renal changes sufficiently reflecting those seen in humans, they can be comparatively used for preclinical drug screening. Among the different models of diabetes, STZ-induced hyperglycemia is the most extensively studied model of diabetic nephropathy. In this model, which is associated with reliable and consistent structural and functional deficits, hyperglycemia occurs because of the toxin-induced destruction of pancreatic Beta-islet cells [43]. This is a type I diabetes chemically induced model, but the development and progression of diabetic nephropathy has been widely demonstrated to be closely associated with hyperglycemia. From this perspective, diabetic nephropathy development does not significantly differ between the two main types of diabetes and the use of this unique reproducible and well-validated animal model of diabetic nephropathy to obtain significant results represents the best ethical choice. The herein protocol describes the multiple low doses approach. Indeed, it was demonstrated that the delayed onset of hyperglycemia, obtained with this method, is not due to a direct, rapid, toxic action of the drug [83], with a response that more closely resembles the Type I diabetes pathogenesis. Moreover, mice do not experience the severe acute renal toxicity induced by a single high-dose STZ injection. The model herein reported led to the development of diabetic nephropathy within 30 weeks, depending on the strain selected (*see* **Note 1**), with animals showing sustained hyperglycemia and longitudinal survival without requirements for exogenous insulin [84, 85]. Prolonged experimental follow-up will drastically affect animal survival. For the purpose of these studies mice should be aged 6–8 weeks old.

1. Design the experiment taking into account the desired power of the study, the attrition rate due to diabetes-long term induced mortality (*see* **Note 5**).
2. House the desired number of animals at 24 °C ± 1 °C and 55% ± 5% humidity, with a 12-h light-dark cycle (light on at 8:00 and off at 20:00) and allow them free access to food and water for at least 5 days before the experiments begin.
3. Accurately determine the body weight of each mouse prior to the study by using a digital scale, and randomly divide mice into different treatment groups according to the experimental design.
4. On experimental day 1, remove all food from cages for all groups 4 h prior to intraperitoneal injection treatment. Provide water as normal.
5. Immediately prior to injection, prepare the buffers and solutions as described in Sect. 2.1.
6. Place one mouse in the isoflurane drop jar, according to the local IACUC anesthesia standards.
7. Remove mouse when breathing has slowed and animal is anesthetized.
8. Using 1-mL syringes and 25-G needles, intraperitoneally inject the appropriate amount of the STZ solution so the final dosage is 50 mg/kg.
9. Allow mouse to awaken and place back in cage, providing free access to normal food and Sucrose water (*see* Sect. 2.1), to avoid sudden hypoglycemia post-injection.
10. Repeat the procedure from step 6 for each animal of the diabetes group(s).
11. Repeat the procedure from step 6 for each animal of the control group intraperitoneally administrating them an equal volume of citrate buffer instead of STZ solution.
12. Each mouse should be given one injection for 5 days consecutively.
13. On experimental day 6, replace the sucrose water with regular water.

3.1.1 Six-Hour Fasting Glucose Determination

Six-hour fasting blood glucose levels are considered an accurate diagnostic tool for diabetes; therefore, there is no need to measure blood insulin levels or to perform the Oral Glucose Tolerance Test (OGTT; not described here).

- On experimental day 14 (9 days after the last STZ injection), and then fortnightly, measure 6 h fasting glycemic level with a Glucometer.

- Remove all food from all cages for 6 h (e.g., from 7:00 to 13:00; *see* **Note 6**). Provide water as normal.
- Place one mouse in a restrainer.
- Hold the hind foot around the ankle. The medial dorsal pedal vessel is located on the top of the foot.
- Clean the foot with absolute alcohol.
- Insert a blood glucose test strip in the provided allocation within the glucometer.
- Puncture the dorsal pedal vein with a 23G/27G needle.
- As soon as drops of blood appear (*see* **Note 7**) on the skin surface, apply the blood glucose test strip holding the Test Strip opening to the drop until it has absorbed enough blood to begin the test and record the value displayed by the device. The animals are considered diabetic when the blood glucose levels of the STZ-injected mice are >150 mg/dL (8.3 mM) and/or statistically higher than in the control mice. A severe glycemia is defined as blood glucose levels >300 mg/dL (16.7 mM). When mice display glycemic level over 600 mg/dL (33.3 mM) in two consecutive measurements insulin treatment should be considered. In animals with severe hypoglycemia (<54 mg/dL or 3 mM) the subcutaneous administration of glucose 5% should be performed.
- Apply a little pressure to stop bleeding and place back in cage, providing free access to normal food and water.
- Repeat the procedure for each animal.

3.2 Renal Function Assessment

The kidney is a key organ for homeostatic, regulatory, and excretory imbalance. Monitoring its function is essential to define renal disease etiopathogenesis and discover new therapeutic approaches. More than a century after the first development of an assay for evaluating kidney function, the scientific community has not yet reached a consensus on the correct method to evaluate the function of this organ [56]. The major challenge is still represented by the standardization of the techniques adopted. Among the current tools used to evaluate renal function the biochemical measurements are the most commonly used. Some of the most relevant methods and parameters to assess the renal function are described below.

3.2.1 Urine Collection

Collection of urine is a basic requirement to evaluate renal function. A small quantity of urine will suffice for qualitative urinalysis, which includes the measurement of urinary pH, protein, glucose, bilirubin, hemoglobin, ketone, urobilinogen, and creatinine levels. However, a quantitative excretion analysis requiring the collection of timed urine samples (e.g., 24 h samples) is useful for

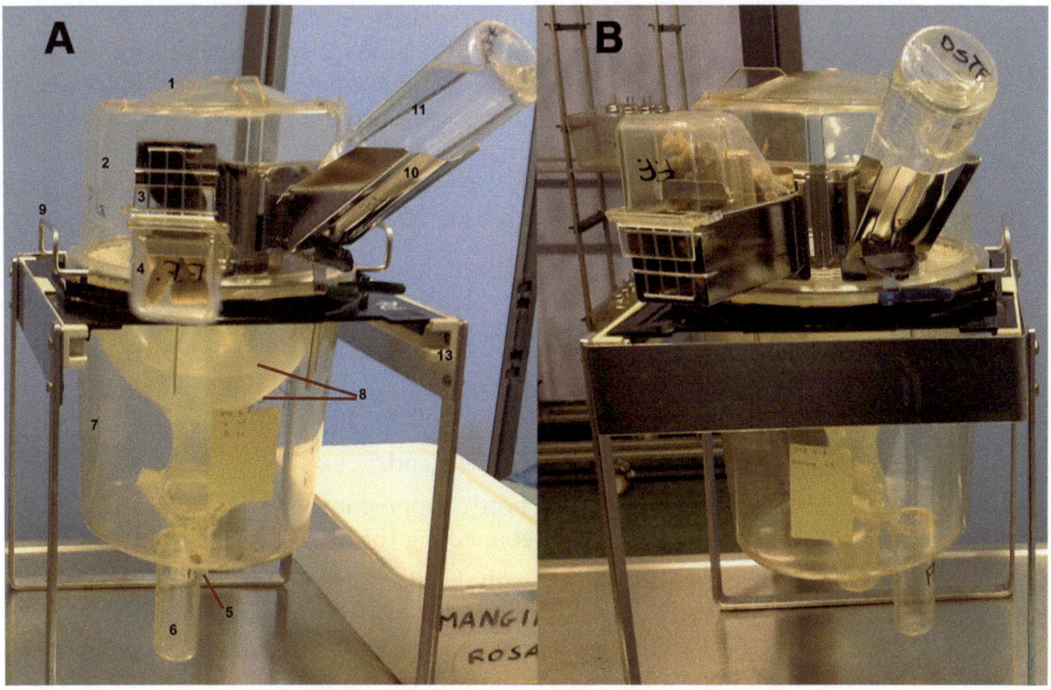

Fig. 1 Metabolic cages. (**a**) Representative image of an assembled metabolic cage; 1 = cover, 2 = Upper chamber, 3 = Feeder chamber, 4 = Feeder drawer, 5 = Feces collection Tube, 6 = Urine collection tube, 7 = Lower chamber, 8 = Collection funnel and separating cone, 9 = Support grid, 10 = Water bottle support, 11 = Water bottle, 12 = Stand. (**b**) Representative image of a metabolic cage with the feeder chamber and drawer horizontally flipped, see Note 2

ascertaining the result of any experimental manipulation, such as drug treatment, that the animal has been subjected to [46]. The optimal 24 h urine collection is performed using metabolic cages (Fig. 1). The intent of a metabolic cage is to collect urine and separate it from feces. Basically, the principle of a metabolic cage is to confine the rodent in an enclosure with a wire grid floor through which urine flows down into the middle of the funnel and further into the collection vial. The feces fall down separately into another vial. To avoid contamination, feeding and watering compartments are cleverly incorporated outside the cage. Although this is a noninvasive collection method, evidence exists to suggest altered neurohumoral control in rodents housed in metabolic cages [47–50] and a sustained change in cardiovascular function has been demonstrated, which could potentially affect renal function [51]. This could be due, at least in part, to the grid floor and lack of nesting material which may influence the animal negatively [86]. Moreover, one of the major problems is the isolation implied in the use of a metabolic cage since the animal is placed by itself without any possibility for social contact. Social isolation is thought to be stressful for mice and rats [87, 88].

For these reasons some researchers recommend the housing of more than one mouse in a metabolic cage, the housing time in a metabolic cage should be minimized and the resort to spot urine analysis for comparison is warranted. There are numerous commercial rodent metabolic cages available to collect urine; here, we reported the example of the Techniplast® metabolic cages for mice & rats, which can be used for up to a three mice group.

1. Insert the collection funnel and the separating cone in the lower chamber.
2. Place support grid floor above the collection funnel.
3. Attach the upper chamber to the lower chamber above the support grid.
4. Place the system in the stand.
5. Insert the water bottle support into the provided space of the upper chamber, connecting the water spillage tube.
6. Fill water bottle with distilled H_2O and attach it to the holder. Water consumption can be monitored by weighing the water-filled bottles before and after the study and/or taking advantage of the graduation on the bottle.
7. Fill the feeder drawer with rodent diet (e.g., rodent chow) (*see* **Note 2**). Slide the filled drawer cautiously into the food chamber. Food consumption can be monitored by weighing food drawer and the food inside before and after the study.
8. Insert the feeder drawer in the SS feeder chamber and allocate it into the provided space of the upper chamber.
9. Place both the urine and feces collection tubes in the lower chamber of the cage.
10. Determine body weight of each mouse prior to study by using a digital scale.
11. Determine the 6 h fasting glycemia of each mouse prior to study by using a glucometer (*see* Sect. 3.1).
12. Put single mouse into the upper chamber on the support grid (*see* **Note 8**).
13. Close the upper chamber of the metabolic cage with the cover.
14. After 24 h mice are removed from the cages and the body weight and the amount of water consumed and urine produced recorded (*see* **Note 9**).
15. Discharge the feces, disassemble and wash accurately the cages.
16. Transfer the collected urine in a centrifuge tube.
17. Centrifuge the urine for 10 min at 10,000 × *g* (RT) to remove solid contaminants.

18. Record the urine pH by using pH test strips.
19. Transfer an amount of urine into 1.5 mL tubes taking care to not transfer any urine sediment.
20. Centrifuge the urine for 10 min at 10,000 × *g* (RT).
21. Transfer to new tubes taking care to not transfer any urine sediment and store sample at −80 °C for long-term storage. Avoid repeated freeze–thaw cycles (*see* **Note 10**).

3.2.2 Blood Collection

Blood sample collection should be performed in keeping with the national and international regulatory agencies and guidelines (for Europe: Directive 2010/63/UE, D.M. 116/92-European Guidelines on protection of animals used for experimental and other scientific purpose), in keeping with European law. On average, the total blood volume in the mouse is 6–8% of its body weight, or 6–8 mL of blood per 100 g of body weight. Blood volume is restored in 24 h, but erythrocytes and reticulocytes may not return to normal levels for up to 2 weeks. Therefore, the maximum amount of 10% of total circulating blood can be withdrawn only once every 2 weeks (1.0% of an animal's total blood volume can be removed every 24 h) [89]. Blood collection can be achieved with different methods, taking into account that both the source and method of blood collection can affect blood parameters, caused to stress induction. Indeed, increases in blood hormone and glucose levels are directly related to stressful methods of blood collection. Blood collection from both saphenous vein and dorsal pedal vein does not require anesthesia and is usually performed to test the glycemic tolerance and the fasting glucose levels with a glucometer (*see* Sect. 3.1). Alternatively, blood samples can be taken from the tail vein, the orbital sinus, the jugular vein, or with a temporary cannula. The cardiac puncture, herein described, as well as blood collection from posterior vena cava, axillary vessel, or orbital sinus are procedures to be performed as terminal procedures [89]. Adequate training is required for blood collection using any method in any species. For the cardiac puncture the three possible approaches, the ventral, left lateral, or open, are described below. The collected blood can be further processed to obtain the plasma, which is suitable for different parameters analysis such as blood creatinine, but also circulating cytokine measurements by different ELISA kit assays and other methods.

1. Properly anesthetize animal, according to the local IACUC anesthesia standards.
2. Subcutaneously administer heparin 20 UI/mice (*see* **Note 3**), to avoid blood clotting and to maximize the amount of blood collected.
3. Test for reaction by corneal reflex and toe pinch.

Ventral Approach

1. Place the animal on the back in a dorsal recumbent position.
2. Palpate the heart.
3. Insert the needle slightly left of and under the sternum directed toward animal's head. Needle and syringe should be held horizontally 20–30°.
4. Insert the needle into the heart.
5. Gently apply a negative pressure on syringe plunger and check for blood appearance. Heart chamber may collapse if the negative pressure is too great. Do not move the needle side-to-side during the procedure as this could lacerate the heart or vena cava. If no blood appears, slowly withdraw the needle so that it remains just under the skin or the diaphragm and redirect in a slightly different direction. If blood stops flowing, slowly rotate needle or move it slightly in or out.
6. Collect the desired blood amount and withdraw the needle after blood has been collected. The blood volumes expected at exsanguination are about the 3% of Body Weight (e.g., for a 25 g mouse about 0.75–1 mL).
7. Perform a secondary method of euthanasia to ensure that animal is dead.

Left Lateral Approach

1. Place the animal on the right side so that it has a right lateral recumbent position.
2. Palpate the heart on left lateral thoracic wall, approximately at point of flexed elbows, between the 5th and 6th ribs.
3. Slowly insert the needle between the ribs and perpendicular to the body, therefore into the heart.
4. Proceed from step 5 of the Ventral Approach (Sect. 3.2.2).

Open Approach

1. Place the animal on the back in a dorsal recumbent position.
2. Swab mouse with 70% alcohol to wet the fur, and thus to minimize the risk for blood to come in contact with mouse's fur.
3. Make a V-cut through the skin and abdominal wall about 1 cm caudal to the last rib.
4. Move the internal organs to the side.
5. Carefully insert the needle through the diaphragm and into the vena cava or the heart.
6. Proceed from step 5 of the Ventral Approach (Sect. 3.2.2).

Blood Sample Processing for Serum

1. Transfer the blood samples obtained as described above into a 1.5 mL centrifuge microtube.
2. Keep blood samples at RT for 30 min to allow the blood to clot.
3. Remove the clot by centrifugation at 1000–2000 × *g* for 10 min at 4 °C.
4. Immediately transfer the supernatant (serum) into a clean 1.5 mL centrifuge microtube using a Pasteur pipette, taking care to not withdraw any cellular component of the pellet. The samples should be maintained at 2–8 °C while handling. If the serum is not analyzed immediately, the serum can be aliquoted and stored at −20 °C for long-term storage. It is important to avoid freeze-thaw cycles to avoid serum component degradation (*see* **Note 10**).

3.2.3 Urinary Protein Determination

The total protein content of urine is a good and reliable index of renal function, proteinuria being the result of both glomerular and tubular dysfunction. Glomerular dysfunction is due to an increase in the passage through glomerular capillaries and is characterized by a loss in plasma proteins with similar or larger size. Tubular dysfunction is due to a decrease of the tubular absorption capacity. A semiquantitative test such as a dipstick for urine protein can be used to screen the general population for the presence of protein in the urine as part of a routine urinalysis. However, this method has been designed for human urine samples. Mice urine has been previously reported to have a considerable quantity of proteins [55, 56]. Therefore, the dipstick test may not be accurate, while a standard colorimetric assay could be run. Herein, we report the protocol to measure proteinuria according to the Bradford method, as the bicinchoninic acid assay (BCA) is significantly affected by the urea content in urine, and the Lowry method also is not accurate for protein determination in urine as ammonium salts interfere with the latter assay. In contrast, the Bradford reagent is compatible with urea. Different Bradford reagents are commercially available and the method should be adjusted to the specific product used (*see* **Note 4**). The following procedure is used for Bradford reagent from Sigma Aldrich, which is a ready to use reagent. The test can be performed in microwell plate formats.

1. Prepare a standard curve with BSA, the linear concentration range for the reagent is 0.1–1.4 mg/mL of protein.
2. Pipette 3 μL of each standard into a 96 multi-well plate.
3. Pipettte 3 μL of each urine sample into the 96 multi-well plate.
4. Add 90 μL of Bradford reagent into each well.

5. Gently mix and shake the plate on a rocker shaker for 5 min at RT.
6. Measure the absorbance at 595 nm with a compatible plate reader.
7. Use the standard curve to determine, for comparison the protein concentration in the urine samples. Calculate as protein concentration per 24 h.

3.2.4 Urinary Albumin Determination

Different dipsticks exist for a semiquantitative analysis of albuminuria. However, its determination by immunoassays is the most commonly used method for laboratory mice, although this method might significantly underestimate albumin and the HPLC method is an alternative (90). However, most of the methods for albumin quantification are immunoassay-based. Notably, not all immunoassays perform equally and whether modified albumin is measured appears to depend on assay design, in particular whether polyclonal or monoclonal antibodies are used. The *Animal Models of Diabetic Complications Consortium* strongly support and suggest the use of the Albuwell M kit. Herein, we describe the protocol to perform the assay using the mouse albumin ELISA quantitation set (Bethyl Laboratories, Inc). Albuminuria can be used to determine not only albumin excretion rate but also the ACR.

1. Design the experimental scheme for a 96 multi-well plate taking into account the standard curve of at least eight points (blank included) and that each sample has to be run in duplicate, standards included.
2. Dilute the Affinity purified goat anti-mouse albumin coating antibody in ELISA coating buffer (*see* Sect. 2.2.4) at the final concentration of 10 μg/mL.
3. Dispense 100 μL/well of the diluted affinity purified antibody, and incubate overnight at 4 °C. Cover the microplate with a TopSeal. If a lower coating time is desired incubation at higher temperature can be performed (e.g., 1 h at 20–25 °C).
4. Wash the wells from the excess non-labeled coating solution. To do this discharge the remaining coating solution from the wells, fill each well with at least 200 μL of ELISA wash solution (*see* Sect. 2.2.4), and discharge. Repeat the procedure four additional times for a total of five washes. Blot plate onto paper towels or other absorbent material. Take care that no bubbles are present at the bottom of the well.
5. Block any nonspecific binding by adding 200 μL of ELISA blocking solution (*see* Sect. 2.2.4). Take care that no bubbles are present in each well.
6. Incubate the plate for 30 min at RT. Cover the microplate with a TopSeal.

7. Remove the ELISA blocking solution and wash each well five times as described in step 4.
8. Dilute the mouse reference serum into sample diluent (*see* Sect. 2.2.4). The standard curve should be in the range 500–0 ng/mL (eight-point curve, blank included).
9. Dilute the urine specimens in Sample Diluent, based on the expected albumin concentration (*see* **Note 11**).
10. Pipette 100 μL of standards and samples into the wells and incubate the plate for 1 h at RT. Cover the microplate with a TopSeal.
11. Remove the excess unbound samples and standards and wash each well five times as described in step 4.
12. Dilute the HRP conjugated goat anti-mouse albumin detection antibody in sample diluent at the dilution of 25 ng/mL (*see* **Note 12**).
13. Pipette 100 μL of diluted HRP detection antibody to each well and incubate the plate for 1 h at RT covering the microplate with a TopSeal.
14. Remove the excess unbound HRP detection antibody and wash each well five times as described in step 4.
15. Pipette 100 μL of TMB Substrate Solution into each well containing the peroxidase reaction and let the enzymatic color reaction develop in the dark at RT for 15 min (the substrate reaction should produce a blue solution due to the dimer formation and can be read on a spectrophotometer at 650 nm).
16. Stop the reaction by adding an equal amount of Stop Solution (*see* Sect. 2.2.4). Addition of sulfuric acid stop solution changes the color to yellow (absorbance maximum at 450 nm), stabilizing the color development to enable accurate measurement of the intensity at 450 nm using a spectrophotometer or plate reader.
17. Gently mix the plate on a rocker shaker.
18. Measure the absorbance on a plate reader at 450 nm. Duplicate absorbance values should be within 10% of each other.
19. Use the standard curve to determine the unknown specimen concentration. Take into account the dilution of the sample.

3.2.5 Creatinine Determination

Creatinine is a by-product of muscle metabolism and is eliminated almost exclusively in urine. The conversion of creatine to creatinine is a non-enzymic process that proceeds at a constant rate; animals with high muscle mass excrete more creatinine in their urine since urinary creatinine output is proportional to body mass. For mice with similar body mass, the protein to creatinine ratio thus provides a simple correction for urine dilution [91]. The measurement of creatinine should be performed by HPLC. Indeed, the more commonly used Jaffe alkaline picrate method overestimates creatinine values approximately double that of HPLC-determined values [92]. More importantly, glucose and bilirubin inhibit the reaction between creatinine and alkaline picrate. Glucose slowly reduces picric acid to picrate, while the bilirubin present in a sample is oxidized to biliverdin under alkaline conditions. This leads to a decrease in absorbance at 520 nm. Therefore, the HPLC method for creatinine determination is described below.

Urine Processing for Creatinine Extraction

1. Mix and centrifuge the urine samples collected as described in Sect. 3.1. If storing of the samples is required, take care to maintain them at 2–8 °C while handling.
2. Transfer 5 μL of urine to each 1.5 mL microtube containing 100 μL of ACN (*see* Sect. 2.2.5) and vortex for about 15 s to extract the creatinine into the ACN.

Plasma Processing for Creatinine Extraction

1. Mix and centrifuge the plasma samples collected as described in Sect. 3.1. If storing of the samples is required take care to maintain them at 2–8 °C while handling. Squeeze any clots using a wooden applicator stick, then centrifuge (minimum 850 × *g* for 10 min at 4 °C) if necessary.
2. Transfer 25 μL of serum to each 1.5 mL microtube containing 100 μL of ACN and vortex for about 15 s to extract the creatinine into the ACN.

Creatinine Extraction

1. Let the extraction run for about 15 min at −20 °C to aid precipitation and freezing the aqueous precipitate avoids carry-over and undissolved particles.
2. Centrifuge at 9500 × *g* for 10 min at 4 °C.
3. Transfer the supernatant to a new 1.5 mL microtube. The volume should be very close to 125 μL taking great care to not transfer any of the precipitate that should be on the wall or bottom of the tube.
4. Evaporate the ACN to dryness using a stream of dry nitrogen (*see* **Note 13**).
5. Remove the tubes and reconstitute to 25.0 μL with filtered mobile phase (*see* Sect. 2.2.5 and **Note 14**). Mix to dissolve the residue containing creatinine using the pipettor.
6. Transfer the liquid containing the creatinine to new 1.5 mL microtubes and centrifuge at 500 × *g* for 10 min at 4 °C.
7. Carefully remove the vials from centrifuge.

8. Connect the column.
9. Prime the pump with the mobile phase. An overnight priming is recommended.
10. Set the instrument to run the column at 45 °C and at a flow rate of 0.30 ± 0.02 mL/min. Detect at 225 nm (UV). The runtime should be set at 10 min.
11. Run the samples, injecting them in an appropriate amount on the basis of the specific loop (*see* **Note 15**). Under this task, fully prime the Hamilton syringe by aspirating and dispensing Mobile phase before filling the syringe with the desired amount of sample. Dispense the final sample volume into the loop injector and rinse the syringe with ACN before proceeding with the following sample.
12. Prepare and inject a standard creatinine curve from 0.003 to 1 mg/dL by serial dilutions.
13. Compare the retention time to pure standard of creatinine for identification. Use the standard curve to determine the unknown specimen's concentration. Take into account any eventual dilution of the sample.
14. Estimate the ACR by the formula: ACR = U[BSA]/U[Cr] and express in μg/mg.
15. Estimate the creatinine clearance by the formula: GFR = U[Cr]∗[Volume]/P[Cr]∗[Time]

where U[Cr]: urinary creatinine concentration in mg/dL; U[Volume]: urine volume in ml; P[Cr] plasmatic creatinine concentration in mg/dL; [Time] in h

3.3 Renal Morphology Assessment

Renal function is strictly correlated to the morphology integrity. Therefore, a morphological analysis is mandatory to assess the entity of renal damage and the efficacy of therapeutic strategy. The standard procedures necessary to characterize the renal integrity are reported herein.

3.3.1 Tissue Collection and Processing

The procedures of organ excision, fixation, and processing profoundly influence the quality of data. In particular, the excision of the kidney from the abdomen should be quickly and accurately carried out and the preservation of the organ in a state most closely resembling its in vivo morphology requires the use of chemical or physical fixation method. The fixation procedure should be carried out as soon as possible after the removal of the organ, as poorly fixed tissues are inadequately protected against the physical and chemical agents of processing [93]. The incorrect fixation of the kidney is known to result in a swelling of the cells lining proximal tubules and in an obliteration of proximal tubule lumens and glomeruli [94]. Where the best possible morphology is required, animals should be anesthetized and subjected to vascular system perfusion through cardiac puncture with saline, followed by a fixative flush, but this approach does not allow us to perform biochemical and functional studies on the tissue. For routine stains where perfusion is not recommended, the fixation is achieved by immersing the specimen in the fixative (immersion fixation) solution, whose volume should be 20 times that of tissue on a weight per volume. For some specialized histochemical procedures fixatives can be occasionally applied in the vapor form. Fixative solutions may contain a single fixative agent dissolved in water or ethanol or more commonly a buffer solution to stabilize pH. Most of the fixative solutions contain several different fixing agents in combination, the rationale being that the defects in one agent can be compensated for by the addition of another. The widely used fixative for paraffin-embedded tissues is neutral buffered formalin-based liquid. Duration of the fixative process determines the extent of tissue stabilization and consequently reactivity in histological and immunohistochemical procedures. Under-fixed tissues are inadequately protected against processing reagents and exhibit artifacts, while prolonged exposure to fixatives may impair tissue reactivity, particularly in immunohistochemical investigations [95]. While samples may be sectioned following a range of preparatory freezing methods, tissues are more commonly taken through a series of reagents and finally infiltrated and embedded in a stable medium, as the paraffin, which, when hard, provides the necessary support for microtome. This treatment is termed tissue processing; the first step is dehydration. Ethanol is the most commonly used dehydrating agent, because it is colorless, miscible with water and, when anhydrous, with most organic solvents. In addition, ethanol also acts as a secondary fixative during tissue processing. As many dehydrating agents are immiscible with embedding medium, an intermediate step, known as clearing, is needed before the infiltration. The clearing is carried out using solvents miscible with both dehydrating and embedding medium to facilitate the transition between dehydration and infiltration steps. The term clearing arises because some solvents have high refractive indices and, on immersion, anhydrous tissues are rendered transparent or clear. Among the different clearing agents, xylene is the most frequently employed. Although it tends to harden tissue if left in too long, it rapidly clears and tissues are rendered transparent, facilitating clearing endpoint determination. After the clearing process, tissue is infiltrated by immersion in a substance fluid when hot and solid when cold to saturate the tissue cavities. This process is known as infiltration and the substance used is generally, but not always, the medium in which the samples are finally embedded. Paraffin wax, a polycrystalline mixture of solid hydrocarbons, is the most widely used medium for embedding. It is traditionally marketed by its melting points that range from 39 to 68 °C and its crystalline morphology altered by incorporating additives which result in a less brittle, more homogeneous wax with good cutting characteristics [95]. The embedding process guarantees that the tissue is surrounded by a medium, which, solidified, provides sufficient external support during sectioning.

Sample Collection

1. At the end of the experimental period, anesthetize the animal.
2. Perform an incision in the cranio-caudal direction throughout the abdomen of the animal, to hold it open and get to the kidney.
3. Clamp and cut the blood vessels connecting to the kidney.
4. Cut the ureter between the bladder and the kidney.
5. Excise the kidney from the abdomen.
6. Rinse the kidney in PBS to remove blood.
7. Sacrifice the animal (eventually by cervical dislocation).
8. Quickly remove from the kidney any eventual surrounding tissue.
9. For classical histological evaluations, place the kidney on dental wax and cut it transversally with two blades, separating it into two portions of comparable volume (*see* **Note 16**).
10. Place the sample into a small plastic cassette that holds it while it is being processed to a paraffin block. Do not forget to identify the sample and label its cassette side in pencil (*see* **Note 17**).

Sample Fixation

1. Place the cassettes into a beaker with a fixative solution and incubate for 4 h at RT (*see* **Note 18**).
2. Change the fixative solution and incubate overnight at 4 °C to avoid over-fixation (*see* **Note 19**).
3. Rinse the cassettes in PBS 1×.

Sample Processing

1. Dehydration from aqueous fixatives: submerge the cassettes in 50% ethanol for 30 min at RT. Change the solution and repeat the procedure under the same conditions.
2. Cover the cassettes with an excess of 75% ethanol for 1 h at RT.
3. Submerge the cassettes in 95% ethanol for 1 h at RT. Change the solution and repeat the procedure under the same conditions (*see* **Note 20**).
4. Submerge the cassettes in absolute ethanol for 1 h at RT. Change the solution and repeat the procedure for 1 h maximum (*see* **Note 21**).

5. Clearing process: cover the cassettes with an excess of xylene for 1 h at RT. Change the solution and repeat the procedure for 1 h (*see* **Note 22**).
6. Infiltration process: melt 500 g of paraffin wax in an oven at 58 °C for at least 4 h.
7. Place the entire cassettes in the melted paraffin and incubate at 58 °C overnight.
8. Embedding process: open the tissue cassette and select a mold most appropriate to the size of the tissue (*see* **Notes 23** and **24**). Discard cassette lid.
9. Fill the mold with molten paraffin wax.
10. Using warm forceps transfer the tissue into mold, taking care that it does not cool in the air.
11. Orientate the tissue with the surface to be cut facing down in the mold and secure it into the wax with warmed forceps.
12. Quickly chill the mold on the cold plate, ensuring that the correct orientation is maintained and the tissue surface to be sectioned is kept flat.
13. Insert the identifying label.
14. If necessary, fill cassette with paraffin while cooling, keeping the mold full until solid.
15. Paraffin should solidify in 30 min. When the wax is completely cooled and hardened (30 min) the paraffin block can be easily popped out of the mold.

Sample Sectioning

Once embedded, the tissues must be cut into sections that can be placed on a microscopic slide for the staining. This procedure is carried out with a microtome, which is nothing more than a sharp knife with a mechanism for advancing a paraffin block standard distances across it. The preparation of high-quality sections for histopathology requires skill and experience. Some tissues are more difficult to section than others. Hard tissue or cavernous tissues present special challenges when sectioning. In addition, less than ideal fixation and embedding techniques can make it difficult.

1. Turn on the dd H_2O bath and check that the temperature is 37 °C.
2. Remove excess of paraffin with a razor blade so that the tissue, surrounded by paraffin, stands out from the block.
3. Trim the upper and lower edges of the block face so that they are parallel.
4. Trim the lateral surfaces so that the resultant face resembles a trapezoid. The tissue should be surrounded by about 1 mm of paraffin.

5. Clamp the block in the microtome carrier that the upper and lower surfaces are parallel with the knife edge.
6. Select the angle of the blade at 20 °C. Move the blade toward the block so that it just clears the block and locks the blade so it does not move.
7. Set thickness of sections at 5 μm (*see* **Note 25**).
8. Move the blade toward the block so that it just clears the block and lock the blade.
9. Unlock the wheel and start to rotate it.
10. The block face will gradually be cut completely and the sections will come off as trapezoids.
11. The sections should form ribbons as they are cut (*see* **Notes 26** and **27**).
12. Cut four sections (*see* **Note 28**) and pick them up with forceps or a fine paint brush and float them on the surface of the 37 °C water bath (*see* **Notes 29** and **30**). The sections should spread and flatten out.
13. Float the sections onto the surface of clean microscope slides (*see* **Note 31**), taking care to carefully arrange the ribbon in the center of the slide parallel to the long axis of the slide.
14. Drain off the excess dd H_2O with a paper towel.
15. Let the slides dry for at least 12 h before staining, storing them preferably overnight at 45 °C in an oven.
16. Slides can then be stored at RT.

3.3.2 H/E Staining

The H/E is the most extensively used staining technique in histology and histopathology, because of its ability to demonstrate a wide range of physiological and pathological tissue components and yet it is a relatively simple stain to carry out on both paraffin and frozen sections. Renal structural alterations, as tubular atrophy, mesangial expansion, commonly termed diffuse diabetic glomerulosclerosis, immune infiltration cells, can be demonstrated by H/E staining [57]. Hematoxylin is not classified as a dye since the molecule possesses no chromophore and its in situ oxidation is effected by the addition of a strong oxidant to the stain, as with sodium iodate. Hematoxylin oxidation product, the hematin, exhibits indicator-like properties, being blue and less soluble in aqueous alkaline conditions, and red and more soluble in alcoholic acidic conditions; in the latter condition, hematin binds to lysine residues of nuclear histones by linkage via a metallic ion mordant, such as aluminum. The over-staining of the tissues with excess nonspecific background coloration is selectively removed by soaking in an alcoholic acidic solution, a process known as differentiation. This process is arrested by returning to an alkaline condition, whereupon the hematin takes on a blue hue, known as blueing-up.

The hematin demonstrates cell nuclei. Full cellular detail is obtained by counterstaining with eosin, a red dye resulting from the action of bromine on fluorescein. Color enhancement is achieved by fortifying the stain with phloxine, a chemical member of the same family as eosin. The best staining is obtained by applying the dye in acidic conditions, whereby more intense specific colorations are obtained, the more acidic tissue components taking up the dye to a greater extent. Eosin is used to stain cell cytoplasm, collagen, and muscle fibers. There are a large number of H/E protocols available for staining cells and tissue. For most tissues, these approaches can be used interchangeably, and selection of a particular protocol will be based upon the particular needs of the investigator. Primary differences are dye composition, staining protocol, and intensity of blue dye. Staining contrast for a particular tissue differs depending upon the approach that is used. The reported protocol is selected to stain renal tissue sections.

1. To deparaffinize the sections put the microscope slides in xylene for 10 min. Change the xylene to remove the paraffin dissolved and repeat the passage (*see* **Note 32**).
2. Put the microscope slides in absolute ethanol for 5 min. Change the ethanol to remove the xylene dissolved and repeat the passage.
3. Put the microscope slides in a graded series of alcohols: 95% ethanol for 5 min, 70% ethanol for 5 min and 50% ethanol for 5 min, and then dd H_2O for 5 min.
4. Stain in Harris hematoxylin solution for 10 min (*see* **Note 33**).
5. Rinse in running tap water for 5 min.
6. Differentiate in 0.3% acid ethanol for 5 s (*see* **Note 34**).
7. Rinse with dd H_2O for 1 min.
8. Counterstain in eosin working solution for 30 s (*see* **Note 35**).
9. To dehydrate the sections put the microscope slides in 95% ethanol for 5 min, then absolute ethanol for 5 min. Change the ethanol to remove the dissolved water and repeat the procedure.
10. To clear the tissue sections put the microscope slides in xylene for 5 min. Change the xylene to remove the dissolved ethanol and repeat (*see* **Note 32**).
11. Mount with xylene-based mounting medium.

3.3.3 PAS Reaction

The PAS reaction is a histochemical method for the demonstration of polysaccharides. The main polysaccharide identified in human tissue sections is glycogen, which is present in numerous organs, including kidney. The PAS reaction is also used to demonstrate tissue basement membrane, whose thin layers of reticular connective tissue anchor and support epithelium. In renal pathophysiology PAS staining is performed to detect GBM and tubular basement membrane (TBM) thickening, and to evaluate mesangial expansion, predominantly due to an increase in mesangial matrix, arteriolar hyalinosis, brush border (microvillus border) of the proximal convoluted tubules, and eventual CAST formation [57]. The principle of the reaction is based on the oxidization of the carbon-to-carbon bonds. Indeed, polysaccharides are composed of monosaccharide units joined by covalent bonds. The first reaction involves periodic acid acting as an oxidizing agent to oxidize the carbon-to-carbon bonds between two adjacent hydroxyl groups. This produces Schiff reactive aldehyde groups. In the second reaction, the tissue section reacts with Schiff reagent, a mixture of basic fuchsin, hydrochloric acid, and sodium metabisulfite. The basic fuchsin in the mixture reacts with newly formed aldehyde groups in the tissue to produce a bright magenta color, whose intensity is proportional to the concentration of hydroxyl groups originally present in the monosaccharide units. Hematoxylin is then typically used as a counter stain to visualize other tissue elements.

1. De-paraffinize and rehydrate sections (*see* Sect. 3.3.2, steps 1–3).
2. Add PAS solution to staining dish for 10 min.
3. Rinse carefully with several exchanges of dd H_2O, because the sections may wash off.
4. Add Schiff Reagent and incubate for 25 min (*see* **Note 36**).
5. Rinse with three exchanges of sulfurous water of 3 min each.
6. Rinse in tap water for 10 min.
7. Rinse in dd H_2O for 5 min.
8. Counterstain nuclei in hematoxylin solution for 1 min.
9. Differentiate in running tap water for 10 min.
10. Rinse with dd H_2O for 1 min.
11. To dehydrate the sections put the microscope slides in a graded series of ethanol: 50% ethanol for 5 min, 75% ethanol for 5 min, 95% ethanol for 5 min, and absolute ethanol for 5 min. Change the ethanol to remove the eventual dissolved water and repeat the procedure.
12. To clear the tissue sections put the microscope slides in xylene for 5 min. Change the xylene to remove the dissolved ethanol and repeat the procedure (*see* **Note 32**).
13. Mount with xylene based mounting medium.

3.3.4 Astra Blue Staining

Astra blue is a cationic dye able to determine GAG. The astra blue staining method is used in clinical diagnosis and in research studies to demonstrate mast cells, due to its affinity for GAG of the mast cell granule. Mast cells, directing innate and adaptive immune responses, modulate inflammation and potentially induce tissue repair and direct fibrosis. However, they also play a role in tissue remodeling, being significant participants in chronic progressive kidney disease [96] and their presence and degranulation extent is associated with fibrosis and functional loss. The properties of mast cell granules, and their consequent ability to be stained by astra blue, are profoundly influenced by the fixation method. An optimal fixation will result in precipitation of GAG leaving polyanionic sites available for binding of dye. Failure to demonstrate mast cells in fixed tissues may be due either to dissolution of non-precipitated GAG, or to blocking of polyanions by cationic proteins [97]. Unfortunately, the widely used fixative for human biopsies, formalin-based fixative, does not permit the detection of mast cells in the tissue and has to be substituted by Mota fluid.

1. De-paraffinize and rehydrate sections (*see* Sect. 3.3.2, steps 1–3).
2. Add astra blue solution and incubate for 60 min.
3. Rinse for 30 s with washing solution.
4. De-hydrate the sections (*see* Sect. 3.3.3, steps 11–12).
5. Mount with xylene-based mounting medium.

3.3.5 Picro-Sirius Red Staining

Picro-sirius red staining is a commonly used technique for collagen histochemistry [98]. The collagen fibers demonstrated by the staining appear red in light microscopy on a pale yellow background. This method, technically very easy to perform, can be applied to paraffin-embedded tissue sections and represents staining of the extracellular matrix components, especially helpful in studying tissue remodeling, particularly in the case of connective tissue pathologies [99]. The dye molecule intercalates into the tertiary groove in the structure of collagen types I and III and imparts a pink stain to most tissues when observed under white light [100]. Although some authors suggested that picro-sirius red is not selective for collagen also binding to other proteins containing basic amino acids, and the staining to a large extent is influenced by electrostatic forces [101], its use is widely accepted by scientific community for the visualization of collagen and a recent study described an analysis method to quantify renal fibrosis using picro-sirius red staining [102].

1. De-paraffinize and rehydrate sections (*see* Sect. 3.3.2, steps 1–3).
2. Apply an adequate picro-sirius red solution to completely cover the tissue section and incubate for 60 min (*see* **Note 37**).
3. Rinse slide quickly in two changes of acetic acid solution.
4. Rinse slide in absolute ethanol for 30 s.

5. Dehydrate with absolute ethanol for 5 min. Change the ethanol and repeat the process.
6. Mount with xylene-based mounting medium.
7. Let the mounting medium dry for at least 4 h.
8. Under light microscopy, choose magnification of 200× and randomly take five photos per section, taking care not to pass by the same structure or modify camera parameters. Overlay the scale bar.
9. Qualitative analysis of the staining can be performed, evaluating its optical density and its area.
10. Launch ImageJ software, freely available at this link: http://imagej.nih.gov/ij/download.html.
11. Open all the images collected.
12. Choose Analyze; Set Measurements and select Integrated density and Limit to threshold option. Then click OK.
13. To set the scale, use the straight line selection tool to drag out a line across the scale bar over-impressed on the photo. Select Analyze and then Set Scale. The distance measured in pixels will be displayed. Enter the known distance (corresponding to that shown in the scale bar) and the unit of length. Then select Global, to maintain the scale across all the images.
14. To set the threshold, select Image; Adjust and then Threshold. Adjust the correct level of threshold, which covers the entire surface of dark red stain and select Apply. Then choose Analyze; Measure.
15. Select each photo and choose Analyze; Measure.
16. Analyze the outputs with a statistical software package.

3.3.6 Electron Microscopy

A detailed morphological analysis of renal specimens, based on immunofluorescence and electron microscopic evaluations and associated with clinico-pathological correlation, is frequently mandatory to reliably obtain a differential diagnosis among the different renal diseases [103]. Electron microscopy has been used for the morphological diagnosis of glomerular diseases since the 1970s, and its value has been widely recognized [104]; 85% of renal biopsies utilized electron microscopy for diagnostic confirmation [105]. Indeed, morphological features of some renal pathological conditions undetected via light microscopy can almost exclusively be characterized by electron microscopy. In particular, focusing attention on the morphological abnormalities associated with diabetic nephropathy, some parameters could be evaluated by electron microscopy: (1) thickening of the GBM [106]; (2) the thickening of TBM; (3) the degree of mesangial expansion, due to extracellular matrix deposition and increased mesangial cellularity; (4) the podocytopenia [107, 108] associated with foot process effacement; (5) electron dense hyalinosis areas, often visible in sclerotic regions. The use of animal models to perform ultrastructural analysis of nephron architecture can represent a valid tool to understand the pathophysiological mechanisms leading to diabetic nephropathy and can play an important role in new target and drug discovery. For technical details, refer to Chap. 10, Sect. 3.6. Herein, only the procedures for sample collecting and fixation are described, which differ from those reported in Chap. 10.

Collection and Fixation of Tissue Sample

1. For ultrastructural examinations, place the kidney on dental wax and cut frontally with two blades. From the cortical and medullar area, cut fragments to less than 1 mm^3 of tissue (*see* **Note 38**).
2. Gently pipette 2 mL of Karnovsky's Glutaraldehyde fixative (*see* Chap. 10, Sect. 2.5) in a glass tube and submerge the specimens.
3. Incubate for at least 8 h at RT or overnight at 4°C.
4. Rinse the sample with 2 mL of Washing buffer (*see* Sect. 2.5) and repeat washes three times. The specimens can be stored for 4 days at 4 °C in a Washing buffer.
5. Do not use metal tools because metal ions react with aldehydes.
6. Post-fix the specimens with phosphate-buffered 1% osmium tetroxide solution (*see* Chap. 10, Sect. 2.5 and **Note 30**) for 1 h at RT.
7. Gently rinse the specimens in 0.5% NaCl solution.
8. Follow the procedure as reported in Chap. 10, Sects. 3.6.2–3.6.7.

4 Notes

1. On the basis of the hierarchical differences (DBA/2 < C57BL/6 < BALB/c) in STZ sensitivity among strains, when inbred mice are used the DBA/2 strain should be the preferred choice. However, it has to be taken into account that a different strain will require a pilot STZ dose-finding study or a second readministration of STZ after 7 weeks of diabetes induction.
2. Although the feeder drawer is not designed for food in pellet form, the problem can be circumvented by adjusting the Feeder Drawer vertically (*see* Fig. 1b); otherwise, the mice will take the pellet to the Support Grid and urine and feces will be contaminated by food.

3. Heparin is suitable when non-hematological downstream applications are required. It offers the advantage that it can be administrated both to living mice maximizing the amount of blood for collection or to be used by precoating the syringe just before the puncture drawing it up in a syringe with the needle used for the puncture, and pulling the plunger all the way back to coat the syringe before discharging the excess into the collecting tube. If hematological downstream applications are desired, an EDTA 0.5 M solution can be used precoating the syringe as previously described or using commercially available precoated sample tubes.
4. Although the Bradford reagent is commercially available and ready-to-use solutions can be purchased, the Reagent can be prepared starting from Coomassie brilliant blue G-250. For this purpose a 5× concentrate Bradford reagent can be prepared by dissolving 100 mg of Coomassie brilliant blue G-250 in 47 mL of methanol 100%. Then, add 100 mL of phosphoric acid 85% and adjust volume to 200 mL with dd H_2O. For the test use 2.5 μL of protein sample diluted in 400 μL of water and 100 μL of the prepared Bradford reagent (final volume 500 μL).
5. The minimum sample size can be determined by applying a power analysis using the Fleiss test. Help can be found at the website http://www.openepi.com/Menu/OE_Menu.htm. To set the parameters, the percent of exposed with outcome (renal impairment) can be set at 50% when the result is unknown, while the percent of unexposed with outcome can be set at 1%. Confidence interval was 95%, and the power was at 80%. If DBA mice are used a 40% of attrition should be considered to avoid that diabetes-induced mortality that could decrease the power of the study.
6. Overnight fasting nearly depletes liver glycogen stores in the mouse. This has the advantage of reducing variability in baseline blood glucose. However, mice have a unique metabolic response to prolonged fasting that contrasts with the response seen in humans. Specifically, a prolonged fast impairs insulin-stimulated glucose utilization in humans, but enhances it in normal mice [109, 110] as well as in some strains of transgenic mice [111, 112]. Therefore, overnight fasting is useful for studies where the focus is on glucose utilization (e.g., effects on muscle uptake of glucose). Otherwise, a 5- to 6-h fast is sufficient to assess insulin action within a more physiological context [113].
7. The quantity of blood required depends on the glucometer used, but for most of them a few μl is sufficient. Do not allow blood clotting before application to the Test Strip. Take care to

use whole blood and not plasma as it can differ from plasma glucose levels by up to 11% (plasma higher).

8. The metabolic cages are usually intended to be used for single mouse urine and feces collections; however, some models allow up to three mice housing, thus avoiding stressful social isolation. If more than one mouse is housed, the animals should be matched for baseline characteristics such as glycemic status and weight. The number of mice/cage has to be taken into account when urinalysis is performed.
9. In diabetic animals, urine may over flow capacity of the collection tube and spill in the lower chamber of mouse cage. Larger containers can be used.
10. For storage, the stability of the analytes should be considered. Albumin is stable for at least 1 week when stored at either 4 or 20 °C [114]. Freezing at −20 °C causes fragmentation, and a single freeze-thaw cycle may cause apparent albumin loss (i.e., from urine, 40% is lost after a single freeze-thaw cycle) although the effect varies with storage duration and between individual samples [115]. If prolonged storage is required, freezing at −80 °C appears to preserve albumin integrity when measured by immunoassay [116]. Creatinine is also stable for at least 1 week at either 4 or 20 °C and is unaffected by freezing at either −20 or −80 °C. When thawing, inspect the sample for clarity and centrifuge if visibly cloudy.
11. A dilution tritiation may be recommended before performing the assay. Notably, the concentration of urine is strictly dependent on the volume of urine excreted; therefore in the diabetic nephropathy model after a 24 h urine collection control mice show the highest concentration, but the lowest total amount of albumin when adjusted for the volume. The urine from control animals should be used to select the best dilution. Importantly, differences exist between strains: for DBA/2 mice a higher dilution is generally required than for the C57BL/6 counterparts (1:1000 *versus* 1:500, respectively).
12. A dilution tritiation may be recommended before performing the assay. The dilution has to be optimized to obtain absorbance values for the high standard of 1.8–2.2 and the reading of the low standard should be above background (blank).
13. Creatinine is stable for at least 1 week at either 4 or 20 °C and unaffected by freezing, samples can be dryed and stored. If long-term storage is desired, freeze samples at −20 °C before reconstitution.
14. The quantity of filtered Mobile Phase used to reconstitute the sample may be adjusted for technical reasons. Indeed, if an excessively high sample loop is used (e.g., 20 μL) the use of a double amount of mobile phase is recommended to avoid

injection of insoluble particles on the bottom or the wall of the tube. The amount of mobile phase in respect to the amount of sample used for the extraction has to be taken into account to determine the proper dilution factor for data analysis.

15. The injection of large amounts of sample due to high capacity loop can dramatically affect the efficiency of the column, depending on the length of the column itself. Eventually, the injection of Mobile phase only between each experimental sample should be considered to ensure the maintenance of column efficiency.
16. Sagittal sections of the kidney are performed to study the relationship of the renal vessels, renal pelvis, and renal pyramids, but transversal sections are preferred to evaluate the nephron structures, especially in the cortical area.
17. Do not use pen, because the ink will be dissolved in the ethanol during the dehydration process.
18. The incubation for some hours at RT allows the fixation fluid to better penetrate into the sample tissue.
19. At low temperatures, structural elements of tissues are stabilized against the destructive effects of solvent changes.
20. The dehydration passage in 95% ethanol can be prolonged up to 12 h without affecting the process quality.
21. The time in absolute ethanol should be minimal. Progressive removal of bound water from carbohydrates and proteins during prolonged immersion in absolute ethanol causes tissues to harden excessively and become brittle.
22. Be careful as xylene is neurotoxic. Synthetic nontoxic solvents are commercially available.
23. A margin of at least 2 mm of paraffin surrounding all sides of the tissue gives optimum cutting support.
24. Disposable plastic molds, which become an integral part of the block and serve as the block holder in the microtome, are commercially available.
25. The section required thickness should be around 5 μm, but a range from 4 to 12 μm is acceptable for histological analysis. The quantification of the staining is negatively affected by the thickness of slice.
26. If the ribbon is crooked, the upper and lower edges of the block face should be parallel to each other or to the knife edge.
27. If the block is not ribboning well place it on the ice to cool the paraffin surface.
28. A slow, uniform cutting stroke is required. Do not ever stop and start a cut mid-way through a section. Some time dedi-

cated to developing the sectioning rhythm on practice blocks before attempting to cut valuable tissue is advisable.

29. If the sections are compressed or folded, the knife may not be sharpened sufficiently or is incorrectly angled. It is also possible that the selected thickness of sections is too thin.
30. If the specimen crumbles, the tissue could be inadequately dehydrated or cleared (dissolve off the paraffin, rehydrate, and clear) or it could be too hard and compact (soak it in water or 70% ethanol to soften it).
31. Do not float your tissue sections any longer than needed to remove their wrinkled appearance, as longer time may affect morphology.
32. To deparaffinize samples, xylene could be substituted with toluene or synthetic histoclear. Take care to consider an extra incubation time when histoclear is used.
33. The length of time necessary to overstain the tissues depends upon fixation and the type of hematoxylin employed. The time reported herein is adjusted for renal tissues.
34. Differentiation with acid ethanol requires some practical experience to choose the correct end-point, since the acid solution alters the color of the tissue to red. The correct end-point is when, after blueing up, the background is almost colorless. For renal tissue sections, two quick dips in 0.3% acid ethanol are enough.
35. The length of time necessary to stain the tissues depends on the type of eosin employed and the kind of tissue sample. For renal tissue sections, 30 s is enough. Eosin is highly soluble in water. Over-staining is removed by washing in dd H_2O.
36. The length of incubation of Schiff reagent depends on the kind of tissue sample. For renal tissue sections at least 25 min is needed.
37. A "near-equilibrium staining" is established with 60 min of incubation. The color intensity does not increase with longer times.
38. The tissue size should be kept small. Blocks should be cut to less than 1 mm^3 to ensure thorough and quick penetration of fixatives and embedding solutions.

References

1. Becker GJ, Hewitson TD (2013) Animal models of chronic kidney disease: useful but not perfect. Nephrol Dial Transplant 28:2432–2438
2. Rak-Raszewska A, Hauser PV, Vainio S (2015) Organ in vitro culture: what have we learned about early kidney development? Stem Cells Int 2015:959807
3. Kim S, Takayama S (2015) Organ-on-a-chip and the kidney. Kidney Res Clin Pract 34: 165–169
4. Giraud S, Favreau F, Chatauret N et al (2011) Contribution of large pig for renal ischemia-reperfusion and transplantation studies: the preclinical model. J Biomed Biotechnol 2011:532127

5. Feng M, DiPetrillo K (2009) Non-invasive blood pressure measurement in mice. Methods Mol Biol 573:45–55
6. Park F (2007) Lentiviral vectors: are they the future of animal transgenesis? Physiol Genomics 31:159–173
7. Kim J, Zarjou A, Traylor AM et al (2012) In vivo regulation of the heme oxygenase-1 gene in humanized transgenic mice. Kidney Int 82:278–291
8. Hewitson TD, Ono T, Becker GJ (2009) Small animal models of kidney disease: a review. Methods Mol Biol 466:41–57
9. Kurts C, Panzer U, Anders HJ et al (2013) The immune system and kidney disease: basic concepts and clinical implications. Nat Rev Immunol 13:738–753
10. Brady HR, Singer GG (1995) Acute renal failure. Lancet 346:1533–1540
11. Lassnigg A, Schmidlin D, Mouhieddine M et al (2004) Minimal changes of serum creatinine predict prognosis in patients after cardiothoracic surgery: a prospective cohort study. J Am Soc Nephrol 15:1597–1605
12. Foundation NK et al (2002) K/DOQI clinical practice guidelines for chronic kidney disease: evaluation, classification, and stratification. Am J Kidney Dis 39:S1–266
13. Mann JF, Gerstein HC, Pogue J et al (2001) Renal insufficiency as a predictor of cardiovascular outcomes and the impact of ramipril: the HOPE randomized trial. Ann Intern Med 134:629–636
14. Jones CA, Francis ME, Eberhardt MS et al (2002) Microalbuminuria in the US population: third National Health and Nutrition Examination Survey. Am J Kidney Dis 39:445–459
15. Muntner P, Coresh J, Klag MJ et al (2002) History of myocardial infarction and stroke among incident end-stage renal disease cases and population-based controls: an analysis of shared risk factors. Am J Kidney Dis 40:323–330
16. Hovind P, Tarnow L, Rossing P et al (2004) Predictors for the development of microalbuminuria and macroalbuminuria in patients with type 1 diabetes: inception cohort study. BMJ 328:1105
17. Rossing P (2005) The changing epidemiology of diabetic microangiopathy in type 1 diabetes. Diabetologia 48:1439–1444
18. Steffes MW, Bilous RW, Sutherland DE et al (1992) Cell and matrix components of the glomerular mesangium in type I diabetes. Diabetes 41:679–684
19. Katz A, Caramori ML, Sisson-Ross S et al (2002) An increase in the cell component of the cortical interstitium antedates interstitial fibrosis in type 1 diabetic patients. Kidney Int 61:2058–2066
20. Singh AP, Junemann A, Muthuraman A et al (2012) Animal models of acute renal failure. Pharmacol Rep 64:31–44
21. Sanz AB, Sanchez-Nino MD, Martin-Cleary C et al (2013) Progress in the development of animal models of acute kidney injury and its impact on drug discovery. Expert Opin Drug Discov 8:879–895
22. Pickering JW, Endre ZH (2014) The definition and detection of acute kidney injury. J Renal Inj Prev 3:21–25
23. Pickering JW, Endre ZH (2014) Acute kidney injury urinary biomarker time-courses. PLoS One 9:e101288
24. Wei Q, Dong Z (2012) Mouse model of ischemic acute kidney injury: technical notes and tricks. Am J Physiol Renal Physiol 303:F1487–F1494
25. Ucero AC, Benito-Martin A, Izquierdo MC et al (2014) Unilateral ureteral obstruction: beyond obstruction. Int Urol Nephrol 46:765–776
26. Ucero AC, Goncalves S, Benito-Martin A et al (2010) Obstructive renal injury: from fluid mechanics to molecular cell biology. Open Access J Urol 2:41–55
27. Thiel G, Wilson DR, Arce ML et al (1967) Glycerol induced hemoglobinuric acute renal failure in the rat. II. The experimental model, predisposing factors, and pathophysiologic features. Nephron 4:276–297
28. Curry SC, Chang D, Connor D (1989) Drug- and toxin-induced rhabdomyolysis. Ann Emerg Med 18:1068–1084
29. Remick DG, Newcomb DE, Bolgos GL, Call DR (2000) Comparison of the mortality and inflammatory response of two models of sepsis: lipopolysaccharide vs. cecal ligation and puncture. Shock 13:110–116
30. Yang HC, Zuo Y, Fogo AB (2010) Models of chronic kidney disease. Drug Discov Today Dis Models 7:13–19
31. Kashtan CE (2002) Animal models of Alport syndrome. Nephrol Dial Transplant 17:1359–1362
32. Ortiz A, Sanchez-Nino MD, Izquierdo MC et al (2015) Translational value of animal models of kidney failure. Eur J Pharmacol 759:205–220
33. Diwan V, Mistry A, Gobe G et al (2013) Adenine-induced chronic kidney and cardio-

vascular damage in rats. J Pharmacol Toxicol Methods 68:197–207

34. Nguy L, Johansson ME, Grimberg E et al (2013) Rats with adenine-induced chronic renal failure develop low-renin, salt-sensitive hypertension and increased aortic stiffness. Am J Physiol Regul Integr Comp Physiol 304:R744–R752
35. Sanchez-Fructuoso AI, Cano M, Arroyo M et al (2002) Lead mobilization during calcium disodium ethylenediaminetetraacetate chelation therapy in treatment of chronic lead poisoning. Am J Kidney Dis 40:51–58
36. Taylor FB Jr, Tesh VL, DeBault L et al (1999) Characterization of the baboon responses to Shiga-like toxin: descriptive study of a new primate model of toxic responses to Stx-1. Am J Pathol 154:1285–1299
37. Granger JP, LaMarca BB, Cockrell K et al (2006) Reduced uterine perfusion pressure (RUPP) model for studying cardiovascular-renal dysfunction in response to placental ischemia. Methods Mol Med 122:383–392
38. Li J, LaMarca B, Reckelhoff JF (2012) A model of preeclampsia in rats: the reduced uterine perfusion pressure (RUPP) model. Am J Physiol Heart Circ Physiol 303:H1–H8
39. Reutens AT, Atkins RC (2011) Epidemiology of diabetic nephropathy. Contrib Nephrol 170:1–7
40. Ghaderian SB, Hayati F, Shayanpour S et al (2015) Diabetes and end-stage renal disease; a review article on new concepts. J Renal Inj Prev 4:28–33
41. Krolewski M, Eggers PW, Warram JH (1996) Magnitude of end-stage renal disease in IDDM: a 35 year follow-up study. Kidney Int 50:2041–2046
42. Ritz E, Orth SR (1999) Nephropathy in patients with type 2 diabetes mellitus. N Engl J Med 341:1127–1133
43. Schlatzer DM, Dazard JE, Dharsee M et al (2009) Urinary protein profiles in a rat model for diabetic complications. Mol Cell Proteomics 8:2145–2158
44. Tay YC, Wang Y, Kairaitis L et al (2005) Can murine diabetic nephropathy be separated from superimposed acute renal failure? Kidney Int 68:391–398
45. Kong LL, Wu H, Cui WP et al (2013) Advances in murine models of diabetic nephropathy. J Diabetes Res 2013:797548
46. Kurien BT, Everds NE, Scofield RH (2004) Experimental animal urine collection: a review. Lab Anim 38:333–361
47. Gil MC, Aguirre JA, Lemoine AP et al (1999) Influence of age on stress responses to metabolic cage housing in rats. Cell Mol Neurobiol 19:625–633
48. Armando I, Carranza A, Nishimura Y et al (2001) Peripheral administration of an angiotensin II AT(1) receptor antagonist decreases the hypothalamic-pituitary-adrenal response to isolation Stress. Endocrinology 142: 3880–3889
49. Eriksson E, Royo F, Lyberg K et al (2004) Effect of metabolic cage housing on immunoglobulin A and corticosterone excretion in faeces and urine of young male rats. Exp Physiol 89:427–433
50. Armando I, Volpi S, Aguilera G et al (2007) Angiotensin II AT1 receptor blockade prevents the hypothalamic corticotropin-releasing factor response to isolation stress. Brain Res 1142:92–99
51. Hoppe CC, Moritz KM, Fitzgerald SM et al (2009) Transient hypertension and sustained tachycardia in mice housed individually in metabolism cages. Physiol Res 58:69–75
52. Beynon RJ, Hurst JL (2004) Urinary proteins and the modulation of chemical scents in mice and rats. Peptides 25:1553–1563
53. Breyer MD, Qi Z (2010) Better nephrology for mice—and man. Kidney Int 77:487–489
54. Meyer MH, Meyer RA Jr, Gray RW et al (1985) Picric acid methods greatly overestimate serum creatinine in mice: more accurate results with high-performance liquid chromatography. Anal Biochem 144:285–290
55. Breyer MD, Bottinger E, Brosius FC et al (2005) Mouse models of diabetic nephropathy. J Am Soc Nephrol 16:27–45
56. Rodrigues WF, Miguel CB, Napimoga MH et al (2014) Establishing standards for studying renal function in mice through measurements of body size-adjusted creatinine and urea levels. Biomed Res Int 2014:872827
57. Fioretto P, Mauer M (2007) Histopathology of diabetic nephropathy. Semin Nephrol 27:195–207
58. Vallon V (2011) The proximal tubule in the pathophysiology of the diabetic kidney. Am J Physiol Regul Integr Comp Physiol 300:R1009–R1022
59. Harris RD, Steffes MW, Bilous RW et al (1991) Global glomerular sclerosis and glomerular arteriolar hyalinosis in insulin dependent diabetes. Kidney Int 40:107–114
60. Najafian B, Kim Y, Crosson JT et al (2003) Atubular glomeruli and glomerulotubular junction abnormalities in diabetic nephropathy. J Am Soc Nephrol 14:908–917
61. Sedor JR, Abboud HE (1984) Actions and metabolism of histamine in glomeruli and

tubules of the human kidney. Kidney Int 26:144–152
62. Abboud HE, Ou SL, Velosa JA et al (1982) Dynamics of renal histamine in normal rat kidney and in nephrosis induced by aminonucleoside of puromycin. J Clin Invest 69:327–336
63. Roberts IS, Brenchley PE (2000) Mast cells: the forgotten cells of renal fibrosis. J Clin Pathol 53:858–862
64. Morgan TK, Montgomery K, Mason V et al (2006) Upregulation of histidine decarboxylase expression in superficial cortical nephrons during pregnancy in mice and women. Kidney Int 70:306–314
65. Beaven MA, Jacobsen S, Horakova Z (1972) Modification of the enzymatic isotopic assay of histamine and its application to measurement of histamine in tissues, serum and urine. Clin Chim Acta 37:91–103
66. Moore TC, Thompson DP, Glassock RJ (1971) Elevation in urinary and blood histamine following clinical renal transplantation. Ann Surg 173:381–388
67. Ichikawa I, Brenner BM (1979) Mechanisms of action of hisamine and histamine antagonists on the glomerular microcirculation in the rat. Circ Res 45:737–745
68. Janoff A (1966) Effect of an antihistamine on the increased vascular permeability induced by leucocyte lysosome fractions. Nature 212:1605–1606
69. Wilson CB, Gushwa LC, Peterson OW et al (1981) Glomerular immune injury in the rat: effect of antagonists of histamine activity. Kidney Int 20:628–635
70. Tanda S, Mori Y, Kimura T et al (2007) Histamine ameliorates anti-glomerular basement membrane antibody-induced glomerulonephritis in rats. Kidney Int 72:608–613
71. Gutzmer R, Diestel C, Mommert S et al (2005) Histamine H4 receptor stimulation suppresses IL-12p70 production and mediates chemotaxis in human monocyte-derived dendritic cells. J Immunol 174:5224–5232
72. Kurata H, Fujii T, Tsutsui H et al (2006) Renoprotective effects of l-carnosine on ischemia/reperfusion-induced renal injury in rats. J Pharmacol Exp Ther 319:640–647
73. Markle RA, Hollis TM, Cosgarea AJ (1986) Renal histamine increases in the streptozotocin-diabetic rat. Exp Mol Pathol 44:21–28
74. Gill DS, Thompson CS, Dandona P (1990) Histamine synthesis and catabolism in various tissues in diabetic rats. Metabolism 39:815–818
75. Alkan M, Machavoine F, Rignault R et al (2015) Histidine decarboxylase deficiency prevents autoimmune diabetes in NOD Mice. J Diabetes Res 2015:965056
76. Sinclair RJ, Bell RD, Keyl MJ (1974) Effects of prostaglandin E2 (PGE2) and histamine on renal fluid dynamics. Am J Physiol 227:1062–1066
77. Banks RO, Fondacaro JD, Schwaiger MM et al (1978) Renal histamine H_1 and H_2 receptors: characterization and functional significance. Am J Physiol 235:F570–F575
78. Schwertschlag U, Hackenthal E (1982) Histamine stimulates renin release from the isolated perfused rat kidney. Naunyn Schmiedebergs Arch Pharmacol 319:239–242
79. Veglia E, Grange C, Pini A et al (2015) Histamine receptor expression in human renal tubules: a comparative pharmacological evaluation. Inflamm Res 64:261–270
80. Rosa AC, Grange C, Pini A et al (2013) Overexpression of histamine H(4) receptors in the kidney of diabetic rat. Inflamm Res 62:357–365
81. Pini A, Chazot PL, Veglia E et al (2015) H3 receptor renal expression in normal and diabetic rats. Inflamm Res 64:271–273
82. Dunn SR, Qi Z, Bottinger EP et al (2004) Utility of endogenous creatinine clearance as a measure of renal function in mice. Kidney Int 65:1959–1967
83. Ganda OP, Rossini AA, Like AA (1976) Studies on streptozotocin diabetes. Diabetes 25:595–603
84. Rossini AA, Williams RM, Appel MC et al (1978) Complete protection from low-dose streptozotocin-induced diabetes in mice. Nature 276:182–184
85. George M, Ayuso E, Casellas A et al (2002) Beta cell expression of IGF-I leads to recovery from type 1 diabetes. J Clin Invest 109:1153–1163
86. Heidbreder CA, Weiss IC, Domeney AM et al (2000) Behavioral, neurochemical and endocrinological characterization of the early social isolation syndrome. Neuroscience 100:749–768
87. Greco AM, Gambardella P, Sticchi R et al (1989) Effects of individual housing on circadian rhythms of adult rats. Physiol Behav 45:363–366
88. Nagy TR, Krzywanski D, Li J, Meleth S et al (2002) Effect of group vs. single housing on phenotypic variance in C57BL/6J mice. Obes Res 10:412–415
89. Parasuraman S, Raveendran R, Kesavan R (2010) Blood sample collection in small labo-

ratory animals. J Pharmacol Pharmacother 1:87–93

90. Martin H (2011) Laboratory measurement of urine albumin and urine total protein in screening for proteinuria in chronic kidney disease. Clin Biochem Rev 32:97–102
91. Rodrigues GR, Lewis DR (2014) Establishing auditory steady-state response thresholds to narrow band CE-chirps((R)) in full-term neonates. Int J Pediatr Otorhinolaryngol 78:238–243
92. Brosius FC 3rd, Alpers CE, Bottinger EP et al (2009) Mouse models of diabetic nephropathy. J Am Soc Nephrol 20:2503–2512
93. Hopwood D (1996) Fixation and fixatives In: Bancroft J, Stevens A (eds) Theory and practice of histological techniques. Churchill Livingstone, New York
94. Andrews PM, Coffey AK (1984) A technique to reduce fixation artifacts to kidney proximal tubules. Kidney Int 25:964–968
95. Winsor L (1994) Tissue processing. In: Woods AE, Ellis RC (eds) Laboratory histopathology: a complete reference, vol 1. Churchill Livingstone, New York
96. Holdsworth SR, Summers SA (2008) Role of mast cells in progressive renal diseases. J Am Soc Nephrol 19:2254–2261
97. Strobel S, Miller HR, Ferguson A (1981) Human intestinal mucosal mast cells: evaluation of fixation and staining techniques. J Clin Pathol 34(8):851–858
98. Vogel B, Siebert H, Hofmann U et al (2015) Determination of collagen content within picrosirius red stained paraffin-embedded tissue sections using fluorescence microscopy. MethodsX 2:124–134
99. Lattouf R, Younes R, Lutomski D et al (2014) Picrosirius red staining: a useful tool to appraise collagen networks in normal and pathological tissues. J Histochem Cytochem 62(10):751–758
100. Grimm PC, Nickerson P, Gough J et al (2003) Computerized image analysis of Sirius Red-stained renal allograft biopsies as a surrogate marker to predict long-term allograft function. J Am Soc Nephrol 14:1662–1668
101. Nielsen LF, Moe D, Kirkeby S et al (1998) Sirius red and acid fuchsin staining mechanisms. Biotech Histochem 73:71–77
102. Street JM, Souza AC, Alvarez-Prats A et al (2014) Automated quantification of renal fibrosis with Sirius Red and polarization contrast microscopy. Physiol Rep 2:pii: e12088
103. Alsaad KO, Herzenberg AM (2007) Distinguishing diabetic nephropathy from other causes of glomerulosclerosis: an update. J Clin Pathol 60:18–26
104. Spargo BH (1975) Practical use of electron microscopy for the diagnosis of glomerular disease. Hum Pathol 6:405–420
105. Tighe JR, Jones NF (1970) The diagnostic value of routine electron microscopy of renal biopsies. Proc R Soc Med 63:475–477
106. Drummond K, Mauer M, International Diabetic Nephropathy Study G (2002) The early natural history of nephropathy in type 1 diabetes: II. Early renal structural changes in type 1 diabetes. Diabetes 51:1580–1587
107. Steffes MW, Schmidt D, McCrery R et al (2001) Glomerular cell number in normal subjects and in type 1 diabetic patients. Kidney Int 59:2104–2113
108. Dalla Vestra M, Masiero A, Roiter AM et al (2003) Is podocyte injury relevant in diabetic nephropathy? Studies in patients with type 2 diabetes. Diabetes 52:1031–1035
109. Heijboer AC, Donga E, Voshol PJ et al (2005) Sixteen hours of fasting differentially affects hepatic and muscle insulin sensitivity in mice. J Lipid Res 46:582–588
110. Ayala JE, Bracy DP, McGuinness OP et al (2006) Considerations in the design of hyperinsulinemic-euglycemic clamps in the conscious mouse. Diabetes 55:390–397
111. Ren JM, Marshall BA, Mueckler MM et al (1995) Overexpression of Glut4 protein in muscle increases basal and insulin-stimulated whole body glucose disposal in conscious mice. J Clin Invest 95:429–432
112. Halseth AE, Bracy DP, Wasserman DH (1999) Overexpression of hexokinase II increases insulinand exercise-stimulated muscle glucose uptake in vivo. Am J Physiol 276:E70–E77
113. Ayala JE, Samuel VT, Morton GJ et al (2010) Standard operating procedures for describing and performing metabolic tests of glucose homeostasis in mice. Dis Model Mech 3:525–534
114. Schachtel BP (1983) Effect of an antihistamine-decongestant on otitis media. J Pediatr 102:319–321
115. Brinkman JW, de Zeeuw D, Duker JJ et al (2005) Falsely low urinary albumin concentrations after prolonged frozen storage of urine samples. Clin Chem 51:2181–2183
116. Brinkman JW, de Zeeuw D, Lambers Heerspink HJ et al (2007) Apparent loss of urinary albumin during long-term frozen storage: HPLC vs immunonephelometry. Clin Chem 53:1520–1526

Chapter 12

Methodological Approaches to Investigate the Effects of Histamine Receptor Targeting Compounds in Preclinical Models of Breast Cancer

Diego J. Martinel Lamas, Melisa B. Nicoud, Helena Sterle, Graciela P. Cricco, Gabriela A. Martin, Graciela A. Cremaschi, Hubert G. Schwelberger, Elena S. Rivera, and Vanina A. Medina

Abstract

Numerous studies demonstrated the pivotal role of histamine in breast cancer development and progression. This chapter aims to describe different preclinical breast cancer models, including in vitro soft agar clonogenic assay and in vivo chemically induced breast tumors in rats, human triple negative breast cancer (TNBC) xenograft, and murine TNBC syngeneic graft in mice. All these models could be useful and complementary to assess the role of histamine receptor ligands in breast cancer, which could originate advances in novel therapeutics to treat this disease. This chapter also describes the gold standard radiometric techniques to evaluate the activity of histamine metabolizing enzymes in breast cancer specimens.

Key words Allograft, Breast cancer, Carcinogenesis, Clonogenic assay, Proliferation, Syngeneic model, Tumor growth, Xenogeneic model, Xenograft

1 Introduction

Cancer continues to be a major health burden, causing now more deaths than all heart diseases [1]. Particularly, breast cancer is the most frequent cause of cancer death in women in less developed regions while it is the second cause of cancer death in more developed countries [2]. Breast cancer is a heterogeneous disease in terms of presentation, histopathology, molecular and genetic profiles, and clinical response to anti-cancer therapies [3, 4]. Thus, an important area of cancer research is focused on the discovery of more specific and effective treatments. Both basic science studies and clinical trials are pivotal constituents of the cancer therapeutic development [5].

Histamine plays a central role in the physiological and pathological conditions of mammary gland [4, 6–10], and several studies

Ekaterini Tiligada and Madeleine Ennis (eds.), *Histamine Receptors as Drug Targets*, Methods in Pharmacology and Toxicology, DOI 10.1007/978-1-4939-6843-5_12, © Springer Science+Business Media LLC 2017

support the involvement of histamine and histamine receptors (HR) in breast cancer [4, 6, 7, 11–23].

To predict the clinical utility of histamine receptor ligands and other potential therapeutics, different preclinical breast cancer models can be investigated. They include in vitro human cell lines, chemically induced breast tumors in rats, human xenograft, and murine allograft in mice [5, 16, 24–27]. In these models, tumor volume or survival (in vivo mouse or rat models) or cell proliferation (in vitro cell lines) is compared between the untreated control group and the histamine/histamine receptor ligands' treatment group.

Colony formation assay is a cell survival assay that relies on the capacity of a single cell to proliferate forming a colony, which is defined as an aggregate of at least 50 cells. This assay basically analyzes individual cells for their ability to undergo unlimited division. It is considered the gold standard to determine cell reproductive death after the treatment with ionizing radiation [28] and has proven predictive value in the chemosensitivity testing of standard and experimental anti-tumoral agents [25]. Colony assay techniques in soft agar may be used to assess in vitro surviving cells in tumors from animals that have been subjected to treatments in vivo, and also for studying in vitro the effects of drugs on clonogenic growth of primary cultures or cancer cell lines [29, 30]. The tumor clonogenic assay could be considered a secondary assay in the approach to discover anti-cancer drugs [25]. Nevertheless, growth in semisolid agar can evaluate only a tumor cell's ability to perform one step in the multistep carcinogenenic process [31]. Thus, animal models using transplantable tumors or chemically induced cancers are the standard preclinical systems for analyzing the efficacy of anti-cancer agents.

Chemically induced mammary tumors in female rats constitute a standard laboratory model for studying biology, prevention, and treatment of breast cancer. The developed tumors mimic the most frequently diagnosed breast cancer in women in relation to the epithelial origin, histopathology, ovarian hormone responsiveness, and gene expression.

These experimental tumors originate from terminal end buds, structures corresponding to the terminal ductal lobular unit in humans, which is the accepted site of origin of ductal human carcinoma. Histological analysis mostly shows locally invasive adenocarcinomas with cribriform, papillary, and comedo patterns that express estrogen (ER) and progesterone (PR) receptors [26, 27, 32, 33].

The chemical carcinogens most usually used for breast cancer induction in rats are N-methyl-N-nitrosourea (NMU) and 7,12-dimethyl-benzanthracene (DMBA). NMU is most widely used since it is water-soluble, does not require metabolic activation, has a shorter half-life and induced tumors are more estrogen dependent and aggressive than the ones developed with DMBA. DMBA needs metabolic activation (tumorigenicity can be altered by agents changing its pharmacokinetics), causes a higher proportion of benign tumors, and tumors are more prolactin dependent and less aggressive [34, 35].

Chan et al demonstrated that NMU-injected rats develop multiple and heterogeneous tumors, arising from different initiated cells, with a molecular gene expression pattern similar to ER-positive, low to intermediate grade human breast cancer [36]. Gullino et al first described the dose, via and interval for administration of NMU to female rats. They reported three intravenous (i.v.) NMU injections at monthly intervals, the first dose administered between 50 and 55 days of age [37]. Later, other researchers demonstrated that intraperitoneal (i.p.) administration (a simpler route that does not require great technical ability) provides similar results [38–42]. This experimental model proved to be useful to evaluate preventive and therapeutic agents for human breast cancer, and also for studying malignant progression, allowing the understanding of processes of mutation, oxidative stress, and inflammation that occur during carcinogenesis [43–46]. In addition, NMU-induced tumors express H1R and H2R in membrane fractions and this model has been successfully used to evaluate the action of H1R and H2R antagonists on tumor growth and histamine role as an autocrine growth factor [14, 16, 17].

However, NMU-induced mammary carcinoma is a relatively time-consuming model, there is some variability and the hosts are rats, a larger animal compared with mice [43]. Also, reports on metastasis are variable and as the tumor micro-environment is rat tissue, this model not fully represents the complexity of human tumors [39, 47].

The discovery that tumor tissue could be xenografted into the mutant athymic "nude" mouse strain opened a new research area for experimental studies of human tumors, including the analysis of their proliferative and metastatic properties [31]. This preclinical cancer method involves genuine human cancer cells or solid tumors, which are transplanted into a host mouse, and represents a more clinically relevant tumor model [48–50]. The host mice have impaired immune systems in order to avoid rejection of foreign cells from the human species. These transplants may be subcutaneous, placed just beneath the mouse's skin or may be orthotopic, meaning that the tumor is placed in the site it would be expected to naturally develop. The main advantage of human xenograft is that the tumor carries human genetic material, being more representative of the characteristics and mutations of the human cancer. On the other hand, because of the use of an immunodeficient host, it may not mimic the actual clinical situation and it is not possible to evaluate the role of the immune system in tumor progression and response to anti-cancer treatments. Other disadvantages include a higher cost compared with syngeneic models, the stromal and other micro-environment components of the tumors are rodent; therefore, there are instances in which the model is inappropriate as a likely predictor of clinical outcome (e.g., anti-angiogenic strategies as the vasculature is of murine origin) [31, 48–51].

Triple-negative breast cancers (TNBC), which lack ER, PR, and epidermal growth factor receptor 2 expressions, represent 15–20% of all breast carcinomas, and are associated with poor prognosis and aggressiveness and are refractory to targeted systemic therapy [3, 52]. One of the most widely used TNBC animal models is the human MDA-MB-231 cells xenografted mice and is useful to assess new therapeutic and adjuvant agents. Several variables affect the occurrence of metastasis, including the health and housing conditions, the routes of tumor cell inoculation, and the intrinsic tumor characteristics. Many human breast tumors can proliferate when injected subcutaneously into nude mice and less frequently produce lung and lymph node metastases. However, the implantation of human breast cancer cells into anatomically appropriate (orthotopic) sites has favored metastatic potential [53].

The expression of histamine receptor subtypes has been demonstrated in cell lines derived from human mammary gland [21, 22, 54]. Histamine modulated the proliferation of the TNBC cell line MDA-MB-231 in a dose-dependent manner [21, 23]. MDA-MB-231 xenograft tumors in immune-deficient nude mice exhibited moderate expression of H4R and high expression of a proliferation marker (PCNA). In vivo treatments with histamine or H4R agonists diminished the tumor growth rate [55] and thus, this is a useful preclinical model to investigate the therapeutic potential of histamine receptor ligands. In this model, histamine enhanced anti-tumor effects of ionizing radiation and doxorubicin, two conventional treatments for breast cancer [11, 56].

In addition, there is increasing evidence that supports the immunomodulatory roles of histamine under different cytokine environments [57]. Breast cancer has not usually been considered a cancer to be treated with immunotherapeutic approaches. However, recent studies have shown that the presence of tumor-infiltrating lymphocytes (TILs) is a prognostic marker for higher responses to neoadjuvant chemotherapy and better survival, particularly in triple negative and HER2-positive early breast cancer [58]. In addition, experiments in syngeneic breast cancer induced in histamine-free (HDC knock-out) and wild-type mice demonstrated that endogenous histamine stimulates the growth of breast adenocarcinoma tumor implants by suppressing anti-tumor immunity accompanied by a predominantly Th2-polarized cytokine pattern [59].

Syngeneic tumor graft systems, also known as syngeneic models, consist of tumor tissues derived from the same genetic background as a given mouse strain. An interesting animal model that can be used to study the effects of histamine and histamine receptor ligands on the anti-tumor immune response in TNBC is the 4T1 cell line. This tumor is an animal model that resembles stage IV human breast cancer. It can be grown in vivo as a primary tumor in BALB/c mice. In order to more closely imitate human clinical disease, the orthotopic transplant into the mammary fat pads is recommended. It was originally isolated from a spontaneously arising mammary tumor in BALB/cfC3H mice [60]. It can spontaneously metastasize from the primary tumor in the mammary gland via the hematogenous route to multiple distant sites including lymph nodes, blood, liver, lung, brain, and bone [61–63]. It induces a leukemoid reaction, characterized by bone marrow hyperplasia, a rapidly evolving granulocytosis that occurs without significant lymphopenia, and splenomegaly caused by massive granulocytic infiltrates [64]. It offers several undeniable advantages, including a normal host immune system, which may more closely represent the clinical characteristics of the tumor's microenvironment, is relatively low cost, and reproducible. The main disadvantages of syngeneic tumor models are that the tumor cells are rodent, and therefore express the mouse homologues of the desired targets and do not always have a clinical predictive value [5].

None of the preclinical cancer models have the power to mimic exactly the extremely complex process of human carcinogenesis, leading to translational limitations. Nonetheless, experimental tumors developed in animal, particularly in rodents, remain a unique source of in vivo data for evaluating novel diagnostic and therapeutic anti-cancer drugs before translation to clinical settings [5, 24].

In this regard, the use of different cancer preclinical models could complement and reinforce the results to better predict the clinical efficacy of anti-cancer agents.

The therapeutic success of new drugs has been limited because of breast cancer heterogeneity, which occurs in part as a consequence of the dysregulation of numerous oncogenic pathways [2, 3]. Thus, the study of the modulation of proto-oncogene products is of great importance. Histamine stimulates Ets-1(v-ets erythroblastosis virus E26 oncogene homolog 1) synthesis in human melanoma cells, which is associated with an epithelial-to-mesenchymal transition (EMT) and cancer progression [65]. However, a previous study was unable to demonstrate any significant effect of histamine agonists on mRNA and protein levels of proto-oncogenes involved in cell growth and differentiation, including c-fos, fosB, c-myc, and c-jun in human breast epithelial cells [54]. On the other hand, recent data reveal that histamine may modify activated-Src levels, a non-receptor tyrosine kinase proto-oncogene involved in cell growth, differentiation and EMT processes [66], in MDA-MB-231 and MCF-7 breast cancer cell lines (Cricco, in press).

In addition, both the enzyme involved in histamine metabolization (histidine decarboxylase, HDC) and all the histamine receptor subtypes are present in breast cancer cells [4, 6, 7, 9, 10, 15, 16, 18, 21, 22], which highlight the important role of histamine as a modulator of diverse biological responses related to breast cancer growth, including cell proliferation, migration, apoptosis and also tumor invasion, immunity, and metastatic potential [4, 6]. Histamine concentration in breast cancer tissues was found to be higher than that in normal tissues of healthy controls by means of an increase in the activity of HDC [12, 13], while polymorphisms of HDC gene seemed to be associated with breast cancer risk [67].

This chapter aims to cover a range of different preclinical breast cancer models, including in vitro soft agar clonogenic assay and in vivo chemically induced breast tumors in rats, the human TNBC xenograft, and the murine TNBC syngeneic graft in mice. All models could be useful and complementary to assess the role of histamine receptor ligands in breast cancer progression, which could originate novel breast cancer treatments.

This chapter also describes the gold standard radiometric techniques to evaluate the activity of histamine metabolizing enzymes in breast cancer specimens.

2 Materials

2.1 N-Methyl-N-Nitrosourea-induced Rat Breast Cancer Model

- Female Sprague-Dawley rats, with known date of birth.
- N-methyl-N-nitrosourea (e.g., Sigma Chemical Co.).
- Sterile distilled water or saline.
- Acetic acid to adjust pH.
- Sterile glass vials.
- Sterile syringes and 27-G 3/8-inch-long hypodermic needles.
- Animal weighing scale.
- Vernier caliper.
- 10% Neutral buffered formalin.
- Sterile instruments for necropsy and surgery (forceps, scissors, and 12-mm wound clips).

2.2 Human Breast Cancer Xenograft Model

- Human breast cancer cell line MDA-MB-231 (ATCC® HTB-26TM), free of Mycoplasma and murine pathogenic viruses.
- 6–8-week-old female nude (NIH nu/nu) mice.
- RPMI 1640 with 10% FBS.
- Glutamine 200 mM.
- Gentamicin 1000× (40 g/L).

- Trypsin-EDTA: 0.25% (w/v) trypsin, 0.02% (w/v) EDTA in PBS.
- 10-cm tissue culture plates or T25 or T75 culture flasks.
- 37 °C tissue culture incubator, 5% CO_2.
- 15 mL conical tubes.
- Bench top centrifuge.
- 1 mL sterile tuberculin syringe and 27-G hypodermic needles.
- Sterile instruments for necropsy and surgery (forceps, scissors, and 12-mm wound clips).
- Sterile gauze squares, 2- and 4-inches sterile cotton swabs (used for surgical procedures).
- Anesthesia: combination of xylazine (10 mg/kg) and ketamine (100 mg/kg).
- Vernier caliper.
- Hemocytometer or Neubauer's chamber.
- 0.4% Trypan blue solution.
- 10% Neutral buffered formalin.
- 70% Ethanol.

2.3 Murine Breast Cancer Syngeneic Model

- Mouse breast cancer cell line 4T1 (ATCC® CRL-2539), free of Mycoplasma and murine pathogenic viruses.
- RPMI 1640 with 10% FBS.
- Glutamine 200 mM.
- 100× Penicillin (10,000 U) and streptomycin (10 mg/mL) solution.
- Trypsin-EDTA: 0.25% (w/v) trypsin, 0.02% (w/v) EDTA in PBS.
- 6–8-week-old female BALB/c mice.
- 10-cm tissue culture plates or T25 or T75 culture flasks.
- 37 °C tissue culture incubator, 5% CO_2.
- 15 mL conical tubes.
- Benchtop centrifuge.
- 1 mL sterile tuberculin syringe and 27-G hypodermic needles.
- Vernier caliper.
- Hemocytometer or Neubauer's chamber.
- Metallic mesh.
- 70 μm cell strainer.
- 0.4% Trypan blue solution.
- Flow Cytometry Staining Buffer: PBS with 1% FBS and 0.02% azide.

- Lysis buffer: NH_4Cl 0.15 M, K_2CO_3 10 mM, EDTA 0.13 mM.
- Dissociation solution: RPMI medium supplemented with 10% FBS, Collagenase type I (200 U/mL) and DNase I (100 μg/mL).
- Polystyrene round bottom 12 × 75 mm^2 Falcon tubes or Eppendorf tubes.
- Cell Surface Staining Antibodies for flow cytometry.
- Flow cytometer and analysis software.
- 10% Neutral buffered formalin.

2.4 *Ex Vivo* Methodologies

2.4.1 Histidine Decarboxylase (HDC) Activity

- Phosphate-buffered saline (PBS) pH 6.5.
- L-histidine.
- L-[carboxyl-^{14}C]-histidine.
- Pyridoxal-5′-phosphate (PDP).
- α-monofluoromethyl-histidine (MFMH).
- Plastic tubes with rubber caps.
- Wire clips.
- Filter paper.
- Organic quaternary ammonium base solution (e.g., Protosol®).
- Trichloroacetic acid (TCA).
- Parafilm M® precut rolls.
- Biodegradable liquid scintillation cocktail.
- Mechanical homogenizer.
- Refrigerated centrifuge.
- 20 mL plastic vials.
- Liquid scintillation analyzer and software.

2.4.2 Radiometric Histamine-N-Methyltransferase (HMT) Assay

- Homogenization buffer: 20 mM Bis-Tris–HCl pH 7.0, complete protease inhibitor cocktail (e.g., Roche Diagnostics, Austria; added immediately before use), 5 mM 1,4-dithiothreitol (DTT, added immediately before use).
- 1 M NaH_2PO_4 (pH 7.5).
- Alkaline stop: 500 mM H_3BO_3, 1 M NaOH (pH 13.9, unadjusted).
- Toluene/Isoamylalcohol/PPO: 500 mL toluene, 500 mL isoamylalcohol, 0.17% w/v 2,5-diphenyloxazole (PPO).
- 500 μM Histamine (stock solution: 100 mM histamine dihydrochloride).
- ^{14}C-SAM: 80 μL S-adenosyl-L-[methyl-^{14}C]-methionine (~60 Ci/mol; 25 μCi/mL), 200 μL 5 mM S-adenosyl-L-methionine, 1720 μL H_2O.

- Mechanical homogenizer.
- Refrigerated centrifuge.
- 6 mL plastic vials.
- Liquid scintillation analyzer and software.
- 2 mL screw-capped centrifuge tubes.

2.4.3 Radiometric Diamine Oxidase (DAO) Assay

- Homogenization buffer: 20 mM Bis-Tris–HCl pH 7.0, complete protease inhibitor cocktail (e.g., Roche Diagnostics, Austria; added immediately before use), 5 mM 1,4-dithiothreitol (DTT, added immediately before use).
- 1 M NaH_2PO_4, pH 7.0.
- 10% (1 M) $HClO_4$.
- Alkaline stop: 0.6 M $NaHCO_3$ pH 12.2.
- Toluene/PPO: 500 mL toluene, 0.17% (w/v) 2,5-diphenyloxazole (PPO).
- 500 μM Histamine (stock solution: 100 mM histamine dihydrochloride).
- ^{14}C-Putrescine: 200 μL [1,4-^{14}C]-putrescine.2HCl (ca. 100 Ci/mol, 50 μCi/mL), 4.5 μL putrescine (1,4-diaminobutane), 10 mL H_2O.
- Mechanical homogenizer.
- Refrigerated centrifuge.
- 6 mL plastic vials.
- Liquid scintillation analyzer and software.
- 2 mL screw-capped centrifuge tubes.

2.4.4 Histamine content in breast cancer

- 0.5 N $HClO_4$.
- ^{125}I-Radioimmunoassay kit for histamine determination.
- Polystyrene flat-bottom P24 culture dish.
- Hank's balanced salt solution.
- Mechanical homogenizer.
- Refrigerated centrifuge.
- Capillary tubes coated with heparin.
- Microcentrifuge.
- Gamma scintillation spectrometer.

2.4.5 Primary culture in soft agar: colony formation assay

- Sterile scalpels.
- 15 mL centrifuge sterile tubes.
- 35 mm sterile dishes.
- Sterile transfer pipettes.

- Centrifuge.
- 0.01% Pronase E.
- 0.012% DNAse.
- Syringes with 21G needles.
- 0.4% Trypan Blue solution.
- Sterile Hank's balanced salts solution (HBSS).
- Sterile McCoy's medium.
- Fetal calf serum (FCS).
- 0.22 mg/mL Sodium pyruvate.
- 42 μg/mL L-serine.
- 2.9 μg/mL Glutamine.
- 4.5 mg/mL Sodium bicarbonate.
- Penicillin and streptomycin.
- 66 or 100 μg/mL L-asparagine.
- 250 or 375 μg/mL DEAE-dextran.
- 7.5 mg/mL Tryptic soy broth.
- 444 μg/mL Calcium chloride.
- 2 units/mL Insulin.
- 53 μg/mL Ascorbic acid.
- 0.4 μg/mL β-Mercaptoethanol.
- Agar.
- Biological safety cabinet.
- Hemocytometer.
- Microwave.
- Water bath.
- Inverted phase microscope.
- 37 °C incubator with a 5% CO_2 humidified atmosphere.

3 Methods

3.1 N-Methyl-N-Nitrosourea-induced Rat Breast Cancer Model

3.1.1 Tumor Induction

All rats have to receive three i.p. injections of 50 mg NMU per kg of body weight at 50, 80, and 110 days of age according to the following procedure (Fig. 1) (*see* **Note 1**).

1. Weigh each rat; calculate volume to inject 50 mg/kg of body weight from a 10 mg/mL solution (*see* **Note 2** for recommended housing conditions).
2. Prepare a 10 mg/mL fresh solution of NMU in sterile distilled water, or in sterile saline adjusted to pH 5 with acetic acid in a glass vial. Protect solution from light (*see* **Note 3**).

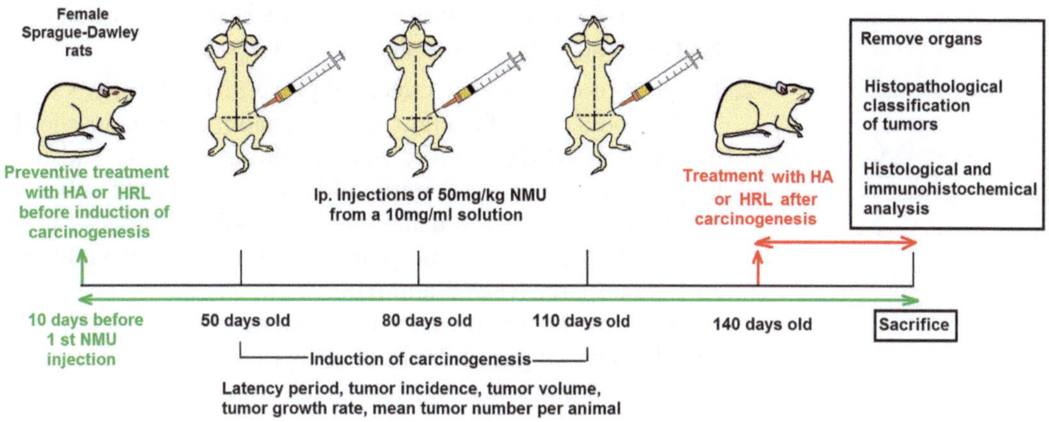

Fig. 1 N-Methyl-N-Nitrosourea (NMU)-induced rat breast cancer model. NMU is a chemical carcinogen widely used for breast cancer induction in rats. Histamine (HA) or histamine receptor ligands (HRL) may be studied as preventive treatments or curative or palliative treatments after carcinogenesis induction

3. Inject the calculated volume of NMU solution intraperitoneally into the ventral midline of the animal halfway between the third and fourth pairs of mammary glands (Fig. 1). In order to reduce the possibility of piercing an organ, use a sterile syringe with a 27-G 3/8-inch-long needle. Inject age-matched control animals with vehicle.

3.1.2 Tumor Development

1. After carcinogen administration, record animals' weight weekly until the completion of treatments.
2. After 3 weeks of the first NMU injection monitor the tumor onset three times a week by palpating mammary gland chains. Record the first date of detection of each tumor and its location (*see* Sect. 3.1.4).
3. When tumors become palpable, measure tumor diameters with Vernier calipers twice a week until the completion of treatments. Make two measurements of the tumor that are perpendicular to each other. Calculate tumor volume (*see* Sect. 3.1.4).

3.1.3 Treatments

1. In order to evaluate the therapeutic effects of treatments on developed tumors, rats should be treated when at least one tumor per animal reaches a volume of 0.5 cm^3. The route of administration could be s.c., i.p., oral administration (p.o.) depending on the compound (for reference *see* **Note 4**).

   Sacrifice animals after 4–6 weeks of treatment, when the tumor volume reaches 2 cm^3 or when animals become moribund (when they showed signs of suffering, hypothermia, and slow locomotion), according to Guide for the Care and Use of Laboratory Animals (*see* **Note 1**), and harvest tumors and organs of interest (lungs, liver, spleen, kidney, lymph nodes) (*see* **Note 5**). Perform histological classification of tumors (*see* **Note 6**) and histopathological analysis of organs.

2. In order to evaluate the effects of preventive treatments or to study modulators of malignant progression, treatments should be initiated 10 days before the 1st NMU injection and prolonged for 4 months or until animals show signs of suffering (*see* **Note 1**). To assess malignant progression, animals can be sacrificed at different time points to excise mammary glands and organs (*see* **Notes 5** and **6**).

Response to treatments may be assessed by the evolution of animal body weight and tumor growth parameters (*see* Sect. 3.1.4).

3.1.4 Tumor Growth Parameters

The following tumor growth parameters may be determined to compare different treatments [42].

- *Latency period*: days between first NMU injection and appearance of the first tumor.
- *Tumor incidence*: Percentage of animals that develop at least one tumor.
- *Mean tumor number per animal* or *tumor multiplicity*: average number of tumors per tumor-bearing rat.
- *Tumor volume (V)*: may be calculated using the following equation [66]:

$$V = \left(\frac{\pi}{6}\right).\text{length}.\text{width}^2$$

- *Tumor growth rate*: evaluate the time course of tumor volume after 1st NMU injection to represent tumor evolution.

3.2 Human Breast Cancer Xenograft Model

3.2.1 MDA-MB-231 Human Breast Cancer Cell Cultures and Preparation for Injection

1. Culture MDA-MB-231 TNBC cells in RPMI 1640 supplemented with 10% FBS, 2 mM glutamine, gentamicin (0.04 g/L), in 10-cm tissue culture plates or T25 or T75 culture flasks and incubated at 37 °C, in a humidified atmosphere containing 5% CO_2, until 90% confluence.
2. Split cultures two to three times per week.
3. To harvest MDA-MB-231 cells for injection first discard culture medium from the tissue culture plate or flask.
4. Wash with serum-free medium.
5. Add 1 mL trypsin-EDTA solution and cover entire plate. Let trypsin-EDTA solution incubate in the plate at room temperature for 5 min.
6. Add 5–7 mL serum-free medium to harvest trypsinized cells from plate and transfer to 15 mL conical tube.

7. Centrifuge cells 5 min at 400 × *g*, room temperature, in a benchtop centrifuge.
8. Discard the supernatant and resuspend the pellet in saline.
9. Place the suspension in ice and proceed to determine cell numbers using a Neubauer's chamber or a hemocytometer.

3.2.2 MDA-MB-231 Xenograft Tumor Development

1. Dilute cells in 100 μL of serum-free medium to the final concentration of 1 × 10^7 cells (*see* **Note 7**).
2. To inject the tumor cells, use a sterile 1 mL tuberculin syringe with a 27-G needle.
3. Anesthetize 6-week-old female nude (NIH nu/nu) mice, until breathing is slow and regular and there is no toe-pinch reflex (*see* **Note 8**).
4. Place the mouse on its left side on the work area, and clean the skin on the right flank with 70% ethanol (*see* **Note 9**).
5. Inoculate the nude (NIH nu/nu) mouse with 100 μL of MDA-MB-231 tumor cell suspension subcutaneously (s.c.) in the left flank by gently penetrating the skin, with the bevel of the needle facing up (Fig. 2).
6. Monitor the tumor onset daily by palpating injection area with the fingers for the presence of a tumor.
7. When developed tumor's volume reaches 8 mm of diameter, animals should be euthanized with CO_2 or anesthetic overdose followed by cervical dislocation and the tumor must be excised (*see* **Note 1**) (Fig. 2).
8. Place the tumor in a sterile plate, wash the tumor excised with saline, cut it into 25–30 mm³ pieces (*see* **Note 10**) (Fig. 2).
9. Anesthetize mice, until their breathing is slow and regular and there is no toe-pinch reflex (*see* **Note 8**).
10. Place the mouse on the work area and clean the skin on one flank (right or left) with 70% ethanol.
11. Make a 5 mm incision through the skin, using forceps and scissors, and introduce the piece of tumor, and close the incision with wound clips (*see* **Note 9**) (Fig. 2).
12. Monitor closely to ensure recovery from the surgery and anesthesia. Remove the wound clips 7 days after surgery (*see* **Note 11**).

3.2.3 Treatments and Tumor Growth Evaluation

1. In order to evaluate the therapeutic effects of histamine receptor ligands' treatment, animals should be treated when the graft volumes reach 100–150 mm³ with s.c. daily injection on the dorsal flank (for reference *see* **Note 12**). When the tumor becomes palpable measure tumor diameters with Vernier calipers two to three times a week. Make two measurements of the tumor that are perpendicular to each other. The tumor size

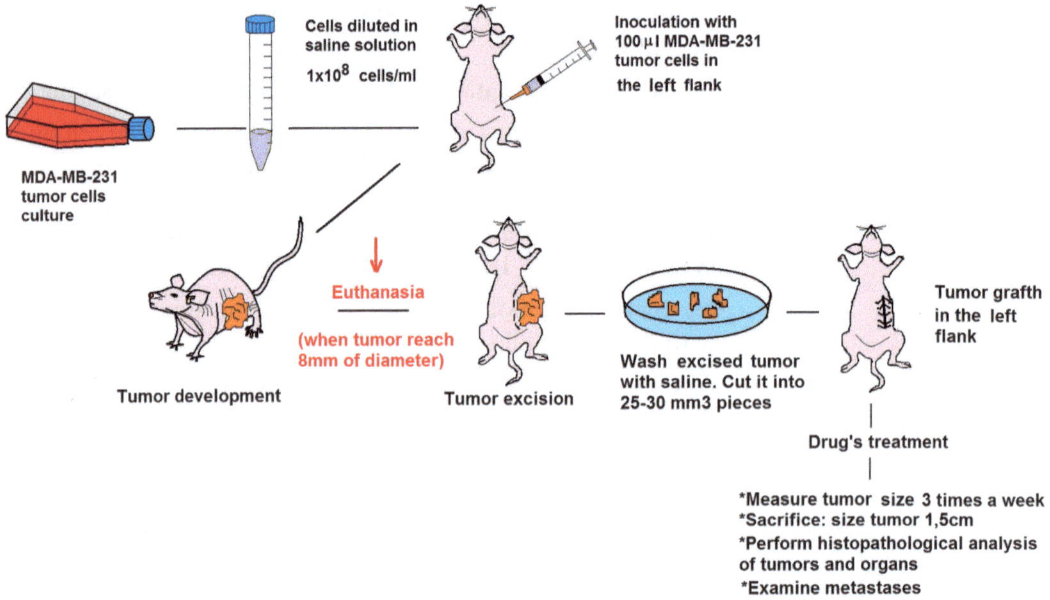

Fig. 2 Human breast cancer xenograft model development. MDA-MB-231 TNBC cells are first injected subcutaneously into immunodeficient mice. The formed tumor is then excised and inoculated in female nude mice to evaluate histamine receptor ligands' treatment

may be calculated as sphere volume according to the following formula (*see* **Note 13**):

$$\text{Tumor volume}\left[mm^3\right] = \frac{4}{3}\pi\left[\frac{(\text{large diameter} + \text{small diameter})}{4}\right]^3$$

Also, tumor volume may be calculated as previously indicated [68] (*see* Sect. 3.1.4).

2. At euthanasia (when tumors are 2 cm³ or 6 weeks after tumor implantation), perform necropsy and examine lungs and abdominal organs for metastases. Fix organs in formalin buffer for histopathological studies (*see* **Note 5**).

3.3 Murine Breast Cancer Syngeneic Model

3.3.1 4T1 Murine Breast Cancer Cell Cultures and Injection

1. Culture 4T1 TNBC cells in RPMI supplemented with 10% FBS, 2 mM glutamine, 100 U penicillin, and 100 µg/mL streptomycin, in 10-cm tissue culture plates or T25 or T75 culture flasks and incubated in a 37 °C, 5% CO_2 tissue culture incubator.
2. Split cultures two to three times per week.
3. To harvest 4T1 tumor cells for injection first discard culture medium from the tissue culture plate or flask (*see* **Note 14**).
4. Wash with serum-free medium.

5. Add 1 mL trypin-EDTA solution and cover entire plate. Let trypsin/EDTA solution incubate in the plate at room temperature for 2 min.
6. Add 5–7 mL serum-free medium to harvest trypsinized cells from plate and transfer to 15 mL conical tube.
7. Centrifuge cells 5 min at 400 × *g*, room temperature, in a benchtop centrifuge.
8. Discard the supernatant and resuspend the pellet in saline (*see* **Note 7**).
9. Determine cell number using a Neubauer's chamber or a hemocytometer.
10. Dilute cells with saline to the final concentration of 1×10^6 cells/mL (Fig. 3).
11. To inject the tumor cells, use a 1 mL tuberculin syringe with a 27-G needle.
12. Inoculate the 6–8-week-old female BALB/c mice with 100 μL of 4T1 tumor cell suspension subcutaneously (s.c.) and orthotopically in the mammary gland by gently penetrating the skin, with the bevel of the needle facing up (Fig. 3).
13. Monitor the tumor onset daily by palpating injection area with the fingers for the presence of a tumor (*see* **Note 15**).
14. When the tumor becomes palpable measure tumor diameters with Vernier calipers every 3–4 days. Make two measurements of the tumor that are perpendicular to each other. Calculate the tumor volume using the following equation [68] (*see* **Note 16**):

$$V = \left(\frac{\pi}{6}\right).\text{length.width}^2$$

3.3.2 Treatments

Mice should be treated when the tumors have reached a volume of 0.1–0.2 cm^3 (*see* Sect. 3.2.3). Sacrifice animals after 2–3 weeks of treatment or when the tumor volume reaches 2 cm^3 (*see* **Note 1**), and harvest tumors and organs of interest (lungs, liver, spleen, kidney, lymph nodes) (*see* **Note 5**). Perform histopathological analysis of organs and tumors and proceed with the following assessments (Fig. 3).

3.3.3 Preparation of Draining Lymph Nodes

1. Remove the draining lymph node and place it in a tissue culture dish containing supplemented medium.
2. Mechanically dissociate the lymph node by pressing it with the plunger of a 1 mL syringe on a metallic mesh.
3. Pass cell suspension through a 70 μm cell strainer to eliminate clumps and debris.
4. Collect cell suspension in a 15 mL conical tube.

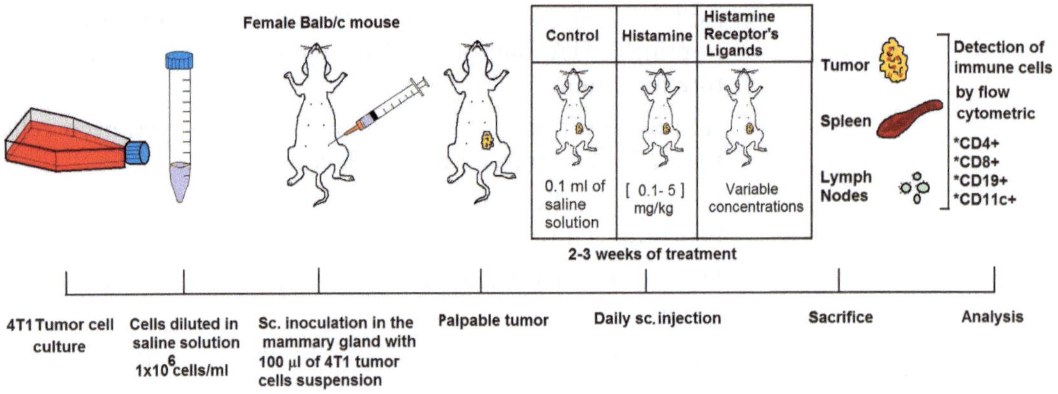

Fig. 3 Murine breast cancer syngeneic model development. 4T1 TNBC cells are injected orthotopically into fad pads of BALB/c mice to evaluate the role of histamine or histamine receptor ligands in tumor immunity

5. Centrifuge cells 5 min at 400 × *g*, room temperature, in a benchtop centrifuge and then discard supernatant.
6. Resuspend the cell pellet and perform a cell count and viability analysis in a Neubauer's chamber by staining the cells with Trypan Blue solution.
7. Centrifuge cells as in step 5 and resuspend the pellet in an appropriate volume of Flow Cytometry Staining Buffer so that the final cell concentration is 6.6×10^7/mL.

3.3.4 Preparation of Spleens

1. Remove the spleen and place it in a tissue culture dish containing supplemented medium.
2. Mechanically dissociate the spleen by pressing it with the plunger of a 1 mL syringe on a metallic mesh.
3. Collect cell suspension in a 15 mL conical tube.
4. Centrifuge cells for 5 min at 400 × *g*, room temperature, in a benchtop centrifuge and then discard supernatant.
5. To lyse red blood cells, resuspend the cell pellet in 2–4 mL of lysis buffer.
6. Incubate the cells for 5 min at 4 °C.
7. Add 8–10 mL of supplemented medium to stop the lysis.
8. Centrifuge the cells as in step 4 and resuspend the pellet in 2–4 mL of Flow Cytometry Staining Buffer.
9. Pass the cell suspension through a 70 μm cell strainer to eliminate clumps and debris.
10. Perform a cell count and viability analysis in a Neubauer's chamber by staining the cells with Trypan Blue solution.
11. Centrifuge cells as in step 4 and resuspend the pellet in appropriate volume of Flow Cytometry Staining Buffer so that the final cell concentration is 6.6×10^7/mL.

3.3.5 Preparation of Tumor Infiltrating Lymphocytes (TILs)

1. Remove the tumor and place it in a tissue culture dish containing supplemented medium.
2. Quickly cut the tumor with scalpels or scissors in small pieces (<3 mm), fragments small enough to be aspirated into a 5 mL pipette without getting stuck.
3. Incubate the pieces in dissociation solution for 30 min with shaking on 37 °C. Use 5 mL of dissociation solution for a tumor size of 1 cm^3. Repeatedly pipette or vortex the tumor cell suspension every 10 min during the incubation to further dissociate cells (*see* **Note 17**).
4. After incubation, pass the cell suspension through a 70 μm cell strainer.
5. Centrifuge the cell suspension at 400 × *g* at 4 °C for 5 min.
6. Resuspend the pellet in 2–4 mL of lysis buffer for 5 min at 4 °C to deplete red blood cells (*see* **Note 18**).
7. Add 8–10 mL of supplemented medium to stop the lysis and centrifuge the cells (step 5).
8. Resuspend cells in Flow Cytometry Staining Buffer, pass cell suspension through a 70 μm cell strainer, and centrifuge at 400 × *g* at room temperature for 5 min.
9. Perform a cell count and viability analysis in a Neubauer's chamber by staining the cells with Trypan Blue solution.
10. Resuspend the pellet in an appropriate volume of Flow Cytometry Staining Buffer so that the final cell concentration is 6.6×10^7/mL.

3.3.6 Cell Staining for Flow Cytometry

1. Prepare the fluorochrome-conjugated antibodies at any appropriate concentration in Flow Cytometry Staining Buffer (*see* **Notes 19** and **20**).
2. Mix 15 μL of the antibody preparation with 15 μL of cell suspension in polystyrene round-bottom 12 × 75 mm^2 Falcon tubes or Eppendorf tubes. This should be done at 2–8 °C with minimal exposure to light. Prepare 1 tube with cells with no antibody as an autofluorescence control, and add 15 μL of Flow Cytometry Staining Buffer. When using a mixture of two or more antibodies, prepare one tube of cells with each antibody alone to further perform the fluorescence compensation.
3. Gently vortex the cells.
4. Incubate the cells during 30 min at 4 °C.
5. After the incubation wash the cells two times by centrifugation at 400 × *g* for 5 min and resuspend them in 500 μL to 1 mL of ice cold Flow Cytometry Staining Buffer. Keep the cells in the dark on ice or at 4 °C in a fridge until the analysis is performed. For best results, analyze the cells on the flow cytometer as soon as possible.

6. If you need to wait longer than an hour, cells should be fixed. For this, after the last centrifugation resuspend the pellet in 300 μL of PBS and add 100 μL of 4% paraformaldehyde while gently vortexing. This will stabilize the light scatter and inactivate most biohazardous agents.

3.3.7 Flow Cytometric Analysis

For the detection of immune cell subsets it is recommended to use a flow cytometer with two or more lasers and at least four detectors (*see* **Note 21**). Any flow cytometer with these characteristics can be used.

1. Run flow cytometry for lymph node or spleen samples first and fix a gate for lymphocytes in a particular FSC and SSC (*see* **Note 22**).
2. Run the autofluorescence tube first and then the individual fluorochromes to perform the fluorescence compensation.
3. Run the lymph node and spleen samples and determine the gates for each immune subset.
4. To analyze the TILs use the same lymphocyte gate you have fixed in step 1. A small population of TILs should be seen, together with a high number of tumor cells, which generally have higher FSC and SSC than lymphocytes.
5. Determine subsequent gating for each immune subset.

3.4 Ex Vivo Methodologies

3.4.1 Histidine Decarboxylase (HDC) Activity

Histidine decarboxylase (HDC; EC 4.1.1.22) is a member of the pyridoxal phosphate-dependent amino acid decarboxylases' family and is the enzyme that specifically catalyzes the reaction that produces histamine by α-decarboxylation of its precursor histidine in mammals and other eukaryotic organisms [69, 70]. The assay that was first described in 1966 and then modified in 1976 is based on trapping of $^{14}CO_2$ produced during incubation of the HDC enzyme with the substrate ^{14}C-histidine [71, 72].

HDC activity can be evaluated in NMU-induced tumors or grafted tumors according to the following protocol, which is a modification of the method of Hakanson et al [72, 73].

Preparation of Tissue

1. Sacrifice female Sprague-Dawley rats bearing NMU-induced tumors (*see* **Notes 1** and **5**).
2. Remove tumors and use immediately.
3. Homogenize tumor masses in ice-cold 50 mM PBS, pH 6.5, to a final concentration of 100 mg (wet weight) per 0.2 mL, employing a mechanical device.
4. Centrifuge homogenates during 15 min at 2000 × *g*, 4 °C.
5. Remove supernatants for further processing, keep on ice.

Protein Determination

1. Determine protein concentration in supernatants (*see* **Note 23**).

Carbon Dioxide Trapping System

1. Assemble a simple and efficient system to trap carbon dioxide forcing a wire clip through the center of the rubber cap of a tube as shown in Fig. 4.
2. Fold a rectangular piece of filter paper (1 × 3 cm).
3. Dip the paper into a strong organic quaternary ammonium base (e.g., Protosol®) and allow it to drip dry.
4. Clamp the paper firmly into the loop of the clip.

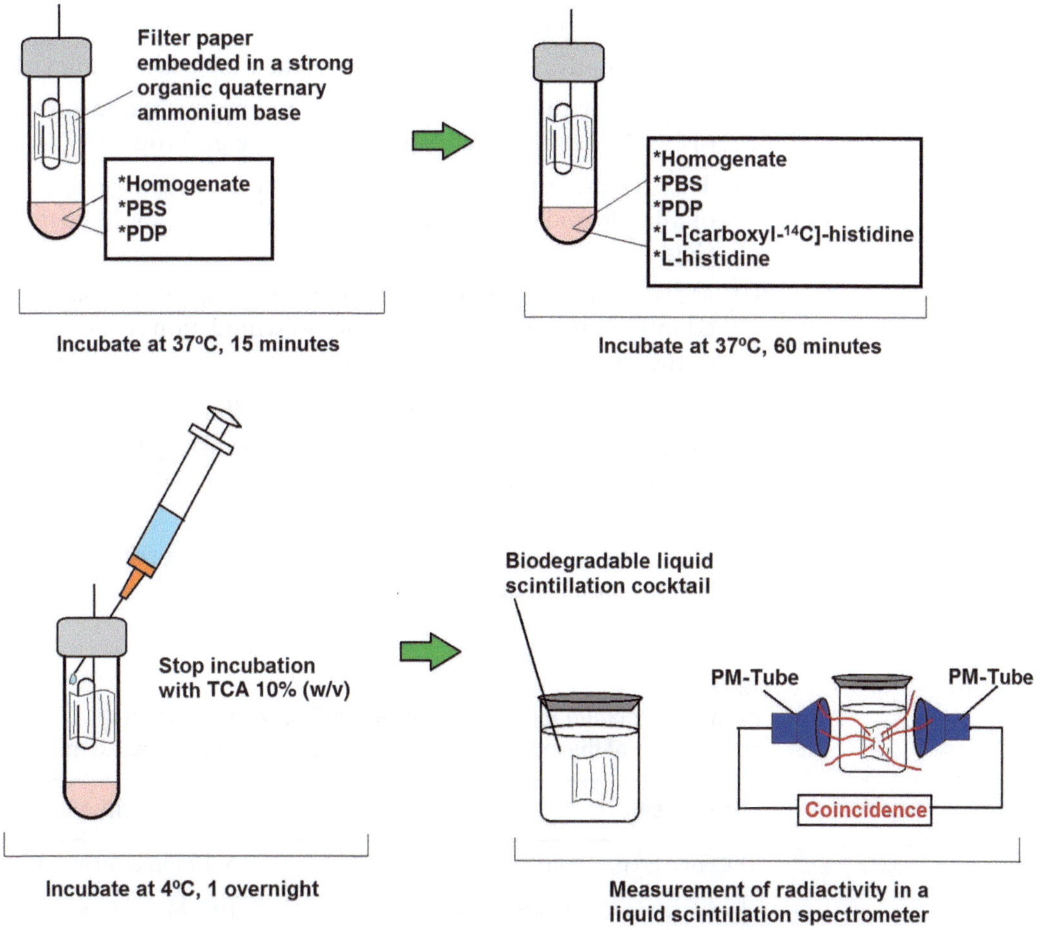

Fig. 4 Schematic representation of the sequential steps to evaluate histidine decarboxylase activity. The $^{14}CO_2$ trapping system is shown

HDC Activity Assay

1. Add 0.2 mL supernatant of centrifuged homogenates, 0.2 mL PBS pH 6.5, and 0.01 mL PDP into the plastic tubes with rubber caps (Fig. 4) (*see* **Note 24**).
2. Prepare blanks for each sample adding 10^{-5} M MFMH (HDC inhibitor) in the incubation mixture.
3. Incubate tubes at 37 °C during 15 min.
4. Add 0.1 mL of a mix containing L-[carboxyl-^{14}C]-histidine (Activity: 3.7 kBq) and L-histidine to each tube to start the enzymatic reaction (*see* **Notes 25** and **26**) (Fig. 4). Final concentrations of components of the mixture are shown in Table 1.
5. Incubate all the tubes at 37 °C for 1 h.
6. Stop incubations by acidification with 0.5 mL TCA (10% w/v). Inject the acid through the rubber cap with a 23-gauge disposable needle (Fig. 4).
7. Seal promptly the hole in the cap of the tube with Parafilm M®.
8. Keep plastic tubes at 4 °C overnight to improve the adsorption of $^{14}CO_2$ into the filter paper wetted in, e.g., Protosol®.
9. Transfer the papers to 20 mL plastic vials containing 3–4 mL of a biodegradable liquid scintillation cocktail (e.g., HiSafe 2) (Fig. 4).
10. Measure the radioactivity of unknown samples and blanks as counts per minute (CPM) in a liquid scintillation spectrometer in the ^{14}C-channel (*see* **Note 26**).
11. Determine counting efficiency for each sample.
12. Determine radioactivity of samples and blanks by liquid scintillation counting in the ^{14}C-channel using a DPM calculation program.
13. Calculate the mean value of blanks in DPM to further discount it from sample values.

Table 1
Incubation mixture for HDC activity assay. Final concentration of components of the mixture are shown. Total reaction volume: 0.5 mL/tube

Components	Final concentration
Enzyme preparation	6–10 mg protein/mL
Pyridoxal-5′-Phosphate	10^{-5} M
PBS pH 6.5	50 mM
L-histidine	50 mM
L-[carboxyl-^{14}C]-histidine	3.7 kBq

14. Calculate the Specific Activity (SA) of HDC employing the following equation, in which an enzyme unit (U) catalyzes the formation of 1 nmol of product per h (*see* **Notes 27–29**) [74].

$$SA\left[\mathrm{U}/mg\right]=\left(DPM_{S}\quad DPM_{0}\right).\frac{1}{4440\left[DPM/\mathrm{nmol}\right]}.\frac{1}{t\left[\mathrm{h}\right]}.\frac{1000}{Ps\left[mg/ml\right].Vs\left[\mu L\right]}$$

DPM_S = Activity of the sample
DPM_0 = Mean activity of blanks for each sample
P_S = Protein concentration of sample
V_S = Volume of sample

3.4.2 Radiometric Histamine-N-Methyltransferase (HMT) Assay

Histamine can be inactivated by two alternative enzymes one of which is histamine N-methyltransferase (HMT, EC 2.1.1.8). HMT catalyzes the transfer of a methyl group from S-adenosylmethionine (SAM) to the imidazole ring of histamine forming N-methylhistamine, which is further oxidized by monoamine oxidase [75]. The assay is based on the HMT catalyzed methylation of histamine with ^{14}C-SAM to Nt-methyl-histamine. At alkaline pH the reaction product can be efficiently extracted into toluene/isoamylalcohol/PPO, which is used as a cocktail for liquid scintillation counting as well.

Preparation of Tissue

1. Remove the tumor and place it in a tissue culture dish containing supplemented medium.
2. Quickly cut the tumor with a scalpel or scissors into small pieces (15 mg) (*see* **Note 30**).
3. For homogenization transfer the tissue to a 2 mL microfuge tube, add 1 mL of homogenization buffer (*see* **Note 31**).
4. Homogenize tissue in benchtop homogenizer (e.g., TissueLyser II, Qiagen) for 3 × 20 s with 20 s cooling intervals on ice.
5. Centrifuge the samples 2 min at 4000 × *g* at 4 °C. Discard pellet.
6. Transfer supernatant to new microfuge tube and spin 10 min at 20,000 × *g* at 4 °C.
7. Transfer supernatant to new microfuge tube. Save an aliquot to determine protein concentration at −20 °C.

HMT Activity Assay

1. To determine HMT activity, the assay must be performed in disposable 2 mL screw-capped centrifuge tubes. In each tube add:

   – H_2O (70-X μL).

- 1 M NaH_2PO_4 pH 7.5 (10 μL).
- 500 μM histamine/H_2O (control) (10 μL).
- Sample (X μL).

2. Mix, spin briefly, and start reaction by the addition of ^{14}C-SAM (500 μM; 2 Ci/mol; 1 nCi/μL) (10 μL) (*see* **Note 32**).
3. Mix and incubate for 30 min at 37 °C.
4. Stop reaction by the addition of alkaline stop (60 μL).
5. Mix and place on ice for 5 min.
6. At room temperature add 1.6 mL Toluene/Isoamylalcohol/PPO mixture.
7. Mix by vortexing vigorously for 30 s, centrifuge 2 min at 10,000 × *g*.
8. Transfer 1.4 mL of Toluene/PPO to a 6 mL vial.
9. Determine radioactivity by liquid scintillation counting in the ^{14}C-channel using a DPM calculation program (*see* **Note 26**).
10. The specific activity (SA) of HMT is calculated according to the following formula where 1 unit (U) converts 1 μmol of substrate per minute (*see* **Notes 29** and **33**):

$$SA\left[mU / mg\right] = \frac{\left(DPMs - DPM_0\right)}{0.77} \cdot \frac{1}{4440\left[DPM / \text{nmol}\right]} \cdot \frac{1}{t\left[\text{min}\right]} \cdot \frac{1000}{Ps\left[mg / mL\right].Vs\left[\mu L\right]}$$

DPM_S = Activity of the sample

DPM_0 = Activity of the blank

P_S = Protein concentration of sample

V_S = Volume of sample

0.77 = Extraction factor

3.4.3 Radiometric Diamine Oxidase (DAO) Assay

Histamine is also catalyzed by the enzyme diamine oxidase (EC 1.4.3.6), which oxidatively deaminates the primary amino group of histamine forming imidazole acetaldehyde. The assay is based on the DAO catalyzed conversion of ^{14}C-putrescine to γ-aminobutyraldehyde, which is converted quantitatively to Δ_1-pyrroline by a spontaneous non-enzymatic cyclization. Whereas putrescine is totally insoluble in toluene, the product can be efficiently extracted into toluene/PPO, which is used as a cocktail for liquid scintillation counting as well [75].

Preparation of Tissue

1. Proceed as indicated in Sect. 3.4.2.

DAO Activity Assay

1. To determine DAO activity the assay must be performed in disposable 2 mL screw-capped centrifuge tubes. In each tube add:
   - H_2O (80-X μL).
   - 1 M Na-phosphate pH 7.5 (10 μL).
   - Sample (X μL).
2. Mix, spin briefly, and start reaction by the addition of ^{14}C-putrescine (4.5 mM; 0.222 Ci/mol; 1 nCi/μL) (10 μL) (*see* **Note 34**).
3. Mix and incubate for 30 min at 37 °C.
4. Stop reaction by the addition of 10% $HClO_4$ (10 μL).
5. Mix, adjust pH by the addition of 0.6 M $NaHCO_3$ pH 12.2 (50 μL).
6. Mix, add Toluene/PPO mixture (1.6 mL).
7. Mix by vortexing vigorously for 30 s, centrifuge for 2 min at 10,000 × *g*.
8. Transfer 1.4 mL of Toluene/PPO to a 6 mL vial.
9. Determine radioactivity by liquid scintillation counting in the ^{14}C-channel using a DPM calculation program (*see* **Note 26**).
10. The specific activity (SA) of DAO is calculated according to the following formula where 1 unit (U) converts 1 μmol of substrate per minute (*see* **Notes 29** and **35**):

$$SA\left[mU/mg\right]=\frac{\left(\mathrm{DPM}s-DPM_0\right)}{0.748}\cdot\frac{1}{493\left[DPM/\mathrm{nmol}\right]}\cdot\frac{1}{\mathrm{t}\left[\mathrm{min}\right]}\cdot\frac{1000}{Ps\left[mg/mL\right].Vs\left[\mu L\right]}$$

DPM_S = Activity of the sample
DPM_0 = Activity of the blank
P_S = Protein concentration of sample
V_S = Volume of sample
0.748 = Extraction factor

3.4.4 Histamine Content

Histamine in tissue, plasma, or culture medium is quantitatively evaluated by ^{125}I-radioimmunoassay (RIA) or by enzyme-linked immunosorbent assay (ELISA). Histamine level in NMU tumor-bearing rats is determined as described in [76].

Histamine Content in Tissues

1. Homogenize tissues with 0.5 N $HClO_4$ on ice, employing a mechanical device (*see* **Note 36**).
2. Centrifuge homogenates for 10 min at 12,000 × *g* and 4 °C.

3. Perform appropriate dilution of supernatants employing 50 mM PBS pH 7.5 (*see* **Note 37**).
4. Use diluted samples to calculate the nanomolar concentration of histamine (X) in the unknown samples employing the curve-fitting technique recommended by the ^{125}I-RIA kit instructions.
5. Express histamine content in tissues using the following equation:

$$\text{Histamine content in tissue}\left(\mu g / \text{g tissue}\right) = \text{X}.111.10^{-6}.DF$$

X: Nanomolar concentration of histamine
111: Histamine molecular weight
10^{-6}: Correction factor for expressing histamine concentration as μg/g tissue
DF: Sample dilution factor

Histamine Content in Plasma

1. Collect blood samples from rats (*see* **Note 38**).
2. Centrifuge and separate the plasma of each blood sample.
3. Dilute plasma from 1:100 to 1:2000 in PBS.
4. Use plasma samples to determine the nanomolar concentration of histamine (X) employing the curve-fitting technique recommended by the ^{125}I-RIA kit instructions.
5. Express histamine content in plasma using the following equation:

$$\text{Histamine in plasma}\left(\mu M\right) = \text{X}.DF.10^{-3}$$

X: Nanomolar concentration of histamine
DF: Sample dilution factor
10^{-3}: Correction factor for expressing plasma histamine concentration in μM.

Histamine Secretion from Explants in Culture Medium

1. Put 100 mg tissue explants in 0.5 mL Hank's medium in polystyrene flat-bottom P24 culture dish.
2. Keep the culture dish with explants in the incubator at 37 °C and 5% CO_2.
3. After 6 h remove and use medium from each well to calculate the nanomolar concentration of histamine (X) employing the curve-fitting technique recommended by the commercial ^{125}I-RIA kit instructions (*see* **Note 39**).

4. Express histamine secreted in culture medium using the following equation:

$$\text{Histamine}\left(\mu g / \text{g tissue}\right) = \frac{\text{X.111}.DF.10^{-6}.0.5}{m}$$

X: Nanomolar concentration of histamine
111: Molecular weight of histamine
DF: Sample dilution factor
10^{-6}: correction factor for expressing histamine concentration as μg/g tissue.
0.5: Incubation volume
m: Explants mass

3.4.5 Primary Culture in Soft Agar: Colony Formation Assay

The clonogenic method in soft agar requires that cells grow in an anchorage independent manner, which is a characteristic of cancer cells and it analyzes the capacity of a tumoral cell to undergo unlimited division. In contrast, normal cells are not able to grow into colonies. It is considered the gold standard method to determine cell reproductive death after treatment with cytotoxic agents and can be employed to investigate the effects of histamine receptor ligands' treatment on clonogenic growth of breast tumors.

Enzymatic Disaggregation of Tumor

1. Tumor must be excised in sterile conditions and collected into sterile 60 mm dishes containing HBSS (*see* **Note 40**).
2. Trim tumor of debris, large vessels, and necrotic areas and cut them into small fragments using sterile scalpels.
3. Rinse the pieces with HBSS until wash liquids are clean using a sterile transfer pipette.
4. Transfer the pieces to a new sterile dish and mince the pieces into smaller ones (roughly 1 mm^3) using a sterile scalpel.
5. Add 4 mL of a sterile solution of 0.01% pronase E and 0.012% DNase in HHBS and incubate at 37 °C in a humidified atmosphere of 5% CO_2 for 2 h. Stir every 20 min.
6. Transfer the medium to a 15 mL centrifuged sterile tube. Wash the remaining tissue fragments with 4 mL of fresh HBSS and transfer the wash liquid to the centrifuge tube.
7. Centrifuge at 900 × *g* for 5 min. Discard the supernatant.
8. Wash the pellet in 2 mL of fresh HBSS. Centrifuge at 900 × *g* for 5 min. Repeat this step. Discard the supernatant.
9. Resuspend the pellet in 1 mL of enriched McCoy's upper layer medium without agar as described (*see* **Note 41**) [77] using a syringe with a 21G needle to obtain a single-cell suspension.

Viable Cell Counting Using Trypan Blue Dye

1. Mix equal volumes of cell suspension, obtained as previously described, and 0.4% Trypan blue dye and leave for 5 min at room temperature (*see* **Note 42**).
2. Count cells using a hemocytometer to determine the percentage of dead or damaged cells.
3. Dilute the single-cell suspension with enriched McCoy's medium (upper layer) to obtain a suspension containing 3.0–4.0 × 10^4 viable cells in 0.5 mL and keep at 37 °C.

Culture in Soft Agar

Cells are cultured in a bilayer soft-agar system.

1. Prepare the bottom layer by diluting 1% agar in pre-warmed 2× enriched McCoy's medium to give a final mixture of 0.5% agar (*see* **Notes 43** and **44**).
2. Dispense immediately 1 mL of the mixture prepared in 1. into 35 mm dishes (Fig. 5).
3. Leave dishes at room temperature until bottom layers become solid.
4. Prepare the upper layer by diluting 1.2% agar in pre-warmed 2× enriched McCoy's medium to give a final mixture of 0.6% agar (*see* **Notes 41** and **44**).
5. Mix equal volumes of 0.6% agar and cell suspension (3.0–4.0 × 10^4 viable cells in 0.5 mL) (*see* **Note 45**).
6. Dispense immediately 1 mL of the final cell suspension in 0.3% agar on the top of the solid lower layer (*see* **Notes 46** and **47**) (Fig. 5).
7. Leave dishes at room temperature until upper layers become solid.
8. Incubate the dishes at 37 °C in a 5% CO_2 humidified atmosphere for 21 days and feed cells with enriched McCoy's medium (upper layer) twice a week.

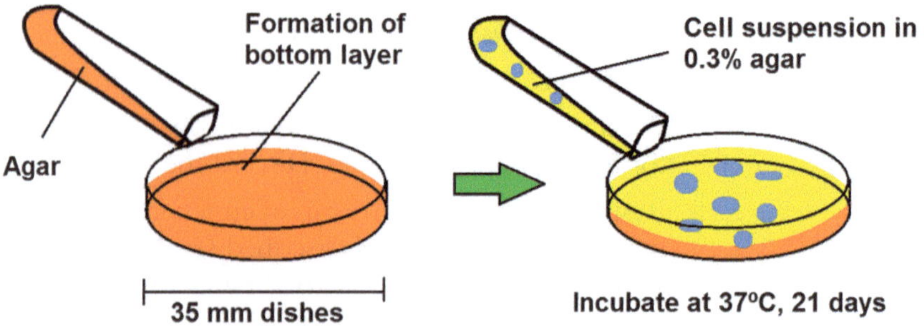

Fig. 5 Cultured cells in a bilayer soft-agar system are shown

Colony Counting

1. Count colonies (>50 cells) using an inverted phase microscope.
2. Alternatively, dishes may be stained with 0.5 mL of 0.04% crystal violet and 2% ethanol in PBS for 1 h before counting cells.

4 Notes

1. All procedures using animals (housing conditions, experimentation, surgical procedures, euthanasia, anesthesia, etc.) must first be reviewed and approved by an Institutional Animal Care and Use Committee (IACUC) and must follow officially approved procedures for the care and use of laboratory animals. This committee is in compliance with international and national guidelines and requirements for the Care and Use of Laboratory Animals (e.g., recommendations from the Guide for the Care and Use of Laboratory Animals of the National Research Council, USA, 1996). Also, all studies involving animals should be reported in accordance with the ARRIVE guidelines for reporting experiments involving animals [78, 79]. Therefore, experimental design should assure the well-being of the animals and use appropriate procedures to reduce pain and suffering and the number of animals involved. In the context of this chapter this means carefully monitoring the development of tumor burden, adequate animal handling and surgical protocols, and the humanitarian use of euthanasia.
2. Animals should be kept in an animal room with 22–23 °C air temperature, 55±10% humidity, a 12 h light-dark cycle and standard rodent pelleted diet and tap water ad libitum.
3. NMU is a light and temperature-sensitive compound and should be carefully stored following provider's instructions. NMU solutions must be freshly prepared, immediately used and discarded. NMU is a flammable solid, toxic if swallowed, carcinogenic and teratogenic in animals and may be a carcinogen and a teratogen in humans. It should be handled and disposed as a hazardous material following local regulations.
4. Treatments and route of administration: Histamine (0.1–1 mg/kg/day, 0.1 mL, s.c.), Ranitidine (50 mg/kg/day, p.o. in drinking water), Cimetidine (2.5 mg/kg/day, p.o., in drinking water), Loratadine (2.5 mg/kg/day, p.o., in drinking water), Astemizol (2.0 mg/kg/day, p.o., in drinking water) [16].
5. Immediately after euthanasia excise all palpable tumors, free them from debris and necrotic areas, and cut in sections. Some sections can be frozen in liquid nitrogen for later use or fixed in 10% neutral buffered formalin for routine histological evaluation or immunohistochemical analysis. Tumors can also be

processed for enzymatic activities, primary cultures, or immunological studies.

6. All tumors must be classified histologically as recommended by Russo and Russo [26], since benign and malignant tumors of stromal and epithelial origin may develop in the mammary gland of NMU-injected rats. Establishing histological characteristics of the tumors is necessary for the thorough interpretation of the results of the experiment. The incidence of spontaneous tumors of the mammary gland in Sprague-Dawley female rats is low (<0.5%) in young animals.
7. To avoid nonspecific immune reaction, cells must be diluted in serum-free medium or in saline.
8. Anesthesia employed is a combination of xylazine (10 mg/kg) and ketamine (100 mg/kg) administered, intraperitoneally, 20 min before the surgical procedure. When using anesthesia on nude mice take precautions to prevent hypothermia. If necessary use a warming pad or lamp during the recovery phase, but do not let the mouse overheat either.
9. Working with immunodeficient animals such as nude mice requires special housing conditions (e.g., Specific Pathogen Free Barrier Facility). All procedures should be performed in sterile isolated conditions, using laminar airflow work stations or an area of exclusive work with immunodeficient animals and using sterile coveralls, caps, masks, shoe covers, and gloves.
10. Immediately after euthanasia excise tumors, free them from debris and necrotic areas, and cut in sections. These xenografts showed large central areas of necrotic tissue.
11. Xenograft tumor can also be developed by the injection of tumor cells (5×10^6) in 50 μL of sterile saline solution with 100 μL of Matrigel Growth Factor Reduced in all the mice [80]. However, to avoid culturing a high number of tumor cells and get higher tumor efficiency you may proceed as described in Sect. 3.2.2.
12. Treatments may be subcutaneously injected on the dorsal flank: histamine (1–5 mg/kg/day), clozapine (1 mg/kg/day), JNJ28610244 (10 mg/kg/day), JNJ10191584 (10 mg/kg/day), JNJ10181457 (10 mg/kg/day) [55]. Use vehicle for control group. The method consists in tenting the skin between the shoulder blades and inserting the needle bevel up in the pocket created.
13. Tumor growth data may be expressed as relative tumor volume (tumor volume measured with respect to initial tumor volume at the beginning of treatment) along time. The equation for exponential growth is: $Yt = Y_0 \times e^{(k \times t)}$, where Y_0 is the initial relative tumor volume that increased exponentially with a rate

constant, k. The tumor doubling time may be calculated as 0.69/k [55].

14. Cells that have been maintained in vitro for more than 2 months should not be used for primary tumor growth because they may be less malignant and metastatic in vivo than earlier passaged cells.
15. Tumor growth and tumor immune response are greatly affected by the housing temperature. At thermo-neutral ambient temperature (30–31 °C) a striking reduction in tumor formation, growth rate, and metastasis has been observed, when compared to animals maintained at standard housing temperature for laboratory mice in research facilities which is between 20 and 26 °C [81, 82]. For this reason, special attention has to be paid to maintaining the temperature conditions between experiments.
16. 4T1 tumors become palpable approximately at day 10 post-inoculation and they reach a volume of approximately 1 cm^3 at day 30 [83, 84].
17. The grade of Collagenase (I-IV) will depend on the cell population to be isolated; myeloid cell isolation is best with type IV, whereas lymphocyte yield is higher using type I.
18. Observe the cell suspension under a microscope to determine whether red blood cells are depleted completely. If there are still too many red blood cells, add more lysis buffer until there are very few red blood cells.
19. Ice-cold reagents and solutions should be used, as low temperature prevents the modulation and internalization of surface antigens. Internalization can cause loss of fluorescence intensity.
20. Subsets of immune cells are positive for the following markers:
    - T lymphocytes: CD3+.
    - T helper lymphocytes: CD4+.
    - T cytotoxic lymphocytes: CD8+.
    - B lymphocytes: CD19+.
    - Natural killer (NK) cells: CD56+ CD3-.
    - Myeloid-derived suppressor cells (MDSC): CD11b+ Gr1+.
    - Dendritic cells: CD11c+.
    - Macrophages: CD68+, CD163+, F4/80.
21. To facilitate the detection, when more than one marker is used, it is important to choose antibodies that are conjugated to fluorochromes with non-overlapping emission spectra.

22. FSC (Forward SCatter) and SSC (Side SCatter) parameters allow distinguishing cells based on size and internal complexity. Along the X-axis is the FSC parameter that measures the amount of the laser beam that passes around the cell, giving a relative size of the cell. Along the Y-axis is the SSC parameter that measures the amount of the laser beam that bounces of particulates inside the cell. Using a known control or standard such as beads with a known size, one can determine the relative size of the cells based on the size of the control or standard.
23. Protein concentration in NMU-induced tumors varies from 1.5 to 2.5 mg per 0.1 mL after homogenization, according to Bradford assay.
24. All samples must be run at least in triplicate.
25. Validity of assay: the reaction proceeds at a linear rate in the experimental conditions and the optimum pH for the reaction is 6.5.
26. Counting efficiency in liquid scintillation must be determined for each sample because of quenching phenomenon, which is different in every sample. To calculate the activity DPM you should apply the appropriate counting efficiency (expressed as a decimal) to the CPM value:

$$DPM = \frac{CPM}{Efficiency}$$

27. Equivalence of the Activity units: 2.22×10^6 DPM = 1 μCi = 37 kBq.
28. This procedure allowed the differentiation between substrate and product, not considering endogenous histamine. Over the years different techniques for the determination of HDC activity emerged and were modified to improve the assay. In the last decade, other protocols were developed to evaluate HDC activity by quantifying histamine on an HPLC equipped with o-phthalaldehyde (OPA) derivatization system [85].
29. The employment of radioactive nuclides should be carried out according to local rules and in accordance with the international regulations, about licensing, personnel training, and waste management. All personnel working with sources of ionizing radiation must be instructed in the basic principles of radiation protection and the potential risks of using radionuclides (Radiation Protection and Safety of Radiation Sources: International Basic Safety Standards, IAEA; 2007 and Recommendations of the International Commission on Radiological Protection. ICRP Publication 103. Ann. ICRP 37 (2–4), 2007).

30. HMT activity may be determined later; in that case store the samples in microfuge tubes at −75 °C. Before the activity determination, the frozen samples must be thawed on ice for 10–20 min.
31. To determine HMT activity in cell culture (>5 × 10^6 cells), cells must be trypsinized and centrifuged 2000 × *g*, 5 min at 4 °C. Save the pellet and resuspend in 500 μL of homogenization buffer and follow the protocol from step 6.
32. This solution is 500 μM SAM and contains 1 nCi/μL ^{14}C-SAM with a specific radioactivity of 2 Ci/mol.
33. To determine the blank activity, sample volume must be replaced by distilled water to a final volume of 70 μL.
34. This solution is 4.5 mM putrescine and contains 1 nCi/μL ^{14}C-putrescine with a specific radioactivity of 0.222 Ci/mol.
35. To determine the blank activity, sample volume must be replaced by distilled water to a final volume of 80 μL.
36. Use a dilution 1/20 W/V for NMU-induced tumor homogenization.
37. For NMU tumors, dilute supernatants from 1:20,000 to 1:40,000 employing 50 mM PBS pH 7.5 [76].
38. Procedure for dorsal pedal vein blood sample collection [86]:
    - Keep the animal in a restrainer.
    - The hind foot around ankle is held and medial dorsal pedal vessel is located on the top of the foot.
    - Clean the foot with absolute alcohol and puncture dorsal pedal vein with 23G/27G needle.
    - Collect drops of blood that appear on the skin surface in a capillary tube and apply a little pressure to stop the bleeding.
39. When investigating histamine secretion from tissues, it is important to verify whether histamine detected is not due to mast cell degranulation. Immunohistochemical staining with specific antibodies for mast cells can be employed.
40. All procedures should be performed in sterile conditions, working in a laminar flow hood or a biological safety cabinet and all solutions and media should be sterilized by filtration through a 0.22 μm filter.
41. The upper layer consists of McCoy's 5A medium enriched with fetal calf serum (10%), calcium chloride (444 μg/mL), insulin (2 units/mL), ascorbic acid (53 μg/mL), penicillin (100 units/mL), streptomycin (100 μg/mL), DEAE-dextran (250 μg/mL), β-mercaptoethanol (0.4 μg/mL), L-asparagine (66 μg/mL), and 0.3% agar.

42. Trypan blue is a vital stain, which does not interact with the cell unless the cell membrane is damaged. Undamaged cells exclude the dye, damaged cells absorb the dye and become blue, and therefore, it selectively colors dead tissues or cells.
43. The bottom layer consists of 0.5% agar and McCoy's 5A medium enriched with fetal calf serum (10%), sodium pyruvate (0.22 mg/mL), L-serine (42 μg/mL), glutamine (2.9 μg/mL), sodium bicarbonate (4.5 mg/mL), penicillin (100 units/mL), streptomycin (100 μg/mL), L-asparagine (100 μg/mL), DEAE-dextran (375 μg/mL), and tryptic soy broth (7.5 mg/mL).
44. Histamine receptors' ligands to be tested should be added in the appropriate concentration to both layers during preparation.
45. After plating and before incubation, dishes should be observed with an inverted phase microscope looking for aggregates that can be confused with colonies.
46. Experiments should be performed using at least triplicate dishes for each experimental condition.
47. When a large number of dishes are to be prepared, the cell suspension in 0.3% agar (upper layer) should be kept warm (40 °C) with continuous stirring.

References

1. World Health Organization (2011). Global Health Observatory Data Repository Number of deaths (World) by cause. Available from: http://apps.who.int/gho/data/node.main.CODWORLD?lang=enaccessed 31.10.2013
2. Ferlay J, Soerjomataram I, Dikshit R et al (2015) Cancer incidence and mortality worldwide: sources, methods and major patterns. Int J Cancer 136:E359–E386
3. Sharma S, Barry M, Gallagher DJ et al (2015) An overview of triple negative breast cancer for surgical oncologists. Surg Oncol 24:276–283
4. Medina VA, Rivera ES (2010) Histamine receptors and cancer pharmacology. Br J Pharmacol 161:755–767
5. Voskoglou-Nomikos T, Pater JL, Seymour L (2003) Clinical predictive value of the in vitro cell line, human xenograft, and mouse allograft preclinical cancer models. Clin Cancer Res 9:4227–4239
6. Medina VA, Coruzzi G, Martinel Lamas DJ et al (2013) Histamine in cancer. In: Stark H (ed) Histamine H4 receptor: A novel drug target in immunoregulatory and inflammatory diseases. Versita, London
7. Martinel Lamas DJ, Rivera ES, Medina VA (2015) Histamine H4 receptor: insights into a potential therapeutic target in breast cancer. Front Biosci (Schol Ed) 7:1–9
8. Davio CA, Cricco GP, Martin G et al (1994) Effect of histamine on growth and differentiation of the rat mammary gland. Agents Actions Spec No:C115–7
9. Maslinski C, KierskaD FW et al (1993) Histamine: its metabolism and localization in mammary gland. Comp Biochem Physiol C 105:269–273
10. Wagner W, Ichikawa A, Tanaka S et al (2003) Mouse mammary epithelial histamine system. J Physiol Pharmacol 5:211–223
11. Martinel Lamas DJ, Cortina JE, Ventura C et al (2015) Enhancement of ionizing radiation response by histamine in vitro and in vivo in human breast cancer. Cancer Biol Ther 16:137–148
12. Sieja K, Stanosz S, von Mach-Szczypiński J et al (2005) Concentration of histamine in serum and tissues of the primary ductal breast cancer in women. Breast 14:236–241
13. von Mach-Szczypiński J, Stanosz S, Sieja K et al (2009) Metabolism of histamine in tissues of primary ductal breast cancer. Metabolism 58:867–870
14. Cricco G, Davio C, Martín G et al (1994) Histamine as an autocrine growth factor in an

experimental mammary carcinoma. Agents Actions 43:17–20

15. Davio C, Cricco G, Bergoc R et al (1995) H_1 and H_2 histamine receptors in experimental carcinomas with an atypical coupling to signal transducers. Biochem Pharmacol 50:91–96
16. Rivera E, Davio C, Cricco G et al (1993) Histamine regulation of tumour growth. Role of H_1 and H_2 receptors. In: Histamine in normal and cancer cell proliferation. Advances in the Bioscience, 89, 299–317. M. García-Caballero, L. Brandes and S. Hosoda. Eds. Pergamon Press, Oxford. ISBN: 0080422020 9780080422022
17. Rivera ES, Cricco GP, Engel NI et al (2000) Histamine as an autocrine growth factor: an unusual role for a widespread mediator. Semin Cancer Biol 10:15–23
18. Davio C, Cricco G, Andrade N et al (1993) H_1 and H_2 histamine receptors in human mammary carcinomas. Agents Actions 38:C172–C174
19. Lemos B, Davio C, Gass H et al (1995) Histamine receptors in human mammary gland, different benign lesions and mammmary carcinomas. Inflamm Res 44:68–69
20. Parshad R, Hazrah P, Kumar S et al (2005) Effect of preoperative short course famotidine on TILs and survival in breast cancer. Indian J Cancer 42:185–190
21. Medina V, Cricco G, Nuñez M et al (2006) Histamine-mediated signaling processes in human malignant mammary cells. Cancer Biol Ther 5:1462–1471
22. Medina V, Croci M, Crescenti E et al (2008) The role of histamine in human mammary carcinogenesis: H_3 and H_4 receptors as potential therapeutic targets for breast cancer treatment. Cancer Biol Ther 7:27–35
23. Medina VA, Brenzoni PG, Martinel Lamas DJ et al (2011) Role of histamine H4 receptor in breast cancer cell proliferation. Front Biosci (Elite Ed) 3:1042–1060
24. Mak IWY, Evaniew N, Ghert M (2014) Lost in translation: animal models and clinical trials in cancer treatment. Am J Transl Res 6:114–118
25. Fiebig HH, Maier A, Burger AM (2004) Clonogenic assay with established human tumour xenografts: correlation of in vitro to in vivo activity as a basis for anticancer drug discovery. Eur J Cancer 40:802–820
26. Russo J, Gusterson BA, Rogers AE et al (1990) Comparative study of human and rat mammary tumorigenesis. Lab Invest 62:244–278
27. Russo J, Russo IH (2000) Atlas and histologic classification of tumors of the rat mammary gland. J Mammary Gland Biol Neoplasia 5(2):187–200
28. Hall EJ, Giaccia AJ (2012) Clinical response of normal tissues. In: Hall EJ, Giaccia AJ, Williams, Wilkins (eds) Radiobiology for radiobiologists, 7th edn. Lippincott, Philadelphia
29. Pavelic PZ, SlocumHK RYM et al (1980) Colony growth in soft agar of human melanoma, sarcoma, and lung carcinoma cells disaggregated by mechanical and enzymatic methods. Cancer Res 40:2160–2164
30. Manni A, Wright C (1983) Assessment of mitogenesis of the hormone-responsive NMU rat mammary tumor grown in culture in soft agar, using ^{3}H-thymidine incorporation into DNA. Breast Cancer Res Treat 3:287–292
31. Price JE, Polyzos A, Zhang RD et al (1990) Tumorigenicity and metastasis of human breast carcinoma cell lines in nude mice. Cancer Res 50:717–721
32. Russo J, Russo IH (1996) Experimentally induced mammary tumors in rats. Breast Cancer Res Treat 39:7–20
33. Hamaguchi T, Matsuoka Y, Kawaguchi H et al (2004) Terminal endbuds and acini as the respective major targets for chemical and sporadic carcinogenesis in the mammary glands of human c-Ha-rasprotooncogene transgenic rats. Breast Cancer Res Treat 83:43–56
34. Perše M, Cerar A, Injac R et al (2009) N-methylnitrosourea induced breast cancer in rat, the histopathology of the resulting tumours and its drawbacks as a model. Pathol Oncol Res 15:115–121
35. Saminathan M, Rai RB, Dhama K et al l (2014) Histopathology and immunohistochemical expression of n-methyl-n-nitrosourea (NMU) induced mammary tumours in sprague-dawley rats. Asian J Anim Vet Adv 9:621–640
36. Chan MM, Lu X, Merchant FM et al (2005) Gene expression profiling of NMU-induced rat mammary tumors: cross species comparison with human breast cancer. Carcinogenesis 26:1343–1353
37. Gullino PM, Pettigrew HM, Grantham FH (1975) N-nitrosomethylurea as mammary gland carcinogen in rats. J Natl Cancer Inst 54:401–414
38. Thompson HT, Adlakha H (1991) Dose-responsive induction of mammary gland carcinomas by the intraperitoneal injection of 1-methyl-l-nitrosourea. Cancer Res 51: 3411–3415
39. Rivera ES, Andrade N, Martin G et al (1994) Induction of mammary tumors in rat by intraperitoneal injection of NMU: histopathology and estral cycle influence. Cancer Lett 86:223–228
40. Martin G, Melito G, Rivera E et al (1996) Effect of tamoxifen on intraperitoneal

N-nitroso-N-methylurea induced tumors. Cancer Lett 100:227–234

41. Martin G, Rivera E, Daivo C et al (1996) Receptors characterization of intraperitoneally N-nitroso-N-methylurea-induced mammary tumors in rats. Cancer Lett 101:1–8
42. Martin G, Davio C, Rivera E et al (1997) Hormone dependence of mammary tumors induced in rats by intraperitoneal NMU injection. Cancer Invest 15:8–17
43. Sporn MB, Dowsett SA, Mershon J et al (2004) Role of raloxifene in breast cancer prevention in post menopausal women: clinical evidence and potential mechanisms of action. Clin Ther 26:830–840
44. Tsubura A, LaiYC MH et al (2011) Animal models of N-Methyl-N-nitrosourea-induced mammary cancer and retinal degeneration with special emphasis on therapeutic trials. In Vivo 25:11–22
45. Kisková T, Jendželovský R, Rentsen E et al (2014) Resveratrol enhances the chemopreventive effect of celecoxib in chemically induced breast cancer in rats. Eur J Cancer Prev 23:506–513
46. Yaacob NS, Yankuzo HM, Devaraj S et al (2015) Anti-tumor action, clinical biochemistry profile and phytochemical constituents of a pharmacologically active fraction of *S. crispus* in NMU-induced rat mammary tumour model. PLoS One. doi:10.1371/journal.pone.0126426 2015
47. McCormick DL, Adamowski CB, Fiks A et al (1981) Lifetime dose-response relationships for mammary tumor induction by a single administration of N-methyl-N-nitrosourea. Cancer Res 41:1690–1694
48. Kelland LR (2004) "Of mice and men": values and liabilities of the athymic nude mouse model in anticancer drug development. Eur J Cancer 40:827–836
49. Graham C, Tucker C, Creech J et al (2006) Evaluation of the antitumor efficacy, pharmacokinetics and pharmacodynamics of the histone deacetylase inhibitor depsipeptide in childhood cancer models in vivo. Clin Cancer Res 12:223–234
50. Kerbel RS (2003) Human tumor xenografts as predictive preclinical models for anticancer drug activity in humans: better than commonly perceived—but they can be improved. Cancer Biol Ther 2:S134–S139
51. Bibby MC (2004) Orthotopic models of cancer for preclinical drug evaluation: advantages and disadvantages. Eur J Cancer 40:852–857
52. Badve S, Dabbs DJ, Schnitt SJ et al (2011) Basal-like and triple-negative breast cancers: a critical review with an emphasis on the implications for pathologists and oncologists. Mod Pathol 24:157–167
53. Pierce JE (1990) Xenograft models in immunodeficient animals. I. Nude mice: spontaneous and experimental metastasis models. In: S.A. Brooks and U. Schumacher© Humana Press Inc (ed) Methods in Molecular Medicine, vol 58: Metastasis Research Protocols, Totowa NJ (ed) Cell Behavior In Vitro and In Vivo Vol. 2. pp 205–213.
54. Davio C, Mladovan A, Lemos B et al (2002) H_1 and H_2 histamine receptors mediate the production of inositol phosphates but not cAMP in human breast epithelial cells. Inflamm Res 51:1–7
55. Martinel Lamas D, Croci M, Carabajal E et al (2013) Therapeutic potencial of histamine H_4 receptor agonists in triple-negative human breast cancer experimental model. Br J Pharmacol 170:188–199
56. Martinel Lamas DJ, Nicoud MB, Sterle HA et al (2015) Selective cytoprotective effect of histamine on doxorubicin-induced hepatic and cardiac toxicity in animal models. Cell Death Discov 1:15059
57. Kmiecik T, Otocka-Kmiecik A, Górska-Ciebiada M et al (2012) T lymphocytes as a target of histamine action. Arch Med Sci 8:154–161
58. Dushyanthen S, Beavis PA, Savas P et al (2015) Relevance of tumor-infiltrating lymphocytes in breast cancer. BMC Med 13:202
59. Hegyesi L, Colombo E, Pállinger S et al (2007) Impact of systemic histamine deficiency on the crosstalk between mammary adenocarcinoma and T cells. J Pharmacol Sci 105:66–73
60. Dexter DL, Kowalski HM, Blazar BA et al (1978) Heterogeneity of tumor cells from a single mouse mammary tumor. Cancer Res 38:3174–3181
61. Pulaski BA, Ostrand-Rosenberg S (1998) Reduction of established spontaneous mammary carcinoma metastases following immunotherapy with major histocompatibility complex class II and B7.1 cell-based tumor vaccines. Cancer Res 58:1486–1493
62. Lelekakis M, Moseley JM, Martin TJ et al (1999) A novel orthotopic model of breast cancer metastasis to bone. Clin Exp Metastasis 17:163–170
63. Heppner GH, Miller FR, Shekhar PM (2000) Nontransgenic models of breast cancer. Breast Cancer Res 2:331–334
64. DuPre' SA, Hunter KW Jr (2007) Murine mammary carcinoma 4T1 induces a leukemoid

reaction with splenomegaly: association with tumor-derived growth factors. Exp Mol Pathol 82:12–24

65. Hegyesi H, Horváth B, Pállinger E et al (2005) Histamine elevates the expression of Ets-1, a protooncogen in human melanoma cell lines through H_2 receptor. FEBS Lett 579:2475–2479
66. Parsons SJ, Parsons JT (2004) Src family kinases, key regulators of signal transduction. Oncogene 23:7906–7909
67. He G, Lin J, Cai W et al (2014) Associations of polymorphisms in histidine decarboxylase, histamine N-methyltransferase and histamine receptor H_3 genes with breast cancer. PLoS One 9(5):e97728
68. Frick LR, Rapanelli M, Arcos ML et al (2011) Oral administration of fluoxetine alters the proliferation/apoptosis balance of lymphoma cells and up-regulates T cell immunity in tumor-bearing mice. Eur J Pharmacol 659:265–272
69. Medina MA, Urdiales JL, Rodriguez-Caso C et al (2003) Biogenic amines and polyamines: similar biochemistry for different physiological missions and biomedical applications. Crit Rev Biochem Mol Biol 38:23–59
70. Medina MA, Correa-Fiz F, Rodriguez-Caso C et al (2005) A comprehensive view of polyamine and histamine metabolism to the light of new technologies. J Cell Mol Med 9:854–864
71. Levine RJ, Watts DE (1966) A sensitive and specific assay for histidine decarboxylase activity. Biochem Pharmacol 5:841–849
72. Hakanson R, Larsson LI, Liedberg G et al (1977) Suppression of rat stomach histidine decarboxylase activity by histamine: H_2-receptor-mediated feed-back. J Physiol 269:643–667
73. Engel N, Cricco G, Davio C et al (1996) Histamine regulates the expression of histidine decarboxylase in NMU-induced tumors in rats. Inflamm Res 45(S1):S64–S65
74. Tran VT, Snyder SH (1981) Histidine decarboxylase. Purification from fetal rat liver, immunologic properties, and histochemical localization in brain and stomach. J Biol Chem 256:680–686
75. Kuefner MA, Feurle J, Petersen J et al (2014) Influence of iodinated contrast media on the activities of histamine inactivating enzymes diamine oxidase and histamine N-methyltransferase in vitro. Allergol Immunopathol 42:324–328
76. Cricco G, Engel N, Crocci M et al (1997) Fluoromethylhistidine inhibits tumor growth without producing depletion of endogenous histamine. Inflamm Res 46:59–60
77. Manni A, Wright C (1983) Effect of tamoxifen and alpha-difluoromethylornithine on clones of nitrosomethylurea-induced rat mammary tumor cells grown in soft agar culture. Cancer Res 43:1084–1086
78. Kilkenny C, Browne W, Cuthill IC et al (2010) NC3Rs reporting guidelines working group. animal research: reporting in vivo experiments: the ARRIVE guidelines. Br J Pharmacol 160:1577–1579
79. McGrath JC, Drummond GB, McLachlan EM et al (2010) Guidelines for reporting experiments involving animals: the ARRIVE guidelines. Br J Pharmacol 160:1573–1576
80. Warin R, Xiao D, Arlotti JA et al (2010) Inhibition of human breast cancer xenograft growth by cruciferous vegetable constituent benzyl isothiocyanate. Mol Carcinog 49:500–507
81. Kokolus KM, Capitano ML, Lee CT et al (2013) Baseline tumor growth and immune control in laboratory mice are significantly influenced by subthermoneutral housing temperature. Proc Natl Acad Sci U S A 110:20176–20181
82. Minton K (2014) Tumour-bearing mice feel the cold. Nat Rev Immunol 14:7
83. Spallanzani RG, Dalotto-Moreno T, Raffo Iraolagoitia XL et al (2013) Expansion of CD11b(+)Ly6G (+)Ly6C (int) cells driven by medroxyprogesterone acetate in mice bearing breast tumors restrains NK cell effector functions. Cancer Immunol Immunother 62:1781–1795
84. Kramer MG, Masner M, Casales E et al (2015) Neoadjuvant administration of Semliki Forest virus expressing interleukin-12 combined with attenuated Salmonella eradicates breast cancer metastasis and achieves long-term survival in immunocompetent mice. BMC Cancer 15:620
85. Nitta Y, Ohshita J, Liu H et al (2010) Expression of recombinant human histidine decarboxylase with full length and C-terminal truncated forms in yeast and bacterial cells. J Biol Macromol 10:73–82
86. Parasuraman S, Raveendran R, Kesavan R (2010) Blood sample collection in small laboratory animals. J Pharmacol Pharmacother 1:87–93

Chapter 13

Evaluation of Histidine Decarboxylase (HDC) Activity and Human Histamine Receptor 3 (H_3R) and HDC mRNA Levels

Carlos Acosta-Andrade, José L. Urdiales, Ignacio Fajardo, and Francisca Sánchez-Jiménez

Abstract

Histamine plays pleiotropic roles in human pathophysiology that are dependent on both its ability to be synthetized in a given environment and the cell-specific combination of histamine receptors expressed in the different human cell types. At present, characterization of the molecular basis of the tissue-specific roles of the histamine metabolism-related elements requires further research efforts to fully explain the multiple roles that histamine plays in human pathophysiology and to develop new intervention strategies derived from this knowledge. In this chapter, we describe some methods used in our laboratory for many years to investigate histidine decarboxylase (HDC) and histamine receptors (HRs) in different human cell types and tissues. These are a radiolabeled method for HDC activity measurement and quantitative real-time polymerase chain reaction (qPCR) methods for quantification and transcript analyses of human HDC and histamine receptor type 3 (H_3R).

Key words Gastric secretion, Histamine, Histamine receptor 3, Histidine decarboxylase expression, Histidine decarboxylase activity, Immune response, Mast cells, Mastocytosis, Nervous system, Neuroblastoma, qPCR

1 Introduction : Distribution of the Histamine Metabolism-Related Elements in the Human Body and Their Physiopathological Roles

Histamine is a pleiotropic amine involved in important physiological processes, as immune response, neurobiology and neuroendocrinology, digestion, and tumor growth, as recently reviewed [1, 2]. Histamine is only expressed in a reduced set of human cell types. The major producing cells accumulate the amine in specific vesicles until they receive the corresponding signal for its extrusion. The highest percentage of histamine production in humans is

Ekaterini Tiligada and Madeleine Ennis (eds.), *Histamine Receptors as Drug Targets*, Methods in Pharmacology and Toxicology, DOI 10.1007/978-1-4939-6843-5_13, © Springer Science+Business Media LLC 2017

carried out by mast cells [3]. These are myeloid cells involved in the allergic response among other inflammatory reactions, immune tolerance, defence against pathogens, etc. [4]. Mast cell precursors migrate from the bone marrow and infiltrate into peripheral tissues where they complete their differentiation processes depending on the local microenvironment [5, 6]. After activation, they release different immune mediators, including histamine and/or other biogenic amines [7, 8]. Basophils can also produce and store histamine; however, other immune cells (for instance, macrophages and platelets) can also be histamine producers, but they lack the possibility of storing the amine in intracellular organelles [9, 10].

Histaminergic neurons are located into the tuberomamillary nucleus and send their axons all over the central nervous system [11]. Histamine is described as being involved in locomotor activity, memory, cognition, anxiety, circadian rhythm, pain perception, food intake, and addition [12]. The presence of histamine in the brain could also be due to the activation of infiltrated immune cells, thus being related to neuroinflammatory diseases [13].

A third type of histamine-producing cells able to store histamine are the gastric enterochromaffin-like cells (ECL), which are able to store and liberate histamine in response to gastrin, as part of the digestive program, as histamine in stomach acts as a paracrine factor inducing acid secretion by parietal cells through binding to parietal cell membrane histamine receptors type 2 (H_2R) [14]. Histamine is also proposed to be an important member of the gut-brain axis [15].

Once released from a histamine producing cell, histamine can be a mediator of different signalling pathways that have a tissue-specific pattern of expression as described in the previous literature and databases [2, 16, 17]. In addition to the four G protein coupled receptors (H_1R-H_4R), histamine has also been described as a ligand of the N-methylaspartate receptor (NMDA) [18]. Information about tissue-specific histamine receptor expression has been included in several recent reviews and books as it is an active research and drug discovery area (for instance [2, 16, 19–26]).

Table 1 provides identification (encoding information) for the specific macromolecules involved in histamine synthesis and signalling in humans, i.e., histidine decarboxylase (HDC), for H_1R-H_4R, and their tissue expression. Information and references about the type of G protein associated with each receptor are also included. This information comes from the National Center for Biotechnology Information (NCBI) and the International Union of Basic and Clinical Pharmacology (IUPHAR) data bases [27]. H_1R and H_2R are expressed in a wide variety of cell types, H_1R and H_4R have a relevant role in inflammation and the immune system in general, and H_3R has a predominant role in neuronal function. There are several molecular aspects in the characterization of these

Table 1
Identification and tissue-specific expression of macromolecules related to histamine synthesis and reception in human cells/tissues

Gene name	Gene symbol (ID)[a]	Protein abbreviation (uniprot code)[a]	G-protein coupled[b]	Expressing cells/tissues[b]
Histidine decarboxylase	HDC (3067)	hHDC (P19113)	–	Mast cells enterochromaffin-like cells; histaminergic neurons; macrophages; monocytes; platelets
Histamine receptor type 1	HRH1 (3269)	H_1R (P35367)	$G_{q/11}$	Lymphocytes; endothelial cells; macrophages; monocytes; dendritic cells; lung; heart; neurons, intestine; liver
Histamine receptor type 2	HRH2 (3274)	H_2R (P25021)	G_s	Gastric mucosa; intestine; adrenal gland; brain; heart; liver; lung; lymph node; muscle; placenta; thyroid gland
Histamine receptor type 3	HRH3 (11255)	H_3R (Q9Y5N1)	$G_{i/0}$	Brain; peripheral nervous system
Histamine receptor type 4	HRH4 (59340)	H_4R (Q9H3N8)	$G_{i/0}$	Immune cells, brain

[a]Information from National Center for Biotechnology Information (NCBI) Databases
[b]Data from Ref. [27]

receptors that deserve special attention, as they are very important to fully understand histamine effects in human health and disease. For example, the existence of different isoforms in different tissues [28], the constitutive activity reported for H_3R and H_4R and the alternative signaling pathways used in the presence or the absence of ligand [29, 30], as well as events of functional cross-talk, protein-protein interactions, and heterodimerization between histamine receptor subunits and dopamine receptor subunits in cell types sensitive to both biogenic amines [31–33].

From present knowledge about the implications of HDC and HRs in many different physiological processes, it can be suspected that alterations in expression and/or activity of any of these elements will be related to a wide spectrum of human pathologies. In fact, after several rounds of computer-assisted text mining searches, using open-source platforms such as SciMiner, Diseases, and DisGeNET [34–37], we were able to collect a list of human diseases in which HDC and HRs are involved. The results are shown in Table 2. It is not an exhaustive list, as sometimes the phenomenological evidence does not allow us to identify a specific histamine metabolism-related element as responsible for the histamine-related effects observed in patients or animal models. Nevertheless, the present list of diseases, which affect an important percentage of the population, claims the attention of researchers working on biomedical problems related to these pathologies especially those working with big sets of "omics" data, which must be further validated with alternative and more reductionist approaches.

Table 3 shows information on the chromosomal location of the different histamine metabolism-related elements mentioned in the previous Tables and some known features on the occurrence of genomic variants associated with human diseases/phenotypes, as well as reported events of alternative splicing during mRNA maturation. This information came from NCBI databases (mainly Gene, PubMed, and ClinVar databases). It will be useful for researchers working on histamine-related diseases, as it can help to discuss the expression results obtained with this or other alternative methods and/or for planning and adapting the methods to specific circumstances (tissue, pathology, etc).

Genes encoding active HDC and HRs are not redundant in the human genome and are located on different chromosomes. This makes it difficult to compensate aberrant expression of any of these proteins, which probably forms the basis of different human pathophenotypes. On the other hand, aberrant expression features can have genetic origins, can be the consequence of an abnormal developmental program (having a different genetic origin), and/or can even have a strong epigenetic contribution. Some examples are provided in Table 3. Thus, from just a single histamine metabolism-related gene, human cells can express different variants with differential characteristics under different circumstances.

Table 2
Human diseases related to dysfunction of histamine synthesis and receptors

Protein[a]	Syndrome/disease	OMIM ID	Reference
HDC	Allergic rhinitis	607154	[68]
	Asthma	600807	[69]
	Atopic dermatitis	603165	[70]
	Mast cell disease	154800	[71]
	Narcolepsy	161400	[72]
	Tourette's syndrome	137580	[73]
H_1R	Allergic rhinitis	607154	[74]
	Atopic dermatitis	603165	[75]
	Crohn disease	266600	[76]
	Myasthenia gravis	159400	[77]
	Motion sickness	158280	[78]
	Asthma	600807	[79]
	Malaria	609148	[80]
	Multiple sclerosis	126200	[81]
	VitD-dependent rickets 2A	277400	[82]
	Familial long QT syndrome	152427	[83]
	Brugada syndrome	601144	[84]
H_2R	Allergic rhinitis	607154	[85]
	Aplastic anaemia	609135	[86]
	Gastroesophageal reflux	109350	[87]
	Juvenile rheumatoid arthritis	604302	[88]
	Schizophrenia	181500	[89]
	Malaria	600807	[80]
	Zollinger-Ellison syndrome	131100	[90]
H_3R	Alzheimer's disease	104300	[91]
	ADHD	143465	[92]
	Hereditary essential tremor	190300	[93]
	Obesity	601665	[25]
	Parkinson's disease	168600	[91]
	Schizophrenia	181500	[94]
	Migraine	157300	[95]
	Narcolepsy	161400	[96]
	Tourette's syndrome	137580	[94]
H_4R	Allergic rhinitis	607154	[97]
	Atopic dermatitis	603165	[26]
	Asthma	600807	[26]
	Breast cancer	114480	[98]
	Parkinson disease	168600	[99]
	Ulcerative colitis	266600	[100]
	Multiple sclerosis	126200	[81]

[a] *HDC* histidine decarboxylase protein, *H1R* histamine receptor 1 protein, *H2R* histamine receptor 2 protein, *H3R* histamine receptor 3 protein, *H4R* histamine receptor 4 protein

Table 3
Chromosomal location of the different histamine metabolism-related genes and some known features on the occurrence of genomic variants associated with human diseases/phenotypes

Gene[a]	Gene location	Type of variation	Pathogenic variation	Related disease/phenotype[b]
HDC	15q21.2 NC_000015.10 (50241945.. ..50266091, complement)	Tourette Syndrome. Single nucleotide variant. G>A—Trp317 changes to STOP	nsv993449	Tics, sensorimotor gating deficiencies, and abnormalities of cortico-basal ganglia circuits. All 9 affected individuals had Tourette syndrome, 4 also had obsessive-compulsive disorder (OCD; 164230), and 1 also had Asperger syndrome Impaired prepulse inhibition of the startle response to an auditory stimulus; Dysregulated binding of dopamine receptors in the substantia nigra
		Copy number loss	nsv869222	Muscular hypotonia
			nsv533138	Developmental delay AND/OR other significant developmental or morphological phenotypes
			nsv916464	Abnormal facial shape
HRH1	3p25 NC_000003.12 (11137093.. ..11263253)	Copy number loss	nsv995278	Seizures
			nsv869341 nsv530002	Developmental delay AND/OR other significant developmental or morphological phenotypes
			nsv530028	Global developmental delay
		Copy number gain	nsv996247	Truncus arteriosus; hyponatremia; decreased urine output
			nsv995408	Seizures; encephalopathy
			nsv916269 nsv869190 nsv869127 nsv817364	Developmental delay AND/OR other significant developmental or morphological phenotypes
			nsv530240	Abnormality of the cerebrum global developmental delay
			nsv530239 nsv530211	Developmental delay AND/OR other significant developmental or morphological phenotypes
			nsv529645	Cleft upper lip; cleft palate

HRH2	5q35.2 NC_000005.10 (175657796.. ..175710756)	Copy number loss	Allele ID 185725	Omphalocele; tetralogy of Fallot; talipes equinovarus; ventriculomegaly; Arnold-Chiari malformation; meningocele. Patient also had duplication chr2:239873381-243006013)
			nsv530862	Global developmental delay
		Copy number gain	nsv533814	Abnormality of cardiac morphology
			nsv995681	Sepsis
			nsv932662	Ventricular septal defect; spasticity; coloboma; growth hormone deficiency; encephalopathy; holoprosencephaly; craniosynostosis; patent ductus arteriosus
			nsv530378	Global developmental delay
			nsv491929	Developmental delay AND/OR other significant developmental or morphological phenotypes
			nsv530862	Global developmental delay
			nsv530579	Abnormal facial shape
			nsv530578	Developmental delay AND/OR other significant developmental or
			nsv530576	morphological phenotypes
HRH3	20q13.33 NC_000020.11 (62214766.. ..62220278, complement)	Copy number gain	nsv993449	Developmental delay AND/OR other significant developmental or
			nsv869222	morphological phenotypes
			nsv533138	
			nsv916464	Autism; global developmental delay; encephalopathy; intrauterine growth retardation; tip-toe gait
			nsv533072	Generalized muscle weakness
			nsv531730	Developmental delay AND/OR other significant developmental or morphological phenotypes
				Abnormality of cardiac morphology

(continued)

Table 3
(continued)

Gene[a]	Gene location	Type of variation	Pathogenic variation	Related disease/phenotype[b]
HRH4	18q11.2 NC_000018.10 (24460568..24487427)	Copy number gain	nsv10676616	Developmental delay AND/OR other significant developmental or morphological phenotypes
			nsv531254	
			nsv531253	
			nsv531251	
			nsv531255	Congenital diaphragmatic hernia
			nsv531249	Encephalocele
			nsv531221	Rocker bottom foot; wide intermamillary distance; polydactyly
			nsv531215	Global developmental delay
			nsv531210	Respiratory distress; intrauterine growth retardation
			nsv932068	Abnormality of cardiac morphology; cataract; talipes equinovarus; macrocephaly
			nsv917340	Developmental delay AND/OR other significant developmental or morphological phenotypes; malformation of the heart and great vessels; low-set ears; abnormal facial shape; premature birth; wide intermamillary distance; cryptorchidism; congenital diaphragmatic hernia; oesophageal atresia; failure to thrive; premature birth; intrauterine growth retardation; tetralogy of Fallot; morphological abnormality of the central nervous system; delayed gross motor development; muscular hypotonia; abnormal facial shape
			nsv917211	Autistic behavior
			nsv996099	Autistic behavior; global developmental delay
			nsv906067	Abnormality of the ear; small anterior fontanelle
			nsv995149	Polyhydramnios; hydrocephalus; macrocephaly
			nsv916842	Intrahepatic cholestasis with episodic jaundice
			nsv492182	Developmental delay AND/OR other significant developmental or morphological phenotypes
			nsv329608	Hydrocephalus; abnormality of cardiac morphology; hypertonia; absent radius; cleft upper lip; abnormal facial shape; cleft palate; Dandy-Walker malformation; developmental delay and/or other significant developmental or morphological phenotypes

[a] *HDC* histidine decarboxylase gene, *HRH1* histamine receptor 1 gene, *HRH2* histamine receptor 2 gene, *HRH3* histamine receptor 3 gene, *HRH4* histamine receptor 4 gene
[b] Data from ClinVar [101] and dbVar [102] databases of genomic structural variation with associated phenotypes

These facts confirm the very complex problems that need the contribution of both systemic (high-throughput technologies and other systems biology approaches) as well as methods for validation of alterations in the structure and/or function of single molecules.

2 H_3R and HDC: Two Difficult Subjects for Molecular Characterization

Molecular characterization of HRs (especially H_3R and H_4R) and HDC still present important difficulties. The receptors are folded and anchored into membranes (7 transmembrane segments), so making even in silico modeling strategies difficult (our own experience). Furthermore, multiple isoforms can be expressed for a single gene with different functional characteristics, and both the receptor activity and the signaling elicited can be modified by heterodimerization events [17]. In addition, the extreme instability of the mammalian HDC protein delayed its structural characterization [38].

The full molecular characterization of these open chapters of histamine research deserves additional efforts, as this knowledge will also help understanding of the clinical variant consequences, and therefore possibilities for prevention and/or intervention. Current high-throughput initiatives, as well as reductionist approaches, require specific methods for quantitative result validation. In this chapter, we will provide several analytical methods that could help in this task. They are quantitative real-time polymerase chain reaction (qPCR) methods for measuring HDC and H_3R mRNA levels, as well as a radiolabeling method for the determination of mammalian HDC activity. These experimental methods have been used in our laboratory for many years and published in more than 20 publications from our group (for instance, [39–42]).

HDC (EC 4.1.1.22) is the enzyme responsible for histamine synthesis [38]. In its active form, mammalian HDC is a homodimeric pyridoxal 5′-phosphate (PLP)-dependent decarboxylase (relative molecular weight over 110 kDa) that has a high degree of homology with mammalian aromatic L-amino acid decarboxylase or L-dopa decarboxylase (DDC), the key enzyme responsible for the synthesis of other biogenic amines such as dopamine, and serotonin and its derivative melatonin [43]. Recently, a direct mutant of the human enzyme bound to a substrate analogue has been solved by X-ray crystallography [44]. Mammalian HDC differs from its paralog DDC in the carboxy-terminus, a fragment around 180 amino acids being absent in DDC that present fragments enriched in proline, glutamic acid, serine and threonine (PEST regions) and endoplasmic reticulum binding motifs related to both the sorting and activation of the enzyme [38]. Mammalian HDC activation requires the removal of a substantial part (~20 kDa) of this C-terminal portion that seems to be involved in the sorting of the active form of the enzyme [38, 45–47]. The kinetic behavior of an active form of mammalian HDC (ratHDC) was first described in 2002 [48], and subsequently enriched [49, 50]. A first model for the mammalian enzyme was obtained in 2003 [43], and further validated by cooperation among different laboratories [49, 51, 52]. The active enzyme is extremely unstable most probably due to the presence of PEST region in the N-terminus and the presence of a flexible loop that is involved in the substrate reception [50].

The H_3R was described in 1983 [53]. It is mainly expressed in the central but also in the peripheral nervous system. It works coupled to $G_{i/0}$ proteins, so negatively regulating adenylate cyclase but activating signaling thought mitogen-activated protein kinases (MAPK) and phosphatidylinositol-4,5-bisphosphate 3-kinase (PI3K) [54]. The H_3R encoding gene is located at chromosome 20 containing up to 4 exonic sequences [55]. Multiple spliced isoforms have been observed, several of them being active, but differing in their ligand affinities and the elicited signaling mechanisms [56]. Isoforms can also exhibit different dimerization patterns, for which regulatory roles are proposed [57]. Sequence differences among variants are located at the N-terminus and exons 3 and 4 [56, 58]. Genetic variants have also been reported, some of them already related to human syndromes, as mentioned above. Further structural and functional information on the receptor can be found in the elegant recently published IUPHAR review on histamine receptors [17]. As far as we know, no three-dimensional structure of this receptor has yet been identified by X-ray crystallography, but it is a promising pharmacological target and is the subject of in silico approaches with the aim of helping in a list of emergent neurological problems [59], a strategy also followed for other histamine receptors [60].

3 HDC Activity Determination

HDC enzymatic activity is measured by following the release of $^{14}CO_2$ from L-[^{14}C(U)]-histidine. The method described here has been extensively used in our laboratory for the quantification of HDC enzymatic activity in different cell types and tissues from different species. These include mouse mast cells at different degrees of differentiation, bone marrow derived mast cells (BMMCs), rat and human basophilic leukaemia cells, human mastocytoma cells, and rat liver [39, 61–63]. The HDC content in these cell types and tissues is very low, making necessary the use of the present radioactive method designed to determine enzymatic activity in a range of histidine concentrations corresponding to first order kinetics (histidine concentration in the reaction is 21 μM, and K_M of mammalian HDC is reported to be 0.2–0.4 mM [38]). This method is very sensitive, and allows the detection of HDC activity even when histamine-producing cells are only a minority in the tissue/organ (e.g., adult mouse liver). However, if working with sources containing higher amounts of active HDC (e.g., transfected cells or purified HDC [42, 48]); the total histidine concentration can be increased up to 3.3 mM by supplementing the reaction with non-radiolabeled histidine (isotopic dilution). In this way, it is possible to achieve saturating concentrations of histidine and perform kinetic calculations (i.e., K_M, k_{cat}, K_i, V_{max}) while saving radiolabeled substrate. We recommend working in a range of concentrations in between 0.021 and 3.3 mM of total histidine, for which the percentage of radiolabeled histidine must be properly adjusted.

3.1 Materials

- Ice-cold phosphate buffered saline (PBS).
- 2× reaction buffer stock solution: 200 mM potassium phosphate buffer pH 6.8, 0.4 mM DTT, 0.02 mM PLP, 20 mg/ml PEG-300).
- Ice-cold reaction buffer: 100 mM potassium phosphate buffer pH 6.8, 0.2 mM dithiothreitol (DTT), 0.01 mM pyridoxal-5′-phosphate (PLP), 10 mg/ml polyethylene glycol 300 (PEG-300) (*see* **Note 1**).
- Tip sonicator, such as the Branson Sonifier 250 equipped with a microtip probe.
- 42 μM L-[^{14}C(U)]-histidine (PerkinElmer; specific activity >300 mCi/mmol) dissolved in reaction buffer (*see* **Note 2**).
- 10 × 1.4 cm glass tube closed with an open-top screwcap equipped with a silicone rubber seal that allows piercing.
- 0.2 ml eppendorf tubes.
- 2 × 0.3 cm strips of Whatman 3MM paper.
- 1 M benzethonium hydroxide.
- Aluminum segment wires (8 cm).
- 5 % perchloric acid.
- 4 ml scintillation vials.
- Scintillation liquid for aqueous solutions (Ultima Gold™, PerkinElmer).
- Scintillation counter.

3.2 Methods

1. Cells are washed with ice-cold PBS and suspended in ice-cold reaction buffer (typically 4 × 10^6 cells in 200 μl) (*see* **Notes 3** and **4**).
2. Cells are homogenized by the application of ultrasonic waves with the use of the tip sonicator (*see* **Note 5**). Usually, the

homogenization is complete after applying only 5–6 pulses of 60 watts (in the Branson Sonifier 250 this is achieved by setting the "duty cycle" dial to 50 and the "output" dial to 2.5).

3. The reaction is started by mixing 40 μl of cell homogenate and 40 μl of 42 μM L-[^{14}C(U)]-histidine dissolved in reaction buffer (*see* **Notes 1** and **2**). The reaction is conducted in a water bath for 1 h at 37 °C in a 10 × 1.4 cm glass tube closed with an open-top screwcap equipped with a silicone rubber seal that allows piercing. To catch the CO_2 released during the reaction, a 0.2 ml eppendorf tube containing a 2 × 0.3 cm strip of Whatman 3MM paper previously soaked in 1 M benzethonium hydroxide is included in the reaction tube, hanging on one end of a piece of wire placed across the silicone rubber seal of the screwcap (*see* **Notes 6** and **7**). The arrangement of the reaction tube is shown in detail in Fig. 1. For each sample, the reaction is preferably conducted in duplicate, and a blank reaction (without cell lysate) must be included.
4. The reaction is stopped by the injection of 200 μl of 5 % perchloric acid into the reaction mixture followed by incubation for 30 min at 37 °C (*see* **Note 8**).
5. The strip of Whatman paper is carefully removed and transferred into a 4 ml scintillation vial containing 4 ml of scintillation liquid.
6. The radioactivity is counted in a scintillation counter.

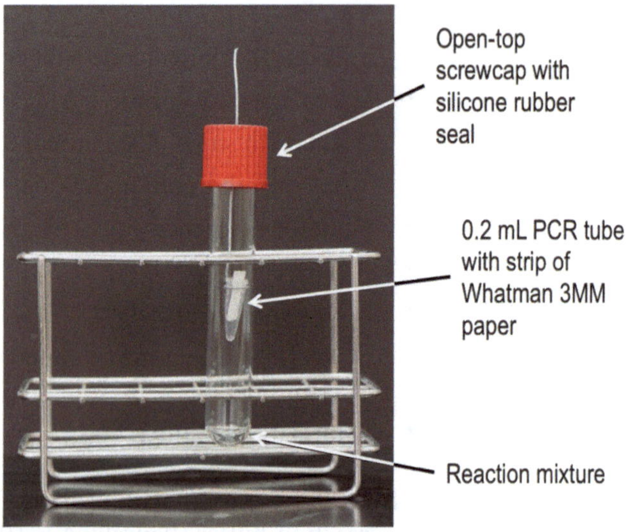

Fig. 1 Arrangement of the reaction tube for the determination of histidine decarboxylase enzymatic activity

7. Results are expressed as pmol of CO_2 released/h/10^6 cells or as pmol of CO_2 released/h/μg of total proteins in the extracts.

Notes

1. The reaction buffer must be prepared freshly. It is important to add the PLP from a freshly prepared solution, since this enzymatic cofactor is quite labile.
2. To prepare the 42 μM L-[^{14}C(U)]-histidine solution it is very convenient to mix one volume of the stock L-[^{14}C(U)]-histidine (usually at a concentration of 167 μM) with one volume of water and two volumes of 2× reaction buffer. The total volume depends on the number of reactions including the blank. It is recommended to prepare sufficient volume for one extra reaction.
3. Cells can be snap-frozen with liquid nitrogen as dry pellets and stored at −80 °C for several months without affecting the HDC enzymatic activity.
4. HDC is a very short-lived enzyme, with an estimated half-life 1–2 h [46, 64]. For this reason, it is extremely important to proceed with the reactions immediately after the preparation of the cell lysates. Everything needed must be prepared (all the buffers and solutions including the 42 μM L-[^{14}C(U)]-histidine solution, and also the reaction tubes provided with the 0.2 ml eppendorf tubes and the strips of Whatmann 3MM paper) prior to the preparation of cell lysates.
5. Homogenization of the cells must be performed keeping the tubes on ice to avoid excessive heat and foaming.
6. The strip of Whatman 3MM paper must be soaked in 1 M benzethonium hydroxide immediately before starting each reaction. It should not be soaked in advance to avoid saturation of benzethonium hydroxide with the CO_2 present in the environment.
7. It is recommended to bore 12–16 holes into the 0.2 ml eppendorf tube containing the strip of Whatman 3MM paper soaked in benzethonium hydroxide to facilitate CO_2 capture.
8. The injection of 5 % perchloric acid can be performed by using a 1 ml syringe fitted with a 23G × 1¼″ (0.6 × 30 mm) or longer needle. Great care must be taken to add the acid to the reaction mixture and not to the strip of Whatman 3MM paper.

4 qPCR of HDC and H_3R

HDC and HRs are expressed throughout the human body. Dependant on the tissue or cell type, we can detect large or small amounts of RNA. Thus appropriate methods must be chosen to quantify the RNA. Conventionally, semiquantitative end point PCR has been performed to detect HDC and HR, often supported by other techniques including western blot and immunocytochemistry. Nevertheless, qPCR represents a suitable approach that presents some advantages such as high sensitivity, high specificity, good reproducibility, and broad dynamic quantification range [65].

Here we describe a qPCR protocol for quantification of human HDC [40] and H_3R (unpublished results). These protocols were used on different cell lines including human mast cell line (HMC)-1, human neuroblastoma cells (Kelly) and human embryonic kidney (HEK)-293 cells.

4.1 RNA Extraction and Quantification

There are many methods of RNA extraction available, the most suitable one for the starting material should be chosen.

1. Cells from cell line cultures are washed with cold PBS, harvested and stored at −80 °C until RNA extraction.
2. Total RNA from the different cells tested is extracted using the RNeasy mini kit (Qiagen) or the GenElute mammalian total RNA miniprep kit (Sigma) according to manufacturer's instructions. All material must be sterilized to prevent possible contamination.
3. RNA is quantified and the quality tested by photometric measurement. RNA samples obtained have a concentration of 0.4–0.6 μg/μl. We only use highly purified RNA ($A_{260}/A_{280} > 1.95$) (*see* **Note 9**).

4.2 cDNA Synthesis

cDNA synthesis is performed using iScript select cDNA synthesis kit (Bio-Rad Laboratories), which contains a recombinant RNase H+ MMLV reverse transcriptase preblended with a recombinant RNase inhibitor. This cDNA synthesis kit allows the use of different strategies for first-strand cDNA priming (oligo(dT) primers only, random primers only, or user-designed gene-specific primers). We employ both random and gene-specific primers strategies (*see* **Note 10**).

1. For cDNA synthesis 1 μg of total RNA is used in a final volume of 20 μl containing (*see* **Note 11**):

Components	Random primers volume	Gene-specific primers volume
Nuclease-free water	Up to 20 μl	Up to 20 μl
5× iScript select reaction mix	4 μl	4 μl
Random primers	2 μl	–
Specific primers (2–20 pmol)		Variable

Components	Random primers volume	Gene-specific primers volume
Gene-specific primer enhancer solution	–	2 μl
RNA sample (1 μg total RNA)	Variable	Variable
iScript Reverse Transcriptase	1 μl	1 μl

2. Reverse transcription is performed by a first step at 25 °C for 5 min, followed by 30–60 min at 42 °C. Reverse transcriptase is heat-inactivated by incubation at 85 °C for 5 min. The first step of incubation (25 °C for 5 min) is omitted when gene-specific primers are used. The cDNA product can be stored at 4 °C for immediate use or at −20 °C for a few days.

4.3 qPCR

Two commercial premixes are used for qPCR amplification, 1× Sybr green supermix (Bio-Rad) used in iCycler iQ optical system (Bio-Rad) and KAPA SYBR fast master mix (2×) universal (KAPA Biosystems) in a Eco™ real-time PCR System (Illumina). Similar results are obtained using both premixes and equipment. qPCR is carried out in a final volume of 20 μl, containing 200 nM of both primers, 1× premix and variable amounts of RT products. Standard curves are prepared by serial dilution of cDNA products. The final range of cDNA used is equivalent to between 400 and 0.4 ng of total RNA. Table 4 shows the primers used for amplification of HDC, H_3R, and glyceraldehyde 3-phosphate dehydrogenase (GAPDH). A 3-step cycling protocol is used:

Step	Temperature	Duration	Cycles
Amplification			
Enzyme activation	95 °C	5 min	Hold
Denaturation Annealing Extension/data acquisition	95 °C Variable[a] 72 °C	5 s 20 s 20 s	30–40
Denaturation (dissociation curve)	95 °C	15 s	Hold
Annealing/dissociation/data acquisition	65 °C	15 s	Increase up to 95 °C

[a] *See* Table 4 for annealing temperature for each gene

Table 4
List of primers used for histidine decarboxylase (HDC), histamine receptor type 3 (H_3R), and glyceraldehyde 3-phosphate dehydrogenase (GAPDH) amplifications

Gene	Accession no	Primer sequence	Annealing temperature (°C)	Amplicon size (bp)
HDC	NM_002112.3	F: GCCCAAGGGAGATGATGGAG R: GGCTGGATGCCCAGGTGAAT	58	339
H_3R	NM_007232.2	F: CCTCCGCACCCAGAACAACTT R: AGCCGTGATGAGGAAGTACCA	55	415
GADPH	BC004109.2	F: TGCACCACCAACTGCTTAGC R: GGCTGGACTGTGGTCATGAG	67.5	88

Notes

9. An important point is to verify the absence of genomic DNA contamination. RNA samples are treated with DNase using On-column DNase I Digestion Set (Sigma-Aldrich) following the manufacturer's recommendations.
10. Primers are designed in silico taking the following into consideration: (a) length between 16 and 28 residues; (b) GC content is 35–65 %; and (c) primer must not contain the same nucleotide in six or more contiguous positions.
11. cDNA synthesis can be performed using either random primers or gene-specific primers. Amplification efficiencies are similar but the crossing point (C_q) values are smaller when gene-specific primers are used (Fig. 2).

5 Concluding Remarks

The methods reported here will be of value to various projects and objectives. HDC expression quantification is useful for the evaluation of the many pathophysiological scenarios. For example, characterization of the relationship between overexpression of HDC in the brain and the increased expression of alpha-synuclein was recently reported using a non-neuronal transfected model [66].

The evaluation of H_3R expression is not only of interest in the many neurological pathologies described above but also for studies on biomedical problems involving histamine signaling elicited by

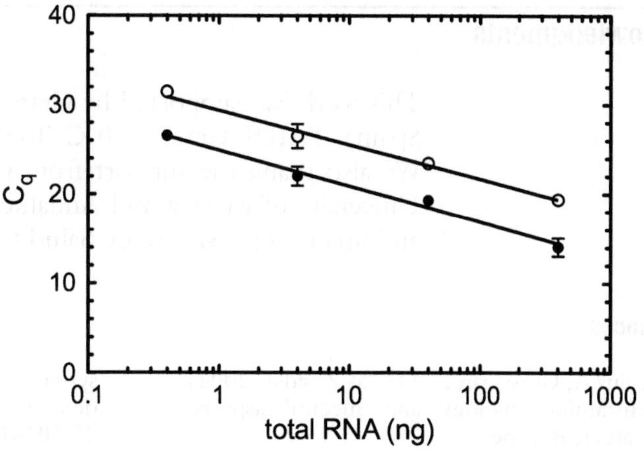

Fig. 2 Standard curve of dilution series of cDNA samples synthetized with gene-specific primers for histamine receptor 3 (*closed circles*) or random primer (*open circles*). The obtained crossing point (*Cp*) values are represented versus the total RNA quantity used for amplifications

peripheral H_3R expressing cells/tissues, e.g., paediatric neuroblastoma cells. A relationship between H_3R and breast cancer cell proliferation has been previously reported and it would be interesting to check the role of this receptor in the neuroblastoma model as it is the most common paediatric malignancy [67].

The present work provides methods for the validation and estimation of alterations in the expression of these two histamine-related macromolecules. The present protocols also allow insights into the occurrence of genotypic and spliced variants taking account of those previously reported. In the case of human HDC, the lack of activity and/or mRNA amplification can suggest either the truncation or the copy number lost associated with human diseases/phenotypes indicated in Table 3. The qPCR method for H_3R quantification, together with the analysis of melting curves of the PCR products, could indicate events of gene amplification or the expression of alternative spliced isoforms (Table 3) [56]. In fact, splicing variants modified in length within the fragment encoding the first 202 amino acids should render different amplification products. For instance, a 42 nucleotides-shorter PCR should be expected after amplification and size analysis of the splicing variant 4 (Uniprot code Q9Y5N1-4).

We expect that the protocols described here will be useful for research groups working on histamine-related diseases, especially those emergent and rare neurological, neuroendocrine, neuroinflammatory diseases, and neoplasias for which a relevant role of both histamine metabolism-related elements (HDC and H_3R) is proposed and/or proven.

Acknowledgments

This work was supported by Grants SAF2011-26518 (MINECO, Spain), PAIDI Grant P10-CVI6585 (Andalusian Government). We also thank the support from CIBERER, as well as from the University of Málaga and Andalucia-Tech facilities. CIBERER is an initiative of Instituto de Salud Carlos III.

References

1. Falus A, Grossman N, Darvas Z (eds) (2004) Histamine: biology and medical aspects. Karger, Budapest
2. Stark H (ed) (2013) Histamine H_4 receptor: a novel drug target for immunoregulation and inflammation. Versita, Berlin
3. Theoharides TC, Valent P, Akin C (2015) Mast cells, mastocytosis, and related disorders. New Engl J Med 373:163–172
4. Landolina N, Gangwar RS, Levi-Schaffer F (2015) Mast cells' integrated actions with eosinophils and fibroblasts in allergic inflammation: implications for therapy. Adv Immunol 125:41–85
5. Gilfillan AM, Austin SJ, Metcalfe DD (2011) Mast cell biology: introduction and overview. Adv Exp Med Biol 716:2–12
6. Valent P, Akin P, Arock M et al (2012) Definitions, criteria and global classification of mast cell disorders with special reference to mast cell activation syndromes: a consensus proposal. Int Arch Allergy Immunol 157:215–225
7. Ringvall M, Rönnberg E, Wernersson S et al (2008) Serotonin and histamine storage in mast cell secretory granules is dependent on serglycin proteoglycan. J Allergy Clin Immunol 121:1020–1026
8. García-Faroldi G, Rodríguez CE, Urdiales JL et al (2010) Polyamines are present in mast cell secretory granules and are important for granule homeostasis. PloS One 5:e15071
9. Schneider E, Rolli-Derkinderen M, Arock M et al (2002) Trends in histamine research: new functions during immune responses and hematopoiesis. Trends Immunol 23:255–263
10. Alcañiz L, Vega A, Chacón P et al (2013) Histamine production by human neutrophils. FASEB J 27:2902–2910
11. Haas H, Panula P (2003) The role of histamine and the tuberomamillary nucleus in the nervous system. Nat Rev Neurosci 4:121–130
12. Schneider EH, Neumann D, Seifert R (2014) Modulation of behavior by the histaminergic system: lessons from HDC-, H3R- and H4R-deficient mice. Neurosci Biobehav Rev 47:101–121
13. Rocha SM, Pires J, Esteves M et al (2014) Histamine: a new immunomodulatory player in the neuron-glia crosstalk. Front Cell Neurosci 8:120
14. Zhao CM, Chen D (2012) The ECL cell: relay station for gastric integrity. Curr Med Chem 19:98–108
15. Buhner S, Schemann (2012) Mast cell-nerve axis with a focus on the human gut. Biochim Biophys Acta 1822:85–92
16. Thurmond RL, Gelfand EW, Dunford PJ (2008) The role of histamine H_1 and H_4 receptors in allergic inflammation: the search for new antihistamines. Nat Rev Drug Discov 7:41–53
17. Panula P, Chazot PL, Cowart M et al (2015) International union of basic and clinical pharmacology. XCVIII. Histamine receptors. Pharmacol Rev 67:601–655
18. Burban A, Faucard R, Armand V et al (2010) Histamine potentiates N-methyl-D-aspartate receptors by interacting with an allosteric site distinct from the polyamine binding site. J Pharmacol Exp Ther 332:912–921
19. Leurs R, Chazot PL, Shenton FC et al (2009) Molecular and biochemical pharmacology of the histamine H4 receptor. Br J Pharmacol 157:14–23
20. Zampeli E, Tiligada E (2009) The role of histamine H^4 receptor in immune and inflammatory disorders. Br J Pharmacol 157:24–33
21. Panula P, Nuutinen S (2011) Histamine and H_3 receptor in alcohol-related behaviors. J Pharmacol Exp Ther 336:9–16
22. Passani MB, Blandina P (2011) Histamine receptors in the CNS as targets for therapeutic intervention. Trends Pharmacol Sci 32:242–249
23. Tiligada E, Kyriakidis K, Chazot PL et al (2011) Histamine pharmacology and new CNS drug targets. CNS Neurosci Ther 17:620–628

24. Chazot PL (2013) Histamine pharmacology: four years on. Br J Pharmacol 170:1–3
25. Provensi G, Blandina P, Passani MB (2016) The histaminergic system as a target for the prevention of obesity and metabolic syndrome. Neuropharmacology 106:3–12
26. Thurmond RL (2015) The histamine H_4 receptor: from orphan to the clinic. Front Pharmacol 6:65
27. Chazot P, Hill SJ, Fukui H et al (2015) Histamine receptors. In: IUPHAR/BPS guide to pharmacology. http://www.guidetopharmacology.org/GRAC/FamilyDisplayForward?familyId=33. Accessed 15 Aug 2016
28. Swan C, Richards SA, Duroudier NP et al (2006) Alternative promoter use and splice variation in the human histamine H_1 receptor gene. Am J Respir Cell Mol Biol 35:118–126
29. Bongers G, Bakker RA, Leurs R (2007) Molecular aspects of the histamine H_3 receptor. Biochem Pharmacol 73:1195–1204
30. Wifling D, Bernhardt G, Dove S et al (2015) The extracellular loop 2 (ECL2) of the human histamine H_4 receptor substantially contributes to ligand binding and constitutive activity. PloS One. 10:e0117185
31. Ferrada C, Ferré S, Casadó V et al (2008) Interactions between histamine H_3 and dopamine D_2 receptors and the implications for striatal function. Neuropharmacology 55:190–197
32. Moreno E, Hoffmann H, Gonzalez-Sepúlveda M et al (2011) Dopamine D_1-histamine H_3 receptor heteromers provide a selective link to MAPK signaling in GABAergic neurons of the direct striatal pathway. J Biol Chem 286:5846–5854
33. Flik G, Folgering JHA, Cremers TI et al (2015) Interaction between brain histamine and serotonin, norepinephrine, and dopamine systems: in vivo microdialysis and electrophysiology study. J Mol Neurosci 56:320–328
34. Hur J, Schuyler AD, States DJ et al (2009) SciMiner: web-based literature mining tool for target identification and functional enrichment analysis. Bioinformatics 25:838–840
35. Pino-Ángeles A, Reyes-Palomares A, Melgarejo E et al (2012) Histamine: an undercover agent in multiple rare diseases? J Cell Mol Med 16:1947–1960
36. Pletscher-Frankild S, Pallejà A, Tsafou K et al (2014) DISEASES: text mining and data integration of disease-gene associations. Methods 74:83–89
37. Piñero J, Queralt-Rosinach N, Bravo A et al (2015) DisGeNET: a discovery platform for the dynamical exploration of human diseases and their genes. Database (Oxford) bav028
38. Moya-Garcia AA, Medina MA, Sanchez-Jimenez F (2005) Mammalian histidine decarboxylase: from structure to function. Bioessays 27:57–63
39. Fajardo I, Urdiales JL, Paz JC et al (2001) Histamine prevents polyamine accumulation in mouse C57.1 mast cell cultures. Eur J Biochem 268:768–773
40. Melgarejo E, Medina MA, Paz JC et al (2006) Real-time RT-PCR analysis of human histidine decarboxylase, a new marker for several types of leukemia and cancer. Oncol Rep 15:193–197
41. Chaves P, Correa-Fiz F, Melgarejo E et al (2007) Development of an expression macroarray for amine metabolism-related genes. Amino Acids 33:315–322
42. Abrighach H, Fajardo I, Sánchez-Jiménez F et al (2010) Exploring polyamine regulation by nascent histamine in a human-transfected cell model. Amino acids 38:561–573
43. Rodríguez-Caso C, Rodríguez-Agudo D, Moya-García AA et al (2003) Local changes in the catalytic site of mammalian histidine decarboxylase can affect its global conformation and stability. Eur J Biochem 270:4376–4387
44. Komori H, Nitta Y, Ueno H et al (2012) Structural study reveals that Ser-354 determines substrate specificity on human histidine decarboxylase. J Biol Chem 287:29175–29183
45. Tanaka S, Nemoto K, Yamamura E et al (1997) Degradation of the 74 kDa form of L-histidine decarboxylase via the ubiquitin-proteasome pathway in a rat basophilic/mast cell line (RBL-2H3). FEBS Lett 417:203–207
46. Dartsch C, Chen D, Håkanson R et al (1999) Histidine decarboxylase in rat stomach ECL cells: relationship between enzyme activity and different molecular forms. Regul Pept 81:41–48
47. Fleming JV, Fajardo I, Langlois MR et al (2004) The C-terminus of rat L-histidine decarboxylase specifically inhibits enzymic activity and disrupts pyridoxal phosphate-dependent interactions with L-histidine substrate analogues. Biochem J 381:769–778
48. Olmo MT, Sanchez-Jimenez F, Medina MA et al (2002) Spectroscopic analysis of recombinant rat histidine decarboxylase. J Biochem 132:433–439
49. Moya-Garcia AA, Ruiz-Pernia J, Marti S et al (2008) Analysis of the decarboxylation step in mammalian histidine decarboxylase. A computational study. J Biol Chem 283:12393–12401

50. Pino-Angeles A, Morreale A, Negri A et al (2010) Substrate uptake and protein stability relationship in mammalian histidine decarboxylase. Proteins 78:154–161
51. Fleming JV, Sánchez-Jiménez F, Moya-García AA et al (2004) Mapping of catalytically important residues in the rat L-histidine decarboxylase enzyme using bioinformatic and site-directed mutagenesis approaches. Biochem J 379:253–261
52. Moya-García AA, Rodríguez-Agudo D, Hayashi H et al (2011) Analysis of mammalian histidine decarboxylase dimerization interface reveals an electrostatic hotspot important for catalytic site topology and function. J Chem Theory Comput 7:1935–1942
53. Arrang JM, Garbarg M, Schwartz JC (1983) Auto-inhibition of brain histamine release mediated by a novel class (H3) of histamine receptor. Nature 302:832–837
54. Lovenberg TW, Pyati J, Chang H et al (2000) Cloning of rat histamine H_3 receptor reveals distinct species pharmacological profiles. J Pharmacol Exp Ther 293:771–778
55. Leurs R, Bakker RA, Timmerman H et al (2005) The histamine H_3 receptor: from gene cloning to H3 receptor drugs. Nat Rev Drug Discov 4:107–120
56. Wellendorph P, Goodman MW, Burstein ES et al (2002) Molecular cloning and pharmacology of functionally distinct isoforms of the human histamine H_3 receptor. Neuropharmacology 42:929–940
57. Bakker RA (2004) Histamine H_3-receptor isoforms. Inflamm Res 53:509–516
58. Cogé F, Guénin SP, Audinot V et al (2001) Genomic organization and characterization of splice variants of the human histamine H_3 receptor. Biochem J 355:279–288
59. Lepailleur A, Freret T, Lemaître S et al (2014) Dual histamine H3R/serotonin 5-HT4R ligands with antiamnesic properties: pharmacophore-based virtual screening and polypharmacology. J Chem Inf Model 54:1773–1784
60. Schultes S, Kooistra AJ, Vischer HF et al (2015) Combinatorial consensus scoring for ligand-based virtual fragment screening: a comparative case study for serotonin 5-HT_3A, histamine H_1, and histamine H_4 receptors. J Chem Inf Model 55:1030–1044
61. Fajardo I, Urdiales JL, Medina MA et al (2001) Effects of phorbol ester and dexamethasone treatment on histidine decarboxylase and ornithine decarboxylase in basophilic cells. Biochem Pharmacol 61:1101–1106
62. Melgarejo E, Medina MA, Sanchez-Jimenez F et al (2007) (−)-Epigallocatechin-3-gallate interferes with mast cell adhesiveness, migration and its potential to recruit monocytes. Cell Mol Life Sci 64:2690–2701
63. Correa-Fiz F, Reyes-Palomares A, Fajardo I et al (2012) Regulatory cross-talk of mouse liver polyamine and methionine metabolic pathways: a systemic approach to its physiopathological consequences. Amino Acids 42:577–595
64. Fleming JV, Wang TC (2000) Amino- and carboxy-terminal PEST domains mediate gastrin stabilization of rat L-histidine decarboxylase isoforms. Mol Cell Biol 20:4932–4947
65. Bustin SA (2000) Absolute quantification of mRNA using real-time reverse transcription polymerase chain reaction assays. J Mol Endocrinol 25:169–193
66. Caro-Astorga J, Fajardo I, Ruiz-Pérez MV et al (2014) Nascent histamine induces α-synuclein and caspase-3 on human cells. Biochem Biophys Res Commun 451:580–586
67. Ruiz-Pérez MV, Medina MA, Urdiales JL et al (2015) Polyamine metabolism is sensitive to glycolysis inhibition in human neuroblastoma cells. J Biol Chem 290:6106–6119
68. Gervasini G, Agúndez JAG, García-Menaya J et al (2010) Variability of the L-histidine decarboxylase gene in allergic rhinitis. Allergy. 65:1576–1584
69. Ohtsu H (2008) Progress in allergy signal research on mast cells: the role of histamine in immunological and cardiovascular disease and the transporting system of histamine in the cell. J Pharmacol Sci 106:347–353
70. Gutowska-Owsiak D, Greenwald L, Watson C et al (2014) The histamine-synthesizing enzyme histidine decarboxylase is upregulated by keratinocytes in atopic skin. Br J Dermatol 171:771–778
71. Krauth MT, Agis H, Aichberger KJ et al (2006) Immunohistochemical detection of histidine decarboxylase in neoplastic mast cells in patients with systemic mastocytosis. Hum Pathol 37:439–447
72. Bastianini S, Silvani A, Berteotti C et al (2015) Histamine transmission modulates the phenotype of murine narcolepsy caused by orexin neuron deficiency. PloS One 10:e0140520
73. Castellan-Baldan L, Williams KA, Gallezot JD et al (2014) Histidine decarboxylase deficiency causes Tourette syndrome: parallel findings in humans and mice. Neuron 81:77–90
74. Dinh QT, Cryer A, Dinh S et al (2005) Transcriptional up-regulation of histamine receptor-1 in epithelial, mucus and inflammatory cells in perennial allergic rhinitis. Clin Exp Allergy 35:1443–1448

75. Ohsawa Y, Hirasawa N (2014) The role of histamine H_1 and H_4 receptors in atopic dermatitis: from basic research to clinical study. Allergol Int 63:533–542
76. Raithel M, Nägel A, Zopf Y et al (2010) Plasma histamine levels (H) during adjunctive H1-receptor antagonist treatment with loratadine in patients with active inflammatory bowel disease (IBD). Inflamm Res 59(S2):S257–S258
77. Lipnik-Stangelj M (2006) Multiple role of histamine H_1-receptor-PKC-MAPK signalling pathway in histamine-stimulated nerve growth factor synthesis and secretion. Biochem Pharmacol 72:1375–1381
78. Carson S, Lee N, Thakurta S (2010) Drug class review: newer antihistamines: final report update 2. In: Drug class review. Oregon Health & Science University. http://www.ncbi.nlm.nih.gov/books. Accessed 15 Mar 2016
79. Rada B, Boudreau HE, Park JJ et al (2014) Histamine stimulates hydrogen peroxide production by bronchial epithelial cells via histamine H_1 receptor and dual oxidase. Am J Respir Cell Mol Biol 50:125–134
80. Beghdadi W, Porcherie A, Schneider BS et al (2008) Inhibition of histamine-mediated signaling confers significant protection against severe malaria in mouse models of disease. J Exp Med 205:395–408
81. Costanza M, Di Dario M, Steinman L et al (2014) Gene expression analysis of histamine receptors in peripheral blood mononuclear cells from individuals with clinically-isolated syndrome and different stages of multiple sclerosis. J Neuroimmunol 277:186–188
82. Pochampally RR, Ylostalo J, Penfornis P et al (2007) Histamine receptor H_1 and dermatopontin: new downstream targets of the vitamin D receptor. J Bone Miner Res 22:1338–1349
83. Leurs R, Church MK, Taglialatela M (2002) H_1-antihistamines: inverse agonism, anti-inflammatory actions and cardiac effects. Clin Exp Allergy 32:489–498
84. Matsuki M, Sato N, Matsuda K et al (2009) Brugada syndrome whose ST-segment changes were enhanced by antihistamines and antiallergenic drugs. Intern Med 48:1009–1113
85. Ciebiada M, Kasztalska K, Gorska-Ciebiada M et al (2014) Histamine type 2 receptor expression on peripheral blood regulatory lymphocytes in patients with allergic rhinitis treated with specific immunotherapy. Am J Rhinol Allergy 28:e130–e135
86. Xia T, Wang QR, Xu YH (2001) Cimetidine inhibits production of interferon gamma and tumor necrosis factor alpha by splenocytes in aplastic anemic mice. Acta Pharmacol Sin 22:239–242
87. Baird DC, Harker DJ, Karmes AS (2015) Diagnosis and treatment of gastroesophageal reflux in infants and children. Am Fam Physician 92:705–714
88. Lindsley CB, Miner PB (1991) Seronegative juvenile rheumatoid arthritis and mast cell-associated gastritis. Arthritis Rheum 34:106–109
89. Meskanen K, Ekelund H, Laitinen J et al (2013) A randomized clinical trial of histamine 2 receptor antagonism in treatment-resistant schizophrenia. J Clin Psychopharmacol 33:472–478
90. Wilcox CM, Hirschowitz BI (2009) Treatment strategies for Zollinger-Ellison syndrome. Expert Opin Pharmacother 10:1145–1157
91. Shan L, Bao AM, Swaab DF (2015) The human histaminergic system in neuropsychiatric disorders. Trends Neurosci 38:167–177
92. Vohora D, Bhowmik M (2012) Histamine H_3 receptor antagonists/inverse agonists on cognitive and motor processes: relevance to Alzheimer's disease, ADHD, schizophrenia, and drug abuse. Front Syst Neurosci 6:72
93. Zoethout RWM, Iannone R, Bloem BR et al (2012) The effects of a novel histamine-3 receptor inverse agonist on essential tremor in comparison to stable levels of alcohol. J Psychopharmacol 26:292–302
94. Rapanelli M, Pittenger C (2015) Histamine and histamine receptors in Tourette syndrome and other neuropsychiatric conditions. Neuropharmacology 106:85–90
95. Alstadhaug KB (2014) Histamine in migraine and brain. Headache 54:246–259
96. Auberson YP, Troxler T, Zhang X et al (2015) From ergolines to indoles: improved inhibitors of the human H_3 receptor for the treatment of narcolepsy. Chem Med Chem 10:266–275
97. Salcedo C, Pontes C, Merlos M (2013) Is the H_4 receptor a new drug target for allergies and asthma? Front Biosci 5:178–187
98. Martinel Lamas DJ, Rivera ES, Medina VA (2015) Histamine H_4 receptor: insights into a potential therapeutic target in breast cancer. Front Biosci 7:1–9
99. Shan L, Liu CQ, Balesar R et al (2012) Neuronal histamine production remains unaltered in Parkinson's disease despite the accumulation of Lewy bodies and Lewy neurites in the tuberomamillary nucleus. Neurobiol Aging 33:1343–1344

100. Fogel WA, Wagner W, Sasiak K et al (2005) The role of histamine in experimental ulcerative colitis in rats. Inflamm Res 54(S1):S68–S69
101. ClinVar Database (2014) National Center for Biotecnology Information, USA. http://www.ncbi.nlm.nih.gov/clinvar. Accessed 2 Dec 2015
102. dbVar Database (2010) National Center for Biotecnology Information, USA. http://www.ncbi.nlm.nih.gov/dbvar/. Accessed 2 Dec 2015

Chapter 14

Cerebrospinal Fluid Markers in Neuroinflammation: The Paradigm of Optic Neuritis

Dimitrios P. Besinis and Maria C. Anagnostouli

Abstract

The central nervous system (CNS) is a complex organ that is isolated from the periphery due to the existence of the blood-brain barrier (BBB). Recently, a large number of biomarkers have been identified, whose presence in the cerebrospinal fluid (CSF) identifies a certain pathology. There are many different types of biomarkers reflecting alterations of the immune system, of BBB disruption, of demyelination, of oxidative stress and excitotoxicity, of axonal/neuronal damage, of gliosis, of remyelination and repair, etc. Neuroinflammation is the specific adaptive response of brain tissue to mechanical damage, hypoxia, and metabolic stress. Optic neuritis, which is the inflammation of the optic nerve, is a specific neuroinflammatory condition that is strongly related to multiple sclerosis (MS) and neuromyelitis optica (NMO). Scientific evidence derived from the experimental model of autoimmune encephalitis (EAE) points out the importance of histamine in the modulation of inflammatory responses in the brain. Related to clinical findings, histamine levels are high in the CSF of patients with MS. Optic neuritis, the inflammation of the optic nerve, is characterized by simultaneous activation of both inflammatory and anti-inflammatory processes. Histamine's effect in the brain is known to be strongly related to receptor activation. In this chapter, we propose a protocol for studying neuroinflammation and identifying an inflammatory profile in patients with optic neuritis, emphasizing mainly in the putative role of histamine in the modulation of demyelinating procedures.

Key words Cerebrospinal fluid (CSF), Histamine, Multiple sclerosis, Neuroinflammation, Optic neuritis

1 Overview of Biomarkers in Central Nervous System Inflammation

The central nervous system (CNS) including the brain and the spinal cord is an extremely complex human organ system, in terms of both structure and function. It is separated from blood circulation via the blood-brain barrier (BBB), which in normal conditions does not allow peripheral immune cells such as T and B cells to penetrate into CNS and have harmful effects. Recently, there has been broad recognition that biomarkers can play a critical role in diagnosis, prognosis, disease monitoring and response to

Ekaterini Tiligada and Madeleine Ennis (eds.), *Histamine Receptors as Drug Targets*, Methods in Pharmacology and Toxicology, DOI 10.1007/978-1-4939-6843-5_14,

treatment, thus enabling the development of personalized therapeutics [1, 2].

Optic neuritis (ON) is the inflammation of the optic nerve which is a clinical component of well-characterized demyelinating diseases like multiple sclerosis (MS) and neuromyelitis optica (NMO) and newly emerged demyelinating disorders, with anti-myelin oligodendrocyte glycoprotein (MOG) positive blood antibodies, which consist of overlapping syndromes in acute disseminated encephalomyelitis (ADEM) and/or NMO spectrum disorders (NMOSD), mainly of young people [3]. A plethora of biomarkers for MS and sequently ON have been discovered giving a tremendous tool towards translational medicine, for clinicians and laboratory researchers. Genomics, epigenomics, neuroproteomics, microarray assessment, magnetic resonance imaging (MRI), evoked potentials, etc., now serve as biomarkers in MS and ON. There are many types of biomarkers: biomarkers reflecting alteration of the immune system, of BBB disruption, of demyelination, of oxidative stress and excitotoxicity, of axonal/neuronal damage, of gliosis, of remyelination and repair, etc. [1, 2].

In this chapter, we describe mainly the neuroinflammatory biomarkers in MS and ON and focus on histamine determination, which plays a key role in both conditions. We present a protocol to approach and study histamine in ON in the well-characterized demyelinating disorders, such as MS and NMO.

2 Neuroinflammation: The Role of Biomarkers and Blood-Brain Barrier

Inflammation in general, as well as inflammation of the optic nerve, has long been considered the body's response to a hostile condition, as an attempt to remove it and begin healing itself to return to the normal state. The word itself comes from the Latin word "*inflammo*" which means "I set alright, I ignite." It can be separated into acute and chronic depending on the onset and the severity of the symptoms.

Inflammation is also considered a specialized immune response of the organism to an invading pathogen, traumatic event, or injurious agent (foreign or self). It involves innate and adaptive immune responses. The innate immune response involves many cells including macrophages, natural killer cells, as well as biochemical processes such as the complement system and cytokines or chemokines. The adaptive immune response involves T and B lymphocytes and antibodies [4].

Neuroinflammation is an adaptive response of brain tissue to mechanical damage, hypoxia, and metabolic stress. Inflammatory processes have been implicated in most acute, autoimmune, neurodegenerative but also some psychiatric disorders. Thus, neuroinflammation plays a crucial role in the development and progression of many of these diseases. Neuroinflammation is a reactive adjustment to damage or to homeostatic disturbances and may initiate repair in the CNS. However, if unregulated, this protective reaction may cause brain damage [5, 6].

It is becoming increasingly evident that glia and in particular microglia and astrocytes are central in mediating the effects of neuroinflammation. Microglial, mesoderm-derived brain macrophages make up the innate immune system of the brain and are key cellular mediators of neuroinflammatory processes. Activated microglia cells and their products are the key mediators of the neuroinflammatory process and may contribute to neuronal damage [7, 8]. Activated microglia cells express major histocompatibility complex (MHC) II antigens (HLA-DR) on their surface, and mediate the neuroinflammatory processes. MHC can be used as a biomolecular marker for activated microglia [9, 10]. Microglia were characterized and named by Rio-Hortega (1882–1945) but the role of activated microglia in the brain of Alzheimer's disease (AD) patients was described in the mid-to late 1980s, when activated microglia were discovered. The term neuroinflammation has come to denote chronic, CNS-specific, inflammation-like glial responses that do not reproduce the classical characteristics of inflammation in the periphery but that may engender neurodegenerative events, including plaque formation, dystrophic neurite growth, and excessive tau phosphorylation. In this way, neuroinflammation has been implicated in chronic unremitting neurodegenerative diseases such as AD and MS [11]. The recognition of microglia as the brain's intrinsic immune system, and the understanding that chronic activation of this system leads to pathological sequelae, has led to the modern concept of neuroinflammation. This new understanding has come from rapid advances in the field of microglial and astrocytic neurobiology over the past 20 years [12].

Microglia can be rapidly activated during systemic infection without the integrity of BBB being compromised. Thus, neuroinflammation has beneficial or detrimental effects. It depends on the duration of the inflammatory response. Neurodegenerative disorders in the CNS are associated with chronic neuroinflammation. Infections, trauma, stroke, toxins, and other stimuli are capable of producing an immediate and short lived activation of the innate immune system in the CNS [12]. Thus, although outside the scope of this article, we should mention the multiple actions of microglia, which constitute 10–15 % of all brain cells. Microglia is involved in neuroinflammation, in neurodegeneration, in viral and bacterial infection, and in aging [13]. Microglia activate the pro-inflammatory cytokines interferon (IFN)-γ, interleukin (IL)-1α, IL-1β and tumor necrosis factor (TNF)-α in the CNS. Microglial cells are also sources of some chemokines and express the monocyte chemoattractant protein (MCP)-1 in particular. Other inflammatory cytokines such as IL-1β and TNF-α, as well as bacterial-derived lipopolysaccharide (LPS), may stimulate microglia to produce MCP-1, macrophage inflammatory protein (MIP)-1α, and MIP-1β. Microglia can express CCR3, CCR5, and CXCL8, CXCR4, and CX3CR1 *in vitro*. Chemokines are pro-inflammatory and therefore contribute to the neuroinflammation process [14].

Acute inflammatory responses involve the activation of the resident innate immune system (microglia), which release anti-inflammatory or pro-inflammatory mediators. An acute insult is typically short-lived and not detrimental to long-term neuronal survival. An acute neuroinflammatory response is typically beneficial to the CNS. Chronic neuroinflammation is a long-standing and often self-perpetuating neuroinflammatory response that persists long after the initial injury or insult. The sustained release of inflammatory mediators perpetuates the inflammatory cycle activating additional microglia and promoting proliferation and further release of inflammatory factors (pro-inflammatory). Chronic neuroinflammation is usually detrimental to the nervous system.

The brain and spinal cord, which make up the CNS, are not usually accessed directly by pathogenic factors in the body's circulation due to a series of endothelial cells known as the BBB. Other resident glial cells, such as astrocytes, or other infiltrated cells, such T or B lymphocytes, are involved in the inflammatory response at later stages.

Studies of neuroinflammatory regulatory mechanisms and their neuroprotective properties in greater detail are vital for the design of therapeutic targets for brain disorders [5]. Under clinical conditions, neuroinflammatory blood or CSF biomarkers are expected to give data on neurochemical mechanisms of brain inflammation. Inflammatory mechanisms appear to be universal; hence, neuroinflammation biomarkers can be studied in any acute or chronic brain disease related to neuroinflammation [5]. Such biomarkers are the pro-inflammatory cytokines, such as TNF-α or IL-1b. Cytokines are known to be the major regulators of neuroinflammation, so their CSF and blood levels can reflect many characteristics of this process. Glutamate excitotoxicity, which activates microglia, appears to be one of the primary pathways that initiate neuroinflammation. In turn, uncontrolled neuroinflammation may result in glutamate excitotoxicity. Glutamate released by oxygen or glucose-deprived neurons was shown to interact with type II glutamate metabotropic receptors (mGluR II) and thus activate nuclear factor (NF)κB in microglial cells. NFκB is a well-known transcription factor responsible for the expression of pro-inflammatory genes [15].

In neuroinflammation, the role of proteases appears to be of special importance. Matrix metalloproteinases (MMP) are a family of secreted neutral proteases and regulate extracellular matrix structure, growth factors availability, and signaling systems at the cell surface. Both constitutive and stress inducible MMPs are expressed in the brain. During neuroinflammation, MMPs play a crucial role in tissue remodeling and repair [16].

One of the ways to assay photeolytic enzyme activity in neuroinflammation is the determination of proteolysis products of brain-specific proteins in blood and CSF. Products of brain-specific proteins in blood and cerebrospinal fluid, such as cleaved Tau and spectrin breakdown products, are of great importance in the neuroinflammation process, reflecting mainly axonal/neuronal damage [17]. Oxidative stress biomarkers, like nitric oxide, nitrotyrosine, 8-isoprostane, and melatonin, are also important in neuroinflammation. Melatonin concentrations greatly increase in CSF but not in blood samples and correlate with glutamate and pyruvate concentration. Melatonin is one of the most multifunctional regulators in the organism. It plays a key role in the control of nerve, endocrine, and immune systems, like the reactions toward autoantigens. In this respect, the subset of T lymphocytes producing IL-17 (Th17) is of special interest, as the Th17 subset plays a key role in neuroinflammation and MS pathogenesis [18]. It is well known that glucocorticoids are one of the major hormones controlling inflammation. Pro-inflammatory cytokines, such as IL-1b and IL-6, strongly induce hypothalamus-pituitary-adrenal axis activation suggesting the presence of negative feedback in the control of inflammation [19]. Adhesion molecules actively regulate BBB permeability and inflammatory cell infiltration. Serum intercellular adhesion molecule (ICAM)-1 and vascular cell adhesion molecule (VCAM) concentrations were shown to predict neurological outcome in stroke. CSF ICAM-1 levels correlate with BBB permeability, lesion volume, and unfavorable outcome in patients with neuroinflammation and MS [5].

On the other hand, concerning MS, increasing evidence shows that many biomarkers, such as semaphorin 7A and ala-β-hisdipeptidase, are associated with the conversion from clinically isolated syndrome (CIS) to clinically definite MS (CDMS) and play a prognostic role. Recently, there are studies regarding semaphoring as a biomarker predicting responsiveness to IFN-β and as a factor for treatment strategy to promote remyelination in all MS-subtypes [20, 21].

Additionally, new data show that natural killer (NK) cell subsets do not increase uniformly in all inflammatory neurological diseases and suggest strongly that regulatory CD56 bright and NK T cells may arise in CSF of MS patients as an attempt to counteract the CNS immune activation characteristic of the disease [4]. An overview, regarding key neuroinflammatory biomarkers in MS, is given extensively in a recent review [2].

The main characteristic of the CNS is its isolation from the periphery through the BBB and the blood neural barrier (BNB) which prevent peripheral inflammatory cells and mediators circulating in the blood to enter the brain [22]. Thus, the CNS has become a very interesting site for studying inflammation. The first study to discover the importance of brain tissue isolation from blood was done by Ehrlich in 1885 with a very simple experiment [23, 24]. He injected a vital dye into the blood circulation of rats and found that brain tissue remained intact. In contrast, if the dye was injected in the ventricular system the brain was stained. Cerebral blood vessels are responsible for the formation of the BBB on the one side. Epithelial cells (ECs) of brain vessels are very close to each other forming tight junctions. In this way, a non-permeable barrier is formed that restricts the passive passage of blood soluble substances into the brain. In addition, several transport systems are present in the BBB promoting active transport. Notably, ECs that belong to the choroid plexus are also involved in the formation of another barrier, the blood-CSF barrier. On the other side of the barrier, neuronal tissue along with glial cells and pericytes including the basal lamina cover the cerebral vessels. Along with the ECs they form the neurovascular unit (NVU) of the BBB.

Brain ECs are very different from other ECs found in vessels outside the CNS. In addition to the tight junctions, they have high metabolic activity that can be concluded by the increased number of mitochondria. Another important characteristic is that membrane receptors expressed in brain ECs are polarized, which adds the ability to control the permeability of soluble compounds and ions [25, 26]. Thus, the BBB provides both mechanical and electrical resistance to blood components.

Cerebral endothelium that forms the basal lamina is now believed to be a key component of the BBB, regulating the interaction of blood and neuronal tissue in physiological and inflammatory states. Along with glial cells, astrocytes, and pericytes the components of the BBB are in close contact with neuronal projections, which in turn have been proven able to change blood flow and vessel dynamics in both health and disease.

Tight intercellular junctions (TJs) found in cerebral ECs are comparable to those found in other tissues. They are also formed by the three common transmembrane proteins, occludin, claudin, and junction associated molecules (JAMs). Additional proteins such as zonula occludens (ZO) which are found in the cytoplasm interact with actin filaments of the cytoskeleton [25]. The stability of the TJs is of major importance for BBB function. Several proteins have been found to regulate TJs. However, cAMP is currently thought to be the primary regulator of TJs in brain ECs. Several alterations such as the phosphorylation of proteins such as occludin and ZO are also involved in the regulation of TJs [26]. Interestingly, VEGF is found to decrease BBB selectivity and filtration. The continuous interaction of components of TJs and Adherens junctions is involved in BBB regulation. For example, extracellular calcium not only regulates Adherens junctions but TJs as well [27]. This interplay, which is currently under investigation, may shed some light on the molecular function of the BBB.

The BBB is very important for the homeostasis of the brain. Taking into consideration that TJs are the most important feature of the BBB, it is easy to understand that whether a blood component can pass the barrier, depends on its molecular weight and lipophilic/hydrophilic characteristics. There are many algorithms that have been constructed in an attempt to predict the permeability of the BBB, but the results are so far not conclusive. Many hydrophilic proteins can pass the BBB through active transport with the help of membrane transporters [28, 29]. The same thing applies to some proteins whose transport is receptor-mediated.

Another major feature is the diapedesis of leukocytes through the BBB. First, the leukocyte needs to bind to the vascular endothelial cell. This happens with tethering followed by rolling and adhesion of the leukocyte [30]. Then leukocytes can pass the basal lamina either through the para-cellular pathway or through the trans-cellular pathway [31]. Even though both types of trans-endothelial migration were proven in vitro and in vivo, the importance of the two different types of transport is not yet clear. There are researchers who believe that both types of transport may help in immune surveillance of the CNS [32].

As noted above, neuroinflammation refers to chronic inflammation of the CNS and mostly refers to neurodegenerative diseases either related to inflammation such as MS, or those related to mostly age-related diseases such as Parkinson's disease (PD) and AD. Dysfunction of the BBB has been proven in all neurodegenerative diseases, not only as an endpoint of the disease itself, but it was recently believed to be implicated in the early pathophysiologic stages.

In normal and healthy conditions, the BBB prevents the infiltration of drugs and immune cells into the brain. Thus, the presence of immune cells is much lower in the brain, compared to other organs of the periphery. In addition, few T cells migrate into the CNS but platelets and other leukocytes are blocked by the ECs. The opposite happens during inflammation. For example in MS immune cells such as T and B lymphocytes migrate into the CNS. Serum proteins that pass the BBB can be detected in the CSF [33].

MS is an autoimmune disease of the brain which affects 0.05–0.15 % of Caucasians. The disease is characterized by inflammation of the white matter (WM) of the CNS and demyelination. Cortical brain tissue is infiltrated with inflammatory cells that are located in demyelinated sites [34]. The demyelinating lesions are located not only near blood vessels but can also affect deeper regions of CNS tissue [35]. During the early stages of inflammation in MS, mainly $CD4^+$ and $CD8^+$ T cells are involved in the demyelinating process.

As inflammation evolves, macrophages migrate into the site and myelin degradation takes place in the presence of astrocytes [36].

One of the important features of the pathophysiology of the disease is believed to be the changes in the BBB in people who have a genetic predisposition [37]. The importance of BBB integrity in MS has been studied for many years using the animal model of autoimmune encephalomyelitis (EAE). Interestingly, many researchers now believe that the severity of MS is linked to the changes in BBB. Furthermore, it is believed that MS can be controlled by controlling the BBB. For example, the onset of symptoms seems to coincide with epigenetic alterations of tight junction proteins such as the dephosphorylation of occludin [38]. These alterations of the BBB, taking place before the demyelination of the brain in MS, can also be seen using MRI [39]. This disruption of the BBB has been linked to MMPs that seem to increase capillary permeability in the brain. Serum MMP-9 in particular is now considered to be a BBB disruption index among MS patients [40].

An interesting theory about the pathophysiology of MS suggests that during the active phases of the disease, ECs increase the production of adhesion molecules in their membrane thus promoting the interaction with cells of the immune system [37]. In that way, monocytes and leukocytes gain access to the CNS through the trans-endothelial pathway. To support this theory it was observed that adhesion molecules such as ICAM-1 and selectin are found in MS lesions [41]. Moreover, INF-β that is broadly used to suppress MS relapses is proven to reduce the expression of adhesion molecules [42]. In line with previous studies, the recently described activated leukocyte cell adhesion molecule (ALCAM) seems to act in series with ICAM-1 and VCAM-1 to increase the permeability of the BBB to leukocytes in the CNS, as shown in the EAE animal model [43]. These findings led to the production of natalizumab (Tysabri®), which blocks the migration of inflammatory cells through the BBB and reduces the size of inflammatory lesions found in MS [44].

Apart from adhesion molecules, reactive oxygen species (ROS) have been proven to disrupt the BBB and allow the entrance of leukocytes in the CNS in MS. ROS produced by macrophages and T cells when connected to the ECs, allow the entrance of immune cells, compromising the BBB. When EAE animals were treated with antioxidants such as luteolin, the permeability of BBB was reduced and the infiltration of immune cells was lower [45].

Recent discoveries shed light on the critical role for certain microRNAs (miRNAs) in controlling the function of the barrier endothelium in the brain (922,181c, 633 human CSF) [46]. In a recent review paper, all the current knowledge on the involvement of BBB dysfunction in MS and the central role that miRNAs play in maintaining BBB integrity under inflammatory conditions is presented [47].

In conclusion, the inflammatory reaction that characterizes most neurodegenerative diseases is called "Neuroinflammation" and consists mainly of elements of the innate immune response, microglia, and astrocytes and of immune blood cells which migrate through the BBB. A wide array of biomarkers in CSF aim at determining several parameters regulating such a complex system, as neuroinflammation, providing new tools towards therapeutics of neuroinflammatory and neurodegenerative diseases, like MS.

3 Optic Neuritis and Neuroinflammation

ON is the inflammation of the optic nerve. Considering which part of the optic nerve is involved ON can be distinguished in three different types: (a) Papillitis, where the inflammation includes the optic nerve head. Consequent optic disc oedema with peripapilary flame shaped hemorrhages is present. In addition, vitreous involvement may be identified with cells present at the posterior vitreous, (b) Retrobulbar neuritis, in which the optic nerve head does not present pathological signs and the inflammation concerns the posterior part of the optic nerve behind the eye up to the chiasm. Retrobulbar neuritis is most commonly found in patients with MS, (c) Neuroretinitis, where the inflamed optic disc is accompanied with inflamed retinal neuronal fiber layer and a macula star. Neuroretinitis is very uncommon in demyelination [48].

Another classification of ON can be performed according to the etiology. In MS and NMO, ON occurs due to demyelination. Parainfectious ON is caused after a viral infection that leads to immunization. Syphilis and Lyme disease cause infectious ON, whereas non-infectious inflammation can be found in autoimmune diseases like sarcoidosis and systemic lupus erythematosous [49].

A typical patient with ON complains about a sudden painful vision loss. The loss in visual acuity may be partial or complete and the patient may describe blurry vision with or without a positive scotoma. Pain is present during eye movement because the inflamed optic nerve is closely related to the cone of muscles behind the eye. Pain may precede visual loss in almost 92.2 % of the patients [50]. Color vision is also compromised and a simple test with Ishihara table may reveal defects in red color detection in the affected eye. Some patients complain about difficulty in stereoscopic vision, commonly known as the Pulrich effect. An increase in body temperature is also capable of worsening the visual symptoms (Uthoff's phenomenon). In contrast, pediatric patients rarely complain about pain in eye movement [51]. Another important clinical sign is the relative afferent pupillary defect (RAPD), which can be found in the affected eye. The difference between the two eyes through the afferent pathway indicates damage to the optic nerve or the retina. In many cases, a patient cannot distinguish the difference in visual acuity and color perception between the two eyes until the patient is instructed to occlude the healthy eye. Most commonly, ON is unilateral but bilateral ON has been described in MS and NMO [52].

ON is always a clinical diagnosis. The optic nerve can be visualized with direct and indirect ophthalmoscopy. In the majority of cases, the optic nerve and the fundus appear completely normal, thus pointing to the diagnosis of retrobulbar neuritis. For the diagnosis of bilateral ON, orbit MRI scan is not necessary but brain MRI scan must be performed to identify an underlying disease [53, 54]. Even though the diagnosis of ON is done clinically, MRI imaging can be helpful in atypical cases. It is also performed routinely to assess the presence of demyelinating lesions that may be the underlying cause of ON, as well as to provide information about patient's risk for developing MS in the future [55].

The most common cause of ON is MS and almost 50 % of MS patients will develop ON at some time point and in 30 % of MS patients the first symptom is ON [56]. Optical coherence tomography (OCT) is also helpful in identifying the remaining functional neural fibers of the optic nerve. In typical bilateral ON no further blood test is necessary. In contrast, bilateral ON should also be examined for NMO and aquaporin4 antibodies in the patient's blood.

In demyelination, myelin is phagocytosed by inflammatory cells and later on supporting cells like astrocytes replace the myelin with fibrous plaques. In that way neuronal signal conduction is disrupted. There are three main demyelinating conditions that may affect the optic nerve. Clinically isolated ON refers to demyelination of the optic nerve with no subsequent evidence of systemic demyelination in other parts of the CNS. MS, as mentioned above, is the most common demyelinating condition related to ON. NMO or Devic's disease, although very rare, is associated with bilateral ON that is followed by demyelination of the spinal cord. A patient with demyelinating ON has certain clinical characteristics. The mean age is about 30 and the patients complain of subacute visual impairment with the presence of phosphenes (flashes and sparkles). In over 90 % there is pain in eye movement along with discomfort and frontal headache. Visual acuity is 6/18 to 6/60 and a relative afferent pupillary defect (RAPD) is always present as a sign of optic nerve impairment and color vision is compromised. As mentioned above demyelinating ON is mainly unilateral with normal disc appearance in the insulted eye. However, disc pallor may be found in the fellow eye as a result of a previous episode of ON. Central positive scotomas are identified in the visual field testing but other atypical defects like altitudinal and arcuate scotomas may be found.

Lumbar puncture should always be performed and cerebrospinal fluid tested for oligoclonal bands (OCB) in electrophoresis to confirm or rule out the diagnosis of MS. Brain MRI is also performed as a means to identify systemic demyelination according to McDonald's criteria [57, 58]. Visually evoked potentials are also abnormal in almost all patients with MS-related ON. If ON affects both optic nerves, further testing for NMO should be considered.

Although ON is multifactorial, there are certain pathways that have been linked to the demyelination of the optic nerve. During an attack of ON, lymphocytes and monocytes infiltrate the optic nerve, an extension of the central nervous system containing a million myelinated fibers. Immune cells directly damage myelin or indirectly cause dysfunction by secreting proteases, nitric oxide, and cytokines that interfere with neuronal function ("conduction block"). Experimental injection of lymphokines into the posterior eye causes an inflammatory response and slowing of visual evoked potentials within hours [59]. Soluble ICAM, a product of activated white blood cells and endothelial cells, is increased in CSF at the first attack of ON [60]. Serum IFN-γ, IL-6 and IL-2 receptors, and CSF IL-2 are increased in patients with ON, indicating that $CD4^+$ and $CD8^+$ T cells are activated and are secreting cytokines in both compartments. These inflammatory cytokines also induce MHC antigens that could provoke chronic inflammation. In six patients who had ON 10 years earlier, mononuclear cells expressed more MHC class II protein than cells from healthy controls [61].

Recent studies suggest that during an acute episode of ON both inflammatory and anti-inflammatory processes take place. For instance, IL-10 is overexpressed and found at high levels in the CSF of ON patients. Interestingly, IL-10 is also increased in blood serum of patients with milder attacks as indicated by shorter symptom duration. These findings that correlate with overexpression of brain-derived neurotrophic factor (BDNF) and glial cell line-derived neurotrophic factor (GDNF) in the CSF of ON patients indicate a simultaneous inflammatory and anti-inflammatory response [62]. These findings are in line with previous studies that have underlined the importance of the anti-inflammatory IL-10 which is associated with the recovery from EAE.

Studies demonstrating the presence of inflammatory cells in brain lesions of MS patients as well as data from animal models have led to the generally accepted hypothesis that disease is mediated by pathogenic T cell responses against myelin antigens, followed by a broader neurodegenerative process [63].

Myelin basic protein-reactive and proteolipid protein-reactive T cells that produce IFN-γ, TNF, or lymphotoxin are increased in the CSF in ON and MS [64, 65]. However, cells secreting the anti-inflammatory and regulatory cytokines, IL-10, IL-4, and transforming growth factor (TGF)-beta are also more frequent, resulting in a complex mix of cytokines, a "cytokine storm". The number of CSF cells producing inflammatory cytokines in ON does not correlate with MRI abnormalities or OCB [66].

The inflammation is reversible. Surprisingly, high expression of the activation markers, HLA-DR and CD45RO, on T cells correlates with fewer OCB in the CSF and with better visual recovery [67]. This indicates the upregulation of protective regulatory T cells, or it may suggest that activated T helper cells are more susceptible to apoptosis. The vitreous is also highly immunosuppressive, so local factors may inhibit inflammation and even enhance repair.

B cells that recognize myelin basic protein are at normal levels in the periphery but are increased 100-fold in the cerebrospinal fluid in both MS and ON, compared to normal controls [68]. In individual patients, this oligoclonal response is often directed against multiple myelin basic protein epitopes, but more frequently against proteolipid protein [69]. In mice transgenic for T cell receptors that recognize MOG, 30 % spontaneously develop ON without any signs of experimental allergic encephalomyelitis [70]. Immunization with oligodendrocyte-specific protein induces an intense ON. ON has appeared in several cases of anti-GQ1b antibody-positive Miller-Fisher syndrome (ophthalmoplegia, ataxia, and areflexia in Guillain-Barré syndrome), suggesting that there is a reaction to this ganglioside that amplifies or causes the neuritis. In MS, anti-myelin basic protein responses are more common than anti-proteolipid protein responses. The antigen-specific response may change over time in demyelinating disease. This suggests there is no single target antigen and that the response to myelin basic protein follows earlier immune activation of unknown cause. In summary, immune changes in ON are similar to those in relapsing-remitting MS.

The OCB are from expanded B cell clones that produce the same type of immunoglobulin from ongoing mutation. This suggests there is an antigen, but a specific ON or MS antigen has not been defined.

Myeloid dendritic cells, which present antigen to T cells, are mature and activated in ON [71]. They induce a Th1 differentiation and T cell proliferation. They are deactivated by simvastatin, but caution must be exercised in the use of statins in conjunction with interferons in demyelinating diseases. Statins increase disease activity when added to ongoing interferon treatment [72, 73] and block interferon signaling in vitro and in vivo.

Markers of axonal injury and nitric oxide metabolites are increased in the plasma of laboratory animals with EAE. Antioxidant enzymes suppress the demyelination in the optic nerves in experimental allergic ON, probably by interfering with the effects of inflammatory monokines [74]. Uric acid, an antioxidant, is reduced in serum of patients with ON, a phenomenon also seen in MS. Functional recovery follows resolution of inflammation and of conduction block, expression of new sodium channels on demyelinated axons, and cord remyelination that can continue for up to 2 years. Immune cells are also capable of secreting neurotrophic factors that induce repair. Previous studies have shown that neurotrophin receptors are present in various cells of the immune system including cell populations of primary and secondary lymphoid tissues. Interestingly, neurotrophins act on lymphocytes increasing the blastogenic response. There may be autocrine and paracrine action of neurotrophins in the immune system [75, 76]. Consequently, there is a major role of neurotrophins in the immune system which can regulate regeneration and remyelination. Neurotrophins such as BDNF can regulate recovery. For instance, BDNF levels in peripheral blood mononuclear cells are higher during the recovery phase of MS. Although elucidating the interplay between neurotrophins and the immune system is difficult, recent studies suggest that neurotrophic factors' pathway should be further investigated to assist with the development of novel treatments [77, 78].

In addition, it has been suggested that during an attack of ON, two distinct inflammatory processes take place. The first concerns trafficking of activated leukocytes which can be distinguished with certain biomarkers such as CXCL13, CXCL10, and MMP-9, which are involved in the breakdown of the BBB and activation of T-cells. The second is involved in tissue damage [79]. Therefore, chitinase 3-like protein (ChI3L), OPN, neurofilament light-chain (NF-L), and myelin basic protein (MBP) represent the degree of optic nerve damage during an ON attack [80].

Magnetic resonance spectroscopy of normal-appearing white matter after ON is the same as in normal controls. If there are visible MRI lesions outside the optic nerve, there are also pathological findings in magnetic resonance spectroscopy [81]. MRI findings are also associated with OCB. Interestingly, the presence of OCB in the CSF strongly correlates with findings in either MRI or visually evoked potentials (VEP). In that way, pathological findings in CSF analysis are expected, if pathological findings have been documented in either MRI or VEP [82].

In other cases, MRI lesions are present in multiple areas of the CNS, suggesting an overlap between the two demyelinating diseases. During recovery of the affected nerve, functional MRI shows extreme activation of areas other than the occipital cortex (extrastriate) including insula, claustrum, thalamus, as well as lateral temporal and posterior parietal cortex [83]. After ON, there is trans-synaptic degeneration in the lateral geniculate nucleus. Fiber tracking with fast marching tractography shows dystrophy and lost connectivity in the optic radiations beyond the lateral geniculate nucleus [84].

Functional MRI shows that ON decreases afferent stimuli to the visual cortex, and reduces functional activation of the cortex [85]. Disruption of the ventral visual stream from the V1 cortical area and the posterior parietal cortex interferes with the construction of the visual world—recognition and identification. At 3 months after the episode, visual activation reverses, and there is more neuronal activity in the occipital and lateral temporal cortices and the hippocampus.

Histologically, in the scattered plaques of MS, axons are usually preserved (although some subtypes of MS differ). In isolated ON, more axons are usually destroyed along with the demyelination, although myelin loss does exceed axonal loss. Ninety-five percent to ninety-nine percent of patients with MS have lesions in the optic nerves at autopsy.

Histamine receptors (HxR) play multiple roles in immune reactions and autoimmune disorders. Histamine may determine, through different receptor activation pathways, a shift in T-helper cell subpopulation, may influence migration of lymphocytes and myeloid cells during CNS invasion, interfere with antigen presentation at the immune synapse level, and determine variations in normal neuronal functions [86–88]. The role of histamine varies according to the specific receptor activation in brain tissues. Activation of H1R and H2R in vitro on DCs modulates cytokine and chemokine production and their ability to drive $CD4^+$ T-cell differentiation to the Th2 phenotype. Interestingly, H4R activation modulates chemotaxis [89]. Histamine can promote Th1 responses through H1R and down-regulate both Th1 and Th2 responses through H2R [90]. Recent evidence suggests an increase in CSF histamine levels in patients with MS [91].

EAE is mediated by myelin-specific T cells, which are activated in the periphery and translocate into the CNS followed by permeabilization of the BBB [92]. However, there are differences between MS and EAE and these have been highlighted by the fact that certain therapies have opposite effects in the two conditions. For example, administration of INF-γ or anti-TNF was protective in EAE, but exacerbated MS [93].

IL-12 is required for the differentiation of Th1 cells in EAE and MS. However, the discovery of IL-23, which is structurally related to IL-12, showed that IL-23 is necessary to drive the induction or expansion of $CD4^+$ T cells that secrete IL-17, termed Th17 cells [94]. Even though IL-23 may not be required for lineage commitment, it is essential for further Th17 development. The IL-17 family of cytokines has a clear pathogenic role in EAE and MS. Although early studies on TH17 cells dismissed a role for Th1 cells, recent studies have suggested that both cell types may play distinct roles in pathology. Th1 cells can access the CNS initially, and this facilitates subsequent recruitment of Th17 cells in EAE [95]. IL-23 is also required for the induction but not the effector phase of the disease [96]. Interestingly, a recent study has identified an enrichment of T cells expressing both IL-12 and INF-γ in brain MS tissue, suggesting that $IL\text{-}12^+$ and $INF\text{-}\gamma^+$ cells may be involved in pathology [97]. Studies in MS patients have provided evidence that Th1 and Th17 cells are active or expanded during diseases, but their contribution to pathology has, understandably, been more difficult to define.

Regulatory T cells (Treg) include both natural and adaptive (also termed inducible) Treg cells. Natural Treg (nTreg) cells express cell surface CD25 and the transcription factor FoxP3 which is essential for directing regulatory function [98]. Adaptive Treg cells, including Tr1, Th3, and subsets of $CD8^+$ Treg cells, are derived from the periphery from uncommitted naive T cells stimulated by antigen under the influence of the immunosuppressive cytokines IL-10 and TGF-β, but also retinoic acid (RA). Studies on human Treg cells, particularly those in disease settings, can be compromised by the fact that many Treg cell markers, including CD25 and FoxP3, may be up-regulated on activated effector cells. For this reason, CD127lo is used in addition to CD25 and FoxP3 to identify human nTreg cells [99]. Tr1 responses have been shown to be reduced in MS patients, reflected in reduced levels of IL-10 [100]. Interestingly, an increased frequency of $CD25^+$ $FoxP3^+$ nTreg cells has been found in the CSF but not the blood in MS patients [101]. Indeed, a more recent study revealed that when CD127lo was used in addition to CD25 to sort Treg cells, there was no reduction in the suppressive function of Treg cells from MS patients compared with controls [102]. The protective effects of $CD4^+$ $CD25^+$ Treg cells appear to be mediated by IL-10, as Treg cells from IL-$10^{-/-}$ failed to confer protection to EAE [103].

Treg cells also appear to play a role in mediating the recovery from actively induced EAE, which is usually self-limiting. Recovery has been associated with induction/activation of TGF-β and IL-10. Indeed in MS, relapse and remission have been correlated with relative decreases and increases in the frequency of Treg cells.

Interestingly, CNS-derived Treg cells were able to suppress INF-γ but not IL-17 [104], suggesting that Th17 cells may be more resistant to suppression. Alternatively, these results might be explained by the recent observation that $FoxP3^+$ Treg cells can produce IL-17, masking any suppressive effect in Th17 cells. $CD4^+$ $CD25^+$ $FoxP3^+$ $CD39^+$ Treg cells do suppress Il-17, whereas total $CD4^+$ $CD25^+$ $FoxP3^+$ human Treg cells fail to suppress IL-17 by responder T cells, due to the fact that $CD39^+$ $CD4^+$ $CD25^+$ $FoxP3^+$ subset produced IL-17, which masked the suppressive effect of the Treg population as a whole [105]. Therefore, it appears that Treg cells can suppress Th17 cells but the suppressive effect of Treg cells cannot be defined by the expression of FoxP3 alone.

Patients with MS have elevated percentages of both CCR5 and CXCR3 expressing T cells vs HC (healthy controls) in blood and vs other neurological diseases (OND) in the CSF. Higher percentages of T cells expressing CCR5 and CXCR3 in blood and in CSF are confined to untreated MS patients, while INF-β-treated MS patients have similar percentages of both CCR5 and CXCR3 expressing T cells vs HC in blood and vs OND patients in the CSF (*see* **Note 1**). Monosymptomatic ON patients, frequently representing early MS, have elevated percentages of CXCR3 expressing T cells vs HC in blood and elevated percentages of CCR5 expressing T cells vs OND patients in CSF [106].

4 A Protocol to Study Neuroinflammation in Optic Neuritis

It is without doubt extremely difficult to identify an inflammatory profile in ON patients, separating them according to the underlying disease. Until now, there is only one definite diagnostic biomarker in ON. The presence of aquaporin-4 antibodies is diagnostic for NMO with a specificity of 99 % [107]. However in order to study inflammatory components of either CSF samples or serum samples certain parameters should be taken into consideration.

1. Groups should be separated according to the disease. It is recommended that the following groups are studied (*see* **Notes 2–3**):
   (a) Patients without any neurological disease who present to the emergency department with CIS ON.
   (b) Patients with already diagnosed MS who present with ON for the first time.
   (c) A third group can be included, ON patients with known NMO disease.
   (d) A further group can be included to compare CSF and serum findings; subjects with OND (*see* **Note 1**) who have undergone lumbar puncture and blood sample analysis can be used as control patients [91, 102].
2. CSF should be examined during presentation and blood/serum samples can be collected regularly in intervals of 1 week (Table 1).
   - Lumbar puncture is routinely performed in patients with ON as a diagnostic tool (*see* **Note 4**). Lumbar puncture is performed at the emergency department as part of the diagnostic procedure. 4 ml is usually collected. One milliliter is stored separately and frozen at −80 °C until analysis. No fasting of patient is necessary for any of the procedures of the protocol (*see* **Note 5**).
   - In contrast, blood samples can be collected more easily since the procedure is less invasive and safer. Blood samples are collected normally at 8.00 a.m. and an effort for every repeat sample to be collected at the same time is made. Blood samples are stored at −20 °C. Analysis should be performed within 1 month of collection (*see* **Note 6**).

5 Notes

1. OND include PD, tension headache, depression, cerebral/cortical atrophy, normal pressure hydrocephalus, cerebrovascular diseases, ataxia, pseudotumor cerebri, neuralgia, and other non-inflammatory conditions.
2. It is of great importance to exclude certain patients from the study to limit external factors that interact with the immune system. Patients with sleep disorders, under statin medication and those with allergic diseases or who have been under medication with anti-histamine drugs and antibiotics during the last month should not be included in any of the groups.
3. In more detail, patients are separated according to the condition. The first group with CIS ON should have no findings suggestive of a demyelinating disease in MRI scan according to McDonald's criteria [57]. The second group comprises patients who are diagnosed with MS, have suggestive lesions in brain MRI scan, and suffer from recent onset ON for the first time. In accordance the third group will have demyelinating lesions indicative of NMO in MRI scan and recent onset ON. The control group that will consist of patients with OND should have no demyelinating lesions. OCB is tested in the CSF of all patients. CSF OCB is tested in each patient with standard methods, as described before [108]. Only patients with CIS ON or MS ON could have OCB in their CSF.
4. In the suggested protocol, no further lumbar puncture should be performed in any of the patients only for research purposes.
5. CSF samples from the lumbar puncture should be collected and analyzed for histamine [109, 110], IL-12, IL-10, IL-17, and IL-23 (ELISA) (Table 1).

Table 1
Neuroinflammation study in patients with optic neuritis

CSF markers in neuroinflammation - Optic neuritis	MRI criteria	OCB (CSF)	Histamine (CSF)	Histamine (blood/serum)	IL-12 (CSF)	IL-10 (CSF)	IL-17 (CSF)	IL-23 (CSF)
CIS ON	(−)	(+) or (−)	Day 1	Days 1,7,14	Day 1	Day 1	Day 1	Day 1
MS + ON	(+)	(+)	Day 1	Days 1,7,14	Day 1	Day 1	Day 1	Day 1
NMO + ON	(+)	(−)	Day 1	Days 1,7,14	Day 1	Day 1	Day 1	Day 1
OND	(−)	(−)	Day 1	Days 1,7,14	Day 1	Day 1	Day 1	Day 1

CIS clinically isolated syndrome, *CSF* cerebrospinal fluid, *IL* interleukin, *MS* multiple sclerosis, *MRI* magnetic resonance imaging, *NMO* neuromyelitis optica, *ON* optic neuritis, *OCB* oligoclonal bands, *OND* other neurological diseases

6. Blood should also be collected at the presentation and every week for the following 2 weeks and analyzed for histamine levels [109, 110] (Table 1).

References

1. Wang KKW, Zhang Z, Kobeissy FH (2014) Biomarkers of brain injury and neurological disorders. CRC Press, Boca Raton, FL
2. Katsavos S, Anagnostouli M (2013) Biomarkers in multiple sclerosis: an up-to-date overview. Mult Scler Int 2013:340508
3. Piccolo L, Woodhall M, Tackley G et al (2016) Isolated new onset "atypical" optic neuritis in the NMO clinic: serum antibodies, prognoses and diagnoses at follow-up. J Neurol 263:370–379
4. Rodriguez-Martin E, Picon C, Costa-Frossard L et al (2015) Natural killer cell subsets in cerebrospinal fluid of patients with multiple sclerosis. Clin Exp Immunol 180:243–249
5. Piskunov AK (2010) Neuroinflammation biomarkers. Clin Neuroc 4:55–63
6. Rosi S, Ramirez-Amaya V, Vazdarjanova A et al (2005) Neuroinflammation alters the hippocampal pattern of behaviorally induced Arc expression. J Neurosci 25:723–731
7. Barger SW, Harmon AD (1997) Microglial activation by Alzheimer amyloid precursor protein and modulation by apolipoprotein E. Nature 388:878–881
8. Barger SW, Basile AS (2001) Activation of microglia by secreted amyloid precursor protein evokes release of glutamate by cystine exchange and attenuates synaptic function. J Neurochem 76:846–854
9. Akiyama H, Itagaki S, McGeer PL (1988) Major histocompatibility complex antigen expression on rat microglia following epidural kainic acid lesions. Neurosci Res 20:147–157
10. Streit WJ, Graeber MB, Kreutzberg GW (1989) Expression of Ia antigen on perivascular and microglial cells after sublethal and lethal motor neuron injury. Exp Neurol 105:115–126
11. McGeer PL, Itagaki S, Tago H et al (1987) Reactive microglia in patients with senile dementia of the Alzheimer type are positive for the histocompatibility glycoprotein HLA-DR. Neurosci Lett 79:195–200
12. Streit WJ, Mrak RE, Griffin WS (2004) Microglia and neuroinflammation: a pathological perspective. J Neuroinflammation 1:14
13. Lawson LJ, Perry VH, Gordon S (1992) Turnover of resident microglia in the normal adult mouse brain. Neuroscience 48:405–415
14. Wood PL (2003) Neuroinflammation: mechanisms and management. Cont Neurosci, 2nd edn. Humana Press, Totowa, NJ
15. Kaushal V, Schlichter LC (2008) Mechanisms of microglia-mediated neurotoxicity in a new model of the stroke penumbra. J Neurosci 28:2221–2230
16. Suehiro E, Fujisawa H, Akimura T et al (2004) Increased matrix metalloproteinase-9 in blood in association with activation of interleukin-6 after traumatic brain injury: influence of hypothermic therapy. J Neurotrauma 21:1706–1711
17. Liu MC, Akle V, Zheng W et al (2006) Extensive degradation of myelin basic protein isoforms by calpain following traumatic brain injury. J Neurochem 98:700–712
18. Kaur C, Ling EA (2008) Antioxidants and neuroprotection in the adult and developing central nervous system. Cur Med Chem 15:3068–3080
19. Canto E, Tintore M, Villar LM et al (2014) Validation of semaphorin 7A and ala-beta-his-dipeptidase as biomarkers associated with the conversion from clinically isolated syndrome to multiple sclerosis. J Neuroinflammation 11:181
20. Nakatsuji Y (2014) Sema4A as a biomarker predicting responsiveness to IFN beta treatment. Rinsho Shinkeigaku 54:972–974
21. Kremer D, Hartung HP, Kury P (2015) Targeting semaphorins in MS as a treatment strategy to promote remyelination: a tale of mice, rats and men. Mult Scler 21:1616–1617
22. Gendelman HE (2002) Neural immunity: friend or foe? J Neurovirol 8:474–479
23. Cipolla MJ (2009) The cerebral circulation. integrated systems physiology: from molecule to function. San Rafael, USA
24. Ehrlich P (1885) Das Sauerstoff-Bedürfniss des Organismus. Eine farbenanalytische Studie. Habilitationsschrift. vol Habilitation. Universität Berlin, Berlin
25. Levanony H, Rubin R, Altschuler Y et al (1992) Evidence for a novel route of wheat storage proteins to vacuoles. J Cell Biol 119:1117–1128
26. Sakakibara A, Furuse M, Saitou M et al (1997) Possible involvement of phosphorylation of occludin in tight junction formation. J Cell Biol 137:1393–1401
27. Rubin LL (1992) Endothelial cells: adhesion and tight junctions. Curr Opin Cell Biol 4:830–833

28. de Lange EC (2004) Potential role of ABC transporters as a detoxification system at the blood-CSF barrier. Adv Drug Deliv Rev 56:1793–1809
29. Begley DJ (2004) ABC transporters and the blood-brain barrier. Curr Pharm Des 10: 1295–1312
30. Greenwood J, Amos CL, Walters CE et al (2003) Intracellular domain of brain endothelial intercellular adhesion molecule-1 is essential for T lymphocyte-mediated signaling and migration. J Immunol 171:2099–2108
31. Carman CV, Springer TA (2008) Trans-cellular migration: cell-cell contacts get intimate. Curr Opin Cell Biol 20:533–540
32. Chavakis T, Preissner KT, Santoso S (2003) Leukocyte trans-endothelial migration: JAMs add new pieces to the puzzle. Thromb Haemost 89:13–17
33. Olsson T, Sun J, Hillert J et al (1992) Increased numbers of T cells recognizing multiple myelin basic protein epitopes in multiple sclerosis. Eur J Immunol 22:1083–1107
34. Lassmann H, Bruck W, Lucchinetti CF (2007) The immunopathology of multiple sclerosis: an overview. Brain Pathol 17:210–218
35. Noseworthy JH, Lucchinetti C, Rodriguez M et al (2000) Multiple sclerosis. N Engl J Med 343:938–952
36. Hafler DA, Slavik JM, Anderson DE et al (2005) Multiple sclerosis. Immunol Rev 204:208–231
37. Frohman EM, Racke MK, Raine CS (2006) Multiple sclerosis--the plaque and its pathogenesis. N Engl J Med 354:942–955
38. Morgan L, Shah B, Rivers LE et al (2007) Inflammation and dephosphorylation of the tight junction protein occludin in an experimental model of multiple sclerosis. Neurosci 147:664–673
39. Waubant E (2006) Biomarkers indicative of blood-brain barrier disruption in multiple sclerosis. Dis Markers 22:235–244
40. Chandler S, Miller KM, Clements JM et al (1997) Matrix metalloproteinases, tumor necrosis factor and multiple sclerosis: an overview. J Neuroimmunol 72:155–161
41. Correale J, Bassani Molinas Mde L (2003) Temporal variations of adhesion molecules and matrix metalloproteinases in the course of MS. J Neuroimmunol 140:198–209
42. Lou J, Gasche Y, Zheng L et al (1999) Interferon-beta inhibits activated leukocyte migration through human brain microvascular endothelial cell monolayer. Lab Invest 79:1015–1025
43. Cayrol R, Wosik K, Berard JL et al (2008) Activated leukocyte cell adhesion molecule promotes leukocyte trafficking into the central nervous system. Nature Immunol 9:137–145
44. Polman CH, O'Connor PW, Havrdova E et al (2006) A randomized, placebo-controlled trial of natalizumab for relapsing multiple sclerosis. N Engl J Med 354:899–910
45. Hendriks JJ, Alblas J, van der Pol SM et al (2004) Flavonoids influence monocytic GTPase activity and are protective in experimental allergic encephalitis. J Exp Med 200:1667–1672
46. Haghikia A, Haghikia A, Hellwig K et al (2012) Regulated microRNAs in the CSF of patients with multiple sclerosis: a case-control study. Neurology 79:2166–2170
47. Kamphuis WWDTC, Reijerkerk A, Romero IA et al (2015) The blood-brain barrier in multiple sclerosis: microRNAs as key regulators. CNS Neurol Disord Drug Targets 14:157–167
48. Khachaturova NK (1973) Classification of optic neuritis. Vestnik Oftalmologii 2:39–42
49. Honan WP, Heron JR, Foster DH et al (1990) Visual loss in multiple sclerosis and its relation to previous optic neuritis, disease duration and clinical classification. Brain 113:975–987
50. Boomer JA, Siatkowski RM (2003) Optic neuritis in adults and children. Semin Ophthalmol 18:174–180
51. Absoud M, Cummins C, Desai N et al (2011) Childhood optic neuritis clinical features and outcome. Arch Dis Child 96:860–862
52. Burman J, Raininko R, Fagius J (2011) Bilateral and recurrent optic neuritis in multiple sclerosis. Acta Neurol Scand 123:207–210
53. Ramanathan S, Prelog K, Barnes EH et al (2016) Radiological differentiation of optic neuritis with myelin oligodendrocyte glycoprotein antibodies, aquaporin-4 antibodies, and multiple sclerosis. Mult Scler 22:470–482
54. Zhang Y, Liang X, Wei S et al (2015) Differential diagnosis for multiple sclerosis-related optic neuritis. Eye Sci 30:23–28
55. Osborne BJ, Volpe NJ (2009) Optic neuritis and risk of MS: differential diagnosis and management (in eng). Clin J Med 76:181–190
56. Szilasiova J, Klimova E, Vesela D (2002) Optic neuritis as the first sign of multiple sclerosis. Cesk Slov Oftalmol 58:259–264
57. Galea I, Freedman MS, Thompson EJ (2011) Cerebrospinal fluid analysis in the 2010 revised McDonald's multiple sclerosis diagnostic criteria. Ann Neurol 70:183
58. Wiendl H, Kieseier BC, Gold R et al (2006) Revision of McDonald's new diagnostic criteria for multiple sclerosis. Nervenarzt 77:1235, 1237–1235, 1245
59. Arezzo JC, Brosnan CF, Schroeder CE et al (1988) Electrophysiological analysis of factors

involved in the primary demyelinating diseases: the rabbit eye model system. Brain Res 462:286–300
60. Petersen AA, Sellebjerg F, Frederiksen J et al (1998) Soluble ICAM-1, demyelination, and inflammation in multiple sclerosis and acute optic neuritis. J Neuroimmunol 88:120–127
61. Kinnunen E, Konttinen YT, Bergroth V et al (1989) Immunological studies on patients with optic neuritis without evidence of multiple sclerosis. J Neurol Sci 90:43–52
62. Tsakiri A, Ravanidis S, Lagoudaki R et al (2015) Neuroprotective and anti-inflammatory mechanisms are activated early in optic neuritis. Acta Neurol Scand 131:305–312
63. Compston A, Coles A (2008) Multiple sclerosis. Lancet 372:1502–1517
64. Soderstrom M, Link H, Sun JB et al (1993) T cells recognizing multiple peptides of myelin basic protein are found in blood and enriched in cerebrospinal fluid in optic neuritis and multiple sclerosis. Scand J Immunol 37:355–368
65. Navikas V, He B, Link J et al (1996) Augmented expression of tumour necrosis factor-alpha and lymphotoxin in mononuclear cells in multiple sclerosis and optic neuritis. Brain 119:213–223
66. Kivisakk P, Tian W, Matusevicius D et al (1998) Optic neuritis and cytokines: no relation to MRI abnormalities and oligoclonal bands. Neurol 50:217–223
67. Roed H, Frederiksen J, Langkilde A et al (2005) Systemic T-cell activation in acute clinically isolated optic neuritis. J Neuroimmunol 162:165–172
68. Soderstrom M, Link H, Xu Z et al (1993) Optic neuritis and multiple sclerosis: anti-MBP and anti-MBP peptide antibody-secreting cells are accumulated in CSF. Neurol 43:1215–1222
69. Sellebjerg F, Madsen HO, Frederiksen JL et al (1995) Acute optic neuritis: myelin basic protein and proteolipid protein antibodies, affinity, and the HLA system. Ann Neurol 38:943–950
70. Bettelli E, Pagany M, Weiner HL et al (2003) Myelin oligodendrocyte glycoprotein-specific T cell receptor transgenic mice develop spontaneous autoimmune optic neuritis. J Exp Med 197:1073–1081
71. Tsakiri A, Tsiantoulas D, Frederiksen J et al (2010) Increased immunopotency of monocyte derived dendritic cells from patients with optic neuritis is inhibited in vitro by simvastatin. Exp Neurol 221:320–328
72. Birnbaum G, Cree B, Altafullah I et al (2008) Combining beta interferon and atorvastatin may increase disease activity in multiple sclerosis. Neurol 71:1390–1395
73. Sorensen PS, Lycke J, Eralinna JP et al (2011) Simvastatin as add-on therapy to interferon beta-1a for relapsing-remitting multiple sclerosis (SIMCOMBIN study): a placebo-controlled randomised phase 4 trial. Lancet Neurol 10:691–701
74. Guy J, Ellis EA, Hope GM et al (1989) Antioxidant enzyme suppression of demyelination in experimental optic neuritis. Curr Eye Res 8:467–477
75. Tabakman R, Lecht S, Sephanova S et al (2004) Interactions between the cells of the immune and nervous system: neurotrophins as neuroprotection mediators in CNS injury. Prog Brain Res 146:387–401
76. Vega JA, Garcia-Suarez O, Hannestad J et al (2003) Neurotrophins and the immune system. J Anat 203:1–19
77. Naghashpour M, Amani R, Sarkaki A et al (2016) Brain-derived neurotrophic and immunologic factors: beneficial effects of riboflavin on motor disability in murine model of multiple sclerosis. Iran J Bas Med Sci 19:439–448
78. Razavi S, Nazem G, Mardani M et al (2015) Neurotrophic factors and their effects in the treatment of multiple sclerosis. Adv Biomed Res 4:53
79. Alvarez E, Piccio L, Mikesell RJ et al (2013) CXCL13 is a biomarker of inflammation in multiple sclerosis, neuromyelitis optica, and other neurological conditions. Mult Scler 19:1204–1208
80. Modvig S, Degn M, Horwitz H et al (2013) Relationship between cerebrospinal fluid biomarkers for inflammation, demyelination and neurodegeneration in acute optic neuritis. PloS One 8:e77163
81. Tourbah A, Stievenart JL, Abanou A et al (1999) Normal-appearing white matter in optic neuritis and multiple sclerosis: a comparative proton spectroscopy study. Neuroradiology 41:738–743
82. Horwitz H, Degn M, Modvig S et al (2012) CSF abnormalities can be predicted by VEP and MRI pathology in the examination of optic neuritis. J Neurol 259:2616–2620
83. Werring DJ, Bullmore ET, Toosy AT et al (2000) Recovery from optic neuritis is associated with a change in the distribution of cerebral response to visual stimulation: a functional magnetic resonance imaging study. J Neurol Neurosurg Psych 68:441–449
84. Ciccarelli O, Toosy AT, Hickman SJ et al (2005) Optic radiation changes after optic neuritis detected by tractography-based group mapping. Hum Brain Map 25:308–316
85. Toosy AT, Hickman SJ, Miszkiel KA et al (2005) Adaptive cortical plasticity in higher

visual areas after acute optic neuritis. Ann Neurol 57:622–633
86. Ferreira R, Santos T, Goncalves J et al (2012) Histamine modulates microglia function. J Neuroinflammation 9:90
87. Liu YW, Li J, Ye JH (2010) Histamine regulates activities of neurons in the ventrolateral preoptic nucleus. J Physiol 588:4103–4116
88. Rosa AC, Fantozzi R (2013) The role of histamine in neurogenic inflammation. Br J Pharmacol 170:38–45
89. Schneider E, Leite-de-moraes M, Dy M (2010) Histamine, immune cells and autoimmunity. Adv Exp Med Biol 709:81–94
90. Jutel M, Klunker S, Akdis M et al (2001) Histamine upregulates Th1 and downregulates Th2 responses due to different patterns of surface histamine 1 and 2 receptor expression. Int Arch Allergy Immunol 124:190–192
91. Kallweit U, Aritake K, Bassetti CL et al (2013) Elevated CSF histamine levels in multiple sclerosis patients. Fluids Barriers CNS 10:19
92. Furtado GC, Marcondes MC, Latkowski JA et al (2008) Swift entry of myelin-specific T lymphocytes into the central nervous system in spontaneous autoimmune encephalomyelitis. J Immunol 181:4648–4655
93. Constantinescu CS, Farooqi N, O'Brien K et al (2011) Experimental autoimmune encephalomyelitis (EAE) as a model for multiple sclerosis (MS). Br J Pharmacol 164:1079–1106
94. Langrish CL, Chen Y, Blumenschein WM et al (2005) IL-23 drives a pathogenic T cell population that induces autoimmune inflammation. J Exp Med 201:233–240
95. O'Connor RA, Prendergast CT, Sabatos CA et al (2008) Cutting edge: Th1 cells facilitate the entry of Th17 cells to the central nervous system during experimental autoimmune encephalomyelitis. J Immunol 181:3750–3754
96. Thakker P, Leach MW, Kuang W et al (2007) IL-23 is critical in the induction but not in the effector phase of experimental autoimmune encephalomyelitis. J Immunol 178:2589–2598
97. Kebir H, Ifergan I, Alvarez JI et al (2009) Preferential recruitment of interferon-gamma-expressing TH17 cells in multiple sclerosis. Ann Neurol 66:390–402
98. Hori S, Sakaguchi S (2004) Foxp3: a critical regulator of the development and function of regulatory T cells. Microbes Infect 6:745–751
99. Liu W, Putnam AL, Xu-Yu Z et al (2006) CD127 expression inversely correlates with FoxP3 and suppressive function of human CD4+ T reg cells. J exp Med 203:1701–1711
100. Martinez-Forero I, Garcia-Munoz R, Martinez-Pasamar S et al (2008) IL-10 suppressor activity and ex vivo Tr1 cell function are impaired in multiple sclerosis. Eur J Immunol 38:576–586
101. Feger U, Luther C, Poeschel S et al (2007) Increased frequency of CD4+ CD25+ regulatory T cells in the cerebrospinal fluid but not in the blood of multiple sclerosis patients. Clin Exp Immunol 147:412–418
102. Michel L, Berthelot L, Pettre S et al (2008) Patients with relapsing-remitting multiple sclerosis have normal Treg function when cells expressing IL-7 receptor alpha-chain are excluded from the analysis. J Clin Invest 118:3411–3419
103. Zhang X, Koldzic DN, Izikson L et al (2004) IL-10 is involved in the suppression of experimental autoimmune encephalomyelitis by CD25+CD4+ regulatory T cells. Int Immunol 16:249–256
104. O'Connor RA, Malpass KH, Anderton SM (2007) The inflamed central nervous system drives the activation and rapid proliferation of Foxp3+ regulatory T cells. J Immunol 179:958–966
105. Fletcher JM, Lonergan R, Costelloe L et al (2009) CD39+Foxp3+ regulatory T Cells suppress pathogenic Th17 cells and are impaired in multiple sclerosis. J Immunol 183:7602–7610
106. Teleshova N, Pashenkov M, Huang YM et al (2002) Multiple sclerosis and optic neuritis: CCR5 and CXCR3 expressing T cells are augmented in blood and cerebrospinal fluid. J Neurol 249:723–729
107. Petzold A, Plant GT (2014) Diagnosis and classification of autoimmune optic neuropathy. Autoimmun Rev 13:539–545
108. Anagnostouli M, Christidi F, Zalonis I et al (2015) Clinical and cognitive implications of cerebrospinal fluid oligoclonal bands in multiple sclerosis patients. Neurol Sci 36:2053–2060
109. Bessinis DP, Dalla C, Daifoti ZP et al (2012) Histamine involvement in visual development and adaptation. Inv Ophthalmol Vis Sci 53:7498–7503
110. Tiligada E, Aslanis D, Delitheos A et al (2000) Changes in histamine content following pharmacologically-induced mast cell degranulation in the rat conjunctiva. Pharmacol Res 41:667–670

Chapter 15

In Vivo Diagnostic Procedures for IgE-Mediated Allergic Disorders

Christopher Koulias, Xenophon Aggelides, Caterina Chliva, and Michael Makris

Abstract

IgE-mediated allergic diseases include atopic diseases, such as eczema or respiratory allergies that are characterized by chronic allergic inflammation, as well as anaphylaxis stemming from clinically important sensitizations to foods, drugs, or venoms, to name the most important categories. It has long been acknowledged that the release of histamine by basophils and mast cells is a hallmark of IgE-mediated diseases. Recent insights into the immunomodulatory role of histamine and its four receptor types and specific aspects of the allergic inflammation have contributed to an increased interest about the mechanisms underlying their interplay. This interest is further fueled by the sharp rise in the prevalence of IgE-mediated diseases in westernized societies during the last decades and the resulting significant increase of the associated socioeconomic burden. *In vivo* diagnostic procedures, including skin testing and provocation tests, have proved to be valuable, yet simple tools for the investigation of allergic diseases both by clinicians and researchers as well as for influencing management decisions. Skin testing for IgE-mediated diseases is extensively used as a surrogate approach for the detection of allergen-specific IgE antibodies, currently being the diagnostic cornerstone for many allergic responses. Furthermore, provocation tests have evolved into an important approach for the diagnostic confirmation or the elucidation of the clinical relevance of suspected allergens, often being the golden standard for allergy diagnosis.

Key words Allergy, Drug provocation test, Hypersensitivity, IgE, In vivo, Intradermal test, Nasal provocation test, Oral food challenge, Skin prick test, Skin testing

1 Introduction

Immunoglobulin E (IgE)-mediated diseases include anaphylactic monoallergies, such as immediate hypersensitivity to foods, drugs and Hymenoptera venoms, as well as classic atopic diseases, such as atopic dermatitis, allergic rhinitis, rhinoconjuctivitis, and asthma, where chronic inflammation leads to tissue injury and remodeling [1–3]. It has long been acknowledged that the release of histamine by basophils and mast cells is a hallmark of IgE-mediated diseases [4, 5]. The recent insights into the role of histamine and the four histamine receptor types in immunoregulation, and the specific

Ekaterini Tiligada and Madeleine Ennis (eds.), *Histamine Receptors as Drug Targets*, Methods in Pharmacology and Toxicology, DOI 10.1007/978-1-4939-6843-5_15, © Springer Science+Business Media LLC 2017

Table 1
In vivo diagnostic methods in IgE-mediated diseases

Skin tests
Skin prick test (SPT)
Intradermal test (IDT)
Provocation tests
Oral provocation test
Oral food challenge (OFC)
Drug provocation test (DPT)
Parenteral provocation test
Organ-specific provocation test
Nasal provocation test (NPT)
Ophthalmic provocation test
Bronchial provocation test

aspects of allergic inflammation have contributed to the currently increased interest in their interplay [6, 7].

The increased prevalence of allergic disorders that was first noted for asthma and allergic rhinoconjuctivitis and the recent sharp rise in hospital admissions due to food allergy, drug hypersensitivity reactions (DHRs), or anaphylaxis (mostly IgE-mediated, rapid onset, multisystem hypersensitivity reaction) of numerous other causes led to the development of more effective symptomatic and disease-modifying treatments and/or to the implementation of preventative measures [2, 3, 8–10]. The first and most important step in the diagnostic algorithm of an allergic disease is the detailed history and the physical examination of the patient. Subsequent ex vivo (referred to as in vitro in everyday clinical practice) and in vivo diagnostic tests aim to identify the allergen against which allergen-specific IgE antibodies (sIgE) have been produced by the immune system [9, 10]. In vivo methods include skin testing and oral, parenteral, or organ-specific provocation tests (Table 1). A positive test indicates the presence of surface-bound sIgEs either on skin and tissue mast cells in the case of skin testing and organ-specific provocations respectively or on basophils and tissue mast cells in the case of oral and parenteral provocation tests. This chapter focuses on skin testing and on oral food challenge (OFC) and nasal (NPT) and drug provocation tests as indicative examples of the in vivo testing procedures commonly used for the diagnosis of IgE-mediated diseases.

2 The Skin as a Site of In Vivo Allergy Diagnostics

2.1 The Skin Response to Histamine and Allergens

The skin is the largest and most easily accessible organ of the human body, serving multiple vital functions through its complexity. Among the numerous cell types, cutaneous mast cells are relatively abundant, their density in normal skin being approximately

7000–10,000 cells/mm^3 [4, 5, 11]. The best-studied mechanism of mast cell activation and the most relevant to the allergic response is mediated through the surface membrane high affinity IgE receptor FcεRI that is stabilized upon IgE binding [4, 5, 12]. Briefly, when a multivalent allergen binds to the FcεRI-bound sIgE, the resulting receptor aggregation initiates a chain of events that leads to the release of mediators, including histamine and tryptase. The actions of histamine and other mediators on the skin are immediate and detectable, thus forming the basis for skin testing for IgE-mediated conditions [9].

Released or introduced histamine into the skin causes an immediate reaction characterized by increased vascular permeability that leads to the formation of a wheal (an evanescent swelling of the skin), and to neural reflex vasodilation that results in flare development (ring of pink erythema). During allergy skin testing, a similar immediate "wheal and flare" reaction is observed, starting approximately 5 min after the introduction of an allergen into the skin, attributed to the degranulation of cutaneous mast cells [9]. The neurogenic mediator substance P, most likely released by histamine from axonal reflexes, contributes to the response by enhancing the reaction *via* positive feedback. Occasionally, a subsequent late phase response reflecting the putative persistent IgE allergic inflammatory milieu is observed 1–2 h after the introduction of the allergen, subsiding within 48 h [13].

Skin testing is the oldest in vivo method that is commonly used for the detection of sIgE against an allergen. It is considered the diagnostic cornerstone for allergies due to its biological relevance, reproducibility, convenience, simplicity, easiness, and rapidness. The introduction of an allergen into the skin of an allergic subject and the resulting immediately observed and measured effects form the basis for the use of skin testing as a surrogate approach for the detection of IgE sensitization. Depending on the method of allergen insertion into the skin, the two main skin tests for immediate hypersensitivity are the skin prick test (SPT) and the intradermal (IDT) or intracutaneous test [14].

2.2 Skin Prick Test (SPT)

SPT is a simple, reliable, quick, and relatively safe method used to identify the presence of sIgE to protein and peptide antigens on the surface of cutaneous mast cells, primarily in IgE-mediated allergic conditions, including allergic rhinoconjuctivitis, asthma, food and latex allergy, and DHRs (Table 2) in adults and children from birth onward [14–17]. SPT involves the introduction of manufactured allergenic extracts into the epidermis skin without inducing bleeding, using a small lancet with a tip. SPTs are also used in some rarer conditions where sIgE might have a pathogenic role, such as eosinophilic esophagitis, in allergic bronchopulmonary aspergillosis, in screening for predisposition to develop atopic diseases, in epidemiological studies and birth cohorts and in preclinical research protocols [18–20].

Table 2
Indications for performing skin prick tests (SPTs)

– Allergic rhinitis, conjuctivitis, rhinoonjuctivitis[a]
– Asthma
– Immediate reactions to food[b]: anaphylaxis, urticaria, acute aggravation of atopic dermatitis
– Insect allergy (Hymenoptera venom allergy)[c]
– Type I hypersensitivity reactions to drugs[c]
– Some types of occupational allergies (e.g., latex allergy[d])

[a]Specificity: 70–95 %, sensitivity 80–97 %
[b]Specificity: 20–60 %, sensitivity: 30–70 %
[c]Only as first step, prior to the main diagnostic intradermal tests
[d]Specificity 100%, sensitivity 93%

2.2.1 Allergen Extracts for SPTs

Allergen extracts utilized for SPTs in respiratory, food, and insect venom allergies are specifically manufactured for this application (e.g., Alk-Abelló, Denmark; Hollister-Stier USA). They are usually solutions of proteins prepared by aqueous extraction of natural allergenic source materials. Glycerol is used as a preservative and contributes to the viscosity of the solution. Venoms are supplied as lyophilized powder to be reconstituted in diluent containing pasteurized human serum albumin (HSA) as a stabilizing agent (e.g., Pharmalgen®, Alk-Abelló, Denmark; Venomil®, Hollister-Stier, USA). Importantly, allergen extracts are stored under controlled conditions, usually at 2–8 °C, and are not left extensively at room temperature.

Being complex mixtures, the allergen extract quality depends on the quality of the source material and on processing, extraction, and storage conditions. Extracts standardized by appropriate biological or in vitro methods should be used whenever possible to ensure allergenic potency or inclusion of adequate concentration of major allergens. However, standardization is performed by in-house methods or by comparison to a U.S. reference standard for potency, thus standardized extracts from different manufacturers are not equipotent. Therefore, extracts from the same manufacturer should be used when direct comparison of the results is desired, as for instance before and after immunotherapy [21, 22].

In addition to the allergen solutions, negative and positive controls are always tested in order to identify hypo- or hyper-reactive skin and to reliably interpret the results. Normal saline or glycerinated HSA serve as the negative control, whereas histamine is commonly used as the positive control. Alternatively, codeine phosphate [9 % (w/v)], causing mast cell degranulation, can also be used [23].

Inhalant Allergens (Aeroallergens)

The panel of allergens tested is relevant to the clinical condition and the exposure pattern. For inhalant allergens, the panel is determined by the geographical region (Table 3), since different species can be clinically important in different parts of the world [23–25]. Local differences are always considered, an indicative example being the extended panel of allergens in the Eastern Mediterranean largely due to the rich flora of the area (Table 4).Moreover,

Table 3
Suggested panel of allergens tested in all patients in Europe (modified from the suggestion of the Global Allergy and Asthma European Network) [23] and important inhaled allergens in North America (suggested by the Immunotherapy Committee and the Allergen Subcommittee of the American Academy of Allergy Asthma and Immunology) [24]

	Europe	North America
Pollen: trees	Birch (*Betula verucosa*) or mixed Betulaceae Plane (*Platanus occidentalis*) Olive (*Olea europaea*) or ash (*Fraxinus exelsior*) Cypress (*Cupressus sempervirens*) or other cypress pollen species	Paper birch (Betula papyrifera) Sycamore/plane (*Platanus occidentalis*) Olive (*Olea europaea*) and white ash (*Fraxinus americana*) Mountain cedar (*Juniperus ashei*) Oaks (white oak, *Quercus alba*; red oak, *Q. rubra*) Elms (elm, *Ulmus americana*; Chinese elm, *U. parvifolia*; Siberian elm, *U. pumila*) Maples (boxelder maple, *Acer negundo*; red maple, *A. rubra* Alder (*Alnus rubra*) Eastern cottonwood (*Populus deltoides*) Black walnut (*Juglans nigra*) Mulberry (*Moras rubra*) Pecan (*Carya illinoensis*)
Pollen: grasses	One species (i.e., *Lolium perenne* or *Phleum pretense*) or mixed grass pollens	Rye (*Lolium perenne*) Timothy grass (*Phleum pretense*) Meadow fescue (*Festuca elatior*) Bermuda grass (*Cynodon dactylon*) Johnson (*Holcus halepensis*) Bahia (*Paspalum notatum*)
Pollen: weeds	Ragweed (*Ambrosia eliator*) Mugwort (*Artemisia vulgaris*) Wall pellitory (*Parietaria officinalis*)	Ragweed (*Ambrosia artemisiifolia*) Mugwort (*Artemisia vulgaris*) English (narrow leaf) plantain (*Plantago lanceolata*) Russian thistle (*Salsola kali*) Burning bush (*Kochia scoparia*) Sheep (common, red) sorrel (*Umex asetosella*) Red root pigweed (*Amaranthus retroflexus*)

(continued)

Table 3
(continued)

	Europe	North America
Moulds	*Alternaria alternata* *Cladosporium album* *Aspergillus fumigatus*[a]	*Alternaria alternata* *Cladosporium* *Aspergillus fumigatus* *Penicillium* (*P. chrysogenum*, *P. expansum*) *Epicoccum nigrum* *Drechslera*
Mites	*Dermatophagoides farinae* *Dermatophagoides pteronyssinus*	*Dermatophagoides farinae* *Dermatophagoides pteronyssinus*
Animals	Cat (*Felix domesticus*) Dog (*Canis familiaris*)	Cat (*Felix domesticus*) Dog (*Canis familiaris*)
Insects	Cockroach (*Blatella* sp.)	Cockroach (*Blatella* sp.)

[a]Not available in all European countries

Table 4
Recommended extended panel of allergens in the Eastern Mediterranean area

Pollen: trees	Olive (*Olea europaea*) Cypress (*Cupressus sempervirens*) Plane (*Platanus occidentalis*) Hazel (*Coryllus avellana*) Oak (*Quercus robur*) Beech (*Fagus sylvatica*) Poplar (*Populus alba*)
Pollen: grasses	Single species (*Lolium perenne* or *Phleum pratense*) or mixed grass pollens Bermuda grass (*Cynodonton dactylon*)[a]
Pollen: weeds	Wall pellitory (*Parietaria officinalis*) Dandelion (*Taraxacum officinale*) Plantain (*Plantago*) Mugwort (*Artemisia vulgaris*) Fat hen (*Chenopodium album*) Russian thistle (*Salsola kali*)
Molds	*Alernaria alternata* *Cladosporium album* *Aspergillus* mix *Penicillium* mix
Dust mites	*Dermatophagoides pteronyssinus* *Dermatophagoides farinae*
Animals	Cat (*Felix domesticus*) Dog (*Canis familiaris*)
Insects	Cockroach (*Blatella* sp.)

[a]Reduced cross-reactivity with temperate-pasture grasses

additional or alternative aeroallergens are clinically important in specific areas, such as, for instance, the pecan tree (*Carya illinoensis*) in Israel [26], *Blomia tropicalis* in tropical regions [27], and Japanese cedar (*Cryptomeria japonica*) in Eastern Asia [28].

Food Allergens

In contrast to most aeroallergens, food extracts are not generally standardized and may be of lower quality due to the variable protein content of source materials and the enzymatic degradation of proteins during manufacturing or storage [29]. Commercial extracts of animal origin (e.g., hen's egg or cod fish) are generally of better quality, whereas reagents with purified proteins have also become available [30]. As a result of the poor outcome obtained with some food extracts, the prick-to-prick technique is commonly employed using material from raw or cooked foods, as a supplementary or alternative method. The prick-to-prick test is a SPT variant that is particularly useful when a relevant commercial extract is not available or when labile or unstable allergens may be involved in the allergic reaction under investigation, as it is the case of the oral allergy syndrome to fruits and vegetables [31].

SPTs for DHRs

Immediate DHRs refer to reactions occurring within 1–6 h after the last drug administration and are not a synonym to IgE-mediated drug allergy. The underlying mechanism is not always identifiable and, therefore, a clinical classification of DHRs is preferred (Table 5). In case of immediate, possibly drug-related symptoms, SPTs and IDTs are recommended (*see* **Note 1**), especially for penicillins and cephalosporins [32]. Positive skin tests are often obtained for muscle relaxants, insulin, protamine, heparin, streptokinase, platinum salt chemotherapeutic agents, such as carboplatin and oxaliplatin [15] and biologics, such as infliximab [33].

Standardized skin test reagents for drugs are commercially available only for penicillins [benzylpenicilloyl poly-L-lysine (PPL) and minor determinant mixture (MDM); Diater SA, Spain]. For

Table 5
Classification of drug hypersensitivity reactions (DHRs) [56]

Immediate DHRs (within 1–6 h after last drug administration)	Urticaria/angioedema, rhinitis, conjunctivitis, bronchospasm, gastrointestinal symptoms (nausea, vomiting, diarrhea, abdominal pain), anaphylaxis, anaphylactic shock
Non-immediate DHRs (these reactions accu rat least 1 h after the initial drug administration)	Delayed urticaria, maculopapular eruptions, fixed drug eruption, vasculitis, Stevens–Johnson syndrome and toxic epidermal necrolysis (TEN), drug reaction with eosinophilia and systemic symptoms (DRESS), acute generalized exanthematous pustulosis and symmetrical drug-related intertriginous and flexural exanthemas; internal organs can be affected either alone or with cutaneous symptoms (DRESS, vasculitis) and include hepatitis, renal failure, pneumonitis, anemia, neutropenia, thrombocytopenia

most drugs, the reagents used for SPTs are solutions or suspensions of parenteral or oral formulations (e.g., tablets, capsules) (Table 6), validation of the appropriate non-irritant concentrations being an ongoing effort [34]. A drug solution/suspension of an oral formulation is prepared by dissolving the tablet or capsule content in normal saline (e.g., 500 mg in 10 ml) at room temperature and the maximum achievable drug concentration is used.

Table 6
Concentrations of β-lactam antibiotics and other selected common drugs used for skin testing (modified from [33])

Drug	SPT	IDT	
β-Lactam antibiotics	Concentration		
Minor determinants	2×10^{-2} mM	2×10^{-2} mM	
Penicilloyl-poly-L-lysine	5×10^{-5} mM	5×10^{-5} mM	
Benzylpenicillin	10,000 IU	10,000 IU	
Amoxicillin	20 mg/ml	20 mg/ml	
Ampicillin	20 mg/ml	20 mg/ml	
Cefuroxime (and most cephalosporins)	2 mg/ml	2 mg/ml	
Anti-inflammatory and analgesic agents			
Aspirin, Diclofenac, Ibuprofen, Mefenamic acid, Meloxicam, Naproxen, Nimesulide	Powder or 1 mg/ml (injectable formulation)	0.1 mg/ml	
Coxibs (Celecoxib, Etoricoxib)	Powder	Not applicable	
Paracetamol and other pyrazolones	Powder	0.1 mg/ml	
Platinum salts			
Carboplatin	10 mg/ml	1 mg/ml	
Oxaliplatin	1 mg/ml	0.1 mg/ml	
Cisplatin	1 mg/ml	0.1 mg/ml	
Monoclonal antibodies			
Adalimumab	50 mg/ml	50 mg/ml	
Infliximab	10 mg/ml	10 mg/ml	
Etanercept	25 mg/ml	5 mg/ml	
Omalizumab	1.25 μg/ml	0.00125 mg/ml	
Perioperative drugs	Maximum concentration	Dilution	Maximum concentration
Atracurium	1 mg/ml	1/1000	0.01 mg/ml

(continued)

Table 6 (continued)

Drug	SPT	IDT	
Cis-Atracurium	2 mg/ml	1/100	0.02 mg/ml
Vecuronium	4 mg/ml	1/10	0.4 mg/ml
Pancuronium	2 mg/ml	1/10	0.2 mg/ml
Suxamethonium	10 mg/ml	1/500	0.1 mg/ml
Midazolam	5 mg/ml	1/10	0.5 mg/ml
Fentanyl	0.05 mg/ml	1/10	0.005 mg/ml
Sufentanil	0.005 mg/ml	1/10	0.0005 mg/ml
Morphine	10 mg/ml	1/1000	0.01 mg/ml
Thiopental	25 mg/ml	1/10	2.5 mg/ml
Propofol	10 mg/ml	1/10	1 mg/ml
Etomidate	2 mg/ml	1/10	0.2 mg/ml
Midazolam	5 mg/ml	1/10	0.5 mg/ml
Ketamine	10 mg/ml	1/10	1 mg/ml
Other agents	Dilution	Dilution	Concentration
Local anaesthetics	Undiluted	1/10	
Iodinated contrast media	Undiluted	1/10	
Heparins and heparinoids	Undiluted	1/10	
Gadolinium derivatives	Undiluted	1/10	
Fluorescein	Undiluted	1/10	
Proton pump inhibitors	Undiluted		40 mg/ml

Testing starts with the minimum concentration and after reading 15–20 min later, tenfold higher concentrations are used until a positive response is observed. When literature and/or experience are lacking, the non-irritant drug concentration is ideally established in 5–10 healthy controls using different dilutions of increasing drug concentration. If possible, instead of the commercial formulations, the active compounds and the excipients should be tested.

2.2.2 Materials for SPTs

- Appropriate allergen extracts (*see* Sect. 2.2.1).
- Sterile single head metal lancet (e.g., Prick Lancet, Stallergenes, France; SPT Lancet, ALK, Denmark) (*see* **Note 2**).
- Histamine dihydrochloride (10 mg/ml; Alyostal Prick, Stallergenes, France) as a positive control.

- Normal saline [0.9% (w/v) NaCl] or glycerinated HSA [50 % (w/v)] as a negative control.
- Transparent ruler marked in mm (preferably circular to quickly assess diameter or caliper).
- Marker pen suitable for marking skin (ball point or felt).
- Alcohol swabs or gauze and alcohol.
- Tissue paper.
- Sharps disposal container.
- Timer with alarm.
- Cellophane tape (optional; to keep a traced copy of the wheal and flare response).
- Flow sheet.
- Medication and equipment for managing allergic reactions (*see* Sect. 4).
- Additional materials for the prick-to-prick test [29] include:
- Food to be tested.
- Single-use food containers.
- Suitable equipment for food slicing and crashing.
- Normal saline (for crushed nuts or other hard solid foods that need to be turned into paste).

2.2.3 Procedure for Performing SPTs

1. The contraindications and the risk, danger and SPT-related factors are considered [35–39] (*see* **Notes 3–4**; Table 7). The subject is advised to have discontinued any interfering medication (Table 8) [25, 29, 39].
2. The procedure is explained to the individual, including possible risks and side effects [40, 41] (*see* **Note 4**).Written informed consent is obtained; intravenous access is established when serious systemic reactions are likely to occur [access to emergency equipment and medication should be available (Fig. 1, Sect. 4)].
3. The number of required SPTs is determined and the order of placement on the skin is planned. For example, cross-reactive pollens are not included in the panel in the case of younger children and infants, where space is limited. Maintaining the same reagent order in all patients renders the test quicker and safer, avoiding potential mix-ups.
4. The tests are performed on healthy clean skin, free of daily care skin products (e.g., emollient, cream, soap). The site for SPTs is commonly the volar surface of the forearm or, if necessary, the upper back depending on the number of SPTs, the co-operation, and age of the subject and the condition of the skin. The reactivity to the allergens is more notable on the upper

Table 7
Factors affecting the skin response to skin prick (SPTs) and intradermal (IDTs) tests that may lead to false-negative or positive results [47–50]

Negative	Positive
– Medication (*see* Table 8) – Technical issues (e.g., no or weak pricking (SPTs); subcutaneous injection (IDTs); inappropriate test site) – Low potency allergen extracts (SPTs) – Chronic illness (e.g., chronic renal failure, cancer); neurological disorders (e.g., diabetic neuropathy, spinal cord injury) – Recent anaphylaxis to the tested allergen[a] – Chronic or acute UV-B radiation of the test site – Age (infants; elderly)	– Dermatographism – Technical issues [e.g., spread of allergen extracts; tests too close (SPTs); intracutaneous bleeding (IDTs)] – Impurities or substances in the allergen extracts causing mast cell degranulation (SPTs)[b]; irritant concentrations (IDTs) – Infection (e.g., respiratory syncytial virus infection)

[a]It is generally recommended to withhold skin testing to insect venoms, food, and drugs for 4–6 weeks after an episode of anaphylaxis, if possible [50]

[b]Raw foods (tomatoes, strawberries, spices, citrus fruits) may have high content of biogenic amines or nonspecific histamine release properties. For the reliable interpretation of the results, testing control subjects with the same materials is recommended. SPTs with any available relevant commercial extract should be performed prior to testing with the raw material

Table 8
Recommended withdrawal period of selected drugs prior to skin testing (modified from [9, 25, 39])

Medication	Withdrawal period
Oral first generation H1 antihistamines	9 Days
Cyproheptadine	5 Days
Hydroxyzine, clemastine	3 Days
Others	
Oral second generation H_1 antihistamines	7 Days
Nasal or ophthalmic formulations of H_1-antihistamines	0
Nasal or inhaled corticosteroids	0
Topical corticosteroids (on test site)	1–3 Weeks depending on the potency[a]
Systemic steroids	0[b]
Omalizumab	4 Weeks
Tricyclic antidepressants	7 Days
Doxepin	2 Weeks
Imipramine	3 Days
Desipramine	
Leukotriene receptor antagonists	0
β-adrenergic agonists	0

(continued)

Table 8 (continued)

Medication	Withdrawal period
Theophylline	0
Topical calcineurin inhibitors	7 Days[a]
Cyclosporin A	0
Topical antihistamines	6 h
Topical capsaicin[c]	3 Weeks

[a]If withdrawal is not possible alternative test sites should be sought

[b]Oral steroids do not normally affect allergy skin prick or intradermal tests, since they do not affect histamine-induced vascular reactivity. Theoretically if administrated for a long period of time (i.e., months), they might compromise the result due to a possible decrease in the number of cutaneous mast cells and a subsequent decrease in the histamine content of the test site. Some authors propose the discontinuation of short-term (<10 days) high-dose (>50 mg prednisolone equivalent) systemic steroids for 1 week and long-term (>10 days) high-dose (>19 mg prednisolone equivalent) systemic steroids for 3 weeks (references). In the authors' experience even high-dose long-term (>10 days) systemic steroids have minimal effect on skin testing for IgE-mediated reactions

[c]Capsaicin abolishes only the associated flare and itch, but not the formation of wheal, therefore withdrawal is not considered an absolute necessity

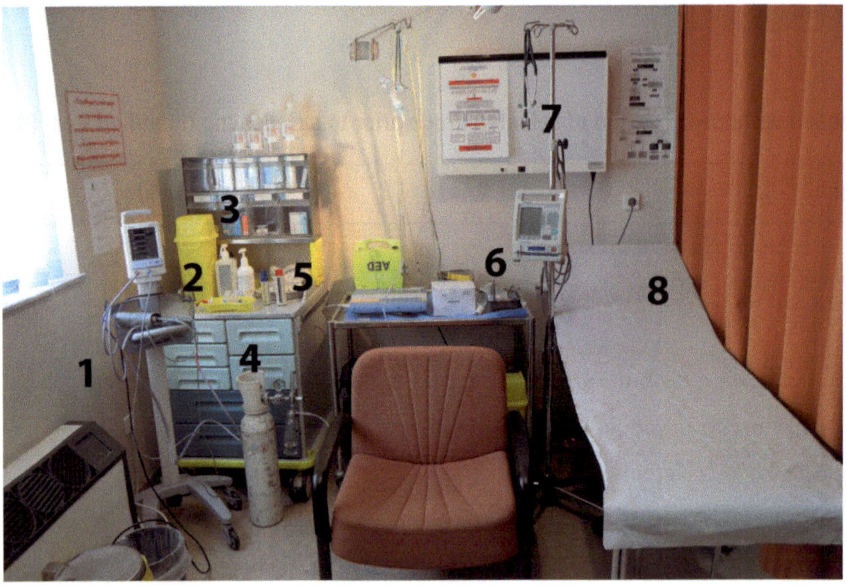

Fig. 1 Indicative equipment for managing anaphylactic reactions that may emerge during in vivo testing for allergic diseases. (1) Sphygmomanometer and pulse oxymeter; (2) tourniquet, syringes, intravenous catheters, and infusion set; (3) appropriate medication: aqueous epinephrine (adrenaline) HCl 1:1000 w/v, glucocorticosteroids for oral and intravenous administration, H_1-antihistamines for oral and intravenous administration, H_2-blockers for intravenous administration, fast-acting β2-agonists for inhalation, infusion solutions (saline/electrolyte solutions, colloidal solutions); (4) equipment to administer oxygen (oxygen supply, oxygen mask/goggles); (5) peak expiratory flow meter (for asthma patients); (6) stethoscope; (7) equipment to maintain an airway appropriate for the supervising physician's expertise and skill; (8) facilities for hospitalization and extension of strict observation period as needed

back than on the forearm, whereas less notable reactivity is observed on the lower back and close to the wrist [42]. When applied at the forearm, the reagents are placed more than 5 cm above the wrist and 3 cm below the antecubital fossa.

5. If the SPTs are to be performed on the forearms, the subject is asked to sit comfortably at a desk facing the investigator; with the arms on the desk so that the volar surface of the forearm is easily accessible. If the site of application is the back, the subject is asked to remove the upper garments and lie down on the examination table. Infants remain seated/held on the lap of the parent or the carer holding firmly their arms (alternatively the upper back could be chosen as the testing site).
6. The reagents to be tested are taken out of the refrigerator (for testing fresh food *see* **Note 5**).
7. The skin is cleaned with alcohol and allowed to dry (in case of dry skin or areas with eczema this step is omitted).
8. The spots where the negative and positive controls and each allergen extract are to be placed are marked with a suitable pen using numbers or appropriate abbreviations for each extract (Fig. 2). Alternatively, a cellophane tape may be used with printed numbers at appropriate points or a test grid. The marks are placed at least 2 cm apart. A double row of SPTs can be performed on each arm in most cases and both arms can be used (Fig. 2). It is common practice to use the area in outer upper arm for controls, especially if multiple allergens are to be tested.

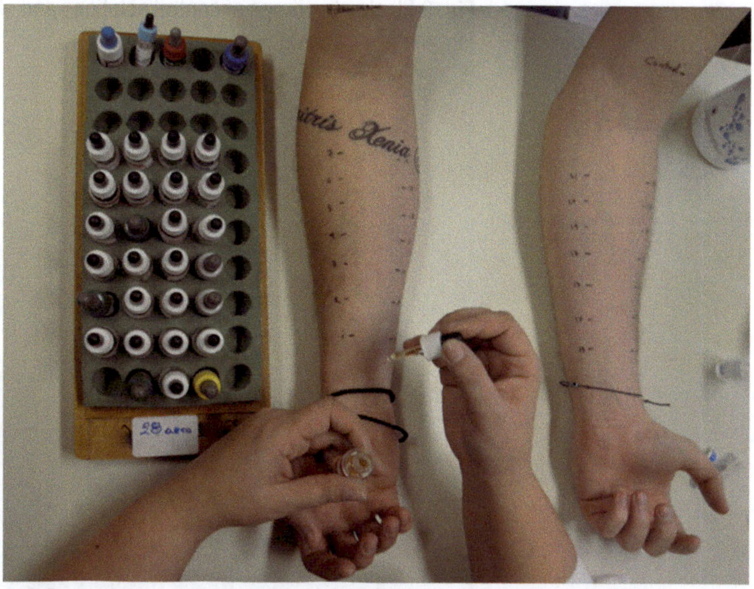

Fig. 2 Preparation and marking of the forearm for skin prick testing

9. The date, plan, and details of the investigator, the patient, and the allergens to be tested are checked on the flow sheet and confirmed.
10. The subject is asked to remain still to avoid cross contamination.
11. A drop of the negative and positive control solutions and of each allergen extract to be tested is placed adjacent to the respective marks using the dropper of the reagent bottle without the tip touching the skin (Fig. 3) (for testing fresh food *see* **Note 5**).
12. A single-head lancet is pressed vertically to the skin (Fig. 4) for 1 s through each drop of allergen extract [43, 44] so that it penetrates the epidermis and upper layer of dermis without

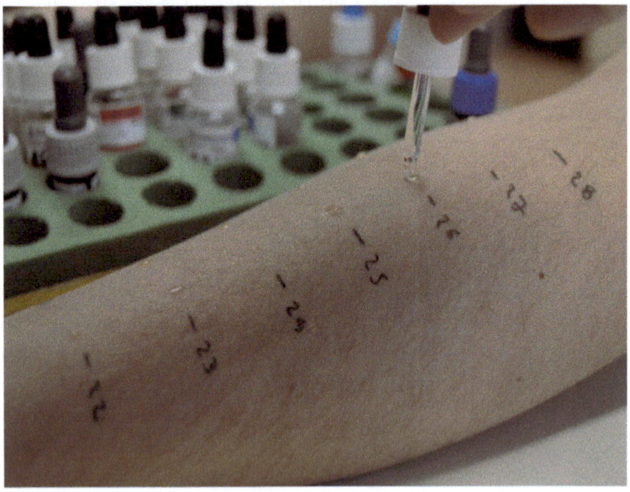

Fig. 3 Placing the drops of control solutions and allergen extracts on the forearm for skin prick testing

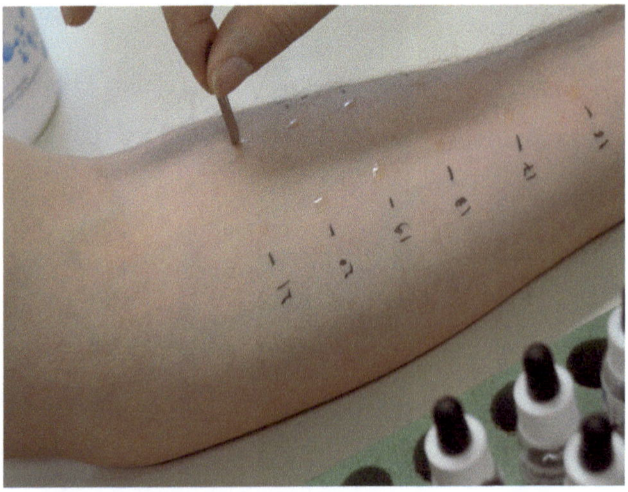

Fig. 4 Pricking through the drops of allergen extracts during skin prick testing

inducing bleeding (*see* **Note 2**). The alternative prick and lift technique, where the lancet (or a needle) is inserted at a low angle and then gently lifted upward to lift part of the epidermis without inducing bleeding, is not recommended as greater result variability is observed. For non-cooperative patients and infants, a set or even one allergen extract is placed on the skin and pricked before proceeding to the next set.

13. Following pricking through each drop of allergen extract, the lancet is discarded. Wiping the lancet with an alcoholic pad and reusing it for pricking through more than one allergen extract increases the risk of injury, carry-over effects, and false-positive results [45].
14. Upon completion of all SPTs, the excess test solutions are blotted by placing a clean tissue vertically onto the skin, pressing gently, and removing vertically without wiping the skin to avoid cross-contamination.
15. The subject is directed not to touch or cover the area until the end of the procedure.
16. The allergen extracts are returned to the storage place.
17. Fifteen minutes after each prick (the use of an alarm timer is strongly advised) the wheal formed on the skin is outlined with a pen under good light conditions (Fig. 5). The size of the wheal is measured in mm using a ruler either directly on the skin or on a recording sheet after blotting the wheal on a cellophane tape (the histamine reaction peaks at 10 min but it continues to be observable at 15 min). The longest wheal diameter (preferably) or the calculated mean diameter is recorded [46].

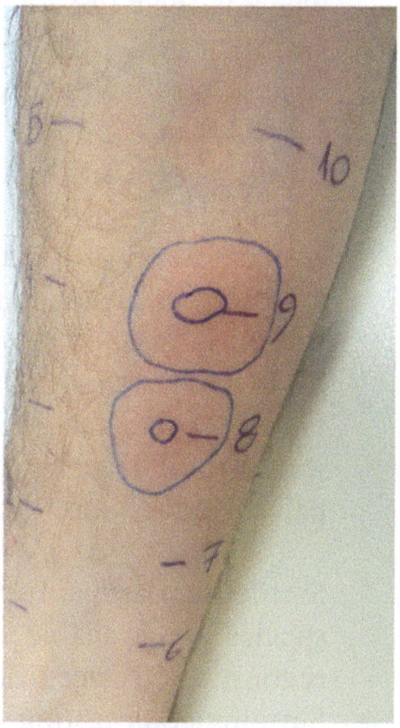

Fig. 5 Recording the skin response in skin prick testing

Any pseudopods that may have arisen are disregarded. The formation of a wheal of ≥3 mm in diameter than the negative control is considered a positive result [39]. If the wheal of the negative control is >3 mm in diameter, the results are evaluated and skin testing is contraindicated.

18. Marks on the skin are removed using an alcohol tab (dry skin might become irritated by alcohol).
19. The subject is monitored for 30 min, especially in the presence of uncontrolled asthma or other risk factors [36, 37] (*see* **Note 4**).
20. The interpretation of the outcome takes into consideration the detailed medical history and the physical examination of the patient as well as all possible factors that may influence the SPT results (Table 8) [47–50].

2.3 Intradermal Tests (IDTs)

IDTs are generally indicated for testing insect venom allergy and immediate DHRs when a parenteral drug formulation is available [34, 51]. Concerning IgE-mediated DHRs, validated in vitro tests are lacking, with the exception of β-lactam antibiotics, and therefore skin testing is extremely important for the investigation of a suspicious reaction before resorting to provocation tests (*see* Sect. 3). However, the sensitivity of skin tests appears to be low for most drugs. In the case of β-lactam antibiotics, perioperative drugs, heparins, platinum salt chemotherapeutics (carboplatin, oxaliplatin), radio-contrast media, and some biologics (e.g., infliximab) skin tests appear to have a moderate to high sensitivity when using non-irritant concentrations that confer high specificity [34]. Additionally, IDTs are useful for the diagnosis of allergic bronchopulmonary aspergillosis by examining hypersensitivity to *Aspergillus* antigens, whereas their use for testing food allergens is not recommended and their value in aerollergen testing is hampered by the high rate of false-positive results [52].

IDTs are performed after the respective STPs and involve injection of a small amount of allergen (0.02–0.05 ml) into the dermis. If no reaction is observed in SPT, the IDT starts at a lower concentration of the allergen and if negative, the concentration is increased in logarithmic steps until the final non-irritating concentration is reached or until a clear reaction is elicited. In general, IDTs carry a slightly higher risk of systemic allergic reactions and fatalities occur mostly in asthmatic patients who had not been subjected to SPTs prior to IDTs. Moreover, IDTs are generally more painful and children tend not to cooperate well.

2.3.1 Allergen Reagents for IDTs

Hymenoptera Venom Extracts

Sterile standardized venom extracts from individual Hymenoptera species are available in the form of lyophilized powder that is reconstituted according to the manufacturer's instructions. Simultaneous testing of more than one Hymenoptera venom is safe [51]. Concentrations of 0.01–100 μg/ml are usually used for the SPT that precedes the IDT, whereas those of the IDT are 0.001–1 μg/ml with a tenfold increase at each sequential step, the sensitivity of 1 μg/ml being >90 %.

IDT Reagents for Testing DHRs

With the exemption of penicillins where specific standardized skin test reagents are commercially available, sterile tenfold dilutions of the parenteral drug solutions are used for IDTs. Water for injection is not used as a diluent as it can be irritant, false-positive reactions, whereas the reported use of non-injectable drug preparations (e.g., capsule powder, tablets) for IDTs is not recommended [53]. Similarly to SPTs, the maximum non-irritant concentration of solutions used in IDTs has been published for selected drug classes (Table 6) but for most drugs data are still lacking (*see* **Note 1**).

2.3.2 Materials for IDTs

All materials are the same as those required for SPTs (*see* Sect. 2.2.2) with the exception of allergen solutions being prepared in sterile containers and the sterile single-head metal lancet being needed only for the positive control (*see* **Note 6**). Additional materials include examination gloves and sterile 1 ml syringes with 26–30-gauge needles, clearly labeled with the name and the concentration of the allergen.

2.3.3 Procedure for Performing IDTs

1. The contraindications and risk, danger, and IDT-related factors are considered (*see* **Notes 1, 3, 4**; Table 7). The subject is advised to have discontinued any interfering medication (Table 8).
2. Appropriate dilutions of the solutions to be used are prepared and syringes are prefilled with 0.05 ml.
3. The procedure is explained to the subject, including possible risks and side effects (*see* **Note 4**). Written informed consent is obtained and intravenous access is established when serious systemic reactions are likely to occur [access to emergency equipment and medication should be available (Fig. 1, Sect. 4)].
4. The maximum number of IDTs that might be required is calculated and the order in which they are to be performed is planned.
5. The testing site on the forearms is determined according to the number of IDTs to be performed and the condition of the skin. The sites for the negative and positive controls as well as for each IDT are marked with a waterproof pen using numbers or the name of the allergen and the respective concentration. The marks are placed more than 5 cm above the wrist and 3 cm below the antecubital fossa and at least 3 cm apart. In case of multiple IDTs (e.g., β-lactam allergy), two rows of IDTs can be performed on each arm and both arms can be used (a constant order is advisable for the same IDTs performed in different subjects on the same day).

6. The date, plan, and details of the investigator, the patient, and the allergens to be tested are checked on the flow sheet and confirmed.
7. All necessary equipment is optimally placed within the reach of the investigator. The investigator washes the hands and wears examination gloves.
8. The subject is asked to sit comfortably at a desk facing the investigator with the arms on the desk, so that the volar surface of the forearm is easily accessible. For infants and children the approach to the examination is determined by their age, level of development, and understanding.
9. The skin is cleansed with an alcohol swab by wiping with a firm circular motion outward from the injection site. The skin is allowed to dry and the subject is asked to remain still.
10. The injection of the prepared allergen solutions is performed by holding the syringe with the dominant hand and removing the needle cap with the non-dominant hand. The skin is pulled with the non-dominant hand and kept stretched over the injection site. The needle is placed nearly in parallel to the skin (bevel side up) and inserted so as the point is seen through the skin. A small volume of the allergen solution (0.02–0.05 ml, usually 0.03 ml) is slowly injected while watching for a small (approximately 3 mm) wheal or bleb to appear (Fig. 6).The needle is then withdrawn at the same angle as it was inserted. If a bleb fails to appear, the procedure is repeated after 20 min has elapsed to avoid increased allergen exposure that might cause a systemic allergic reaction.

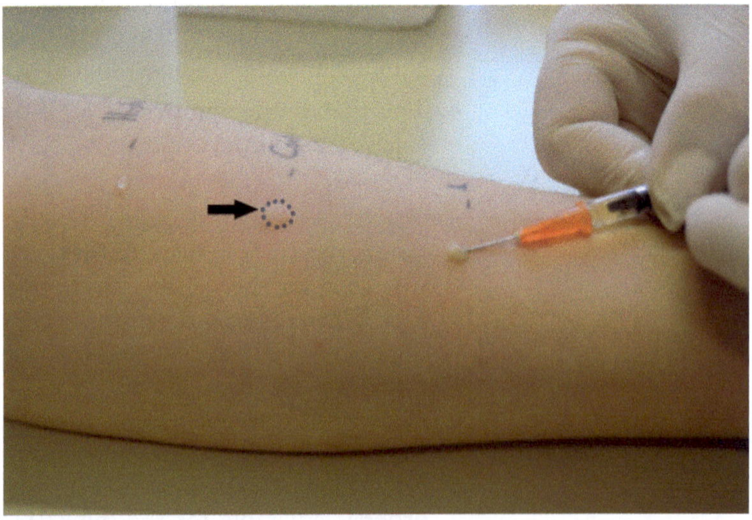

Fig. 6 Performing an intradermal test. The *arrow* indicates the marked borders of the bleb

11. The needle and syringe are discarded in the disposal container.
12. The borders of the bleb are marked with the pen (Fig. 6).
13. The injection of the negative control is performed as described for the allergen solutions in steps 10–12 above.
14. The positive control is performed by SPT as described in **steps 10–14** of Sect. 2.2.3 (*see* **Note 6**).
15. The timer is set at 20 min and the patient is asked not to touch or cover the test area until the end of the procedure.
16. After 20 min, the wheal of the positive control (*see* **step 18** of Sect. 2.2.3) and the borders of the IDT edema are marked with a pen under good light conditions (cross lighting the area, pressing lightly on the test site with a transparent ruler, or gently stretching the skin of the test site may help in defining the borders).
17. The size of the wheals is measured either directly on the skin or on the flow sheet after blotting the wheal on a cellophane tape and transcribing it onto the sheet. The two longest perpendicular wheal diameters are measured with the ruler and the mean is calculated and recorded as a single figure in mm. The test is considered positive when the diameter of the initially formed bleb (*see* **step 12** above) increases by ≥3 mm after 20 min and is associated with a flare.
18. The subject is monitored for 30 min, especially in the presence of uncontrolled asthma or other risk factors (*see* **Note 4**).

Notes

1. In non-immediate DHRs (e.g., maculopapular rush), patch tests and/or late readings of the IDT tests after 24, 48, and 72 h are recommended to investigate the putative implication of a T-cell-dependent mechanism. Systemic reactions following skin testing may also occur (*see* **Note 4**). Skin testing is not indicated or is not useful in other conditions where immunological responses to drugs occur; the value of skin tests in hematological (anemia, thrombocytopenia, leukopenia), renal (glomerulonephritis), or hepatic manifestations (hepatitis) has not been proven, and it is not considered to be helpful in autoimmune diseases (systemic lupus erythematosis, bullous pemphigoid, interstitial lung disease). IDTs are not performed in patients with Stevens-Johnson syndrome, toxic epidermal necrolysis, or leukocytoclastic vasculitis and have to be considered with caution in the drug rash with eosinophilia and systemic symptoms (DRESS) syndrome. Importantly, testing subjects without a prior DHR history is not supported by the available literature and, therefore, it is not recommended by any scientific society.

2. For highly reproducible and fewer false-negative results a single-head metal prick lancet is preferable to other available devices, such as plastic lancets that are associated with lower sensitivity, or multiple-headed lancets that are more painful and prick simultaneously multiple sites leading to increased result variability [43, 44]. The alternative use of an intravenous needle as the pricking device is not recommended due to difficulties in controlling skin penetration depth.
3. For drug testing, it is advised to perform the test 4–6 weeks after the reaction (similarly to food and insect venom anaphylaxis), but not later than the first few months after the reaction. If >6–12 months elapse, tests may be negative thus warranting further evaluation with IDT.
4. In general, SPTs are safe and well tolerated, although they may cause some discomfort mainly due to the wheal-associated itch. Local application of ice or a H_1-antihistamine per os might offer some relief, whereas topical corticosteroids are not indicated. IDTs are generally more painful. Although not very common, adverse events with skin testing may occur, especially when testing for food, latex, venoms, and medications associated with anaphylaxis. They are classified into non-allergic (syncope; near syncope; headache/malaise) [35], and allergic (progressive local late phase reactions; generalized allergic reactions) [36]. Commercially available aeroallergens rarely cause any systemic side effects. Increased risk for allergic reactions due to skin testing is noted in infants [40], active eczema [40], testing foods (especially fresh), latex, hymenoptera venoms or drugs in subjects with a history of anaphylaxis [25], testing when allergy symptoms are present (e.g., during the allergy season) [39], and elevated basal serum tryptase levels [41]. Skin testing is associated with increased danger in pregnant women and in patients with uncontrolled asthma [52] or under medication with β-blockers or/and angiotensin converting enzyme (ACE) inhibitors. Skin testing should be avoided during acute inflammatory illness, severe skin disease, severe dermographism, and/or intake of medications that affect the results of skin testing and cannot be withdrawn. Most systemic reactions occur within the first 30 min. Therefore, monitoring of patients for 30 min after skin testing is recommended [36, 37].
5. Skin reactivity varies depending on the variety, storage, and stages of fruit or vegetable [29]. The prick-to-prick variant may be used for testing fruits and vegetables, and other foods, such as milk, nuts, fish, and shellfish. Before starting the procedure, small pieces of the foods to be tested are cut and placed in separate single-use food containers. Most foods of animal origin (e.g., meat, fish) are cooked (boiled) prior to testing without the addition of any other ingredient. Foods that are especially

hard to prick (e.g., nuts) are crashed using a mortar and turned into paste with the addition of normal saline. To avoid cross-contamination, all equipment and surfaces used for the preparations should be clean. Pricking is similar to SPT, but a piece of food is pricked with an ordinary prick lancet immediately before pricking the skin with the same lancet. Alternatively, a small quantity of the food to be tested is placed on the skin and the skin is pricked through the food with a single move. Care should be taken to remove the excess of food that may increase the risk of systemic reactions in highly sensitized patients. A drop of fresh milk can be used directly on the skin as in SPTs.

6. Using a reported intracutaneous injection of 0.03 ml of 1 % (w/v) histamine as a positive control for IDTs is not recommended, since severe local reactions and itch, as well as anxiety, may occur. Instead, a SPT using histamine dihydrochloride as described in Sect. 2.2.3 is commonly used as the positive control for IDTs.

3 Allergen Provocation Tests

When first-line diagnostics, such as skin testing and ex vivo serum assays, fail to designate the causal association between an allergen and the experienced symptoms, allergen provocation tests under controlled conditions may be the only remaining option [54]. In addition to the diagnostic value, challenging an allergic individual with allergens has increased the understanding of allergic inflammation and tolerance induction and has verified the efficacy of therapeutic interventions, including biologics and allergen immunotherapy [54–56]. Allergen provocation tests are mostly utilized in allergic rhinitis, food allergy, and DHRs, thereby enhancing the diagnostic accuracy and the experimental approach to these pathologies [54]. Other organs, such as the eye or bronchial tree, can also be challenged with allergens, but their clinical or experimental use in humans is currently limited and is not discussed herein.

3.1 Nasal Provocation Test (NPT)

Allergic rhinitis and asthma have become a worldwide concern following the expansion of industrialization, urbanization, and the consequent adaptation of western lifestyle. Therefore, governments, health organizations, and pharmaceutical companies prioritized the development of preventive and therapeutic approaches to restrain this *allergy epidemic* [57–59]. Related research has largely focused on the nasal mucosa mainly due to its advantageous accessibility and less invasiveness for manipulation, examination, and investigation of biomarkers, mediators, and cells [60]. The nasal mucosa is the outermost part of the airways. Besides facilitating olfaction, it constitutes the first line of defense against inhaled particles and external insults. Defense mechanisms include sensory nerve activation and increased blood flow, glandular cell secretion, and vascular permeability that may cause pruritus and sneezing, congestion, and rhinorrhea [59, 60].

In allergic rhinitis, exposure of sensitized individuals to inhalant allergens induces IgE-mediated mast cell and basophil degranulation and release of proinflammatory mediators, such as histamine, leukotrienes, cytokines, and chemokines [4, 5, 59]. During the early phase, histamine released from mast cells leads to immediate symptoms, such as sneezing rhinorrhea and nasal congestion, whereas a late phase reaction is typically manifested as nasal congestion and mucosal hyperreactivity3–11 h after allergen exposure [58–60]. Nasal allergen provocations have proved to be valuable experimental and clinical tools (Table 9) and continue to provide insights into the pathophysiology of the early and late phases of allergic inflammation and into the actions and efficacy of pharmacologically active agents [54, 55, 59, 61–64]. Since the original attempt of Charles Blackley in 1873 to reproduce the symptoms of allergic rhinitis by introducing grass pollen grains into the nose [65], cold dry air and substances such as histamine and metacholine have been used to study nasal reactivity and neuronal hyper-responsiveness [66].

NPTs are a safe and relatively easy tool to investigate allergic rhinitis. They are conducted by trained personnel in a controlled environment and involve the application of progressively increasing allergen doses to the nasal mucosa through one or both nostrils [54, 55, 67]. Besides intrinsic nonspecific nasal hyper-reactivity and the potential nonspecific reactions due to preservatives [54], a limitation of NPTs arises from the false-negative results due to, for instance, the presence of chronic inflammation such as perennial allergy and the priming effect [68].

Table 9
Indications and contraindications for performing nasal provocation tests (NPTs) (modified from [69, 73])

Indications	Contraindications
– Evaluation of the clinical significance of a seasonal allergen upon multiple sensitizations to airborne allergens with overlapping seasons – Evaluation of perennial allergens when the duration of symptoms is unclear – Identification of the most significant allergens for allergen immunotherapy – Confirmation of local allergic rhinitis where the medical history is convincing but the skin and in vitro tests are negative – Confirmation of extranasal symptomatology after allergen exposure – Diagnosis of occupational rhinitis	– Severe lower airway obstruction (FEV1 <60 % of predicted value); uncontrolled asthma; acute rhinitis, sinusitis, or infection of the lower airways – History of severe cardiopulmonary diseases – Patients under treatment with beta-blockers or ACE inhibitors – History of anaphylaxis or significant angioedema to the tested allergen – Current nasal bleeding or recent nasal surgery – Pregnancy (NPTs are safe for breastfeeding women)

ACE angiotensin converting enzyme, *FEV1* forced expiratory volume in one second

3.1.1 Allergen Solutions for NPTs

In most cases, allergen solutions used for NPTs are commercially available allergen extracts that are specifically manufactured for this purpose (e.g., Leti provocation tests, Laboratorios Leti, Spain). However, different manufacturers use different units of allergen concentrations and there is no consensus on the standardization and quantification. Moreover, data on relative potency of the available extracts are lacking and, therefore, comparisons are not feasible [54]. Optimal concentrations may differ between allergens and are individualized for each allergen. If lyophilized, following reconstitution in diluent, 3–4 serial tenfold dilutions (1/1, 1/10, 1/100, 1/1000) are prepared according to the provided instructions. Typically, 0.5 ml is transferred to a vial containing 4.5 ml diluent using a sterile 1 ml syringe to prepare consecutive 1/10 dilutions. The date of reconstitution is marked on the vial since the reconstituted allergen extract maintained at 4 °C usually expires after 6 months.

3.1.2 Materials for NPTs

- Clearly marked vials containing solvent (e.g., monosodium phosphate dehydrate, sodium chloride, phenol, water for injection, human serum albumin) with nasal spray pump and sterile nozzles to prepare the tenfold dilutions of the reconstituted allergen extract (*see* Sect. 3.1.1) to be tested (*see* **Note 7**).
- A clearly marked vial containing the lyophilized allergen extract.
- Sterile 1 ml syringes with 25–27-gauge needles for preparing the diluted solutions.
- Vienna nasal specula [small, medium, and large size; e.g., MeisterHand, Integra® Miltex®, USA) and a light source (e.g., Heine K 100 otoscope, Heine Optotechnik, Germany).
- Youlten peak nasal inspiratory flow meter (Clement Clarke International, UK) with face masks (sizes 3–6) (Fig. 7).
- Spirometer (Jaeger® MasterScreen™, Pneumo, Viasys Healthcare, Germany) with plastic disposable mouthpieces.
- Rhinomanometer for anterior active rhinomanometry (AAR) (e.g., Jaeger® MasterScreen™, Pneumo, Viasys Healthcare, Germany) with facial masks (sizes 3–6) and disposable nose adapters of 12, 15, 18 mm diameter for rhinomanometry.
- Timer.
- Flow sheet.
- Medication and equipment for treating allergic reactions (Fig. 1, Sect. 4).

3.1.3 Procedure for Performing NPTs

1. The contraindications (Table 9) and the limitations are considered, including medication regimens (Table 10) (*see* **Notes 7–10**).
2. The subject receives information on the procedure, the benefits, and the possible risks (*see* **Note 10**). Written informed consent is obtained.

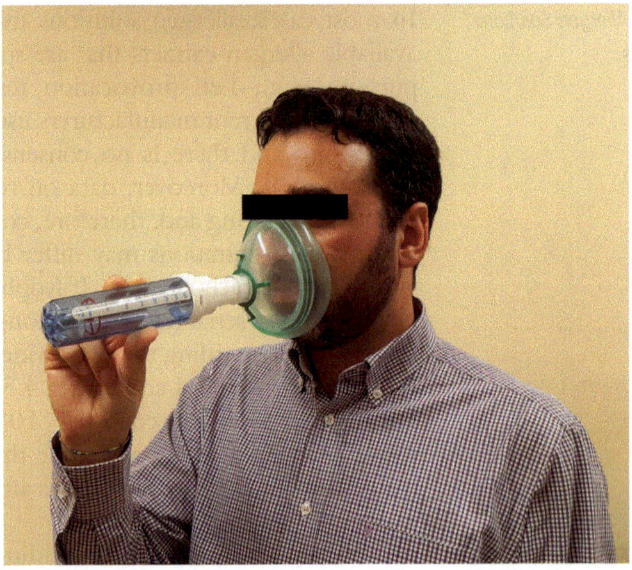

Fig. 7 Measurement of the peak nasal inspiratory flow (PNIF) using a Youlten peak nasal flow meter equipped with a facial mask to assess nasal obstruction and the response to nasal provocation

Table 10
Medications that may interfere with the interpretation of nasal provocation tests (NPTs) (modified from [69, 73])

Drug	Withdrawal period prior to NPTs
H_1-antihistamines	3 Days
Oral	3 Days
Nasal spray	2 Days
Eye drops	
Leukotriene antagonists	5 Days
Steroids	2 Weeks
Oral, intramuscular, intravenous	7 Days
Nasal	
Sodium cromoglycate, nedocromil (oral)	3 Days
Nasal decongestants	2 Days
Non-steroidal antinflammatory drugs	7 Days
Oral H_2 receptor antagonists	3 Days
Tricyclic antidepressants	3 Days

3. A clinical examination of the upper and lower airways (chest auscultation, peak expiratory flow rate, spirometry) and inspection of the anterior nasal cavity with a nasal speculum is performed regardless of the absence of any relevant medical history. The basal measurements of the forced expiratory volume in 1 s (FEV1), peak nasal inspiratory flow (PNIF), anterior active rhinomanometry (AAR), total nasal symptom score (TNSS), and visual analog scale (VAS) are obtained and recorded [69–71].
4. To exclude possible nonspecific nasal hyper-reactivity, nasal provocations begin with the deposition of the diluent (negative control) through the nasal pump to the nasal mucosa. The subject is asked to gently blow the nose and directed to bend the head forward. The nozzle of the nasal spray bottle containing the diluent is placed into the nostril with the best breathing ability. The nozzle tip points away from the septum and toward the unilateral eye (Fig. 8) in order for the solution to be delivered to the inferior and middle turbinate and not to reach the nasopharynx [72]. After allowing a deep breath in, the subject holds the breath and the nasal spray pump is pressed (*see* **Note 11**).
5. After 15 min, the PNIF, AAR, TNSS, and VAS are recorded [69–71, 73] (*see* **Note 12**).
6. When the negative control induces a response with TNSS ≥3, PNIF reduction by 15 %, or airflow reduction during AAR

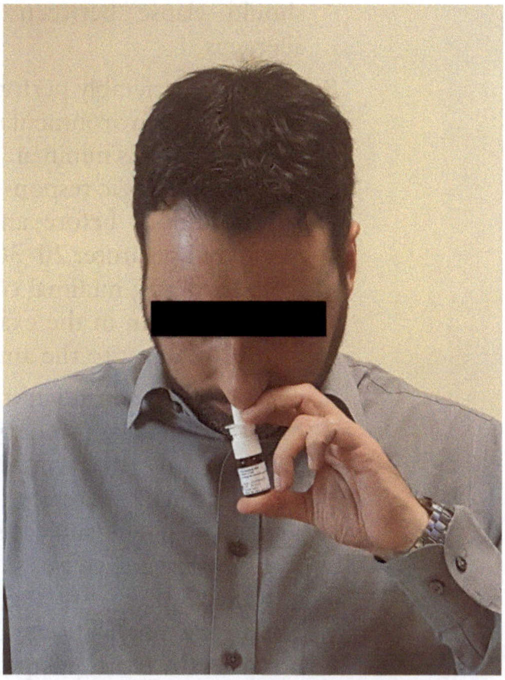

Fig. 8 Use of the nasal spray pump to deliver the allergen

>20 %, the testing is interrupted due to nasal hyper-reactivity and rescheduled.

7. If the negative control does not trigger any response, the administration of the allergen solutions is initiated. The patient is challenged with a dose of the 1/100 dilution by repeating **step 5** and assessed (**step 6**) being closely monitored (the 1/1000 dilution is normally reserved for highly sensitized patients). If no reaction occurs, the patient is challenged with a dose of the 1/10 dilution in the opposite nostril by repeating **step 5** and assessed (**step 6**). If the patient remains asymptomatic, **steps 5–6** are repeated using the original reconstituted solution (*see* Sect. 3.1.1). If no reaction occurs after testing the maximum allergen concentration, the procedure is terminated, a final spirometry is conducted and the patient is monitored for 30 min for safety reasons.
8. The NPT is considered positive and the procedure is concluded when the TNSS is ≥5, the PNIF is reduced by ≤40 % or the flow reduction in AAR under 150 Pa is >40 % [69–71, 73] (*see* **Note 12**).
9. In case of a positive nasal or bronchial reaction, the allergen is washed away by nasal rinsing with normal saline and the subject is treated accordingly (*see* **Note 13**).

Notes

7. Only a single allergen is tested per day. A period of 1 week should elapse between consecutive NPTs with different allergens.
8. NPTs are preferably performed in the morning when exposure to noxious environmental stimuli (e.g., pollution, tobacco smoke, odors) is minimal. To minimize the occurrence of nonspecific or allergic responses due to external factors, the ambient conditions before and during the NPT are controlled (room temperature: 20–30 °C; humidity: 40–60 %; protection from air drafts; minimal concentrations of airborne allergens). Patients remain in the examination room for 30 min prior to testing to adjust to the ambient conditions.
9. The detailed medical history of allergies, comorbidities, and medication intake (15 days prior to the test) by the patient are recorded. To avoid priming, NPTs are conducted at least 1 month after a respiratory tract infection and outside the pollen season [58]. The subject should have been advised to refrain from morning exercise, smoking, and consumption of alcohol at least 12 h prior to the test and to avoid taking potentially interfering medications (Table 10). If these conditions are not met, the test is postponed.

10. The possible adverse events of NPTs are bronchoconstriction (cough, dyspnea, wheezing), pruritus of the pharynx and the soft palate, edema of the uvula and the pharynx, urticaria, or anaphylaxis. The medication and the equipment for managing acute allergic reactions should be readily available (Fig. 1, Sect. 4).
11. The nasal spray pump is considered the most appropriate device for performing NPTs as it delivers evenly into the nasal mucosa a relatively consistent dose (70–100 μl) of the solution in the form of aerosol, whereas the risk of solution leakage to the pharynx is minimal. Alternative methods and devices include instillation into the inferior turbinate using a syringe or a micropipette and paper disks to introduce the allergen to the inferior turbinate [72]. The latter method allows the study of cells and mediators and is reserved for experimental purposes.
12. No single standardized method for evaluating symptoms, nasal airflow, and/or inflammation is available. Positivity criteria for NPTs are based on a relatively wide range of assessment approaches. A combination of subjective (TNSS, VAS) and objective (FEV1, PNIF, AAR) methods is considered the best approach to assess the responsiveness to nasal provocation [69]. Concerning symptom scoring, the TNSS is the most extensively used, whereas using VAS, mild, moderate, or severe responses correspond to marks between 0 and 30 mm, 40–70 mm, or 80–100 mm, respectively [70]. For PNIF with a modified Youlten meter equipped with a facial mask (Fig. 7), values of 100–300 l/min are considered normal, whereas the NPT is postponed when basal PNIF is <80 l/min.
13. Congestion is treated with a topical decongestant, while oral H_1-antihistamines are more appropriate for managing pruritus, sneezing, and rhinorrhea. For asthma, inhaled β-agonists and corticosteroids are first-line treatment options.

3.2 Oral Food Challenge (OFC)

Allergic reactions to foods range from mild to life threatening, whereas misdiagnosis, food avoidance, and incorrect nutritional replacement may lead to malnutrition [74, 75]. IgE-mediated food allergy is the most common and well-recognized form of food hypersensitivity characterized by rapid onset; usually within minutes to 2 h after exposure/ingestion of the offending food allergen [74]. The detailed allergy-focused clinical history of the patient is central to the identification of the potential food allergen [76–78]. Any implication of an IgE-mediated underlying mechanism is demonstrated by the presence of sIgE using ex vivo serum assays, SPTs, and prick-to-prick tests (*see* Sects. 2.2, 2.3 and **Note 5**). In case of inconclusive findings, the oral food challenge (OFC) is the relevant subsequent diagnostic approach (Table 11) [74, 76–81]. OFC involves ingestion of incremental doses of the suspected food over a specific period of time, normally under monitoring and

Table 11
Indications and contraindications for performing oral food challenge (OFC)

Indications	Contraindications
– Confirmation of food allergy diagnosis – Identification of the offending food (in case of multiple food consumption before the allergic reaction) – Monitoring and resolution of food allergy – Confirmation of oral tolerance to a food after prolonged avoidance – Assessment of tolerance status to cross reacting foods – Assessment of the effects of food processing on food tolerability (e.g., safe consumption of baked eggs by a subject with egg allergy) – Determination of the threshold dose of a causative food allergen – Determination whether food allergens associated with chronic conditions (e.g., atopic dermatitis) may cause immediate allergic reactions	– High probability of allergic reaction (as predicted by medical history and skin/serum sIgE testing) – Recent anaphylactic reaction to the offending food (e.g., after accidental exposure); time depending on food and age – Uncontrolled asthma; exacerbation of atopic dermatitis or allergic rhinitis – Acute illness (e.g., recent viral infection) – Conditions that may interfere with allergic reaction treatment (e.g., pregnancy) – Intake of medications that may interfere with interpretation of results (*see* Table 1) – Lack of an experienced trained physician; unavailable allergic reaction management tools (e.g., drugs)

supervision of a board-certified allergist [74, 82]. The procedure can be open, single-blind, or double-blind placebo-controlled (DBPCFD) food challenge based on the potential for bias in the interpretation of the results [78].

3.2.1 Food to Be Tested

Ideally, a single-ingredient food is used (*see* **Note 14**). For open OFCs, the food can be provided by the subject following detailed preparation instructions based on the sensitivity- and allergenicity-related properties of the food and the eating habits of the subject, whereas for blind OFCs the test material is preferably provided by a dietician [78]. When more than one OFC are being conducted in the same area, care should be taken to avoid cross-contamination with other foods. For placebo-controlled OFCs, any food known to be safe or a portion of the same texture, smell, taste, and color that is known to be tolerated by the subject is used to blind the challenge [78, 79].

3.2.2 Materials for OFC

- Safe, clean, and comfortable environment to perform the challenge.
- Clean bench for the preparation of the food doses.
- Flow sheet to record administered doses, symptoms, signs, and treatment, if required.
- Food to be tested.
- Placebo portion (for placebo-controlled OFCs).
- Single-use food containers.
- Plastic plates, cups, and utensils, measuring cups and spoons.

- Equipment suitable for slicing and crashing food (especially for nuts).
- Empty opaque capsules for placing food (for single-blinded OFCs in adults).
- Sterile 1, 5, and 10 ml syringes (for OFCs with liquid food).
- Precision scale (weighing capacity 200 g with 0.01 g readability).
- Microwave oven to warm food as needed.
- Equipment for establishing intravenous access (considered in high-risk patients).
- Medication and equipment for managing allergic reactions (Fig. 1, Sect. 4).

3.2.3 Procedure for Performing OFCs

1. Indications and contraindications are considered (Table 11); a thorough physical examination is conducted and any acute illness is excluded; pre-existing allergic conditions, such as bronchial asthma and atopic eczema, are controlled [82] and medications that might affect the OFC have been discontinued in due time (Table 12); the risks and benefits are discussed

Table 12
Medications that may interfere with the oral food challenge (OFC) (modified from [79])

Drug	Withdrawal period prior to OFCs
Oral H_1-antihistamines[a]	5–7 Days
H_1-antihistamines (nasal spray)[a]	12 h
Oral H_2 receptor antagonist	12 h
Antidepressants	3 Days–3 weeks
Oral/intramuscular/intravenous steroids[a]	3 Days–2 weeks
Leukotriene antagonist	24 h
Short-acting bronchodilator	8 h
Long-acting bronchodilator	24 h
Inhaled cromolyn sodium	48 h
Theophylline (long-acting)	48 h
Ipatropium bromide (inhaled/ intranasal)	4–12 h
Oral short-acting β-agonist	12 h
Oral long-acting β-agonist	24 h

[a]Drugs that are not discontinued include H_1-antihistamine eye drops, inhaled/intranasal corticosteroids, topical steroids, topical immunosuppressants (e.g., tacrolimus, pimecrolimus)

with the subject and/or the carer(s) and written informed consent is obtained (*see* **Note 14**).

2. The food portion quantities (doses) and the time interval between administrations are defined and recorded in the flow sheet (*see* **Note 15**).
3. The appropriate incremental food doses to be administered are prepared with accuracy using an electronic scale to minimize the risk of severe allergic reactions and to clearly identify the lowest provoking dose (*see* **Note 16**).
4. The patient receives the starting dose and remains under the supervision of qualified personnel. The dose and time are recorded on the flow sheet. Food residues on the face or hands are wiped off with water to avoid contact irritant reactions.
5. Any signs indicative of an allergic reaction (Table 13) are recorded. In case of only subjective symptoms being reported, the administration of the next dose is postponed to observe the progress [81]. If symptoms subside, **step 4** is repeated using the same dose to avoid allergen overloading. If no reaction occurs, the next dose is administered (**step 4**) (*see* **Note 16**).
6. The OFC is considered to be negative (oral tolerance) in the absence of any clinical symptoms 2 h after consumption of the last dose. For negative DBPCFCs, an open or appropriate cumulative ingestion of the food is used to substantiate oral tolerance [83]. The OFC is positive when objective clinical reactions occur (Table 13) and it is therefore terminated (*see* **Note 16**). The subject receives appropriate treatment and

Table 13
Symptoms and signs of positive oral food challenges (OFCs)[a]

Subjective symptoms and signs[b]	Objective symptoms and signs
– Nonverbal clues such as ear picking, tongue rubbing, putting a hand in the mouth, or neck scratching (children) – Changes in general demeanor (children) – Itching of the mouth or throat – Abdominal pain – Nausea – General malaise	– *Skin*[c]: flushing, pruritus, urticarial and erythematous rash, angioedema – *Upper respiratory track*: sneezing, nasal pruritus, nasal congestion, rhinorrhea, angioedema, oropharyngeal findings (uvular edema), dry cough, inspiratory wheezing – *Lower respiratory track*: dry cough, wheezing, dyspnea – *Gastrointestinal track*[c]: vomiting, diarrhea – *Cardiovascular system*[d]: pale skin color, weakness, dizziness, tachycardia, mental status change, drop in blood pressure, bradycardia, collapse, unconsciousness

[a]The OFC is terminated when objective signs are present, when no symptoms are evident after the last dose or when subjective symptoms are reported after administration of three doses but not in placebo (in placebo-controlled testing)
[b]Infants and very young children may not be able to describe the experienced symptoms
[c]More common in infants and young children
[d]Mainly in adults

is observed closely for 2 h after the final dose or after the subsidence of elicited symptoms (hospitalization for 24 h may be necessary depending on the severity of the reaction) [84] (*see* **Note 17**). Quantification of serum tryptase and/or histamine may clarify a doubtful OFC outcome [85].

Notes

14. OFCs to different foods are scheduled at least 7 days apart. An OFC starts early in the morning and it is usually completed within 6–8 h. Fasting for at least 4 h prior to testing is required (a light meal could be administered to infants and small children 2 h before the OFC).
15. The total administered dose is 8–10 g for dry food, 16-20 g for meat, chicken, or fish, and 100 ml of wet food or milk, typically divided into 3–6 incremental doubling doses [79, 80]. The starting dose is 0.1–1 % of the total dose, whereas it is smaller in patients at risk for severe reactions. The doses are generally administered every 20–30 min over 3 h.
16. In some cases after a positive OFC, the possibility of development of spontaneous tolerance may warrant repetition of the OFC after an appropriate time interval depending on the age of the individual (child versus adult) and/or the type of food.
17. Upon discharge, patients are instructed to monitor possible late symptoms [80] and not to consume amounts of the tested food that exceed those of the total dose even after a negative OFC.

3.3 Drug Provocation Test for Immediate DHRs

DHR is the preferred term for drug allergy and refers to the clinical manifestations attributed to drugs or their excipients that resemble an allergic reaction (Table 5) [56]. DHRs are type B adverse drug reactions that, according to the World Health Organization, are dose-independent, unpredictable, noxious, and unintended responses to a drug taken at a dose normally used in humans. Parameters such as the route of administration, the immunological effects of drug metabolites, the underlying disease, and co-medication may alter the reaction onset or progression [86].

3.3.1 Immediate Versus Nonimmediate/Delayed DHRs

The vast majority of immediate DHRs develop upon sensitization as a result of the production of sIgEs against the drug antigen (presumably a hapten–protein complex) by antigen-specific B lymphocytes and the subsequent activation of mast cells and basophils [87]. Upon drug re-exposure, the acute response is attributed to the release of preformed mediators (e.g., histamine, tryptase) and occurs within minutes, whereas the late reaction is cytokine-driven and develops after several hours [87]. On the other hand, most nonimmediate/delayed allergic DHRs are T lymphocyte-mediated. In this case, drug antigens are processed by dendritic cells, internalized, transported to the regional lymph nodes, and presented to naive T cells or they may directly stimulate antigen-specific T cells [56]. Furthermore, several drugs may trigger allergic-like reactions through distinct mechanisms, including nonspecific mast cell or basophil histamine release (e.g., opiates, vancomycin), bradykinin accumulation (e.g., ACE inhibitors), complement activation (e.g., protamine), alteration in arachidonic acid metabolism [e.g., non-steroidal anti-inflammatory drugs (NSAIDs)], and bronchospasm induction (e.g., β-blockers, sulfur dioxide). A careful review of the medical history is the first step in DHR evaluation [88, 89], followed by diagnostic procedures, such as in vivo skin testing (*see* Sects. 2.2, 2.3), yet finding a reliable diagnosis is particularly difficult (Fig. 9).

3.3.2 General Principles of the Drug Provocation Test

The drug provocation test, also referred to as drug challenge, incremental test dosing or graded challenge, is the gold standard in confirming or excluding DHR diagnosis (Fig. 9) [56, 90, 91]. Contrary to skin testing (*see* Sects. 2.2, 2.3), drug provocation tests do not provide any direct information on the pathogenesis of the reaction, yet they take into account individual factors such as drug metabolism and intermediate metabolites and personalized disposition of the individual.

The general principle of drug provocation tests is the administration of gradually increasing doses of the offending drug [56, 86, 87]. The procedure usually starts with low doses

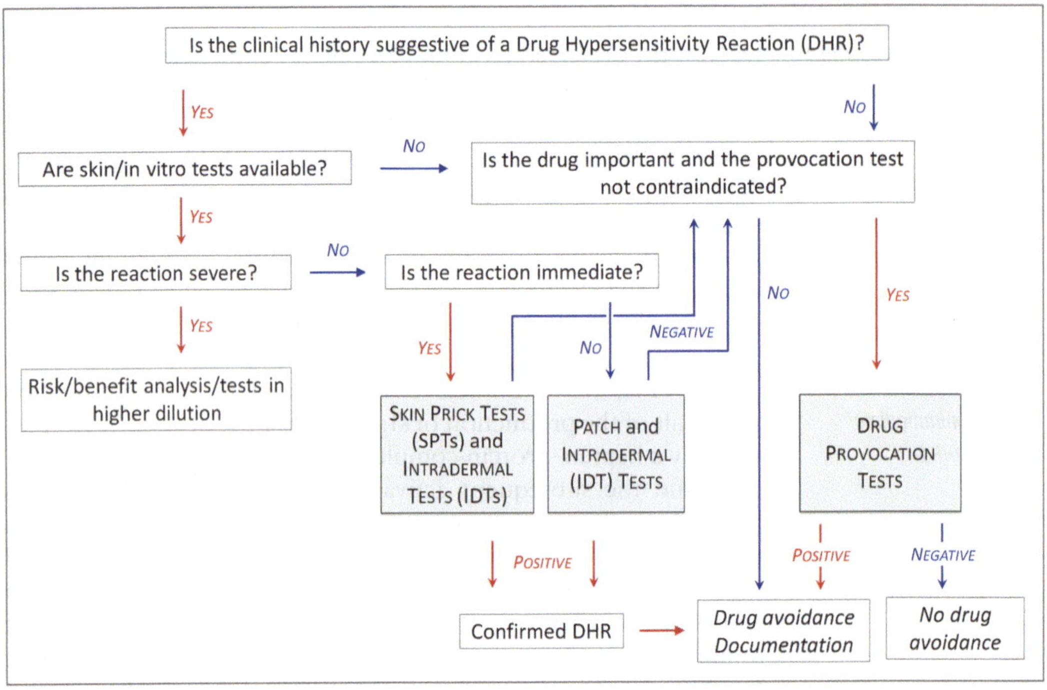

Fig. 9 Diagnostic algorithm for drug hypersensitivity

following by the rapid administration of dose increments until reaching the full therapeutic dose. Practically, the starting dose ranges from 1:10,000 to 1:10 of the therapeutic dose of the tested agent, depending on the severity and the type of reaction (lower starting doses in immediate versus delayed reactions), the route of administration (oral, parenteral, conjunctival, mucosal), and the expected time latency between application and reaction [92]. Sequential doses are incremented by at least 30-60 min time intervals. Smaller dosing intervals of about 20 min can be implemented for parenteral administration due to faster drug absorption. For testing immediate DHRs, drug provocation is usually performed with a maximum of 4–5 incremental doses and is completed in 1 day.

3.3.3 Materials for Drug Provocation Tests

- Safe, clean, and comfortable environment to perform the challenge.
- Clean bench for the preparation of drug reagents.
- Flow sheet to record administered doses, symptoms, signs, and treatments.
- Drug to be tested.
- Empty gelatin capsules of different sizes (for solid oral formulations; e.g., CapsulCN®, China; size 000, 00, 0, 1, 2, 3, 4, 5).
- Precision scale (weighing capacity 200 g with 0.01 g readability).
- Drinkable water (for the dilutions of orally administered drugs).
- Water for injection (for the solutions of parenteral formulations).
- Equipment suitable for crushing tablets.
- Sugar or aspartame (for placebo capsule preparation).
- Sterile 1, 5, and 10 ml syringes (for liquid formulation solutions).
- Portable peak flow meter for peak expiratory flow (PEF) measurements and spirometer (especially in case of asthmatic patients being tested or for procedures involving NSAIDs).
- Infusion pump (for intravenous administration especially in severe cases; e.g., Sigma Spectrum Infusion System, Baxter™, USA).
- Saturation pO_2 and blood pressure monitor with 24 h continuous measurement (for intravenous drug provocation tests and in cases with history of severe reactions).
- Equipment for establishing intravenous access (considered in high-risk patients).
- Medication and equipment for managing allergic reactions (Fig. 1, Sect. 4).

3.3.4 Procedure for Drug Provocation Tests

1. The subject's personal details, medical history (including recent laboratory test and spirometic values), and co-medication regimens are recorded (*see* **Note 18**).
2. The procedure largely depends on the marketed pharmaceutical formulation of the drug under investigation. Depending on the protocol, the orally administered drugs are prepared in capsules or in liquid forms, whereas for parenteral administration drug solutions are prepared in sterile syringes or in infusion pumps (*see* **Note 19**). Indicative protocols for testing drugs administered in capsules or in suspension are illustrated in Figs. 10 and 11, respectively (*see* **Note 20**).
3. Drug provocation tests are considered as being negative when no clinical symptoms are observed upon administration of the final drug dose. Tests are positive when administration of the tested drug results in an immediate allergic reaction (Table 14) commonly characterized by similar symptoms to the initial reaction, even of milder severity. During results interpretation both false-positive and negative reactions are considered (Table 14).

1. The tablet is ground into as small particles as possible.
2. The total weight of the ground particles is recorded [e.g. 650 mg (500 mg active substance + 100 mg excipients)].
3. The individual consecutive doses to be tested (e.g. 1/100, 1/10, 1/3, 2/3, remaining amount) are calculated according to the protocol (e.g. 6.5 mg, 65 mg; 215 mg, 435 mg, 363.5 mg, respectively).
4. Soft capsules are filled with the appropriate doses. For placebo preparation, sugar or aspartame is placed in one or more capsules. Care is taken so as no traces of the capsule content are noticeable.
5. The drug is administered according to the following scheme (symptoms and signs indicative of a positive reaction are recorded and evaluated before proceeding to any subsequent step).

Step	Dose fraction	Weight (mg)		Cumulative dose (mg)	
		Total	Active substance	Total	**Active substance**
0	Placebo	0	0	0	**0**
1	1/100	6.5	5	6.5	**5**
2	1/10	65	50	71.5	**55**
3	1/3	215	165	286.5	**220**
4	Remaining	363.5	280	650	**500**

Fig. 10 Procedure for testing drugs administered in capsules presented as an indicative example of a drug prescribed as 500 mg tablets

1. The individual consecutive doses to be tested (e.g. 1/100, 1/10, 1/3, 2/3, remaining amount) are calculated according to the protocol (e.g. 2.5 mg, 25 mg, 80 mg, 142.5 mg, 212.5 mg, respectively)
2. Comparable, easy to handle suspension volumes are prepared for the different doses, starting with the 1/10 dilution (e.g. 2 ml mixed with 18ml of drinkable water to yield a concentration of 5 mg/ml), followed by the appropriate dilutions using drinkable water.
3. The drug is administered according to the scheme below under strict medical supervision (symptoms and signs indicative of a positive reaction are recorded and evaluated before proceeding to any subsequent step).

Step	Dose fraction	Concentration (mg/ml)	Dose of active substance (mg)	Volume (ml)	**Cumulative dose (mg)**
0	Placebo	Sugar/aspartame	0	-	**0**
1	1/100	5	2.5	0.5	**2.5**
2	1/10	50	25	0.5	**27.5**
3	1/3	50	80	1.6	**107.5**
4	Remaining	50	142.5	2.85	**250**

Fig. 11 Procedure for testing drugs administered in suspension presented as an indicative example of a drug prescribed as 250 mg/ml suspension

Table 14
Considerations in the interpretation of drug provocation tests (modified from [92])

False-positive reactions	False-negative reactions
– Psychological-subjective symptoms – Underlying diseases (e.g., chronic urticaria) – Drug-induced aggrevation of pre-existing symptoms – Self-infliction	– Anti-allergic medications (antihistamines, corticosteroids, omalizumab) – Absence of co-factors (viral infection, exercise, exposure to light, co-medication) – Short time of drug intake and/or observation – Increased time interval from reaction (>1 year) – Low doses of the tested drug – Induction of tolerance during the drug provocation test

4. The subject is monitored for at least 2 h depending on the drug class and/or on the reported reaction. Treatment of adverse events during provocation testing depends on the type and the severity of the reaction (Sect. 4).

Notes

18. Drug provocation tests are not performed in case the reaction to the drug under investigation was experienced within 4–6 weeks prior to testing (at least 5× elimination half time is required for complete drug elimination), as well as in subjects

under H_1-antihistamine or oral steroid medication and/or with active signs of underlying diseases, such as urticaria, uncontrolled asthma (FEV1<70 % of predicted value), uncontrolled cardiac, renal or hepatic disease, or current infection [92]. Pregnancy is generally considered a contraindication unless the drug under investigation is required during pregnancy or delivery [91].

19. For drugs marketed in both oral and parenteral formulations, oral challenge is preferred as it is safer and causes less stress. In case of combination drugs, each active compound and the excipients are tested separately, whereas proof of tolerance is assessed using the commercial preparation [92].

20. Placebo-controlled tests are strongly recommended to eliminate false-positive results for patients with largely subjective reactions. Single-blind placebo-controlled drug challenges are preferred in every-day practice, whereas double-blind tests are reserved for research and clinical trials as they are more complicated and time-consuming.

4 Conclusion

The classification of allergic and hypersensitivity conditions remains an area of active discussion [93]. Yet, in vivo testing is a valuable approach in well-trained and experienced hands for the diagnosis of IgE-mediated allergic disorders [92, 93], despite the recent development of sophisticated in vitro tools, such as the component-resolved diagnostics that promise to decrease the need for provocation testing [92] and to improve the specificity of allergen-specific immunotherapy [10]. Skin testing is extensively used as a surrogate approach for the detection of sIgE antibodies, whereas provocation tests are valuable tools for the diagnostic confirmation or the elucidation of the clinical relevance of the suspected allergen and often provide crucial information that allows optimal management. Although uncommon, in vivo investigations contain a risk to elicit systemic allergic reactions. Therefore, they should be performed in a suitable setting by trained personnel who have access to appropriate management equipment (Fig. 1). According to the World Allergy Organization an anaphylactic reaction should be treated immediately by intramuscular administration of 0.01 ml/kg of 1:1000 adrenalin (epinephrine) that may be repeated after 15–20 min if necessary, administration of a fast-acting β_2 agonist (preferably salbutamol) and supplemental oxygen if there is involvement of respiratory system, corticosteroids (methylprednisolone or prednisolone at 1–2 mg/kg), and H_1 and H_2 antihistamines [94, 95].

References

1. Okada H, Kuhn C, Feillet H et al (2010) The "hygiene hypothesis" for autoimmune and allergic diseases: an update. Clin Exp Immunol 160:1–9
2. Holgate ST, Wenzel S, Postma DS et al (2015) Asthma. Nat Rev Dis Primers 1:15025
3. Iweala OI, Burks AW (2016) Food allergy: our evolving understanding of its pathogenesis, prevention, and treatment. Curr Allergy Asthma Rep 16:37
4. Ghably J, Saleh H, Vyas H et al (2015) Paul Ehrlich's mastzellen: a historical perspective of relevant developments in mast cell biology. Methods Mol Biol 1220:3–10
5. Kakavas S, Zampeli E, Papamichael K et al (2006) The mast cell pathway to inflammation and homeostasis: pharmacological insights. Anti-Inflamm Anti-Allergy Agents Med Chem (5):323–334
6. Chliva C, Aggelides X, Makris M et al (2015) Comparable profiles of serum histamine and IgG4 levels in allergic beekeepers. Allergy 70:457–460
7. Zampeli E, Tiligada E (2009) The role of histamine H_4 receptor in immune and inflammatory disorders. Br J Pharmacol 157:24–33
8. Eder W, Ege MJ, von Mutius E (2006) The asthma epidemic. N Engl J Med 355:2226–2235
9. Chiriac AM, Bousquet J, Demoly P (2014) In vivo methods for the study and diagnosis of allergy. In: Middleton's allergy, 8th edn. Elsevier, Philadelphia
10. Treudler R, Simon JC (2013) Overview of component resolved diagnostics. Curr Allergy Asthma Rep 13:110–117
11. Mikhail GR, Miller-Milinska A (1964) Mast cell population in human skin. J Invest Dermatol 43:249–254
12. Sibilano R, Frossi B, Pucillo CE (2014) Mast cell activation: a complex interplay of positive and negative signaling pathways. Eur J Immunol 44:2558–2566
13. Reshef A, Kagey-Sobotka A, Adkinson N Jr et al (1989) The pattern and kinetics in human skin of erythema and mediators during the acute and late-phase response (LPR). J Allergy Clin Immunol 84:678–687
14. Demoly P, Bousquet J, Romano A (2014) In vivo methods for the study of allergy. In: Adkin-son Jr NF, Bochner BS, Busse WW, Holgate ST, Lemanske Jr RF, FER S (eds) Middleton's allergy, principles and practice, 8th edn. Philadelphia, Mosby Elsevier Inc
15. Leguy-Seguin V, Jolimoy G, Coudert B et al (2007) Diagnostic and predictive value of skin testing in platinum salt hypersensitivity. J Allergy Clin Immunol 119:726–730
16. Crobach MJ, Hermans J, Kaptein AA et al (1998) The diagnosis of allergic rhinitis: how to combine the medical history with the results of radioallergosorbent tests and skin prick tests. Scand J Prim Health Care 16:30–36
17. Cabañes N, Igea JM, de la Hoz B (2012) Latex allergy: position paper. J Investig Allergol Clin Immunol 22:313–330
18. Greenhawt M, Aceves SS, Spergel JM et al (2013) The management of eosinophilic esophagitis. J Allergy Clin Immunol Pract 1:332–340
19. Agarwal R, Aggarwal AN, Gupta D et al (2009) Aspergillus hypersensitivity and allergic bronchopulmonary aspergillosis in patients with bronchial asthma: systematic review and meta-analysis. Int J Tuberc Lung Dis 13:936–944
20. Keil T, Kulig M, Simpson A et al (2006) European birth cohort studies on asthma and atopic diseases: II. Comparison of outcomes and exposures--a GA2LEN initiative. Allergy 61:1104–1111
21. Rhodius R, Wickens K, Cheng S et al (2002) A comparison of two skin test methodologies and allergens from two different manufacturers. Ann Allergy Asthma Immunol 88:374–379
22. Focke M, Marth K, Flicker S et al (2008) Heterogeneity of commercial timothy grass pollen extracts. Clin Exp Allergy 38:1400–1408
23. Blunk JA, Schmelz M, Zeck S et al (2004) Opioid-induced mast cell activation and vascular responses is not mediated by mu-opioid receptors: an in vivo microdialysis study in human skin. Anesth Analg 98:364–370
24. Bousquet J, Heinzerling L, Bachert C et al (2012) Practical guide to skin prick tests in allergy to aeroallergens. Allergy 67:18–24
25. Bernstein IL, Li JT, Bernstein DI et al (2008) Allergy diagnostic testing: an updated practice parameter. Ann Allergy Asthma Immunol 100(Suppl 3):S1–148
26. Rachmiel M, Verleger H, Waisel Y et al (1996) The importance of the pecan tree pollen in allergic manifestations. Clin Exp Allergy 26:323–329
27. Fernandes-Calda E, Puerta L, Mercado D et al (1993) Mite fauna Der p I, Der f I and *Blomia tropicalis* allergen levels in a tropical environment. Clin Exp Allergy 23:292–297

28. Yamada T, Saito H, Fujieda S (2014) Present state of Japanese cedar pollinosis: the national affliction. J Allergy Clin Immunol 133:632–9.e5
29. Henzgen M, Ballmer-Weber BK, Erdmann S et al (2008) Skin testing with food allergens. Guideline of the German Society of Allergology and Clinical Immunology (DGAKI), the Physicians' Association of German Allergologists (ADA) and the Society of Pediatric Allergology (GPA) together with the Swiss Society of Allergology. J Dtsch Dermatol Ges 6:983–988
30. Asero R, Monsalve R, Barber D (2008) Profilin sensitization detected in the office by skin prick test: a study of prevalence and clinical relevance of profilin as a plant food allergen. Clin Exp Allergy 38:1033–1037
31. Webber CM, England RW (2010) Oral allergy syndrome: a clinical, diagnostic, and therapeutic challenge. Ann Allergy Asthma Immunol 104:101–108 quiz 109–10, 117
32. Blanca M, Romano A, Torres MJ et al (2009) Update on the evaluation of hypersensitivity reactions to betalactams. Allergy 64:183–193
33. Benucci M, Manfredi M, Demoly P et al (2008) Injection site reactions to TNF-alpha blocking agents with positive skin tests. Allergy 63:138–139
34. Brockow K, Garvey LH, Aberer W et al (2013) Skin test concentrations for systemically administered drugs—an ENDA/EAACI Drug Allergy Interest Group position paper. Allergy 68:702–712
35. Norrman G, Fälth-Magnusson K (2009) Adverse reactions to skin prick testing in children - prevalence and possible risk factors. Pediatr Allergy Immunol 20:273–278
36. Liccardi G, D'Amato G, Walter Canonica G et al (2006) Systemic reactions from skin testing: literature review. J Investig Allergol Clin Immunol 16:75–78
37. Ruëff F, Bergmann KC, Brockow K et al (2011) Skin tests for diagnostics of allergic immediate-type reactions. Guideline of the German Society for allergology and clinical immunology. Pneumologie 65:484–495
38. Lockey RF, Benedict LM, Turkeltaub PC et al (1987) Fatalities from immunotherapy (IT) and skin testing (ST). J Allergy Clin Immunol 79:660–677
39. Heinzerling L, Mari A, Bergmann KC et al (2013) The skin prick test—European standards. Clin Transl Allergy 3:3
40. Devenney I, Falth-Magnusson K (2000) Skin prick tests may give generalized allergic reactions in infants. Ann Allergy Asthma Immunol 85:457–460
41. Rueff F, Przybilla B, Bilo MBet al (2009) Predictors of severe systemic anaphylactic reactions in patients with Hymenoptera venom allergy: importance of baseline serum tryptase-a study of the European Academy of Allergology and Clinical Immunology Interest Group on Insect Venom Hypersensitivity. J Allergy Clin Immunol 124:1047–1054
42. Nelson HS, Knoezner J, Bucher B (1997) Effect of distance between sites and region of the body on results of skin prick tests. J Allergy Clin Immunol 97:596–601
43. Carr WW, Martin B, Howard RS et al (2005) Comparison of test devices for skin prick testing. J Allergy Clin Immunol 116:341–346
44. Masse MS, Granger Vallée A, Chiriac A et al (2011) Comparison of five techniques of skin prick tests used routinely in Europe. Allergy 66:1415–1419
45. Kupczyk M, Kuprys I, Gorski P et al (2001) Not one lancet for multiple SPT. Allergy 56:256–257
46. Konstantinou GN, Bousquet PJ, Zuberbier T et al (2010) The longest wheal diameter is the optimal measurement for the evaluation of skin prick tests. Int Arch Allergy Immunol 151:343–345
47. Barbee RA, Brown WGH, Kaltenborn W et al (1981) Allergen skin test reactivity in a community population sample: correlation with age, histamine skin reactions and total serum immunoglobulin E. J Allergy Clin Immunol 68:15–19
48. Goldberg A, Confino-Cohen R (1997) Timing of venom skin tests and IgE determinations after insect sting anaphylaxis. J Allergy Clin Immunol 100:183–184
49. Vocks E, Stander K, Rakoski J et al (1999) Suppression of immediate-type hypersensitivity elicitation in the skin prick test by ultraviolet B irradiation. Photodermatol Photoimmunol Photomed 15:236–240
50. Skoner DP, Gentile DA, Angelini B et al (2006) Allergy skin test responses during experimental infection with respiratory syncytial virus. Ann Allergy Asthma Immunol 96:834–839
51. Strohmeier B, Aberer W, Bokanovic D et al (2013) Simultaneous intradermal testing with hymenoptera venoms is safe and more efficient than sequential testing. Allergy 68:542–544
52. Schwindt CD, Hutcheson PS, Leu S-Y et al (2005) Role of intradermal skin tests in the evaluation of clinically relevant respiratory allergy assessed using patient history and nasal

challenges. Ann Allergy Asthma Immunol 94:627–633
53. Romano A, Guéant-Rodriguez RM, Viola M et al (2005) Diagnosing immediate reactions to cephalosporins. Clin Exp Allergy 35:1234–1242
54. Agache I, Bilò M, Braunstahl GJ et al (2015) In vivo diagnosis of allergic diseases—allergen provocation tests. Allergy 70:355–365
55. Rondón C, Fernández J, López S et al (2009) Nasal inflammatory mediators and specific IgE production after nasal challenge with grass pollen in local allergic rhinitis. J Allergy Clin Immunol 124:1005–1011
56. Demoly P, Adkinson NF, Brockow K et al (2014) International consensus on drug allergy. Allergy 69:420–437
57. Bousquet J, Schünemann HJ, Samolinski B et al (2012) Allergic rhinitis and its impact on asthma (ARIA): achievements in 10 years and futureneeds. J Allergy Clin Immunol 130:1049–1062
58. Licari A, Marseglia A, Caimmi S et al (2015) Emerging and future therapies for allergic rhinitis. J Biol RegulHomeost Agents 29(S1):38–46
59. Settipane RA, Schwindt C (2013) Chapter 15: allergic rhinitis. Am J Rhinol Allergy 27(S1):S52–S55
60. Hilberg O, Grymer LF, Pedersen OF (1995) Nasal histamine challenge in nonallergic and allergic subjects evaluated by acoustic rhinometry. Allergy 50:166–173
61. Baroody FM, Shenaq D, DeTineo M et al (2009) Fluticasone furoate nasal spray reduces the nasal-ocular reflex: a mechanism for the efficacy of topical steroids in controlling allergic eye symptoms. J Allergy Clin Immunol 123:1342–1348
62. Baroody FM, Mucha SM, Detineo M et al (2008) Nasal challenge with allergen leads to maxillary sinus inflammation. J Allergy Clin Immunol 121:1126–1132
63. Boot JD, de Kam ML, Mascelli MA et al (2007) Nasal nitric oxide: longitudinal reproducibility and the effects of a nasal allergen challenge in patients with allergic rhinitis. Allergy 62:378–384
64. Erin EM, Zacharasiewicz AS, Nicholson GC et al (2005) Topical corticosteroid inhibits interleukin-4, -5 and -13 in nasal secretions following allergen challenge. Clin Exp Allergy 35:1608–1614
65. Blackley C (1873) Experimental researches on the causes and nature of catarrhus aestivus, Balliere Tindal & Cox, London
66. Naclerio RM, Baroody FM (1992) Response of nasal mucosa to histamine or methacholine challenge: use of a quantitative method to examine the modulatory effects of atropine and ipratropium bromide. J Allergy Clin Immunol 90:1051–1504
67. Airaksinen L, Tuomi T, Vanhanen M et al (2007) Use of nasal provocation test in the diagnostics of occupational rhinitis. Rhinology 45:40–46
68. Wachs M, Proud D, Lichtenstein LM et al (1989) Observations on the pathogenesis of nasal priming. J Allergy Clin Immunol 84:492–501
69. Dordal MT, Lluch-Bernal M, Sánchez MC et al (2011) Allergen-specific nasal provocation testing: review by the Rhinoconjunctivitis Committee of the Spanish Society of Allergy and Clinical Immunology. J Investig Allergol Clin Immunol 21:1–12
70. Ciprandi G, Mora F, Cassano M et al (2009) Visual analog scale (VAS) and nasal obstruction in persistent allergic rhinitis. Otolaryngol Head Neck Surg 141:527–529
71. Clement PA, Gordts F (2005) Consensus report on acoustic rhinometry and rhinomanometry. Rhinology 43:169–179
72. Djupesland PG (2013) Nasal drug delivery devices: characteristics and performance ina clinical perspective-a review. Drug Deliv Transl Res 3:42–62
73. Riechelmann H, Bachert C, Goldschmidt O et al (2003) Application of the nasal provocation test on diseases of the upper airways. Position Paper of the German Society for Allergology and Clinical Immunology (ENT Section) in cooperation with the Working Team for Clinical Immunology. Laryngorhinootologie 82:183–188
74. Sicherer C, Sampson HA (2010) Food allergy. J Allergy Clin Immunol 125(S2):S116–S125
75. Keller M, Shuker M, Heimall J et al (2012) Severe malnutrition resulting from use of rice milk in food elimination diets for atopic dermatitis. IMAJ 14:40–42
76. Boyce J, Assa'ad A, Burks AW et al (2010) Guidelines for the diagnosis and management of food allergy in the United States: Report of the NIAID-Sponsored Expert Panel. J Allergy Clin Immunol 126:S1–S58
77. Sackeyfio A, Senthinathan A, Kandaswamy P et al (2011) Diagnosis and assessment of food allergy in children and young people: Summary of NICE guidance. BMJ 23:342
78. Nowak-Wegrzyn A, Assa'ad AH, Bahna SL et al (2009) Work Group report: oral food

challenge testing. J Allergy Clin Immunol 123:S365–S383
79. Bindslev-Jensen C, Ballmer-Weber BK, Bengtsson U et al (2004) Standardization of food challenges in patients with immediate reactions to foods–position paper from the European Academy of Allergology and Clinical Immunology. Allergy 59:690–697
80. Sampson HA, Gerth van Wijk R, BindslevJensen C et al (2012) Standardizing double-blind, placebo controlled oral food challenges: American Academy of Allergy, Asthma & Immunology-European Academy of Allergy and Clinical Immunology PRACTALL consensus report. J Allergy Clin Immunol 130:1260–1274
81. Ito K (2013) Diagnosis of food allergies: the impact of oral food challenge testing. Asia Pac Allergy 3:59–69
82. Perry TT, Matsui EC, Conover-Walker MK et al (2004) Risk of oral food challenges. J Allergy Clin Immunol 114:1164–1168
83. Vickery BP, Burks AW (2009) Immunotherapy in the treatment of food allergy: focus onoral tolerance. Curr Opin Allergy Clin Immunol 9:364–370
84. Sampson HA, Munoz-Furlong A, Campbell RL et al (2006) Second symposium on the definition and management of anaphylaxis: summary report—second National Institute of Allergy and Infectious Disease/Food Allergy and Anaphylaxis Network symposium. Ann Emerg Med 47:373–380
85. Licari A, De Amici M, Nigrisoli S et al (2015) Tryptase and histamine may support oral food challenge in the diagnosis of allergy. J Biol Regul Homeost Agents 29:1–7
86. Bircher AJ, Scherer Hofmeier K (2012) Drug hypersensitivity reactions: Inconsistency in the use of the classification of immediate and nonimmediate reactions. J Allergy Clin Immunol 129:263–264
87. Park BK, Naisbitt DJ, Demoly P (2012) Drug hypersensitivity. In: Holgate S, Church M, Broide D, Martinez F (eds) Allergy. Elsevier, New York
88. Demoly P, Kropf R, Bircher A et al (1999) Drug hypersensitivity: questionnaire. EAACI interest group on drug hypersensitivity. Allergy 54:999–1003
89. Demoly P, Pichler W, Pirmohamed M et al (2008) Important questions in allergy: 1–drug allergy/hypersensitivity. Allergy 63:616–619
90. Joint Task Force on Practice Parameters; American Academy of Allergy, Asthma and Immunology; American College of Allergy, Asthma and Immunology; Joint Council of Allergy, Asthma and Immunology (2010) Drug allergy: an updated practice parameter. Ann Allergy Asthma Immunol 105:259–273
91. Mirakian R, Ewan PW, Durham SR et al (2009) BSACI guidelines for the management of drug allergy. Clin Exp Allergy 39:43–61
92. Aberer W, Bircher A, Romano A et al (2003) Drug provocation testing in the diagnosis of drug hypersensitivity reactions: general considerations. Allergy 58:854–863
93. Tanno LK, Calderon MA, Demoly P (2016) Optimization and simplification of the allergic and hypersensitivity conditions classification for the ICD-11. Allergy 71:671–676
94. Simons FE, Ardusso LR, Bilò MB et al (2011) World allergy organization guidelines for the assessment and management of anaphylaxis. World Allergy Organ J 4:13–37
95. Simons FE, Ebisawa M, Sanchez-Borges M et al (2015) 2015 update of the evidence base: World Allergy Organization anaphylaxis guidelines. World Allergy Organ J 8:32

Chapter 16

Dermatological Indications of Antihistamines

Chrysovalantis Korfitis, Efstathios Rallis, and Dimitrios Rigopoulos

Abstract

Antihistamines are drugs that exert their biological effects inhibiting the action of histamine by occupying its receptors. They are divided into four subclasses depending on their tendency to bond with H_1, H_2, H_3, or H_4 histamine receptors. H_1 antihistamines are the most commonly used in dermatology for the treatment of urticaria and other pruritic dermatoses.

Key words Antihistamines, Atopic dermatitis, Dermatology, Histamine, Histamine receptors, Pruritus, Urticarial

1 Background Information

1.1 Histamine and Histamine Receptors

Histamine is a mediator distributed into the tissues of the body with its concentration being higher in the skin, lungs, and gastrointestinal tract. It is produced from histidine with the aid of histidine decarboxylase and is localized primarily in mast cells and basophils. Histamine plays a role in inflammation, the permeability of the capillaries to white blood cells, gastric acid secretion, neurotransmission, smooth muscle contraction along with other actions [1–3]. Histamine's tendency to bond with a special class of receptors induces its biological effects that depend on the subtype and the localization of the receptor.

Four types of histamine receptors (H_1–H_4) have currently been found. The H_1 receptor is expressed in many tissues throughout the body and appears to be the main histamine receptor of cutaneous mast cells. H_1 receptors participate in the induction of allergic inflammatory responses in conditions such as urticaria, atopic dermatitis, and asthma [3, 4]. H_2 receptors consist of 358–359 amino acids and play important role in the gastric physiology of acid secretion and the regulation of neuronal functions. Besides their gastric and cerebral abundant expression, H_2 receptors are also found on epithelial and immune system cells as well as smooth muscle cells and chondrocytes [1, 5, 6].

Ekaterini Tiligada and Madeleine Ennis (eds.), *Histamine Receptors as Drug Targets*, Methods in Pharmacology and Toxicology, DOI 10.1007/978-1-4939-6843-5_16, © Springer Science+Business Media LLC 2017

The H_3 receptor is a 445-amino acid polypeptide, with at least 20 isoforms [1]. It is located in the central nervous system inhibiting the release of histamine and interacting with dopaminergic neurotransmission [7]. Lastly, H_4 receptors are expressed on cells of the immune system, the intestine, the lung, the central nervous system, and malignant cells [3]. They mediate calcium mobilization and mast-cell chemotaxis in the process of allergic response [8, 9], along with functions derived from other immune cells, such as Langerhans cells [10], neutrophils [11], eosinophils [12], and T cells [13].

1.2 Antihistamines

Antihistamines are drugs widely used in everyday dermatological practice [14], prescribed commonly for adult and pediatric patients [15]. They bind with histamine receptors preventing histamine from exerting its biological effects. The H_1 alone and secondarily the H_2 receptor blockade in combination with H_1 receptor blockade are targeted in various skin conditions, due to their role in the process of allergic response and inflammation.

H_1 antihistamines are divided into two categories, the first-generation and the low-sedating second-generation antihistamines. The latter do not cross the blood-brain barrier exhibiting minimal soporific action, unlike their first-generation counterparts [16]. Their chemical classification consists of six classes, alkylamines, ethanolamines, ethylenediamines, phenothiazines, piperazines, and piperidines. Examples of each class are shown in Table 1. Antihistamines are available for oral administration as well as intravenous injection, intranasal or ophthalmic formulations, and topical application.

H_2 antagonists are used for the treatment of peptic ulcer and gastroesophageal reflux disease. Agents like cimetidine, the prototypical H_2 antihistamine, ranitidine, and famotidine, although valuable in gastroenterology, play a minimal role in the treatment of dermatological diseases.

Table 1
Chemical classification and examples of H_1 antihistamines available for oral administration

Alkylamines	Brompheniramine, chlorpheniramine, dimethindene	Acrivastine
Ethanolamines	Dimenhydrinate, diphenhydramine	
Ethylenediamines	Mepyramine	
Phenothiazines	Methdilazine	
Piperazines	Hydroxyzine, oxatomide	Cetirizine, levocetirizine
Piperidines	Cyproheptadine, ketotifen	Bilastine, desloratadine, ebastine, loratadine, mizolastine, rupatadine

1.3 Other Histamine Receptor Antagonists

Doxepin is a nonaddictive tricyclic antidepressant for the treatment of depression, anxiety disorders, and insomnia. In addition to its other actions, doxepin also behaves as an H_1 receptor antagonist, 800 times more potent than diphenhydramine [17, 18]. Thus, doxepin is beneficial in pruritus of urticaria and atopic dermatitis and can be administered either orally or topically [18].

Ketotifen is a potent H_1 antagonist and mast cell stabilizer useful in the treatment of chronic and cholinergic urticaria [19–21]. Mast cell stabilizers act by inhibiting signaling molecules responsible for the outflow of calcium from the cell and the initiation of allergic reaction, thus preventing mast cells from releasing clinically relevant mediators, such as histamine, interleukin (IL)-6, IL-8, IL-33, and other mediators [22, 23].

2 Indications of Antihistamines in Dermatology

H_1 antihistamines are widely used in dermatological practice. There are several secondary indications where antihistamines may prove beneficial, alone or concomitantly with other regimens or drugs. However, their main indication is for the treatment of urticaria and related conditions, where they are considered first-line therapy [24].

2.1 Urticaria

Urticaria is characterized clinically by the formation of wheals (Fig. 1) with or without angioedema and histologically by edema and vasodilatation of the dermis. Its pathophysiology depends on the release of histamine along with other mediators derived from activated mast cells [24]. Urticaria is divided into acute and chronic with their distinction being applied after 6 weeks of duration. Chronic urticaria is further identified as spontaneous and inducible with the latter also distinguished in cold, heat contact, delayed pressure, solar, cholinergic, vibratory, aquagenic, and contact urticarias as well as symptomatic dermographism (Fig. 2) [25]. Chronic urticaria has been attributed to causes such as autoimmunity, medications, neurologic factors, stress, infections, and others [26].

Treating urticaria may prove to be an intricate task. Although empirical data suggest that acute urticaria can be treated effectively with H_1 antihistamines [14], in chronic urticarias the initiation of additional drug therapy may be needed. The identification and elimination of any triggering factors is important as an initial step, followed by pharmacotherapy.

In 2013, the EAACI/GA^{2}LEN/EDF/WAO panel consensus published guidelines on the management and treatment of urticaria [24]. Recommending the preference of the second-generation H_1 antihistamines over first-generation antihistamines, in approved doses, as first-line therapy, due to the latter having sedative and anticholinergic effects, they concluded that if no response is

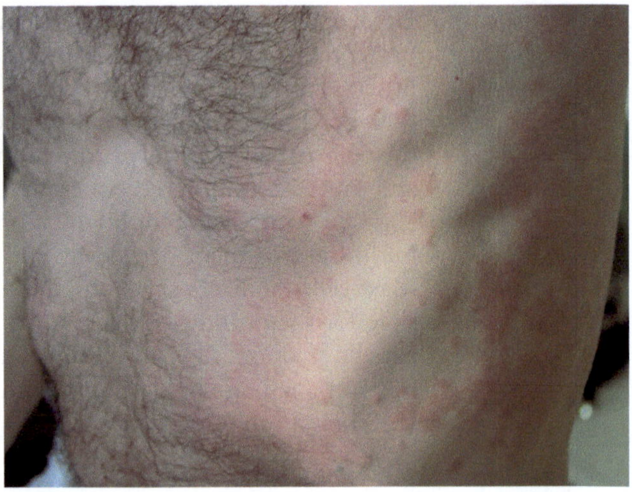

Fig. 1 Urticaria

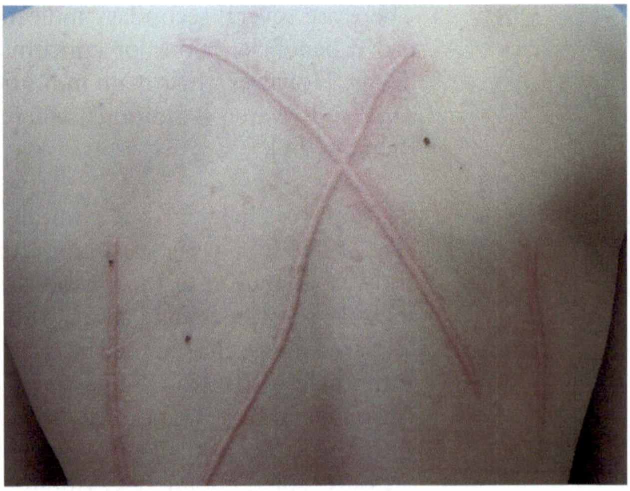

Fig. 2 Dermographism

observed after 2 weeks, then a four-times increase in dosage should be considered for the continuation of the treatment. If, after 4 more weeks, there is no satisfactory result then another medication, such as omalizumab, cyclosporin, or montelukast, should be added. Also, especially in cases of chronic spontaneous urticaria, a short course of corticosteroids may be useful.

In 2014, the Joint Task Force on Practice Parameters (JTFPP) published clinical practice guidelines for acute and chronic urticaria [27]. Their approach in chronic urticaria includes four steps, starting with a second-generation H_1 antihistamine. If the symptoms persist, an increase in the dosage should be made and/or the addition of one or more drugs should be considered. A second H_1

antihistamine, either of first or second-generation, an H_2 antagonist or a leukotriene receptor antagonist, such as montelukast, may be utilized. Next, the administration of hydroxyzine or doxepin is advised, and lastly the addition of omalizumab or immunosuppressive drugs is an option.

In order to assess the efficacy and safety of H_1 antihistamines in chronic spontaneous urticaria, a systematic review of randomized controlled trials was made by Sharma and coworkers [28]. They reviewed the effects of cetirizine, loratadine, desloratadine, levocetirizine and rupatadine versus placebo, and loratadine versus cetirizine, mizolastine, desloratadine, emedastine, and hydroxyzine as compared in various studies, also desloratadine versus levocetirizine, and fexofenadine versus cetirizine. Overall, they concluded that no antihistamine was found more effective than the others, and no differences in withdrawal due to side effects were observed as compared to placebo.

Randomized controlled trials were the subject of another systematic review conducted by Fedorowicz et al., aiming to assess H_2 antihistamines' safety and efficacy in urticaria [29]. The available literature's limited and unreliable evidence prevented the authors from reaching definite conclusions. However, it was reported that combination therapy with ranitidine and diphenhydramine was more effective than diphenhydramine alone and the same was observed with cimetidine and diphenhydramine.

2.2 Atopic Dermatitis

Atopic dermatitis is a chronic inflammatory pruritic dermatosis of unknown etiology [30]. Usually, it starts in early childhood, although an adult-onset form is also described (Fig. 3) [31, 32]. Clinically, the prevalent symptom is intense pruritus with or without signs of dermatitis, while pathology reveals features of dermatitis without specific attributes. Its pathophysiology is complex and evidence suggests the presence of impaired skin barrier along with modified immune response, involving Th2 lymphocytes and mast cells, under the influence of exogenous factors [3, 33].

Although there is lack of evidence regarding their effectiveness, H_1 antihistamines are often employed in the management of atopic dermatitis. Data show that histamine and histamine receptors play a role in the inflammatory response and skin barrier impairment in atopic dermatitis [3, 4, 34]. However, H_1 antihistamines do not seem to interfere with the course of the disease, but at the same time they offer palliation to the intense pruritus, especially the first-generation antihistamines with their sedating action [14, 16, 35]. Recently, some encouraging results have been reported regarding the administration of a novel H_4 receptor antagonist, JNJ39758979, in the treatment of pruritus in patients with atopic dermatitis as well as in healthy individuals after histamine challenge [3, 36, 37]. These findings have added to previous findings in studies in mice with provoked chronic allergic dermatitis [38].

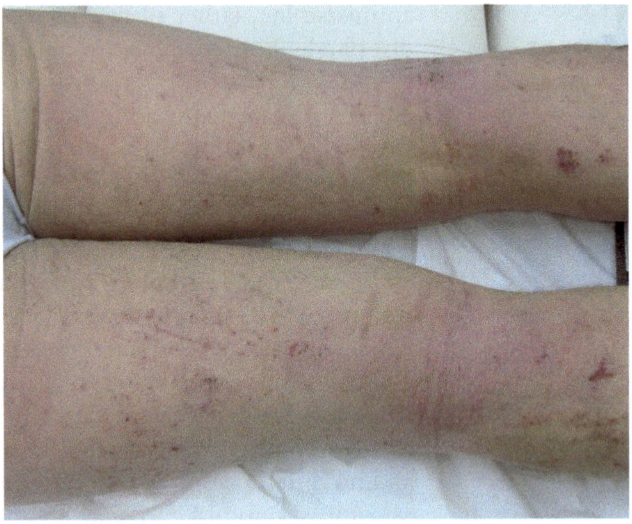

Fig. 3 Atopic dermatitis in an adult

2.3 Other Indications

Antihistamines have become a customary solution in clinical practice whenever a skin condition is accompanied by pruritus. The sedative effect of older H_1 antihistamines may reduce the discomfort caused by pruritus [39, 40]. Also, in many cases, the release of histamine is responsible, mainly or in part, for the symptoms [14], justifying the use of H_1 antihistamines. However, the evidence is not conclusive and additional studies are needed [39]. H_1 antihistamines have been used in a multitude of instances, such as:

- Insect bites (Fig. 4) [14, 41],
- Pruritus in burns by exploiting their soporific action (Fig. 5) [40],
- Hydroxyzine with or without doxepin for pruritus in HIV-1 positive patients [42],
- Doxepin for the pruritus in patients with end-stage renal disease on hemodialysis [43],
- Loratadine, hydroxyzine, and others for urticaria pigmentosa (Fig. 6), cutaneous and systemic mastocytosis, in co-administration with H_2 antihistamines such as famotidine [14, 23].

Further indications have been reported for dimethindene for pruritus in varicella infection [44], as well as doxepin and cimetidine for postherpetic neuralgia [45], and cetirizine or other antihistamines with corticosteroids, antibiotics, or topical agents for eosinophilic cellulitis [46, 47].

There is evidence that H_2 antagonists exhibit immunomodulatory effects [21, 48]. In particular, cimetidine has been used in the

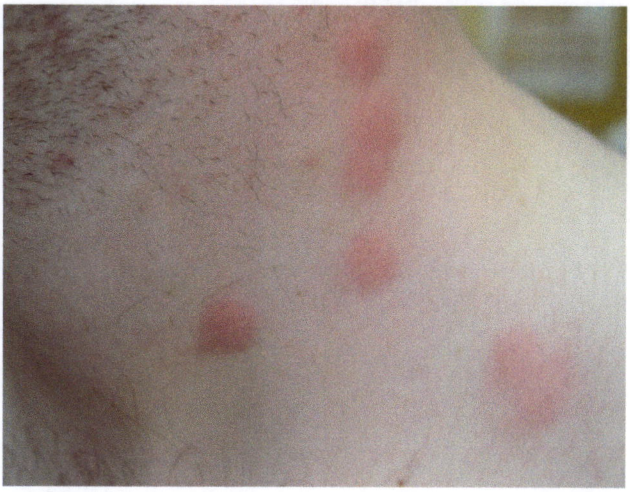

Fig. 4 Insect bites

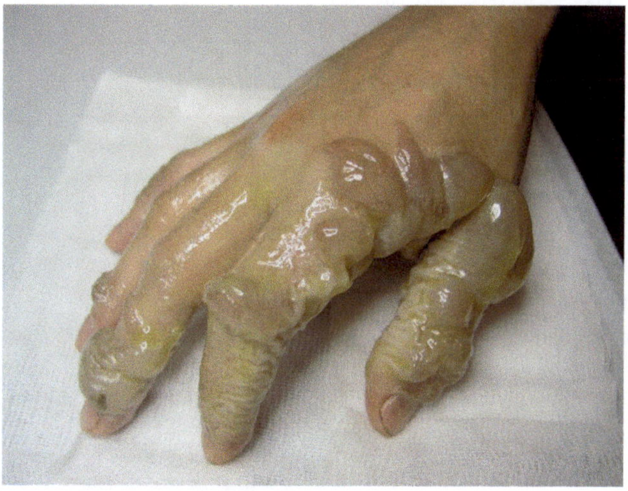

Fig. 5 A burn of the right hand caused by hot water

treatment of infections in which cell-mediated immunity plays a role. Cimetidine and ranitidine were tested in some studies in the treatment of warts (Fig. 7) with moderate results [49, 50], which may be interpreted that H_2 antagonists may be helpful as adjuvant therapy.

Cimetidine was also administered in cases of epidermodysplasia verruciformis [51], herpes zoster (Fig. 8), erythema multiforme (Fig. 9), chronic mucocutaneous candidiasis, Job syndrome, common variable hypogammaglobulinemia, hirsutism [21] and psoriasis in patients with AIDS (Fig. 10) [52].

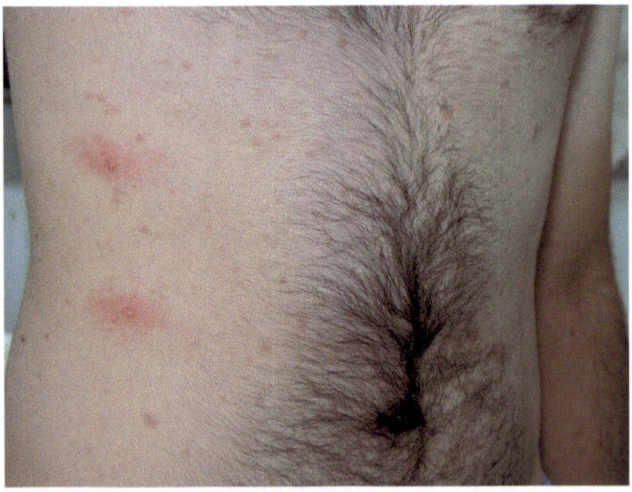

Fig. 6 Urticaria pigmentosa, Darier's sign

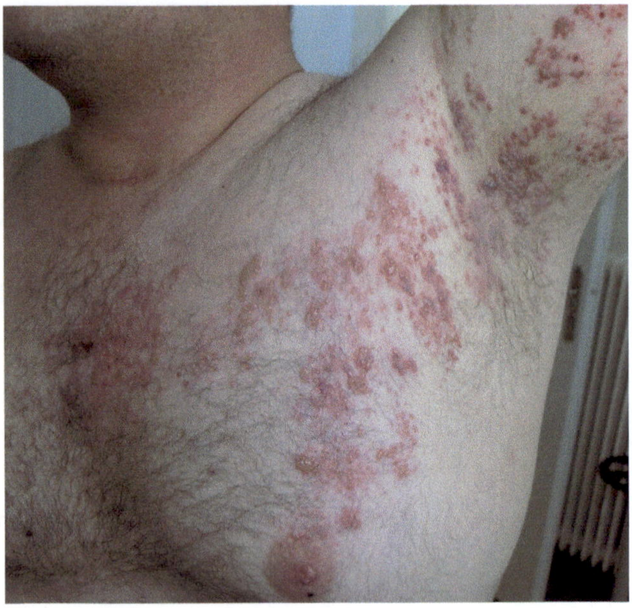

Fig. 7 Warts. Koebner phenomenon after cryosurgery

3 Limitations in Using Antihistamines

3.1 Side Effects

The commonest and most well-known side effect of first-generation H_1 antihistamines is sedation. Although sedation is desirable in many instances of tormenting itching, it is also unwanted in many others since it interferes with [53] or fails to improve [54] normal everyday activity of patients compared to non-sedating H_1 antihistamines. It was soon observed that second-generation H_1

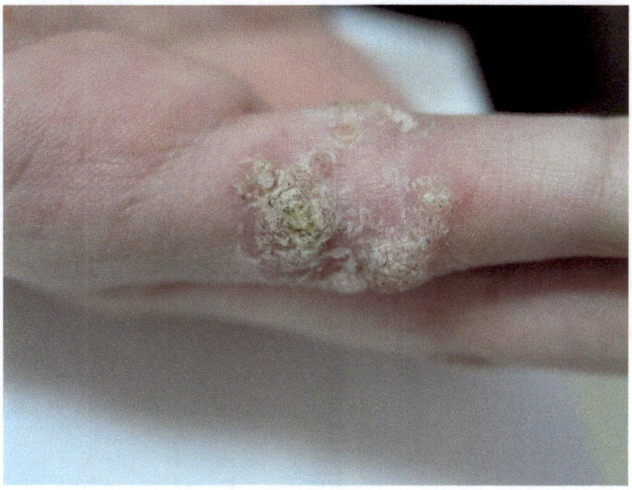

Fig. 8 Varicella zoster virus infection

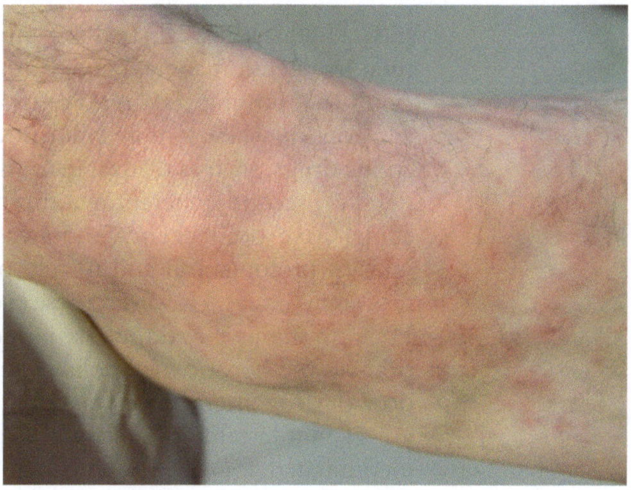

Fig. 9 Erythema multiforme. "Target"-like lesions

antihistamines cause no or minimal somnolence. It was also seen that the feeling of sedation may vary individually and that after a few days of continuous use of classic H_1 antihistamines the soporific effect may subside [55]. More recently, it was discovered that newer H_1 antihistamines showed affinity for P-glycoprotein efflux pump on the endothelial cells comprising the blood-brain barrier [56, 57], a property not possessed by older H_1 antihistamines.

Older H_1 antihistamines may also exhibit anticholinergic effects [24]. Symptoms and signs include dry mouth and eyes, urinary retention, constipation, blurring of vision, glaucoma, etc. [14]. Evidence suggests some second-generation H_1 antagonists, such as desloratadine, fexofenadine, and loratadine, may cause movement dysfunction, like increased choice reaction time or even sedation

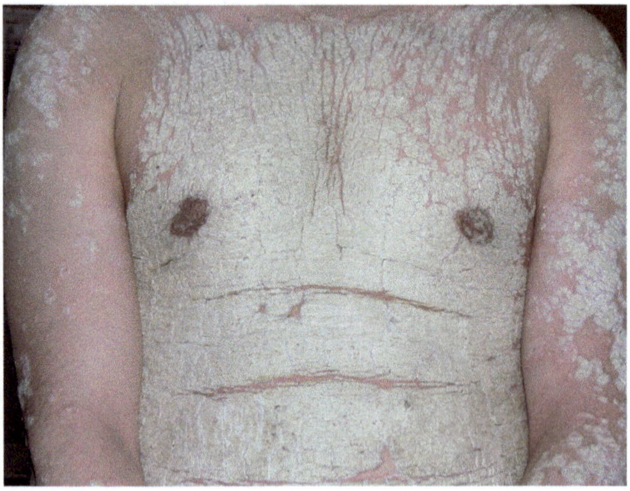

Fig. 10 Severe psoriasis in a HIV (+) patient

[58]. H_1 antagonists also exhibit antiadrenergic actions, such as postural hypotension and appetite stimulation with subsequent weight gain [14], possibly as a reaction to the hypothalamic H_1 receptor antagonism, which is more eminent with second-generation antipsychotic drugs, such as olanzapine and clozapine [59].

Two second-generation antihistamines, astemizole and terfenadine, have both been withdrawn from market because of QT interval prolongation and related potentially life-threatening cardiac arrhythmias. However, these events are considered rare among H_1 antihistamines and they are induced due to insufficient elimination via the hepatic metabolic system, resulting either from overdose or drug interactions [60, 61].

H_2 antihistamines, and more specifically cimetidine has been incriminated for side effects such as gynecomastia [62], sperm count reduction, and antiandrogenic activity in general [63–65]. Although cimetidine is still used today it has been superseded by newer and safer H_2 receptor antagonists.

3.2 Contra-indications and Precautions

Antihistamines should be used with caution under certain circumstances. There is evidence that diphenhydramine may be associated with the development of delirium in individuals at risk [66]. There is also a possibility that the same side effect could be seen with H_2 antagonists as well. However there is no clear evidence for the latter [66]. Furthermore, older patients, especially those with chronic kidney disease, when receiving H_2 antihistamines at standard doses, may be at increased risk of altered mental status. It is suggested that older patients should be initiated on lower doses and increase later, if necessary [67]. Cimetidine may hide the symptoms and delay diagnosis of gastric cancer [68]. The hypothesis that it may also prolong the survival of patients with gastric cancer has not been conclusively confirmed [69], although data from in vitro and in vivo studies exist [70, 71].

Due to anticholinergic effects, H_1 antihistamines are contraindicated in patients with glaucoma, prostatic hypertrophy, and urinary retention and they should be administered with caution. There have been reports of drug-induced hepatotoxicity [72, 73] so special consideration should also be given to patients with hepatic disease. Also, pharmacokinetic studies have shown that elimination of H_1 antihistamines may be prolonged in patients with renal insufficiency [74, 75].

H_1 antihistamines are used as antiemetics and for other symptoms of pregnancy, such as indigestion and nausea [76, 77]. They are given as well for the treatment of pregnancy dermatoses (Fig. 11). Large studies that have been conducted to identify any correlations between antihistamines in pregnancy and birth defects are quite encouraging. Most studies have shown no significant differences between the groups exposed and those not exposed to antihistamines; however, there are a few that found positive associations [76, 77]. Moreover, H_1 antihistamines have been more thoroughly examined than H_2 antagonists in pregnancy. Currently, FDA classifies antihistamines into pregnancy as category B or C [78].

3.3 Drug Interactions

H_1 antihistamines tend to interact with several drugs. The older ones accentuate the depressive effect of alcohol, opioids, benzodiazepines, sedatives, and antianxiety agents [24, 79–82]. The co-administration of chlorpheniramine or brompheniramine with monoaminoxidase inhibitors should be avoided [83]. Cardiotoxicity was reported with terfenadine and astemizole, now withdrawn

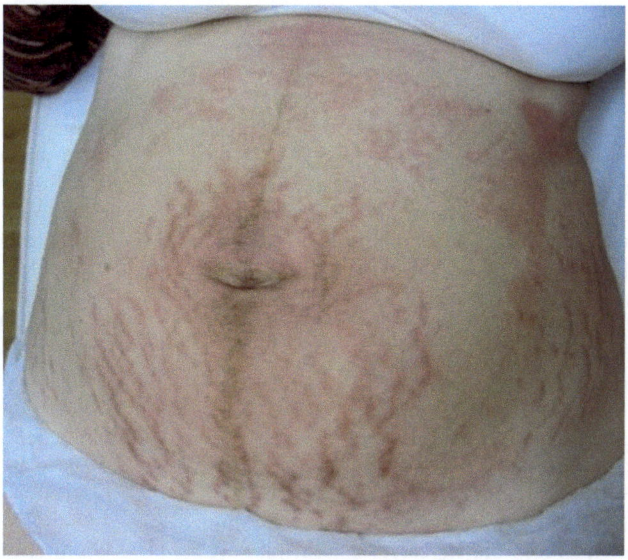

Fig. 11 Pruritic and urticarial papules and plaques of pregnancy (PUPPP)

antihistamines, after interacting with drugs that inhibit isoenzyme CYP3A4 of cytochrome P450, such as ketoconazole, erythromycin, clarithromycin, and isoniazid [60, 61, 84]. For the same reason H_1 antihistamines should not be administered along with fluconazole and itraconazole [85]. Similarly, the H_2 antagonist cimetidine interacts with a multitude of agents, such as calcium channel blockers, carbamazepine, sulphonylureas, warfarin, propranolol, phenytoin, and others [65]. In contrast, famotidine and nizatidine do not interact with cytochrome P450 and do not manifest clinically relevant drug interactions [65].

4 Conclusion

Since the discovery of the very first H_1 antihistamine, piperoxan in 1933 [86], the research concerning antihistamines, histamine, and histamine receptors has achieved great advancements. Disciplines like medicine, pharmacology, biochemistry, or molecular biology have contributed to our current knowledge and much more research on the field is under way. Moreover, the interest in the medical application of antihistamines has been fulfilled with the development of new generation drugs without the proverbial soporific action of the oldest ones, offering more therapeutic options for the patients. Yet, the approaches used in dermatology are essentially empirical and current related research, such as that presented in Chap. 9, is essential to drive therapeutics in dermatology into the twenty-first century. In the future, further understanding of the pathophysiology and the molecular basis of diseases will provide us with more sophisticated and effective treatments such as the novel H_4 receptor antagonists.

References

1. Panula P, Chazot PL, Cowart M et al (2015) Histamine receptors. Pharmacol Rev 67:601–655
2. Smuda C, Bryce PJ (2011) New developments in the use of histamine and histamine receptors. Curr Allergy Asthma Rep 11:94–100
3. Ohsawa Y, Hirasawa N (2014) The role of histamine H_1 and H_4 receptors in atopic dermatitis: from basic research to clinical study. Allergol Int 63:533–542
4. Thurmond RL, Gelfand EW, Dunford PJ (2008) The role of histamine H_1 and H_4 receptors in allergic inflammation: the search for new antihistamines. Nat Rev Drug Discov 7:41–53
5. Hu WW, Chen Z (2012) Role of histamine and its receptors in cerebral ischemia. ACS Chem Nerosci 3:238–247
6. Kopic S, Geibel JP (2013) Gastric acid, calcium absorption, and their impact on bone health. Physiol Rev 93:189–268
7. Ellenbroek BA (2013) Histamine H_3 receptors, the complex interaction with dopamine and its implications for addiction. Br J Pharmacol 170:46–57
8. Hofstra CL, Desai PJ, Thurmond RL et al (2003) Histamine H_4 receptor mediates chemotaxis and calcium mobilization of mast cells. J Pharmacol Exp Ther 305:1212–1221
9. Nijmeijer S, de Graaf C, Leurs R et al (2012) Molecular pharmacology of histamine H_4 receptors. Front Biosci (Landmark Ed) 17:2089–2106
10. Gschwandtner M, Rossbach K, Dijkstra D et al (2010) Murine and human Langerhans cells

express a functional histamine H_4 receptor: modulation of cell migration and function. Allergy 65:840–849
11. Dib K, Perecko T, Jenei V et al (2014) The histamine H_4 receptor is a potent inhibitor of adhesion-dependent degranulation in human neutrophils. J Leukoc Biol 96:411–418
12. Ling P, Ngo K, Nguyen S et al (2004) Histamine H_4 receptor mediates eosinophil chemotaxis with cell shape change and adhesion molecule upregulation. Br J Pharmacol 142:161–171
13. Dunford PJ, O'Donnell N, Riley JP et al (2006) The histamine H_4 receptor mediates allergic airway inflammation by regulating the activation of CD4+ T cells. J Immunol 176:7062–7070
14. Greaves MW (2005) Antihistamines in dermatology. Skin Pharmacol Physiol 18:220–229
15. Del Cuvillo A, Sastre J, Montoro J et al (2007) Use of antihistamines in pediatrics. J Investig Allergol Clin Immunol 17(S2):28–40
16. Simons FE, Simons KJ (2008) H_1 antihistamines: current status and future directions. World Allergy Organ J 1:145–155
17. Richelson E (1979) Tricyclic antidepressants and histamine H_1 receptors. Mayo Clin Proc 54:669–674
18. Singh H, Becker PM (2007) Novel therapeutic usage of low-dose doxepin hydrochloride. Expert Opin Investig Drugs 16:1295–1305
19. Egan CA, Rallis TM (1997) Treatment of chronic urticaria with ketotifen. Arch Dermatol 133:147–149
20. Sokol KC, Amar NK, Starkey J et al (2013) Ketotifen in the management of chronic urticaria: resurrection of an old drug. Ann Allergy Asthma Immunol 111:433–436
21. Paquette D, Rothe MJ (2000) Unapproved dermatologic indications for H_2 receptor antagonists, cromolyn sodium, and ketotifen. Clin Dermatol 18:103–111
22. Finn DF, Walsh JJ (2013) Twenty-first century mast cell stabilizers. Br J Pharmacol 170:23–37
23. Theoharides TC, Valent P, Akin C (2015) Mast cells, mastocytosis, and related disorders. N Engl J Med 373:163–172
24. Zuberbier T, Aberer W, Asero R et al (2014) The EAACI/GA(2) LEN/EDF/WAO Guideline for the definition, classification, diagnosis, and management of urticaria: the 2013 revision and update. Allergy 69:868–887
25. Schoepke N, Doumoulakis G, Maurer M (2013) Diagnosis of urticaria. Indian J Dermatol 58:211–218
26. Sachdeva S, Gupta V, Amin SS et al (2011) Chronic urticaria. Indian J Dermatol 56:622–628
27. Bernstein JA, Lang DM, Khan DA et al (2014) The diagnosis and management of acute and chronic urticaria: 2014 update. J Allergy Clin Immunol 133:1270–1277
28. Sharma M, Bennett C, Cohen SN et al (2014) H1-antihistamines for chronic spontaneous urticaria. Cochrane Database Syst Rev 11:CD006137
29. Fedorowicz Z, van Zuuren EJ, Hu N (2012) Histamine H2-receptor antagonists for urticaria. Cochrane Database Syst Rev 3:CD008596
30. Lee JH, Son SW, Cho SH (2016) A comprehensive review of the treatment of atopic eczema. Allergy Asthma Immunol Res 8:181–190
31. Bannister MJ, Freeman S (2000) Adult-onset atopic dermatitis. Australas J Dermatol 41:225–228
32. Kanwar AJ, Narang T (2013) Adult onset atopic dermatitis: under-recognized or under-reported? Indian Dermatol Online J 4:167–171
33. Novak N, Leung DY (2011) Advances in atopic dermatitis. Curr Opin Immunol 23:778–783
34. De Benedetto A, Yoshida T, Fridy S et al (2015) Histamine and skin barrier: are histamine antagonists useful for the prevention or treatment of atopic dermatitis? J Clin Med 4:741–755
35. Nicolaidou E, Katsambas AD (2003) Antihistamines and steroids in pediatric dermatology. Clin Dermatol 21:321–324
36. Savall BM, Chavez F, Tays K et al (2014) Discovery and SAR of 6-alkyl-2,4-diaminopyrimidines as histamine H_4 receptor antagonists. J Med Chem 57:2429–2439
37. Kollmeier A, Francke K, Chen B et al (2014) The histamine H4 receptor antagonist, JNJ 39758979, is effective in reducing histamine-induced pruritus in a randomized clinical study in healthy subjects. J Pharmacol Exp Ther 350:181–187
38. Ohsawa Y, Hirasawa N (2012) The antagonism of histamine H1 and H4 receptors ameliorates chronic allergic dermatitis via anti-pruritic and anti-inflammatory effects in NC/Nga mice. Allergy 67:1014–1022
39. O'Donoghue M, Tharp MD (2005) Antihistamines and their role as antipruritics. Dermatol Ther 18:333–340
40. Goutos I, Dziewulski P, Richardson PM (2009) Pruritus in burns: review article. J Burn Care Res 30:221–228

41. Juckett G (2013) Arthropod bites. Am Fam Physician 88:841–847
42. Smith KJ, Skelton HG, Yeager J et al (1997) Pruritus in HIV-1 disease: therapy with drugs which may modulate the pattern of immune dysregulation. Dermatology 195:353–358
43. Pour-Reza-Gholi F, Nasrollahi A, Firouzan A et al (2007) Low-dose doxepin for treatment of pruritus in patients on hemodialysis. Iran J Kidney Dis 1:34–37
44. Englisch W, Bauer CP (1997) Dimethindene maleate in the treatment of pruritus caused by varicella zoster virus infection in children. Arzneimittelforschung 47:1233–1235
45. Mamdani FS (1994) Pharmacologic management of herpes zoster and postherpetic neuralgia. Can Fam Physician 40:321–326
46. Verma P, Singal A, Sharma S (2012) Idiopathic bullous eosinophilic cellulitis (Wells syndrome) responsive to topical tacrolimus and antihistamine combination. Indian J Dermatol Venereol Leprol 78:378–380
47. Sinno H, Lacroix JP, Lee J et al (2012) Diagnosis and management of eosinophilic cellulitis (Wells' syndrome): a case series and literature review. Can J Plast Surg 20:91–97
48. Tripathi T, Shahid M, Khan HM et al (2010) Modulation of in vivo immunoglobulin production by endogenous histamine and H1R and H2R agonists and antagonists. Pharmacol Rep 62:917–925
49. Sinha S, Relhan V, Garg VK (2015) Immunomodulators in warts: unexplored or ineffective? Indian J Dermatol 60:118–129
50. Bauman C, Francis JS, Vanderhooft S et al (1996) Cimetidine therapy for multiple viral warts in children. J Am Acad Dermatol 35:271–272
51. Micali G, Nasca MR, Dall'Oglio F et al (2003) Cimetidine therapy for epidermodysplasia verruciformis. J Am Acad Dermatol 48:S9–10
52. Stashower ME, Yeager JK, Smith KJ et al (1993) Cimetidine as therapy for treatment-resistant psoriasis in a patient with acquired immunodeficiency syndrome. Arch Dermatol 129:848–850
53. Staevska M, Gugutkova M, Lazarova C et al (2014) Night-time sedating H1-antihistamine increases daytime somnolence but not treatment efficacy in chronic spontaneous urticaria: a randomized controlled trial. Br J Dermatol 171:148–154
54. Murota H, Kitaba S, Tani M et al (2010) Impact of sedative and non-sedative antihistamines on the impaired productivity and quality of life in patients with pruritic skin diseases. Allergol Int 59:345–354
55. Nicholson AN (1983) Antihistamines and sedation. Lancet 322:211–212
56. Chishty M, Reichel A, Siva J et al (2001) Affinity for the P-glycoprotein efflux pump at the blood-brain barrier may explain the lack of CNS side-effects of modern antihistamines. J Drug Target 9:223–228
57. Hu Y, Sieck DE, Hsu WH (2015) Why are second-generation H1-antihistamines minimally sedating? Eur J Pharmacol 765:100–106
58. Naicker P, Anoopkumar-Dukie S, Grant GD et al (2013) The effects of antihistamines with varying anticholinergic properties on voluntary and involuntary movement. Clin Neurophysiol 124:1840–1845
59. He M, Deng C, Huang XF (2013) The role of hypothalamic H1 receptor antagonism in antipsychotic-induced weight gain. CNS Drugs 27:423–434
60. Woosley RL (1996) Cardiac actions of antihistamines. Annu Rev Pharmacol Toxicol 36: 233–252
61. Rico S, Antonijoan R, Barbanoj M (2009) Ebastine in the light of CONGA recommendations for the development of third-generation antihistamines. J Asthma Allergy 2:73–92
62. Deepinder F, Braunstein GD (2012) Drug-induced gynecomastia: an evidence-based review. Expert Opin Drug Saf 11:779–795
63. Van Thiel DH, Gavaler JS, Smith WI Jr et al (1979) Hypothalamic-pituitary-gonadal dysfunction in men using cimetidine. N Engl J Med 300:1012–1015
64. Schmidt JB (1998) Other antiandrogens. Dermatology 196:153–157
65. Hafeez ZH (1996) Antihistamines and their role in dermatology. J Pak Med Assoc 46:264–267
66. Clegg A, Young JB (2011) Which medications to avoid in people at risk of delirium: a systematic review. Age Ageing 40:23–29
67. Tawadrous D, Dixon S, Shariff SZ et al (2014) Altered mental status in older adults with histamine2-receptor antagonists: a population-based study. Eur J Intern Med 25:701–709
68. Elder JB, Ganguli PC, Gillespie IE (1979) Cimetidine and gastric cancer. Lancet 313:1005–1006
69. Langman MJ, Dunn JA, Whiting JL et al (1999) Prospective, double-blind, placebo-controlled randomized trial of cimetidine in gastric cancer. British Stomach Cancer Group. Br J Cancer 81:1356–1362
70. Jiang CG, Liu FR, Yu M et al (2010) Cimetidine induces apoptosis in gastric cancer cells in vitro and inhibits tumor growth in vivo. Oncol Rep 23:693–700

71. Tønnesen H, Knigge U, Bülow S et al (1988) Effect of cimetidine on survival after gastric cancer. Lancet 332:990–992
72. Pompili M, Basso M, Grieco A et al (2004) Recurrent acute hepatitis associated with use of cetirizine. Ann Pharmacother 38:1844–1847
73. Ekiz F, Yüksel I, Ekiz O et al (2011) Levocetirizine induced hepatotoxicity in a patient with chronic urticaria. Ann Hepatol 10:237–238
74. Paton DM, Webster DR (1985) Clinical pharmacokinetics of H1-receptor antagonists (the antihistamines). Clin Pharmacokinet 10:477–497
75. Zazgornik J, Huang ML, Van Peer A et al (1993) Pharmacokinetics of orally administered levocabastine in patients with renal insufficiency. J Clin Pharmacol 33:1214–1218
76. Gilboa SM, Strickland MJ, Olshan AF et al (2009) National Birth Defects Prevention Study. Use of antihistamine medications during early pregnancy and isolated major malformations. Birth Defects Res A Clin Mol Teratol 85:137–150
77. Gilboa SM, Ailes EC, Rai RP et al (2014) Antihistamines and birth defects: a systematic review of the literature. Expert Opin Drug Saf 13:1667–1698
78. FDA Pregnancy Categories. http://www.drugs.com/pregnancy-categories.html. Accessed 26 Apr 2016
79. Poza J, Caminal P, Vallverdú M et al (2007) Study of the EEG changes during the combined ingestion of alcohol and H1-antihistamines by using the wavelet transform. Conf Proc IEEE Eng Med Biol Soc 2007:23–26
80. Scaglione F (2012) Safety profile of bilastine: 2nd generation H1-antihistamines. Eur Rev Med Pharmacol Sci 16:1999–2005
81. Montoro J, Bartra J, Sastre J et al (2013) H1 antihistamines and benzodiazepines. Pharmacological interactions and their impact on cerebral function. J Investig Allergol Clin Immunol 23(S1):17–26
82. Bartra J, Valero AL, del Cuvillo A et al (2006) Interactions of the H1 antihistamines. J Investig Allergol Clin Immunol 16(1):29–36
83. Stahl SM, Felker A (2008) Monoamine oxidase inhibitors: a modern guide to an unrequited class of antidepressants. CNS Spectr 13:855–870
84. Zhou S, Yung Chan S, Cher Goh B et al (2005) Mechanism-based inhibition of cytochrome P450 3A4 by therapeutic drugs. Clin Pharmacokinet 44:279–304
85. Katz HI (1999) Drug interactions of the newer oral antifungal agents. Br J Dermatol 141(S56):26–32
86. Fourneau E, Bovet D (1933) Recherches sur l' action sympathicolytique d' un nouveau dérivé du dioxane. Arch Int Pharmacodyn Ther 46:178–191

Chapter 17

Histamine Quantification in Human Blood Samples

Ekaterini Tiligada, Maria Kakolyri, and Madeleine Ennis

Abstract

Histamine is a short-acting biogenic amine that elicits pleiotropic actions mainly through binding to four receptor types designated as H_1–H_4. Since its discovery more than a century ago, it has been one of the most studied molecules in biomedical sciences and has provided blockbuster therapeutic drugs for the management of allergies, gastric ulcers, and more recently for narcolepsy. The discovery of the high affinity H_4 receptor at the turn of the millennium revived the interest in histamine research and translational potential, particularly in the expanding field of immunopharmacology. Among the various methods developed for the quantification of histamine in human whole blood, plasma, and serum, the fluorometric assay that was developed more than 65 years ago still remains popular in biomedical and clinical protocols. The common basis of the several available modifications is the reaction of the extracted histamine with *o*-phthalaldehyde (*o*-PT) in an alkaline environment to produce fluorescent condensation derivatives. These are stabilized by acidification commonly 4 min after the addition of *o*-PT and measured using a fluorospectrophotometer at excitation and emission wavelengths of 360 and 450 nm, respectively. The histamine concentration in the unknown sample is read off a standard curve. A number of factors that may potentially influence the level of circulating histamine should be considered when designing the investigation or evaluating the outcome, including patient information and medical history, as well as blood sampling, handling, and storage conditions.

Key words Fluorospectrophotometry, Histamine, Human, Peripheral blood, Plasma, Serum

1 Introduction

Histamine (Fig. 1) is a short-acting biogenic amine formed by the decarboxylation of the basic amino acid L-histidine through the catalytic activity of the rate-limiting enzyme histidine decarboxylase (HDC) [1, 5]. The two major catabolic pathways in man comprise the methylation of the imidazole ring by histamine *N*-methyltransferase (HNMT) and the oxidative deamination of the primary amino group by diamine oxidase (DAO) (Fig. 1) [1]. In mammals, the classical source of histamine is the pluripotent heterogeneous mast cell [6], where it is stored in cytosolic granules and released in response to various immunological and non-immunological stimuli [7, 8]. Histamine release from mast cells

Ekaterini Tiligada and Madeleine Ennis (eds.), *Histamine Receptors as Drug Targets*, Methods in Pharmacology and Toxicology,
DOI 10.1007/978-1-4939-6843-5_17,

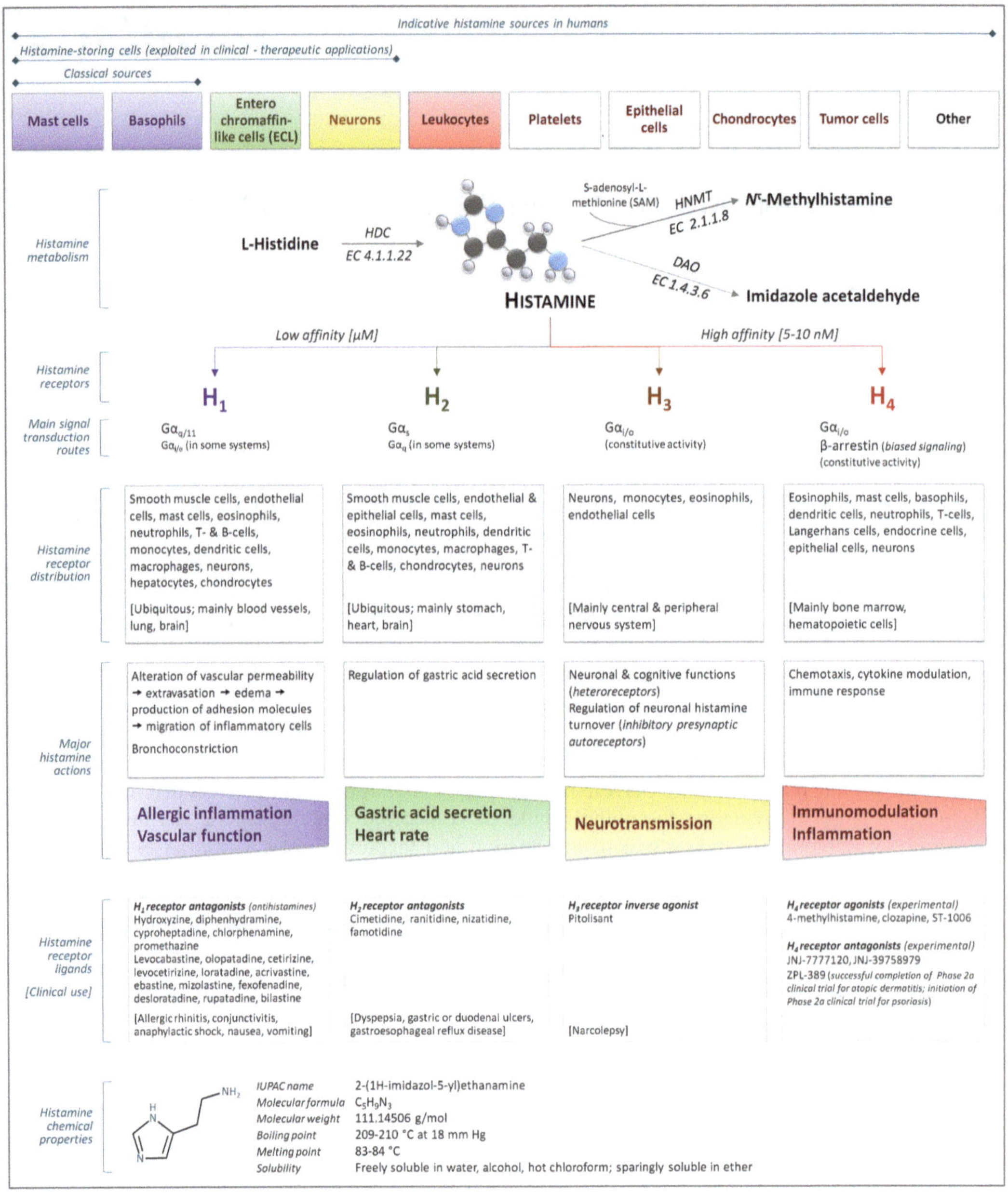

Fig. 1 Overview of histamine properties in mammals. Histamine is formed in various cell types and exerts numerous actions via binding to four receptor types, designated as H_1–H_4. DAO: diamine oxidase, EC: Enzyme Commission number, HDC: histidine decarboxylase (detectable only in cells that actively synthesize histamine), HNMT: histamine-N-methyltransferase, IUPAC: International Union of Pure and Applied Chemistry [1–4]

has been traditionally associated with mild to severe signs and symptoms that characterize hypersensitivity reactions, including erythema, urticaria, itching, tachycardia, hypotension, ventricular fibrillations, bronchospasm, and cardiac and respiratory arrest [9–11]. To date, numerous additional sources have been identified, including basophils [12], gastric enterochromaffin-like cells [13], neurons [14, 15], as well as cancer cells [16].

Since its discovery more than 100 years ago [17], histamine has been one of the most studied molecules in biomedical sciences [2]. In addition to modulating a wide range of physiological processes [3, 18, 19], histamine is implicated in pathological conditions including allergies and anaphylaxis [20–23], asthma and chronic inflammation [24–26], autoimmune [27, 28], cardiovascular [28, 29], neuropsychiatric [14, 15, 30, 31], and endocrine [32, 33] disorders as well as cancer [16, 34, 35] (Fig. 1). Histamine exerts its pleiotropic actions mainly through binding to four types of G-protein-coupled receptors (GPCRs), designated as H_1–H_4 that are differentially expressed in various cell types and exhibit considerable variations among species (Fig. 1) [2, 3, 36]. Notably, receptor-independent effects have also been described in both eukaryotic and prokaryotic organisms [37, 38].

1.1 Current Challenges in Histamine Research and Therapeutic Exploitation

The histaminergic system has been exploited for more than 70 years, providing blockbuster therapeutic H_1 (H_1 antihistamines) and H_2 receptor antagonists for the treatment of allergies and gastric ulcers, respectively [2]. The latest advances in histamine research reflect the ongoing efforts to dissect new key pathways underlying a number of pathologies with high economic and societal impact. An illustrative example is the recent recommendation of the European Medicines Agency (EMA) to grant marketing authorization for the first selective H_3 receptor inverse agonist pitolisant (previously called BF2.649) (Fig. 1) for the management of narcolepsy [39]. Furthermore, the discovery of the high affinity H_4 receptor in 2000 and its constitutive activity and expression mostly on immune cells (Fig. 1) continues to reveal new roles for histamine in inflammation, and greatly contributes to the presently expanding field of immunopharmacology [24, 40]. The translational potential of this new drug target provides attractive novel therapeutic options, as indicated by the successful completion and the initiation of Phase 2a proof of concept studies with the H_4 receptor antagonist ZPL-389 for the management of atopic dermatitis and psoriasis [41]. Further to these successes, the complex pluridimensional rather than linear pharmacology of the H_4 receptor ligands exhibiting biased signaling and exemplified by the prototype molecule JNJ 7777120 is currently under intense investigation, providing a paradigm for the novel approaches governing the pharmacological investigation of GPCRs [42]. Moreover, the continuing challenge to (re)define the translational value of research findings, frequently hampered by the commonly overlooked species differences, seeks to identify and validate novel drug targets and to optimize lead candidates to meet the existing therapeutic challenges [43].

1.2 Methods for Histamine Quantification

The biological significance of histamine and its implication in a number of human pathologies (Fig. 1) underlines the demand for the reliable quantification of this amine in biological samples. A variety of methodologies, ranging from the simple colorimetric and biological tests to the more complex chromatographic and immunoabsorbent assays, have been developed (Table 1). They aim to determine the histamine levels in various tissues and fluids, including plasma, serum, urine, cerebrospinal fluid and hair, as well as in primary cell and tissue cultures and cell lines. The first attempts to measure histamine were based on colorimetric techniques and bioassays. Considering the lack of exploitable light absorption and emission properties of histamine, nonbiological quantification methods rely on chemical derivatization [80]. Colorimetric assays date back to the 1910s, when the use of a diazo reaction was reported [44]. However, their use in biomedical research and clinical applications has been hampered by unsatisfactory recovery for quantitative chemical titration. In contrast, bioassays commonly utilizing isolated guinea pig ileum and blood pressure measurements in cats or dogs have been historically used to determine the biological responses and the pharmacological effects of histamine in living systems [46–51]. Subsequently, numerous methodologies have been developed, including radioenzymatic assays [62–64], chromatographic techniques [65–68], immunological methods, such as radioimmunoassays [71–73] and enzyme-linked immunosorbent assays (ELISA) or enzyme immunoassays (EIA) [75, 76], mass spectrometry [69, 70], and more recently flow cytometry [77–79] or combinations of these techniques [81] (Table 1). Many of them are reserved mainly for the measurement of the histamine content in food, such as fish, meat, and cheese [45, 82–85], as well as in wine and fruit juices [86].

The most common method used for histamine quantification in biomedical protocols is the fluorometric assay that was developed more than 65 years ago [52] and still remains popular [20, 28, 53–57]. Automated fluorescence assays for histamine quantification have also been developed [58, 59] and are still in use largely for in vitro allergy testing [23]. The common basis of the several available modifications of the fluorometric assay is the reaction of histamine with *o*-phthalaldehyde (*o*-PT) in an alkaline environment to produce highly fluorescent condensation derivatives, which are stabilized by the acidification of the solution to pH 2–4 [56, 60]. The fluorophore shows excitation and emission maxima at 360 and 444 nm, respectively, whereas fluorescence intensity reaches a maximum 4 min after the addition of *o*-PT [60, 61].

Table 1
Main analytical methods used for measuring histamine levels in biological samples

Assay outline	Indicative examples and comments
Colorimetric techniques	
Chemical coupling of the extracted/purified histamine typically with a diazo reagent; measurement of the absorbance of the colored derivative using a spectrophotometer [44, 45]	• Limited use in biomedical research (mostly used to measure histamine content in food) • Alternative enzymatic tests use diamine oxidase (DAO), horseradish peroxidase (HRP), and a reagent to visualize the colored compounds resulting upon histamine oxidation
Bioassays	
Physiological responses to histamine used as the final test to determine the tissue histamine equivalent [46–51]	• Simple and sensitive, yet laborious; technical skills required; use of animals • Use of selective agonists and/or antagonists to increase specificity • Dependent on the isolated tissue and/or organ sensitivity; influenced by diurnal variations • Prior histamine extraction/purification required • Interference by endogenous substances, bathing medium components, and experimental drugs
Fluorometric assays	
Reaction of extracted/purified histamine with *o*-phthalaldehyde (o-PT) in alkaline environment; stabilization of the fluorescent condensation derivatives by acidification; measurement using a fluorospectrophotometer [52–61]	• Popular in clinical and biological research • Laborious; prior histamine extraction from the biological sample required • Several modifications reported to date • Automated assays available
Radioenzymatic methods	
Transfer of a radioactive methyl group from [^{14}C]- or [^{3}H]methyl-S-adenosyl-L-methionine (SAM) to histamine using histamine-*N*-methyltransferase (HNMT) to form $N\tau$-[^{14}C]- or [^{3}H]methyl-histamine; separation of the histamine bound radioactive fraction; quantification using a liquid scintillation counter [62–64]	• Double-isotope ([^{14}C]SAM and [^{3}H]histamine); single-isotope single-step ([^{14}C]SAM); single-isotope multiple-step ([^{3}H]SAM) assays developed • Prior histamine extraction not required • Relatively simple but expensive • May be influenced by drugs and/or HNMT substrates
Chromatography and mass spectrometry	
Various methods used including thin-layer chromatography (TLC), high-performance liquid chromatography (HPLC), gas-liquid chromatography and gas chromatography-mass spectrometry (GC-MS) [65–70]	• Commonly but not exclusively used for brain and cerebrospinal fluid (CSF) histamine determination; with or without prior extraction and/or precolumn derivatization • Expensive and laborious; complex separation procedures may be required to avoid cross-reactivity with other biogenic amines • Measurement of the levels of the major metabolites (methylhistamine, imidazoleacetic acid, methylimidazoleacetic acid) in urine

(continued)

Table 1 (continued)

Assay outline	Indicative examples and comments
Immunoassays	
Histamine is too small to serve as an antigen; it is not immunogenic and may not be iodinated. The main limitation is to produce antibodies directed toward histamine itself to take advantage of the specificity of an antigen-antibody reaction [71]	
Radioimmunoassay (RIA)	
Use of antibodies against antigens in which histamine is integrated [71–74]	• Antibody directed against histamine coupled to bovine serum albumin (BSA) using a coupling reagent, such as benzoquinone and [^{125}I]tracer (Immunotech, France) • Coupling canine serum albumin to N^{τ}-methylhistamine (Pharmacia, Sweden); not useful for plasma histamine determination
Enzyme-linked immunosorbent assay (ELISA) & Enzyme immunoassay (EIA)	
Several kits commercially available; no prior histamine extraction/purification; typically based on the competition of an unknown amount of derivatized or non-derivatized histamine (antigen) a fixed amount of enzyme-labeled antigen for the binding sites of the coated antibodies; the developed color intensity read at the appropriate wavelength; histamine levels determined using a standard curve [75, 76]	• Quantitative histamine acylation prior to the completion for the bound antibody binding sites; detection (commonly) by IgG-peroxidase conjugate using 3,3′,5,5′-tetramethylbenzidine (TMB) as substrate (LDN®, Germany; IBL, Germany; Abnova, Taiwan; MyBiosure, USA; Fitzgerald, USA) • Competition between free histamine in the sample and HRP-labeled histamine using TMB as a substrate (Oxford Biomedical Research, UK) • Histamine acylation not required; based on a polyclonal antibody, biotinylated histamine tracer, IgG and HRP conjugated streptavidin (Enzo®, USA) • Competition between unlabeled derivatized histamine and histamine linked to acetylcholinesterase (AChE) as tracer (SPI-BIO, France) • Acylated histamine incubated in coated monoclonal antibody in the presence of alkaline phosphatase acylated histamine conjugate (Immunotech, France)
Flow cytometry	
Analysis of intracellular histamine and release by an enzyme-affinity-fluorochrome method using coupling of diamine oxidase (DAO) to fluorochromes (HistaFlow) [77–79]	• Localization of intracellular histamine in mast cells and basophils to study histamine transport and ultrastructural alterations during degranulation

2 Fluorometric Determination of Histamine Levels in Peripheral Blood

The interest in determining histamine levels in peripheral blood stems from the decisive value of blood biochemical analyses in disease diagnosis and monitoring. Most tests are performed using blood plasma (prepared by collecting whole blood in anticoagulant-containing tubes followed by cell removal by centrifugation; makes up ~55% of the blood) or serum (the clear yellowish liquid fraction that remains after the blood is allowed to clot). Analysis of other body fluids, such as urine and cerebrospinal fluid, is also common [69, 73]. However, measuring histamine levels in human plasma or serum has long been a matter of discussion [54]. Histamine has a short half-life (2–4 min) before being converted to the major metabolite N^{τ}-methylhistamine and in some cases it has to be determined in either or both plasma and serum depending on earlier data or on the need to perform correlation studies with other parameters measured in the respective blood fraction [20, 21, 54]. In a quality-control study performed in 1988, five histamine assays used in different European laboratories to determine clinically relevant histamine concentrations in human plasma (0–45 nmol/l) and aqueous solutions (0–10 nmol/l) were compared [54]. For human plasma, estimating concentrations within the normal range seemed to be the most difficult part.

Basal plasma histamine levels have been reported to be in the upper pM to the lower nM range [21, 54, 63], yet a number of factors (Fig. 2) may potentially influence the level of circulating

- **Sex**
- **Age**
- **Race**
- **Circadian rhythm**
- **Food intake**
- **Body temperature**
- **Medical history – General health**
- **Medication**
- **Dietary supplements** (e.g. vitamins, minerals)
- **Compliance/concordance of the subject with preparatory instructions**
- **Sampling technique**
- **Variations between laboratories**

Fig. 2 Non-exhaustive list of factors that may influence the results of laboratory tests, including histamine determination in human samples [4, 18, 20, 22, 28, 29, 32–35, 54, 87–93] histamine and therefore, they should be considered when designing the investigation or evaluating the outcome (Fig. 3). These include age, sex, and diurnal rhythms [18, 19, 33, 87, 88], pathological conditions [29, 32, 34], allergen tolerance [20], medication regimens [35, 89], as well as sampling techniques [90, 91] and assay methodologies [4, 54, 74, 92]. For instance, histamine skin reactivity has been reported to increase with body mass index (BMI) in adults with allergic nasal symptoms [22], whereas it did not vary throughout the menstrual cycle but was positively correlated with serum sex hormones levels at mid-cycle [93]. Consequently, it is important to gather a complete medical history, including relevant laboratory test results that are often part of a routine checkup (Fig. 3). The system used within our laboratory is detailed below.

2.1 Sample Collection and Handling

2.1.1 Equipment and Materials

- Sample identification form (Fig. 3).
- Labels with identification codes or a durable marker for writing on the tubes.
- Commercially available blood handling tubes (Vacutainer®, Becton Dickinson, USA): red topped for serum samples; purple (EDTA-treated) or light blue (citrate-treated) topped for whole blood and plasma samples (*see* **Notes 1 and 2**).
- Polypropylene tubes for transferring serum or plasma (e.g., Falcon® 15 ml conical tubes, Corning® Inc., USA).
- Polypropylene tubes (2 ml) for storing aliquots (e.g., Eppendorf® Safe-Lock tubes).
- Suitable tube racks.
- Single-use disposable transfer pipettes.
- Precision autoclavable pipettes (volume range 1000–5000 ml) with disposable polypropylene tips.
- Refrigerated centrifuge capable of 3000 × *g*.
- Refrigerator (4 °C).
- Freezer (−20 °C, −80 °C).
- Container with crushed ice for sample transfer (if needed).
- Boxes for tube storage.
- Timer.

2.1.2 Methods

Blood drawing is performed by qualified personnel according to the standard procedures established in the institution [90, 91] (*see* **Notes 1** and **2**).

1. Informed consent is obtained from the donor [94].
2. The identification code, the investigator's and phlebotomist's details, and the sections A, B, C1, C2, and C3 are completed in the sample identification form shown in Fig. 3.

Sample identification code: ....
Investigator/Physician: .... **Phlebotomist** ....

A. Sampling Information

Date: ...... /...... / ...... ☐ Spring (20 Mar -20 Jun) ☐ Summer (21 Jun -21 Sep) ☐ Autumn (22 Sep - 20 Dec) ☐ Winter (21 Dec - 19 Mar)

Time: ...... : ...... ☐ Morning (8am -2pm) ☐ Afternoon (2-8pm) ☐ Night (8pm-8am)

B. Subject Details

Date of Birth: ...... /...... / ...... Age at the time of sampling: ....years

☐ Baby (0-1y) ☐ Toddler (1-3y) ☐ Child (3-13y) ☐ Teenager (13-18y) ☐ Adult (18-65y) ☐ Elderly (>65y)

☐ Male ☐ Female Last menstrual period (LMP) ☐ Pregnant ☐ Nursing

Menstrual cycle phase ☐ Menstrual (day 1-5) ☐ Follicular (day 1-13)

☐ Ovulation (day 14) ☐ Luteal (day 15-28)

Weight (W): ....Kg Height (H): ....cm Body mass index ($BMI=W/H^2$) ....

Comments: ....

C. Medical History

C1. Illnesses & Chronic Medication

Immune system: ....
Allergies: ....
Gastrointestinal track: ....
Endocrine system: ....
Cardiovascular system: ....
Central nervous system: ....
Other: ....

Tobacco use: ☐ No ☐ Yes Cigarettes/day: ...... Years of use: ......
Alcohol use: ☐ No ☐ Yes Units/week: ...... Years of use: ......

C2. Medication Used within 7 Days Prior to Sampling (Formulation - Dose - Hours elapsed since last dose)

Antinflammatory ....
Corticosteroids ....
H_1-antihistamines ....
H_2-antagonists ....
Mast cell stabilizers ....
Antileukotrienes ....
Omalizumab ....
Antidepressants ....
Other (incl. vitamins) ....
....

Comments: ....

C3. Clinical (Medical) Laboratory Tests

White blood cell count (WBC)	....	Lymphocytes	....
Neutrophils	....	Monocytes	....
Basophils	....	Eosinophils	....
Total serum protein	....	C-reactive protein (CRP)	....
Tryptase	....	Immunoglobulin E (IgE)	....

Comments: ....

D. Histamine quantification

Date : ...... /...... / ...... Whole blood levels ....
Date : ...... /...... / ...... Plasma levels .... [commonly in ng/ml]
Date : ...... /...... / ...... Serum levels ....

Comments: ....

General comments: ....
....
....

Boxes checked accordingly

Fig. 3 Template of the sample identification form, including medical history and the most relevant laboratory test results

A *Whole Blood*

3A. Venous whole blood (2 × 3 ml) is collected in a purple or light blue topped tube and placed on ice after collection (*see* **Notes 1** and **2**).

4A. If analysis is not performed on the day of blood collection, the samples are immediately stored at −80 °C (for analyses performed within 3 days, the samples may be kept at −20 °C) (*see* **Note 3**).

B *Serum Preparation*

3B. Venous whole blood (10 ml) is collected in a red topped blood tube.

4B. The blood is allowed to clot at room temperature (RT; 15–24 °C) for 20–30 min.

5B. The samples are centrifuged at 1500 × *g* for 10 min at 4 °C.

6B. The resulting supernatant is carefully collected and immediately transferred into a clean polypropylene tube using a single-use disposable transfer pipette. If not analyzed immediately, serum is divided into 2 ml aliquots and stored at −80 °C until assayed (*see* **Note 3**).

C *Plasma Preparation*

3C. Venous whole blood (10 ml) is collected in a purple or light blue topped tube.

4C. The samples are centrifuged at 2000 × *g* for 15 min at 4 °C as soon as possible (within 20 min after blood collection) to remove cells including platelets.

5C. Plasma is obtained by immediately collecting and transferring the resulting supernatant into a clean polypropylene tube using a single-use disposable transfer pipette. If not analyzed immediately, plasma is divided into 2 ml aliquots and stored at −80 °C until assayed (*see* **Note 3**).

2.2 Histamine Extraction and Quantification

2.2.1 Equipment and Materials

- Screw cap laboratory bottles for solution storage (Pyrex®; capacity 500 ml).
- Screw top amber glass vials (capacity 10, 50 ml).
- Laboratory glassware for the preparation of solutions (Pyrex®; 500 ml graduated measuring cylinders, 400 ml graduated beakers) (Fig. 4).
- Glass test tubes (capacity 15 ml).
- Borosilicate glass test tubes with glass stoppers (QuickFit®, capacity 15 ml; properly balanced).
- Suitable test tube racks.
- Container with crushed ice.
- Adjustable-volume pipettes (100–1000 μl, 500–2500 μl) and suitable disposable polypropylene pipette tips.
- Precision scale (weighing capacity 200 g, 0.001 g readability).
- Laboratory vortex mixer.
- Magnetic stirrer with heating plate and magnetic bar (to accommodate 400 ml glass beakers).

SOLUTIONS FOR HISTAMINE EXTRACTION AND QUANTIFICATION

PERCHLORIC ACID ($HClO_4$: 70 %; d = 1.67 g/ml; MW 100.5)

0.4N $HClO_4$	6.88 ml $HClO_4$	IN	200 ml d.H_2O*

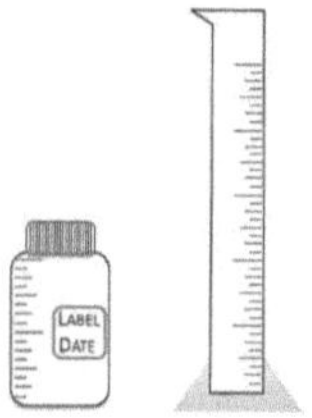

SULFURIC ACID (H_2SO_4 : 95-98%; d=1.84 g/ml; MW 98.08)

2N H_2SO_4	11.2 ml H_2SO_4	IN	200 ml d.H_2O*
0.1N H_2SO_4	1.4 ml H_2SO_4	IN	500 ml d.H_2O*
0.05N H_2SO_4	0.14 ml H_2SO_4	IN	100 ml d.H_2O*

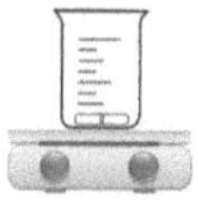

SODIUM CHLORIDE, SATURATED (NaCl; solubility in cold H_2O: 357 g/l)

Sat-NaCl	~110 g NaCl	IN	300 ml d.H_2O

→ stirred well at 24-25 °C for ~ 30 min

SODIUM HYDROXIDE (NaOH; anhydrous pellets; MW 40)

5N NaOH	40 g NaOH	IN	200 ml d.H_2O*
1N NaOH	8 g NaOH	IN	200 ml d.H_2O*
salt-sat 0.1N NaOH	0.8 g NaOH	IN	200 ml filtered sat-NaCl*

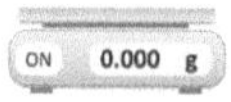

HISTAMINE STOCK SOLUTION#

100 μg/ml 8.3 mg histamine · 2HCl IN 50 ml 0.05N H_2SO_4

HISTAMINE WORKING SOLUTION (freshly prepared in a glass test tube)†

1 μg/ml 0.1 ml histamine stock solution mixed with 9.9 ml 0.1N H_2SO_4

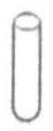

***O*-PHTHALALDEHYDE** (*o*-PT; freshly prepared in a screw top amber glass vial)†

1 % (w/v)	10 mg o-PT	IN	1 ml methanol

*Can be stored in screw cap laboratory bottles at 4°C for up to 3 months

#Only the mass of histamine (MW 111.15) is considered for calculations. Stored in a screw top amber glass vial at 4 °C for up to 2 months. Returned to 4 °C immediately after use.

†Placed on ice until use. Volumes may vary depending on the quantities required for quantification (e.g. microcuvettes or 96-well plates require much smaller quantities than standard cuvettes)

d: density; d.H_2O: distilled water; MW: molecular weight; sat: saturated

Fig. 4 Preparation of solutions used for the in-house extraction and fluorometric determination of histamine in human biological samples

- Glass homogenizers (Pyrex®; capacity 10 ml; properly balanced) with Teflon® pestle.
- Bench mixer stirrer homogenizer [e.g., Tri-R Stir-R, 500–11,000 revolutions per minute (rpm)].
- Refrigerated centrifuge [angle rotor with bucket adaptor to accommodate 15 ml QuickFit® glass test tubes with glass stopper; relative centrifugal force (RCF) 2000 × *g*].
- Laboratory shaker [to accommodate 15 ml QuickFit® glass test tubes with glass stopper].
- Water bath (37 °C).

- Laboratory aspirator pump (attached to a laboratory faucet).
- Fluorescence spectrophotometer (e.g., LS55 Perkin Elmer, USA; calibrated according to the instructions of the manufacturer) and suitable cuvettes.
- Disposable glass Pasteur pipettes.
- Timer.

Chemicals and Reagents

- Distilled water (d.H_2O).
- Perchloric acid ($HClO_4$; 70%; density 1.67 g/ml; MW 100.5).
- Sulfuric acid (H_2SO_4; 95–98%; density 1.84 g/ml; MW 98.08).
- Sodium chloride (NaCl; anhydrous, reagent grade, ≥99%; MW 58.44).
- Sodium hydroxide (NaOH; anhydrous pellets, reagent grade, ≥98%; MW 40).
- Histamine dihydrochloride ($C_5H_9N_3$ 2HCl; analytical grade, ≥99%; MW 184.07).
- *o*-Phthalaldehyde (*o*-PT; analytical grade, ≥99%; MW 134.13).
- Methanol (CH_3OH; MeOH; ≥99%; MW 32.04).
- 1-Butanol [$CH_3(CH_2)_3OH$; ≥99%; MW 74.12].
- n-Heptane [$CH_3(CH_2)_5CH_3$; ≥99%; MW 100.20].
- Solutions (Fig. 4).

2.2.2 Methods

1. The reagents are prepared as shown in Fig. 4.
2. Aliquots of 0.75 g NaCl(s) are prepared and stored at RT until used (*see* **step 6** below).
3. 2 ml of whole blood is placed in a glass homogenizer (*see* **Notes 4** and **5**); 2.1 ml of 0.4 N $HClO_4$ is added and homogenized on ice with a Teflon® pestle for ~30 s using a bench mixer stirrer homogenizer (for plasma and serum this step is omitted).
4. The homogenate is left to stand for 10 min at RT and centrifuged at 1400 × *g*, 4 °C for 10 min (for plasma and serum this step is omitted).
5. 2 ml of the supernatant is transferred into a balanced Quickfit® glass-stoppered test tube (for plasma and serum 2 ml aliquots are used; *see* **Notes 4–6**).
6. 0.25 ml of 5 N NaOH, 0.75 g of NaCl(s), and 5 ml of 1-butanol are added.
7. The tubes are stoppered, vigorously shaken for 5 min, and centrifuged at 1400 × *g*, 4 °C for 10 min.
8. The lower (aqueous) phase is discarded using a glass Pasteur pipette (*see* **Note** 7).
9. 2.5 ml of salt-saturated 0.1 N NaOH is added.

10. The tubes are stoppered, vigorously shaken for 5 min, and centrifuged at 1400 × *g*, 4 °C for 10 min.
11. 4 ml of the upper butanol layer is transferred into a clean and dry, balanced Quickfit® glass-stoppered test tube.
12. 2.5 ml of 0.1 N H_2SO_4 and 7.5 ml of heptane are added.
13. The tubes are stoppered, vigorously shaken for 1 min, and centrifuged at 1400 × *g*, 4 °C for 10 min.
14. The upper organic phase is discarded using a glass Pasteur pipette fitted in an aspirator pump.
15. The remaining aqueous phase (sample) is transferred into a glass test tube.
16. Following derivatization with *o*-PT (Fig. 5), histamine is quantified using a fluorescence spectrophotometer at excitation 360 nm and emission 450 nm.

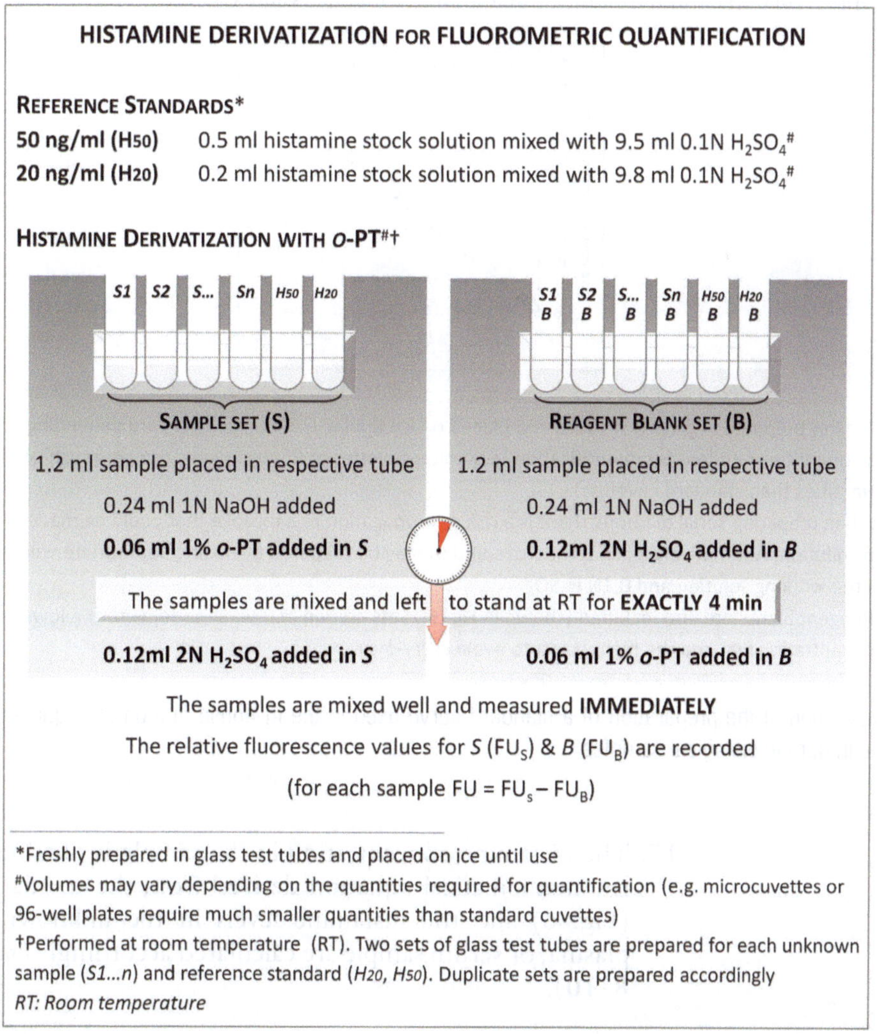

Fig. 5 Outline of the procedure used for the in-house fluorometric quantification of histamine in human biological samples

HISTAMINE STANDARD CURVE

Histamine Standards*

2.5 ml histamine working solution mixed with 7.5 ml 0.1N H_2SO_4 (250 ng/ml)

→ serial 2-fold dilutions (thorough mixing in each step) as shown in the diagram below#

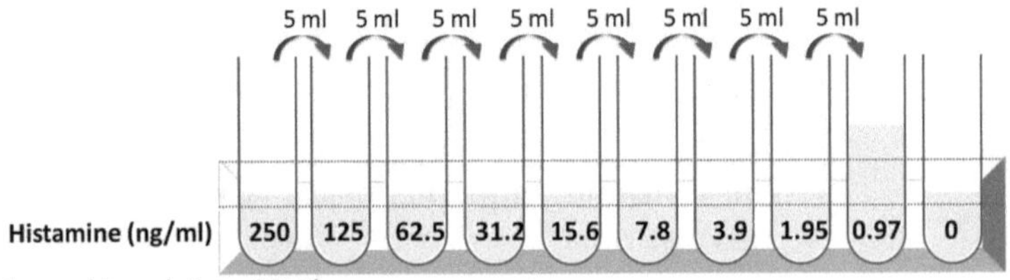

Histamine working solution	2.5 ml										
0.1N H_2SO_4	7.5	5.0	5.0	5.0	5.0	5.0	5.0	5.0	5.0	5.0	ml

→ Histamine is quantified following derivatization with *o*-phthalaldehyde (**Fig. 5**), using a fluorescence spectrophotometer (excitation 360 nm, emission 450 nm)†

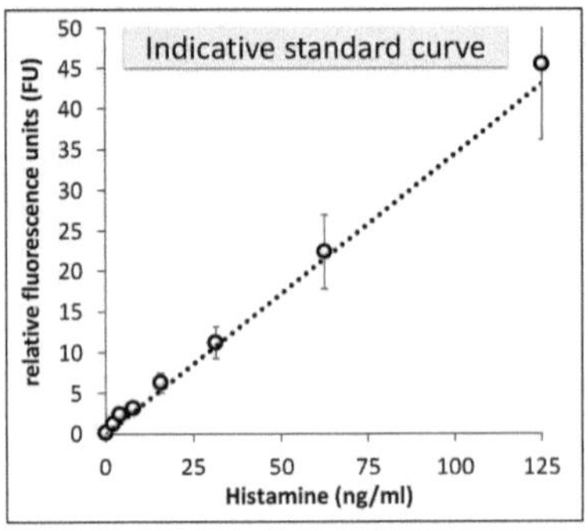

*Freshly prepared in glass test tubes and placed on ice until use. Volumes may vary depending on the quantities required for quantification (e.g. microcuvettes or 96-well plates require much smaller quantities than standard cuvettes)

#When preparing serial dilutions there is a risk of propagation of a mistake that could be made at any dilution. Alternatively, each standard solution may be prepared by mixing appropriate volumes of the working solution and 0.1N H_2SO_4

†Reagent blanks are also included (shown in **Fig. 5**). Sets are run in reverse order with the lowest concentration first and the highest last to avoid carry-over

Fig. 6 Illustration of the preparation of a standard curve used in the in-house fluorometric quantification of histamine in human biological samples

17. The histamine concentration in the sample is obtained using the mathematical equation derived from the standard curve (Fig. 6) and the histamine levels in the unknown blood, plasma, or serum sample are calculated accordingly (*see* **Notes 8–10**).

3 Notes

1. Since skin flora are a common source of contaminants, an antiseptic is used on the donor's sampling area before blood drawing [88]. During sample collection and preparation by venipuncture histamine may be released—mainly but not exclusively—from basophils due to injury, hemolysis, clotting, centrifugation, and storage conditions [54].
2. All tubes are properly labeled with a traceable sample identification code that is unambiguously connected to the donor, the sample, and the phlebotomist. It is recommended to record the information shown in Fig. 3 for each sample. Particular attention is paid to record ingestion of any agents and/or drugs that cause or modify allergic responses, H_1-antihistamines, corticosteroids, and H_2 antagonists 24 h before blood drawing.
3. The samples are maintained in ice while handling and for not more than 30 min. They are transported at <−20 °C avoiding freeze-thaw cycles. The integrity of a specimen is kept from collection until assayed. It is recommended not to use hemolyzed, icteric, or lipemic samples for histamine quantification.
4. There are numerous methods in the literature that have not been tested for reliability under specific laboratory and or field conditions. There is a need for standardization of measurement techniques to provide reproducible results as much as individual patient variation and technique will allow [33, 54, 56]. It is recommended that histamine stability and recovery from whole blood from healthy volunteers ($n = 4$–5) is investigated to optimize blood collection and storage conditions prior to assays [92]. Whole blood and the respective serum and plasma samples are spiked with 0–100 ng/ml histamine dihydrochloride, split into aliquots, and kept at −80, −20, 4 °C or RT until assayed in triplicate following all steps of the extraction procedure (histamine recovery is normally >94%). The precision of the assay is determined by calculating the standard deviation of the repeated measurements and the accuracy by assessing the agreement between the measured and nominal concentrations of the analyzed samples.
5. Frozen samples are rapidly thawed in a water bath (37 °C, ~5 min or until completely thawed under close monitoring), thoroughly and adequately mixed and tested immediately.
6. Complement activation during blood clotting may result in histamine release from basophils. Therefore, serum histamine values may differ from their plasma counterparts that are considered to provide more accurate information on the levels of free circulating histamine [54].

7. Care is taken not to introduce air bubbles to the sample and not to contaminate the upper (organic) phase while sliding slowly down the pipette tip against the wall of the tube.
8. It is helpful to perform a preliminary analysis of the unknown samples before planning the concentration range of the standard curve. Each investigator must run a standard curve four to six times. If histamine determination is performed routinely, a standard curve is prepared every month or more frequently if at least one reagent batch changes, while two standard histamine solutions are included in every assay (Fig. 5).
9. A number of substances may be present in the blood (e.g., tryptamine, putrescine, spermidine, spermine, tyramine) and interfere with the assay [95]. To explore their presence in the extract, appropriate dilutions of the suspected potentially interfering substances are used to examine any cross reactions with the fluorometric assay.
10. The value obtained after reading off the standard curve corresponds to the histamine concentration in the final aqueous layer. In order to calculate the histamine levels in unknown blood, plasma, or serum sample, the dilution factors of all extraction steps have to be taken into consideration.

References

1. Schwelberger HG, Ahrens F, Fogel WA et al (2013) Histamine metabolism. In: Stark H (ed) Histamine H_4 receptor: a novel drug target for immunoregulation and inflammation. Versita, London
2. Parsons ME, Ganellin CR (2006) Histamine and its receptors. Br J Pharmacol 147(S1): S127–S135
3. Panula P, Chazot PL, Cowart M et al (2015) International Union of Basic and Clinical Pharmacology. XCVIII. Histamine Receptors. Pharmacol Rev 67:601–655
4. Windholz M (1976) The Merck Index, 9th ed. Merck & Co., Inc., Rahway, NJ, p 619
5. Ohtsu H (2010) Histamine synthesis and lessons learned from histidine decarboxylase deficient mice. Adv Exp Med Biol 709:21–31
6. Riley JF, West GB (1952) Histamine in tissue mast cells. J Physiol 117:72–73
7. Kakavas S, Zampeli E, Papamichael K et al (2006) The mast cell pathway to inflammation and homeostasis: pharmacological insights. Anti-Inflamm Anti-Allergy Agents Med Chem 5:323–334
8. Ghably J, Saleh H, Vyas H et al (2015) Paul Ehrlich's mastzellen: a historical perspective of relevant developments in mast cell biology. Methods Mol Biol 1220:3–10
9. Afrin LB, Butterfield JH, Raithel M et al (2016) Often seen, rarely recognized: mast cell activation disease - a guide to diagnosis and therapeutic options. Ann Med 48:190–201
10. Fourie P (2016) Kounis syndrome: a narrative review. South Afr J Anaesth Analg 22:72–80
11. Modena BD, Dazy K, White AA (2016) Emerging concepts: mast cell involvement in allergic diseases. Transl Res 174:98–121
12. Falcone FH, Zillikens D, Gibbs BF (2006) The 21st century renaissance of the basophil? Current insights into its role in allergic responses and innate immunity. Exp Dermatol 15:855–864
13. Prinz C, Zanner R, Gratzl M (2003) Physiology of gastric enterochromaffin-like cells. Annu Rev Physiol 65:371–382
14. Haas HL, Sergeeva OA, Selbach O (2008) Histamine in the nervous system. Physiol Rev 88:1183–1241
15. Cacabelos R, Torrellas C, Fernández-Novoa L et al (2016) Histamine and immune biomarkers in CNS disorders. Mediators Inflamm 2016:1924603

16. Falus A, Hegyesi H, Lazar-Molnar E et al (2001) Paracrine and autocrine interactions in melanoma: histamine is a relevant player in local regulation. Trends Immunol 22: 648–652
17. Dale HH, Laidlaw PP (1910) The physiological action of β-imidazolylethylamine. J Physiol 41:318–341
18. Miliani A, Catini C, Filippelli M et al (1993) Daily rhythmic variations in histamine in human blood. Int Arch Allergy Immunol 100: 53–55
19. Bessinis DP, Dalla C, Daifoti ZP et al (2012) Histamine involvement in visual development and adaptation. Invest Ophthalmol Vis Sci 53:7498–7503
20. Chliva C, Aggelides X, Makris M et al (2015) Comparable profiles of serum histamine and IgG4 levels in allergic beekeepers. Allergy 70:457–460
21. Makris M, Aggelides X, Chliva C et al (2015) High baseline blood histamine levels and lack of cross-reactivity in a patient with ranitidine-induced anaphylaxis. J Investig Allergol Clin Immunol 24:361–363
22. Park do Y, Kim YS, Kim JH et al (2015) Association of body mass index and other factors with histamine skin reactivity in adults with allergic nasal symptoms. Am J Rhinol Allergy 29:e160–e163
23. Babina M, Guhl S, Artuc M et al (2016) Phenotypic variability in human skin mast cells. Exp Dermatol 25:434–439
24. Zampeli E, Tiligada E (2009) The role of histamine H_4 receptor in immune and inflammatory disorders. Br J Pharmacol 157:24–33
25. O'Mahony L, Akdis M, Akdis CA (2011) Regulation of the immune response and inflammation by histamine and histamine receptors. J Allergy Clin Immunol 128: 1153–1162
26. Tiligada E (2012) Editorial: is histamine the missing link in chronic inflammation? J Leukoc Biol 92:4–6
27. Stegaev V, Sillat T, Porola P et al (2012) Brief report: first identification of H_4 histamine receptor in healthy salivary glands and in focal sialadenitis in Sjögren's syndrome. Arthritis Rheum 64:2663–2668
28. Kyriakidis K, Zampeli E, Palaiologou M et al (2015) Histamine H_3 and H_4 receptor ligands modify vascular histamine levels in normal and arthritic large blood vessels in vivo. Inflammation 38:949–958
29. Kitakaze M (2016) Clinical evidence of the role of histamine in heart failure. J Am Coll Cardiol 67:1553–1555
30. Tiligada E, Zampeli E, Sander K et al (2009) Histamine H_3 and H_4 receptors as novel drug targets. Expert Opin Investig Drugs 18: 1519–1531
31. Tiligada E, Kyriakidis K, Chazot PL et al (2011) Histamine pharmacology and new CNS drug targets. CNS Neurosci Ther 17:620–628
32. Kakavas S, Tiligada E (2006) Time course of thyroxine on hypothalamic histamine in the rat. Inflamm Res 55(S1):S32–S33
33. Farage MA, Berardesca E, Maibach H (2010) The possible relevance of sex hormones on irritant and allergic responses: their importance for skin testing. Contact Dermatitis 62:67–74
34. Kyriakidis K, Zampeli E, Tiligada E (2009) Histamine levels in whole peripheral blood from women with ductal breast cancer: a pilot study. Inflamm Res 58(S1):73–74
35. Makris M, Gkavogiannakis N, Grosicki M et al (2016) Serum histamine and cytokine levels in cancer patients undergoing desensitization to carboplatin: a pilot study. In: Abstracts of the 45th annual meeting of the European Histamine Research Society, Florence, 11–14 May 2016
36. Bongers G, de Esch I, Leurs R (2010) Molecular pharmacology of the four histamine receptors. Adv Exp Med Biol 709:11–19
37. Walther DJ, Stahlberg S, Vowinckel J (2011) Novel roles for biogenic monoamines: from monoamines in transglutaminase-mediated post-translational protein modification to monoaminylation deregulation diseases. FEBS J 278:4740–4755
38. Kyriakidis DA, Tiligada E (2013) Non receptor-mediated histamine actions. In: Stark H (ed) Histamine H_4 receptor: a novel drug target for immunoregulation and inflammation. Versita, London
39. Dauvilliers Y, Bassetti C, Lammers GJ et al (2013) Pitolisant versus placebo or modafinil in patients with narcolepsy: a double-blind, randomized trial. Lancet Neurol 12: 1068–1075
40. Tiligada E, Ishii M, Riccardi C et al (2015) The expanding role of immunopharmacology: IUPHAR Review 16. Br J Pharmacol 172:4217–4427
41. Ziarco Pharma (2016) Pipeline ZPL-389. http://www.ziarcopharma.com. Accessed 8 Jun 2016
42. Nijmeijer S, Vischer HF, Sirci F et al (2013) Detailed analysis of biased histamine H_4 receptor signalling by JNJ 7777120 analogues. Br J Pharmacol 170:78–88

43. Coruzzi G, Pozzoli C, Adami M et al (2012) Strain-dependent effects of the histamine H_4 receptor antagonist JNJ7777120 in a murine model of acute skin inflammation. Exp Dermatol 21:32–37
44. Koessler KK, Hanke MT (1919) A microchemical colorimetric method for estimating imidazole derivatives. J Biol Chem 39: 497–519
45. Patange SB, Mukundan MK, Ashok Kumar K (2005) A simple and rapid method for colorimetric determination of histamine in fish flesh. Food Control 16:465–472
46. Barsoum GS, Gaddum JH (1935) The pharmacological estimation of adenosine and histamine in blood. J Physiol 85:1–14
47. Code CF (1937) The quantitative estimation of histamine in the blood. J Physiol 89:257–268
48. McIntire FC, Roth LW, Shaw JL (1947) The purification of histamine for bioassay. Fed Proc 6:356
49. Adam HM, Hardwick DC, Spencer KE (1957) A method of estimating histamine in plasma. Br J Pharmacol Chemother 12:397–405
50. Dale MM (1958) An inhibitory effect of acetycholine on the response of the guineapig ileum to histamine. Br J Pharmacol Chemother 13:17–19
51. Mannaioni PF (1991) Bioassays. In: Uvnäs B (ed) Histamine and histamine antagonists. Handbook of experimental pharmacology, vol 97. Springer, Heidelberg, pp 3–8
52. Shore PA, Burkhalter A, Cohn VH Jr (1959) A method for the fluorometric assay of histamine in tissues. J Pharmacol Exp Ther 127: 182–186
53. Stahl Skov P, Norn S, Weeke B (1984) A new method for detecting histamine release. Agents Actions 14:414–416
54. Costing E, Neugebauer E, Keyzer JJ et al (1990) Determination of histamine in human plasma: the European external quality control study 1988. Clin Exp Allergy 20:349–357
55. Lorenz W, Thon K, Neugebauer E et al (1987) Reliability and practicability of the fluorometric-fluoroenzymatic histamine determination in pathogenetic studies on peptic ulcer: detection limits and problems with specificity. Agents Actions 21:1–25
56. Lorenz W, Neugebauer E (1991) Fluorometruc assays. In: Uvnäs B (ed) Histamine and histamine antagonists. Handbook of experimental pharmacology, vol 97. Springer, Heidelberg, pp 9–30
57. Tiligada E, Aslanis D, Delitheos A et al (2000) Changes in histamine content following pharmacologically-induced mast cell degranulation in the rat conjunctiva. Pharmacol Res 41:667–670
58. Siraganian RP, Brodsky MJ (1976) Automated histamine analysis for *in vitro* allergy testing. I. A method utilizing allergen-induced histamine release from whole blood. J Allergy Clin Immunol 57:525–540
59. Ennis M (1991) Automated fluorometric assays. In: Uvnäs B (ed) Histamine and histamine antagonists. Handbook of experimental pharmacology, vol 97. Springer, Heidelberg, pp 31–38
60. Rönnberg AL, Hansson C, Drakenberg T et al (1984) Reaction of histamine with o-phthalaldehyde: isolation and analysis of the fluorophore. Anal Biochem 139:329–337
61. Yoshimura T, Kaneuchi T, Miura T et al (1987) Kinetic analysis of the fluorescence reaction of histamine with orthophthalaldehyde. Anal Biochem 164:132–137
62. Snyder SH, Baldessarini RJ, Axelrod J (1966) A sensitive and specific enzymatic isotopic assay for tissue histamine. J Pharmacol Exp Ther 153:544–549
63. Dyer J, Warren K, Merlin S et al (1982) Measurement of plasma histamine: description of an improved method and normal values. J Allergy Clin Immunol 70:82–87
64. Beaven MA (1991) Radioenzymatic assays in biological fluids. In: Uvnäs B (ed) Histamine and histamine antagonists. Handbook of experimental pharmacology, vol 97. Springer, Heidelberg, pp 39–48
65. Mahy N, Gelpi E (1977) Gas chromatographic separation of histamine and its metabolites. J Chromatogr 130:237–242
66. Yamatodani A, Fukuda H, Wada H et al (1985) High-performance liquid chromatographic determination of plasma and brain histamine without previous purification of biological samples: cation-exchange chromatography coupled with post-column derivatization fluorometry. J Chromatogr 344:115–123
67. Bourgogne E, Mathy FX, Boucaut D et al (2012) Simultaneous quantitation of histamine and its major metabolite 1-methylhistamine in brain dialysates by using precolumn derivatization prior to HILIC-MS/MS analysis. Anal Bioanal Chem 402:449–459
68. Chen R, Deng Y, Yang L et al (2016) Determination of histamine by high-performance liquid chromatography after precolumn

derivatization with o-phthalaldehyde-sulfite. J Chromatogr Sci 54:547–553

69. Kolmert J, Forngren B, Lindberg J et al (2014) A quantitative LC/MS method targeting urinary 1-methyl-4-imidazoleacetic acid for safety monitoring of the global histamine turnover in clinical studies. Anal Bioanal Chem 406:1751–1762
70. Koyama J, Takeuchi A, Tode C et al (2009) Development of an LC-ESI-MS/MS method for the determination of histamine: application to the quantitative measurement of histamine degranulation by KU812 cells. J Chromatogr B Analyt Technol Biomed Life Sci 877:207–212
71. Waldum HL, Sandvik AK, Brenna E et al (1991) Radioimmunoassay of histamine. Scand J Gastroenterol 26(S180):32–39
72. McBride P, Bradley D, Kaliner M (1988) Evaluation of a radioimmunoassay for histamine measurement in biologic fluids. J Allergy Clin Immunol 82:638–646
73. Garbarg M, Pollard H, Trung Tuong MD et al (1989) Sensitive radioimmunoassays for histamine and tele-methylhistamine in the brain. J Neurochem 53:1724–1730
74. Laroche D, Dubois F, Gérard JL et al (1995) Radioimmunoassay for plasma histamine: a study of false positive and false negative values. Br J Anaesth 74:430–437
75. Chevrier D, Guesdon JL, Mazié JC et al (1986) Enzyme immunoassay for the measurement of histamine. J Immunol Methods 94:119–125
76. Morel AM, Delaage MA (1988) Immunoanalysis of histamine through a novel chemical derivatization. J Allergy Clin Immunol 82(4):646–654
77. Dvorak AM, Morgan ES, Schleimer RP et al (1993) Diamine oxidase-gold labels histamine in human mast-cell granules: a new enzyme-affinity ultrastructural method. J Histochem Cytochem 41:787–800
78. Ebo DG, Bridts CH, Mertens CH et al (2012) Analyzing histamine release by flow cytometry (HistaFlow): a novel instrument to study the degranulation patterns of basophils. J Immunol Methods 375:30–38
79. Nullens S, Sabato V, Faber M et al (2013) Basophilic histamine content and release during venom immunotherapy: insights by flow cytometry. Cytometry B Clin Cytom 84:173–178
80. McIntire FC (1966) Determination of histamine by chemical means. In: Rocha e Silva M (ed) Histamine and antihistaminics. Part 1 Histamine. Its chemistry, metabolism and physiological and pharmacological actions. Handbook of experimental pharmacology, vol XVIII/1. Springer, Heidelberg, pp 57–80
81. Withington DE, Aranda JV (1997) Measurement of plasma histamine by high performance liquid chromatography and radioimmunoassay. Inflamm Res 46(S1):S77–S78
82. Muscarella M, Iammarino M, Centonze D et al (2005) Measurement of histamine in seafood by HPLC, CE, and ELISA: comparison of three techniques. Vet Res Commun S2:343–346
83. Saccani G, Tanzi E, Pastore P et al (2005) Determination of biogenic amines in fresh and processed meat by suppressed ion chromatography-mass spectrometry using a cation-exchange column. J Chromatogr A 1082:43–50
84. Self RL, Wu WH, Marks HS (2011) Simultaneous quantification of eight biogenic amine compounds in tuna by matrix solid-phase dispersion followed by HPLC-orbitrap mass spectrometry. J Agric Food Chem 59:5906–5913
85. Luo L, Xu ZL, Yang JY et al (2014) Synthesis of novel haptens and development of an enzyme-linked immunosorbent assay for quantification of histamine in foods. J Agric Food Chem 62:12299–12308
86. Cunha SC, Faria MA, Fernandes JO (2011) Gas chromatography-mass spectrometry assessment of amines in Port wine and grape juice after fast chloroformate extraction/derivatization. J Agric Food Chem 59: 8742–8753
87. Singh S, Bajorek B (2014) Defining 'elderly' in clinical practice guidelines for pharmacotherapy. Pharm Pract (Granada) 12:489
88. Reed BG, Carr BR (2016) The normal menstrual cycle and the control of ovulation. In: De Groot LJ, Beck-Peccoz P, Chrousos G et al (eds) Available via MDText.com, Inc.; 2000-. http://www.ncbi.nlm.nih.gov/books/NBK279054. Accessed 5 Jun 2016
89. Aslanis D, Tiligada E (2001) Effect of fluoxetine on histamine content in the rat conjunctiva. J Fr Ophtalmol 24:169–171
90. World Health Organization (2010) WHO guidelines on drawing blood: best practices in phlebotomy. World Health Organization, Geneva
91. Nikolac N, Supak-Smolcić V, Simundić AM et al (2013) Croatian Society of Medical Biochemistry and Laboratory Medicine: national recommendations for venous blood sampling. Biochem Med (Zagreb) 23: 242–254

92. Thavasu PW, Longhurst S, Joel SP et al (1992) Measuring cytokine levels in blood. Importance of anticoagulants, processing, and storage conditions. J Immunol Methods 153:115–124
93. Yuksel H, Mete N, Bayrak P et al (2004) Is the menstrual cycle affecting the skin prick test reactivity? Asian Pac J Allergy Immunol 22:197–203
94. U.S. Food and Drug Administration (2016) Informed consent information sheet. http://www.fda.gov/RegulatoryInformation/Guidances/ucm404975.htm. Accessed 19 Jun 2016
95. Minois N, Carmona-Gutierrez D, Madeo F (2011) Polyamines in aging and disease. Aging 3:716–732

Index

Ekaterini Tiligada and Madeleine Ennis (eds.), *Histamine Receptors as Drug Targets*, Methods in Pharmacology and Toxicology, DOI 10.1007/978-1-4939-6843-5,

D

E

F

G

H

I

K

S

T

U

V

W

X

Z

MIX
Papier aus verantwortungsvollen Quellen
Paper from responsible sources
FSC® C105338

If you have any concerns about our products,
you can contact us on
ProductSafety@springernature.com

In case Publisher is established outside the EU,
the EU authorized representative is:
Springer Nature Customer Service Center GmbH
Europaplatz 3, 69115 Heidelberg, Germany

Printed by Libri Plureos GmbH
in Hamburg, Germany